# Global Perspectives on Cancer

# Global Perspectives on Cancer

## Incidence, Care, and Experience

### Volume 2: Challenges and Progress in Care across Nations

Kenneth D. Miller, MD, and
Miklos Simon, MD, Editors

Foreword by Sandra M. Swain

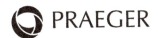 PRAEGER

AN IMPRINT OF ABC-CLIO, LLC
Santa Barbara, California • Denver, Colorado • Oxford, England

Copyright © 2015 by Kenneth D. Miller and Miklos Simon

All rights reserved. No part of this publication may be reproduced, stored in a retrieval system, or transmitted, in any form or by any means, electronic, mechanical, photocopying, recording, or otherwise, except for the inclusion of brief quotations in a review, without prior permission in writing from the publisher.

**Library of Congress Cataloging-in-Publication Data**

Global perspectives on cancer : incidence, care, and experience / Kenneth D. Miller and Miklos Simon, editors ; foreword by Sandra M. Swain.
      p. ; cm.
   Includes bibliographical references and index.
   ISBN 978-1-4408-2857-7 (hardback : alk. paper) — ISBN 978-1-4408-2858-4 (ebook)
I. Miller, Kenneth D., 1956–, editor.   II. Simon, Miklos, 1968–, editor. [DNLM:
1. Neoplasms.   2. Health Services Accessibility.   3. Healthcare Disparities.
4. Socioeconomic Factors.   QZ 200]
   RC263
   616.99'4—dc23       2014024016

ISBN: 978-1-4408-2857-7
EISBN: 978-1-4408-2858-4

19  18  17  16  15     1  2  3  4  5

This book is also available on the World Wide Web as an eBook.
Visit www.abc-clio.com for details.

Praeger
An Imprint of ABC-CLIO, LLC

ABC-CLIO, LLC
130 Cremona Drive, P.O. Box 1911
Santa Barbara, California 93116–1911

This book is printed on acid-free paper ∞

Manufactured in the United States of America

# Contents

# Foreword

As more infectious diseases are controlled and extinguished in different parts of the world, it is clear that cancer is a significant health problem. The estimated number of cancer cases worldwide for 2008 was 12.7 million, with 7.6 million deaths. Predictions for 2030 are staggering, with estimates of 22 million new cases and 12 million deaths.

I am personally gratified that so much attention is being paid to the worldwide problem of cancer. It is very exciting that the United Nations meeting in 2011 placed cancer for the first time on the global health agenda. A new global monitoring framework was agreed upon in November 2012 with input from governments around the world as well as a wide coalition of nongovernmental organizations, led by the NCD Alliance with participation from the American Society of Clinical Oncology, the American Cancer Society, and the Union for International Cancer Control. These agreements are commitments by member states, including the United States, to address the rise of noncommunicable diseases. At the 66th World Health Assembly of the UN held in Geneva in May 2013, the WHO Global NCD Action Plan 2013–2020 was adopted.

This plan is a road map and menu of policy options to achieve nine voluntary global targets, one of which is a 25% relative reduction in premature death because of cancer, cardiovascular diseases, diabetes, or chronic respiratory diseases by 2025. It is thought that 90% of the premature deaths are from low- and middle-income countries. Other targets related to cancer include a 30% relative reduction in tobacco use in people over age 15 years, stopping obesity, and an 80% availability of basic technologies and medicines to treat the diseases. Indicators or metrics that are enumerated include access to palliative care measured by morphine equivalent consumption, vaccines for human papillomavirus, hepatitis B vaccine, and proportion of women screened for cervical cancer.

What was really important in this document was that the overarching principles were articulated, which were essential to implement the plan. These overarching principles include a human rights approach, an equity-based approach, a national action and international cooperation and solidarity, multisectoral action, a life-course approach, empowerment of people and communities, evidence-based strategies, universal health coverage, and management of conflict of interest.

Unfortunately, the infrastructure including the workforce available to combat cancer is severely limited in many countries. However, creative opportunities arise in these situations. Professional medical societies have a big role to collaborate with *other* nongovernmental and governmental organizations to make their members available to share knowledge and expertise. For example, the American Society of Clinical Oncology has a volunteer program for doctors to go to different countries like Bhutan, Costa Rica, Honduras, Paraguay, and Vietnam to train physicians in areas of need and enhance health-care services available. Dr. Surendra Shastri in India has implemented a screening program for cervical cancer utilizing community health workers. These workers are taking on the responsibility of screening and follow-up of women after a short period of training.

These kinds of programs incorporated into a well-thought-out and implemented national cancer program are essential to lower cancer incidence and deaths in low- and middle-income countries.

This book touches on the many aspects of health care around the world and will be an invaluable addition to those health-care professionals who desire to make a difference globally. The more recognition of the differences in various parts of the world, the more knowledge and information that can be disseminated, the more likely will there be changes for the better for all of humanity.

Sandra M. Swain, MD, FACP
*Medical Director, Washington Cancer Institute*
*Medstar Washington Hospital Center*
*Professor of Medicine, Georgetown University*
*Washington, DC*

# Acknowledgments

The primary goal of this textbook is to help improve global cancer care. With this goal in mind, we want to thank each and every author for contributing his or her knowledge, expertise and insight. This book could not have gone to publication without the time and energy that each contributor has made to this immense body of work.

We would each like to acknowledge our coeditor for his commitment to moving this project from concept to reality. We also want to say a special thank you to our editor, Debbie Carvalko, who initiated this project and helped to see it through. Her supreme attention to detail and positive attitude made this project possible.

Finally, we would like to take this opportunity to acknowledge all the health-care professionals who are working to improve cancer care for patients and families across the globe.

Kenneth D. Miller, MD
Miklos Simon, MD

# Part I

# Types of Cancer

# 1

# Head and Neck Cancer

*Franklin W. Huang and Lori J. Wirth*

## INTRODUCTION

Together, the cancers of the head and neck are among the most common cancers diagnosed in the world. An estimated half-million cases were diagnosed in 2008.[1] Cancers of the head and neck are a diverse spectrum of tumors made up of primary malignancies arising within the epithelial linings of the upper aerodigestive tract and salivary glands, thyroid and parathyroid tumors, skin cancers, and other less frequently encountered tumors, such as neuroendocrine tumors and sarcomas. This chapter focuses on squamous cell carcinoma of the head and neck (SCCHN), which accounts for approximately 85% of these cancers. The causes of head and neck cancers are multifactorial and, in part, can be attributed to environmental exposures, including tobacco and alcohol, and infectious disease, such as human papillomavirus (HPV). Two of the three leading risk factors for global disease burden, tobacco and alcohol, are responsible for a significant numbers of SCCHN cases, with tobacco accounting for almost half of the deaths due to SCCHN and another estimated 16% of deaths due to heavy alcohol consumption.[2,3]

At diagnosis, the majority of head and neck cancers are locally advanced by American Joint Committee on Cancer staging guidelines. Because of differences in the natural history and surgical options available, SCCHN treatment approaches are based on the primary site of disease, divided into (1) nasopharynx, (2) nasal cavity and paranasal sinuses, (3) oral cavity, (4) oropharynx, and (5) larynx. Early-stage disease can often be treated and cured with surgery or radiation alone, whereas treatment for locally advanced head and neck cancers is typically multidisciplinary, with need for medical, surgical, and radiation oncology expertise. Patients with locally advanced disease are potentially curable, but multimodality treatment is both time and resource intensive. Moreover, the head and neck regions contain the most complex functional anatomy in the human body. Not only can cancer arising in the region affect significantly the basic human functions of vision, hearing, breathing, speech, and swallowing, but its treatment also frequently results in substantial acute and chronic morbidity. Thus, the impact of head and neck cancers extends beyond that of survival and can result in long-term functional, psychosocial, and other quality of life challenges to the patient and community.

In high-income countries, it is now recognized that a rising proportion of cancers of the head and neck are associated with HPV.[4] This association has significant implications for treatment and prevention. HPV-associated SCCHN carries a better prognosis than similar cancers not associated with HPV. This relatively high cure rate has led to a shift in the focus of research efforts from cure alone to maintaining high cure rates while minimizing the burden of treatment-related morbidity.

In low- and middle-income countries, the major challenges in the field of SCCHN remain prevention by reducing tobacco and alcohol use, as well as providing comprehensive and specialized cancer care services, including radiation therapy and surgical services.

## Epidemiology

Worldwide in 2008 there were an estimated 482,000 new cases of head and neck cancers, with 273,000 deaths.[5] With nearly a quarter million deaths, SCCHN ranks as the eighth most common cause of cancer death in the world.

Tobacco and alcohol have long been recognized as major contributing factors to the development of SCCHN.[6] The World Health Organization estimates that there are currently 1 billion smokers worldwide, 80% of whom live in low- and middle-income countries.[7] Heavy users of both tobacco and alcohol are at highest risk of SCCHN, which is as high as 35-fold greater risk than nonusers in people who smoke two packs of cigarettes and drink four alcoholic beverages per day. The Global Tobacco Surveillance System now tracks smoking prevalence in many parts of the world. In 2012, the Global Adult Tobacco Survey reported on tobacco use in 14 low- and middle-income countries, and from the United Kingdom and the United States.[8] These data show that across the world, smoking remains more prevalent in men than women, with the highest male rates in Russia, China, Ukraine, Turkey, and the Philippines. Among women, smoking rates are highest in Poland, Russia, the United Kingdom, Uruguay, and the United States. Perhaps the most concerning trends are seen in young people, as demonstrated by the Global Youth Tobacco Survey. Of the 100 school sites in countries across the globe that make up this survey, 61 sites reported no change in tobacco use among 13- to 15-year-olds between 1999 and 2008, despite the global tobacco control efforts spearheaded by the World Health Organization.[9] In addition, smoking rates are on the rise among adolescent girls. Tobacco and alcohol cessation programs are critical in modifying these lifestyle risk factors. Even then, however, the risk of developing SCCHN remains high for at least 20 years after cessation. Thus, not only must smoking cessation programs intervene before middle age to avoid the lifetime risk of malignancy for any one individual, but also decades are required for smoking cessation programs to achieve a clinically meaningful impact on the incidence of SCCHN on a population-wide basis.[10]

A strong body of case-control and epidemiologic evidence has now established that infection by high-risk HPV, primarily type HPV16, is tightly associated with the development of oropharyngeal SCCHN arising in tonsillar fossa and base of tongue. The proportion of oropharyngeal cancers caused by HPV varies widely across the world, with the lowest rates reported in developing countries, such as Bangladesh, Central European countries, and Latin American countries. In the developed world, however, the incidence of HPV-associated oropharyngeal cancers has been increasing dramatically over the past three decades.[11] For example, in the United States, the presence of HPV in oropharynx cancers increased from 16% during the 1980s to 72% in the 2000s.[12,13]

Overall, men have a higher incidence rate of HPV-positive SCCHN than women, with a ratio ranging from 2:1 to 15:1.[14] While both HPV-negative and HPV-positive oropharyngeal cancers predominate in men, HPV-positive cancers occur at a younger age of onset (3 to 5 years earlier than HPV-negative cancers), and are not associated with tobacco and alcohol use, but rather show strong associations with sexual behaviors, consistent with sexual transmission of HPV. The reasons behind this changing pattern of increasing HPV-predominant oropharyngeal cancer in the developed world are not yet fully understood, but it is thought that an increase in viral exposure as a birth cohort effect may be acting in concert with changing sexual behaviors in the population over time.

Like HPV, Epstein–Barr virus (EBV) is also closely associated with a distinct subtype of SCCHN, nasopharyngeal carcinoma (NPC). The majority of non-keratinizing and undifferentiated NPCs harbor EBV. NPC is rare globally, with an incidence of less than 1/100,000, but the incidence reaches as high as 20/100,000 in endemic areas of the world, such as southern China.[15,16] The incidence of EBV-associated NPC is also high in parts of Southeast Asia, the Arctic, the Middle East and North Africa, and the Mediterranean basin.[17] Interestingly, the incidence of NPC is decreasing in some endemic parts of the world, such as Hong Kong. This trend, plus the fact that EBV-associated NPC is less common among Chinese born in North America as compared to Chinese immigrants to North America, suggests an etiologic role beyond EBV and genetic susceptibility and implicates environmental cofactors that may be mitigated over time.[18,19]

## ETIOLOGY

### Environment/Exposures

#### Tobacco

Nearly half of cancers of the head and neck can be associated with the use of tobacco. According to the WHO, if current trends continue, by 2020 tobacco will be responsible for nearly 8 million deaths per year and the vast majority of these deaths will occur in low- and middle-income countries.[20] Worldwide, tobacco is used in many different forms. In addition to the smoking of cigarettes, cigars, bidis, and pipes, various smokeless oral products, including chewing tobacco, are consumed. Smokeless tobacco products also cause cancer, particularly oral cavity cancers, though they do not significantly increase the risk of lung cancer. One fundamental problem with tobacco is its ingredient, nicotine. Nicotine is a sympathomimetic stimulant that binds to the nicotinic acetylcholine receptor, resulting in one of the most challenging addictions known in humans. The burning of tobacco and its additives at high temperatures produces an estimated 7,000 chemical compounds, many of which are toxic and directly trigger injury, inflammation, and carcinogenesis. Tobacco toxins include at least 45 known or suspected human carcinogens, including aldehydes, toxic metals, nitrosamines, benzene, and polonium.[21] Passive exposure to secondhand smoke exposes many more people beyond the smokers themselves to these toxins. Chronic exposure to tobacco can result in field cancerization, in which the mucosa of the upper aerodigestive tract becomes condemned by multiple genetic alterations. Clonal evolution can arise out of initiating events in one or more sites and lead not just to one cancer, but to synchronous, metachronous, or second tobacco-related cancers arising within the same individual.[22]

Of increasing alarm is the rising rate of tobacco use and tobacco-related cancers in the developing world, which will impact significantly the incidence of head and neck cancers.[8] The rising burden of cancer in the developing world will likely significantly strain health-care systems that are poorly equipped to manage cancer.

Alcohol is another major contributor to the development of SCCHN.[23] Approximately half of the worldwide adult population consumes alcohol at a per capita rate of 6.1 liters, indicating the enormous potential impact alcohol has on public health.[24] Patterns of alcohol exposure vary substantially across the world. For example, North Africa, the Middle East, and South Asia have the highest percentage of lifetime abstainers (greater than 80%), whereas southern Latin America and Australasia have the lowest percentage of abstainers (9%). Of the worldwide population, 6% are heavy consumers of alcohol, defined as greater than 40 g of alcohol per day for women and 60 g for men. The countries of Eastern and Central Europe contain the greatest numbers of heavy drinkers (15% to 18%).

Alcohol by-products, including acetaldehyde and reactive oxygen species, are considered genotoxic. An even greater effect from alcohol appears to be the multiplicative effect of tobacco. This may be in part due to the role of alcohol as a solvent of tobacco carcinogens. Tobacco increases the risk of head and neck cancers by greater than 5-fold. This risk is increased to as much as 35-fold by concurrent alcohol use. Recent studies have confirmed this multiplicative effect of alcohol and tobacco use on the risk of head and neck cancers.[25] Although studies of its independent effect are challenging due to the confounding use of alcohol and tobacco, it appears that contrary to earlier conclusions, alcohol at any level of consumption, not just heavy drinking, increases the risk of cancers in sites such as the pharynx that come into direct contact with alcohol.[26,27]

### Betel Nut

Betel nut is the seed of the areca palm (*Areca catechu*) and is widely chewed in Asia. Betel nut is actually a misnomer and it is so called since the predominant preparation in Asia is the areca nut wrapped in betel leaf with slaked lime and chewed together. This preparation is called "betel quid." The role of betel nut as a carcinogen has been recognized by the International Agency for Research in Cancer and is thought to account in part for the higher incidence rates of oral cavity cancers in Asia compared to Western nations. It is estimated that up to 10% of the world's population may be chewing areca nut or betel quid. The chewing of areca nut or betel quid has been associated with an increased risk of cancers of the oral cavity and, like alcohol, has synergistic effects with tobacco.

### Viral: HPV and EBV

At least 25% of head and neck cancers are not related to exposure to tobacco or alcohol and may be related to viral exposures, such as HPV.[28]

The incidence of HPV-associated cancers is increasing rapidly in the developed world, and parts of the developing world are mirroring these trends. Most adults, where studied, have been exposed to HPV. Considering genital infections alone, the rate of lifetime exposure is more than 80% in women and 60% in men.[29,30] Lifetime rates for oral infections are not known, but evaluation of the point prevalence for oral HPV in healthy people in the United States showed a rate of infection in 4% of woman and 10% of men.[4] The majority of these infections are transient and cleared by the host, but in a small number of people, the HPV viral genome becomes integrated into the host tissue genome, which is considered an essential first step in carcinogenesis.

Following viral integration into the host genome, viral proteins E6 and E7 dysregulate tumor suppressor pathways and cell proliferation, which can result in genomic instability and the accumulation of mutations and lead to oncogenesis.[31] HPV viral proteins act in a number of processes normally regulated by p53 and Rb, co-opting cellular factors involved in cell cycle checkpoint and genome stability.

Similar to HPV, EBV infection is common around the world. Therefore, it is thought that it is not variable exposure that accounts for the varying incidence of NPC across subpopulations. Rather, the etiology of endemic NPC seems to be associated with other factors beyond EBV infection, including dietary factors (such as salted fish and other preserved foods high in nitrosamines), other potentially genotoxic substances, smoke exposure by virtue of poor ventilation, and genetic susceptibility. The mechanisms of EBV-related carcinogenesis are complex and are not yet fully understood. However, it is known that EBV can latently infect nasopharyngeal tissue and express a limited range of viral proteins, namely EBNA1, LMP1, and LMP2. Virus-encoded small RNAs and microRNAs are also expressed. Among these viral factors, LMP1 is thought to be a key player in the development of NPC. LMP1 possesses the capability to immortalize B cells and transform epithelial cells, as well as promote cell growth and immortality. In addition, the expression of LMP1 upregulates cellular features contributing to distant metastasis, consistent with the typical clinical presentation of the disease.[32]

## EGFR

SCCHN results from an accumulation of multiple genetic and epigenetic alterations influencing a variety of cellular pathways with complex interactions. Similar to other epithelial cancers, in head and neck cancers, the epidermal growth factor receptor (EGFR) is recognized as playing a significant role in carcinogenesis. EGFR, a member of the ErbB/HER family of receptor tyrosine kinases, activates a number of signaling pathways including the PI3-kinase-AKT pathway, the ras-MEK-ERK pathway, and STAT proteins that drive a number of oncogenic processes including cellular proliferation and cell invasion. Because EGFR is over-expressed in a large majority of SCCHN tumors and its over-expression correlates with poor prognosis, EGFR has emerged as a leading target for the development of new therapeutic strategies in SCCHN.[33-36] Despite over-expression of EGFR in SCCHN, targeted therapy directed against EGFR has had limited efficacy. EGFR-independent mechanisms have been posited to play a role in resistance to EGFR inhibitors. Nevertheless, cetuximab, a monoclonal antibody against EGFR, is approved for use in head and neck cancers. However, the efficacy of cetuximab as a single-agent in head and neck cancers is modest. When added to radiation, cetuximab does improve locoregional control and overall survival in locally advanced SCCHN, but no studies have compared cetuximab plus radiation to chemoradiotherapy, which is an established standard of care for the disease.[37] Thus, cetuximab and radiotherapy have not replaced chemoradiotherapy in the treatment of locally advanced SCCHN.

## Genomic Insights into SCCHN

Recently, two studies have reported on large-scale exome sequencing of SCCHN tumors, demonstrating that the majority of mutations in SCCHN occur as inactivating mutations in tumor suppressor genes, including *TP53*, *CDKN2A*, and *NOTCH1–3*, while activating mutations in oncogenes that are more readily targetable are less common.[38,39] For example, inactivating mutations in *TP53* are found in approximately half of all SCCHN tumors. Inactivation of the protein product, p53, allows for cell proliferation despite the presence of damaged DNA and the accumulation of additional genetic mutations, facilitating unchecked cell division and tumor progression. Unfortunately, this common genetic alteration and other tumor suppressor inactivating mutations seen in SCCHN are not easily druggable, because restoring a vital cell function is far more challenging than blocking a function that is constitutively turned on by an activating oncogene mutation.

The exome sequencing studies have further demonstrated that HPV-associated SCCHN differs markedly at the molecular level from HPV-negative SCCHN, suggesting distinct biological differences in the etiology and pathogenesis of these cancers.[39] First, the mutation rate of HPV-positive SCCHN is approximately half that of HPV-negative tumors. In addition, *TP53* mutations are limited to HPV-negative cancers. And more recently, there is evidence that *PIK3CA* mutations may be enriched in HPV-associated SCCHN.[40]

## Prevention

The etiologic shift that is currently under way in SCCHN, from cancers arising out of the field cancerization effects of chronic tobacco and alcohol exposure to oropharyngeal malignancies resulting from the oncogenic virus, HPV, has important implications for the prevention of SCCHN.

### *Tobacco*

Tobacco use remains the leading cause of preventable death worldwide. Although HPV is emerging as a frequent cause of SCCHN, the potential impact tobacco cessation can make on SCCHN prevention globally is enormous, particularly because of the rising use of tobacco and smoking in low- and middle-income countries. For instance, in China, there are an estimated 350 million smokers. In India, the world's second most populous country,

14% of the population smokes. There is, however, reason for optimism, as there are proven, cost-effective means to combat tobacco use, and antismoking campaigns have had some success.[41] Perhaps the most comprehensive approach to tobacco cessation is the WHO's MPOWER campaign. This program, established in 2008, calls for the implementation of six evidence-based tobacco control measures: (1) monitoring tobacco use and prevention policies, (2) protecting people from tobacco smoke, (3) offering people help in quitting tobacco use, (4) warning people of the dangers of tobacco, (5) enforcing bans on tobacco advertising, and (6) raising taxes on tobacco.[42] Progress has indeed been made; 2.3 billion people living in 92 countries are now protected by at least one MPOWER measure, up from 1.3 billion people in 48 countries as of 5 years ago. Still, much of the progress made has been in small low- and middle-income countries. More progress is necessary, including in high-population and high-income countries, in order to protect the multitude of lives at risk for death by tobacco over the next century.

## HPV Vaccine

HPV vaccines against the prevalent HPV serotypes associated with cervical cancer and anal cancer were recently approved for use based on the efficacy of reducing cervical cancer rates. The two commercially available vaccines include a bivalent vaccine directed against HPV serotypes 16 and 18 and a quadrivalent vaccine directed against HPV serotypes 6, 11, 16, and 18. At the time of FDA approval, there was no data on whether these vaccines would prevent against oral HPV infection. However, a recent study performed in Costa Rica demonstrated a 93.3% reduction in oral HPV infection in vaccinated women aged 18 to 25 four years after vaccination compared to a control unvaccinated group.[43] It is presumed that this decline in infection would also translate into decreased oropharyngeal cancer rates. It is not known for how long an individual would be protected from oral HPV with these vaccines. At this time, two high-risk HPV vaccines are available. The quadrivalent vaccine (Gardasil) provides protection against oncogenic HPV types 16 and 18, as well as types 6 and 11, which are associated with genial warts. The second vaccine (Cervarix) protects against HPV types 16 and 18. These two vaccines are highly effective at preventing HPV-associated premalignant cervical lesions in women, genital warts, and anal premalignant lesions in high-risk men.[44-48] Although it is still unclear what the impact of the HPV vaccine will be on the future incidence of SCCHN, the HPV vaccines are expected to be protective against HPV-associated oropharyngeal cancers. For vaccine efficacy, administration must occur before adolescents become sexually active, as viral transmission may occur soon after the initiation of sexual activity. The U.S. Centers for Disease Control and Prevention thus currently recommends routine HPV vaccination for girls and boys, from age 11 up to 26. Surprisingly, the current vaccine rate of vaccine completion in girls in the United States is only 25%. This falls far short of the goal of 80% vaccination by 2020, established to ensure herd immunity and promoted by the federal government's Healthy People campaign.[49] When the reasons behind this lack of vaccination were surveyed, a large proportion of parents indicated no intention to vaccinate their adolescent daughters against HPV, despite the high disease prevalence.[50] This trend suggests that making the vaccine available in the United States is not enough and that a major need for additional interventions, such as global public health education campaign, exists. Despite the regional differences in HPV-associated oropharyngeal carcinoma, HPV is the most common sexually transmitted infection worldwide. Therefore, the rationale for widespread administration of HPV vaccination is strong. Fortunately, the Global Alliance for Vaccines and Immunization (GAVI Alliance), whose mission is to increase access to immunization in the developing world, has added the HPV vaccine to its program for subsidized vaccination in low-income countries. In addition, manufacturer pricing has incorporated tiered pricing for HPV vaccines, making widespread vaccination more feasible.

## TREATMENT

Optimal treatment of head and neck cancers involves a multidisciplinary team, including medical oncologists, surgeons, radiation oncologists, nurses, nutritionists, and speech and swallow therapists. In general, all patients without distant metastatic disease are considered potentially curable, even when the disease is locally advanced, stage IV. Limited disease, that is, stage I or II, can typically be treated with a single modality, such as surgery or radiotherapy. The optimal choice of therapy depends on the primary site of disease, as well as the functional impact of treatment. For example, a stage I or II oral cavity cancer is almost always resectable with acceptable morbidity in terms of speech and swallowing, whereas even a small laryngeal primary tumor is often treated with radiation as an organ sparing alternative to surgery. There are laryngeal sparing surgical approaches that may adequately treat an early-stage larynx cancer without total laryngectomy, but these advanced surgical techniques are not available at all centers. Five-year survival ranges from 70% to 90% in patients with early-stage disease, while in locally advanced stage III–IV disease, 5-year survival is approximately 50%.

### Surgery

In the developed world, surgery or definitive radiation treatment is the primary treatment for early-stage or localized cancers of the oral cavity, pharynx, and larynx. Surgery is also employed in locally advanced stage III and

IV disease in select cases, and in the absence of distant metastasis. There have been great advancements in the field of head and neck surgery over the last two decades, which have significantly transformed functional and cosmetic outcomes for patients and allowed for acceptable outcomes even in advanced disease. Examples include free tissue transfer techniques for reconstruction following tumor ablation, transoral laser microsurgery for tumor resection with preservation of laryngopharyngeal function, and, most recently, transoral robotic surgery that facilitates exposure of the oropharynx without requiring a hemimandibulectomy. Surgery is the initial modality of therapy considered in essentially all oral cavity cancers, sinonasal cancers, and in select other primary sites. The challenges to appropriate surgical services for head and neck cancers are, however, significant in low- and middle-income countries. As an example, in Africa, there is an estimated deficit of nearly 4,700 otolaryngology surgeons; 9 out of 18 African countries surveyed had 10 or fewer otolaryngology surgeons.[51]

## Chemotherapy

Platinum agents form the basis of chemotherapy for head and neck cancers and are used both concurrently with radiotherapy and in metastatic disease. For patients with locally advanced SCCHN, an alternative to primary site surgery is concurrent chemoradiotherapy, which can offer cure rates similar to those seen with surgery, but also allows primary site preservation. This alternative treatment to surgery can allow for critical improvements in quality of life, such as when chemoradiotherapy is utilized in place of laryngectomy in laryngeal and hypopharyngeal primary tumors.[52] When chemoradiotherapy is employed in the upfront treatment of SCCHN, surgery is generally reserved for the salvage of persistent or recurrent disease. Multiple large randomized clinical trials have demonstrated the superiority of chemoradiotherapy over radiation alone as an organ preservation approach to locally advanced SCCHN.[53-55] Although not all studies have used the same chemotherapy, concurrent cisplatin, given either weekly or in higher doses every 3 weeks during radiation, is a commonly used and feasible regimen.

While distant metastasis is present in a minority of SCCHN patients at presentation, approximately 50% of patients initially treated for locally advanced SCCHN will develop locoregionally recurrent and/or distant metastatic disease. Only those patients in whom salvage surgery can encompass the entire disease are potentially curable. The remainder of patients can be considered for palliative chemotherapy, but gains in improving overall survival have, to date, been modest. The most active regimen studied thus far is a combination of cisplatin (or carboplatin), 5-fluorouracil, and the EGFR monoclonal antibody, cetuximab, which is shown in the EXTREME trial to increase overall survival from 7 months with cisplatin and 5-fluorouracil alone to 10 months with the three drugs.[56] Although the use of cetuximab-containing regimens is a standard of care in the developed world, the cost and availability of cetuximab in low- and middle-income countries remain a challenge, and in low-income countries cetuximab is likely not available at all. Moreover, the benefit of multiagent chemotherapy in the palliative setting needs to be weighed against the downside of added toxicity, and many patients with recurrent/metastatic SCCHN do not have a good enough performance status to tolerate combined chemotherapy. In this case, single agents, including taxanes, 5-fluorouracil, and methotrexate, can be considered.

## Radiation Therapy

Radiotherapy is a vital and essential component of treatment for SCCHN. Radiotherapy is used as curative therapy alone for early-stage disease and in combination with concurrent chemotherapy in locally advanced disease. Doses of 66 to 72 Gray (Gy) in 2-Gy fractions to gross disease are typically employed in the upfront setting. When radiotherapy is administered in the adjuvant setting following surgery, the dose ranges from 60 to 66 Gy. Radiotherapy is also an essential component of treatment of localized and locally advanced NPC. The lack of sufficient radiation therapy in developing countries limits the ability to sufficiently care for patients with head and neck cancers. In addition, it is important to consider the addition of platinum chemotherapy when high-risk features, such as positive surgical margins and extranodal extension, are present.[57,58]

In high-income countries, recent advancements in radiotherapy for SCCHN include improvements in defining the fields covered by treatment and in radiation delivery. In the former, improvements in targeting with better anatomic staging by CT, MRI, and positron emission tomography imaging have resulted in more precisely defined target tissues and delineation of adjacent normal structures for radiation sparing. Thus, a tighter correlation between radiation dose and extent of disease can be achieved. In the latter realm of advancements in radiotherapy, intensity-modulated radiation therapy (IMRT) has been the most widely adopted improvement. IMRT improves the radiation's ability to conform to concave tissue structures by the use of multileaf collimator technology and highly tailored computer algorithms to sculpt the delivery of radiation, maximizing dose to the tumor while sparing normal tissues. One of the most compelling examples of the benefits of IMRT in treating SCCHN is the ability to spare the major salivary glands. This approach has led to improvements in xerostomia-related complications, such as dental injury, and improvements in quality of life for SCCHN survivors. Unfortunately, widespread adoption of IMRT is limited not only by the high equipment costs but also by the expertise required to implement the technology. With IMRT, the radiation oncologist must be an expert in head and neck anatomy, as he or she must manually delineate the treatment fields one CT image at a time through the entire disease site. Following this step, radiation physicists and dosimetrists must be available to create the treatment plan. The lack of sufficient radiotherapy in developing countries limits the ability to sufficiently care for patients with head and neck cancers. For example, in Africa, where radiation therapy services are most lacking, demand far exceeds supply and was estimated that 21% of the population had no access to radiation therapy services at all.[59]

## CONCLUSION

Although most patients with SCCHN present at a locoregionally advanced stage, it is important to understand that these cancers are potentially curable. The challenge to curative therapy for SCCHN is that optimal treatment requires complex multimodality expertise and that specialty care is also necessary for survivors to overcome the chronic toxicities of therapy. Although the multimodality care needed for comprehensive treatment of SCCHN is challenging for many low-income countries that lack medical oncologists, radiation facilities, and surgeons, SCCHN is a cancer for which curative therapy can be achieved despite advanced presentations.

The main epidemiologic drivers of SCCHN include global tobacco, alcohol, and HPV. In 2011, nearly 80% of the 6 million deaths due to tobacco use occurred in low- and middle-income countries. The WHO estimates that more than 8 million people per year will die from tobacco-related causes by 2030 and that 80% of these premature deaths will occur in low- and middle-income countries. High rates of smoking in low- and middle-income countries remain a sobering reminder that the trend of SCCHN as a major public health problem will persist. Nevertheless, opportunities for major progress are provided by efforts in prevention. Prioritization of tobacco and alcohol prevention programs would make the greatest impact on death due to SCCHN around the world. The major shift occurring in SCCHN with the rise of HPV-positive SCCHN presents another major opportunity for prevention through the adoption of vaccine strategies. Coupling these prevention strategies to the development of comprehensive cancer care in low- and middle-income countries should remain a top priority in order to prevent and treat SCCHN.

## REFERENCES

1. Jemal A, Bray F, Center MM, Ferlay J, Ward E, Forman D. Global cancer statistics. CA *Cancer J Clin* 2011 Mar–Apr; 61(2): 69–90.

2. Danaei G, Vander Hoorn S, Lopez AD, Murray CJ, Ezzati M, Comparative Risk Assessment Collaborating Group (Cancers). Causes of cancer in the world: comparative risk assessment of nine behavioural and environmental risk factors. *Lancet* 2005 Nov 19; 366(9499): 1784–93.

3. Lim SS, Vos T, Flaxman AD, et al. A comparative risk assessment of burden of disease and injury attributable to 67 risk factors and risk factor clusters in 21 regions, 1990–2010: a systematic analysis for the Global Burden of Disease Study 2010. *Lancet* 2012 Dec 15; 380(9859): 2224–60.

4. Gillison ML, Broutian T, Pickard RK, et al. Prevalence of oral HPV infection in the United States, 2009–2010. *JAMA* 2012 Feb 15; 307(7): 693–703. doi:10.1001/jama.2012.101. Epub Jan 26, 2012.

5. Ferlay J, Shin H, Bray F, Forman D, Mathers C, Parkin DM. Estimates of worldwide burden of cancer in 2008: GLOBOCAN 2008. *Int J Cancer* 127(12); 2010 Dec 15: 2893–917.

6. Blot WJ, McLaughlin JK, Winn DM, et al. Smoking and drinking in relation to oral and pharyngeal cancer. *Cancer Res* 1988 Jun 1; 48(11): 3282–87.

7. Available at http://www.who.int/mediacentre/factsheets/fs339/en/.

8. Giovino GA, Mirza SA, Samet JM, et al. Tobacco use in 3 billion individuals from 16 countries: an analysis of nationally representative cross-sectional household surveys. *Lancet* 2012 Aug 18; 380(9842): 668–79. doi:10.1016/S0140-6736(12)61085-X.

9. Warren CW, Lea V, Lee J, Jones NR, Asma S, McKenna M. Change in tobacco use among 13–15 year olds between 1999 and 2008: findings from the Global Youth Tobacco Survey. *Glob Health Promot* 2009 Sep; 16(2 Suppl): 38–90.

10. Available at http://www.iarc.fr/en/publications/pdfs-online/wcr/2008/wcr_2008.pdf.

11. Chaturvedi AK. Epidemiology and clinical aspects of HPV in head and neck cancers. *Head Neck Pathol* 2012 Jul; 6(Suppl 1): S16–24. doi:10.1007/s12105-012-0377-0. Epub Jul 3, 2012.

12. Shiboski CH, Schmidt BL, Jordan RC. Tongue and tonsil carcinoma: increasing trends in the U.S. population ages 20–44 years. *Cancer* 2005; 103: 1843–49.

13. Chaturvedi AK, Engels EA, Pfeiffer RM, et al. Human papillomavirus and rising oropharyngeal cancer incidence in the United States. *J Clin Oncol* 2011 Nov 10; 29(32): 4294–301.

14. Mehanna H, Paleri V, West CML, Nutting C. Head and neck cancer—part 1: epidemiology, presentation, and prevention. *BMJ* 2010; 341: c4684.

15. Black RJ, Bray F, Ferlay J, Parkin DM. Cancer incidence and mortality in the European Union: cancer registry data and estimates of national incidence for 1990. *Eur J Cancer* 1997 Jun; 33(7): 1075–107.

16. Cao SM, Simons MJ, Qian CN. The prevalence and prevention of nasopharyngeal carcinoma in China. *Chin J Cancer* 2011 Feb; 30(2): 114–19.

17. Chang ET, Adami HO. The enigmatic epidemiology of nasopharyngeal carcinoma. *Cancer Epidemiol Biomarkers Prev* 2006 Oct; 15(10): 1765–77.

18. Lee AW, Foo W, Mang O, et al. Changing epidemiology of nasopharyngeal carcinoma in Hong Kong over a 20-year period (1980–99): an encouraging reduction in both incidence and mortality. *Int J Cancer* 2003 Feb 20; 103(5): 680–85.

19. Dickson RI, Flores AD. Nasopharyngeal carcinoma: an evaluation of 134 patients treated between 1971–1980. *Laryngoscope* 1985 Mar; 95(3): 276–83.

20. Murray CJL, Lopez AD. Alternative projections of mortality and disability by cause 1990—2020: Global Burden of Disease Study. *Lancet* 1997 May 24; 349(9064): 1498—504.

21. Fowles J, Dybing E. Application of toxicological risk assessment principles to the chemical constituents of cigarette smoke. *Tob Control* 2003 Dec; 12(4): 424–30.

22. Partridge M, Emilion G, Pateromichelakis S, Phillips E, Langdon J. Field cancerisation of the oral cavity: comparison of the spectrum of molecular alterations in cases presenting with both dysplastic and malignant lesions. *Oral Oncol* 1997 Sep; 33(5): 332–37.

23. Sturgis EM, Wei Q, Spitz MR. Descriptive epidemiology and risk factors for head and neck cancer. *Semin Oncol* 2004 Dec; 31(6): 726–33.

24. Shield KD, Rylett M, Gmel G, Gmel G, Kehoe-Chan TA, Rehm J. Global alcohol exposure estimates by country, territory and region for 2005—a contribution to the Comparative Risk Assessment for the 2010 Global Burden of Disease Study. *Addiction* 2013 May; 108(5): 912–22.

25. Hashibe M, Brennan P, Chuang SC, et al. Interaction between tobacco and alcohol use and the risk of head and neck cancer: pooled analysis in the International Head and Neck Cancer Epidemiology Consortium. *Cancer Epidemiol Biomarkers Prev* 2009 Feb; 18(2): 541–50.

26. Freedman ND, Schatzkin A, Leitzmann MF, Hollenbeck AR, Abnet CC. Alcohol and head and neck cancer risk in a prospective study. *Br J Cancer* 2007 May 7; 96(9): 1469–74.

27. Bagnardi V, Rota M, Botteri E, et al. Light alcohol drinking and cancer: a meta-analysis. *Ann Oncol* 2013 Feb; 24(2): 301–8.

28. Curado MP, Boyle P. Epidemiology of head and neck squamous cell carcinoma not related to tobacco or alcohol. *Curr Opin Oncol* 2013 May; 25(3): 229–34.

29. Schiffman M, Wacholder S. Success of HPV vaccination is now a matter of coverage. *Lancet Oncol* 2012 Jan; 13(1): 10–12.

30. Schabath MB, Villa LL, Lazcano-Ponce E, et al. Smoking and human papillomavirus (HPV) infection in the HPV in Men (HIM) study. *Cancer Epidemiol Biomarkers Prev* 2012 Jan; 21(1): 102–10.

31. Miller DL, Puricelli MD, Stack MS. Virology and molecular pathogenesis of HPV (human papillomavirus)-associated oropharyngeal squamous cell carcinoma. *Biochem J* 2012 Apr 15; 443(2): 339–53.

32. Yoshizaki T, Kondo S, Wakisaka N, et al. Pathogenic role of Epstein–Barr virus latent membrane protein-1 in the development of nasopharyngeal carcinoma. *Cancer Lett* 2013 Aug 28; 337(1): 1–7.

33. Dassonville O, Formento JL, Francoual M, et al. Expression of epidermal growth factor receptor and survival in upper aerodigestive tract cancer. *J Clin Oncol* 1993 Oct; 11(10): 1873–78.

34. Grandis JR, Tweardy DJ. Elevated levels of transforming growth factor alpha and epidermal growth factor receptor messenger RNA are early markers of carcinogenesis in head and neck cancer. *Cancer Res* 1993 Aug 1; 53(15): 3579–84.

35. Reuter CW, Morgan MA, Eckardt A. Targeting EGF-receptor-signalling in squamous cell carcinomas of the head and neck. *Br J Cancer* 2007 Feb 12; 96(3): 408–16.

36. Vokes EE, Seiwert TY. EGFR-directed treatments in SCCHN. *Lancet Oncol* 2013 Jul; 14(8): 672–73.

37. Bonner JA, Harari PM, Giralt J, et al. Radiotherapy plus cetuximab for squamous-cell carcinoma of the head and neck. *N Engl J Med* 2006 Feb 9; 354(6): 567–78.

38. Agrawal N, Frederick MJ, Pickering CR, et al. Exome sequencing of head and neck squamous cell carcinoma reveals inactivating mutations in NOTCH1. *Science* 2011 Aug 26; 333(6046): 1154–57.

39. Stransky N, Egloff AM, Tward AD, et al. The mutational landscape of head and neck squamous cell carcinoma. *Science* 2011 Aug 26; 333(6046): 1157–60. doi:10.1126/science.1208130. Epub 2011 Jul 28.

40. Nichols AC, Palma DA, Chow W, et al. High frequency of activating PIK3CA mutations in human papillomavirus-positive oropharyngeal cancer. *JAMA Otolaryngol Head Neck Surg* 2013 Jun; 139(6): 617–22.

41. McAfee T, Davis KC, Alexander RL Jr, Pechacek TF, Bunnell R. Effect of the first federally funded US antismoking national media campaign. *Lancet* 2013 Sep 6. pii: S0140–6736(13)61686–4.

42. Available at http://www.who.int/tobacco/global_report/2013/en/.

43. Herrero R, Quint W, Hildesheim A, et al. Reduced prevalence of oral human papillomavirus (HPV) 4 years after bivalent HPV vaccination in a randomized clinical trial in Costa Rica. *PLoS One* 2013 Jul 17; 8(7): e68329.

44. Brown DR, Kjaer SK, Sigurdsson K, et al. The impact of quadrivalent human papillomavirus (HPV; types 6, 11, 16, and 18) L1 virus-like particle vaccine on infection and disease due to oncogenic nonvaccine HPV types in generally HPV-naive women aged 16–26 years. *J Infect Dis* 2009 Apr 1; 199(7): 926–35.

45. Muñoz N, Kjaer SK, Sigurdsson K, et al. Impact of human papillomavirus (HPV)-6/11/16/18 vaccine on all HPV-associated genital diseases in young women. *J Natl Cancer Inst* 2010 Mar 3; 102(5): 325–39.

46. Giuliano AR, Palefsky JM, Goldstone S, et al. Efficacy of quadrivalent HPV vaccine against HPV infection and disease in males. *N Engl J Med* 2011 Feb 3; 364(5): 401–11.

47. Palefsky JM, Giuliano AR, Goldstone S, et al. HPV vaccine against anal HPV infection and anal intraepithelial neoplasia. *N Engl J Med* 2011 Oct 27; 365(17): 1576–85.

48. Lehtinen M, Paavonen J, Wheeler CM, et al. Overall efficacy of HPV-16/18 AS04-adjuvanted vaccine against grade 3 or greater cervical intraepithelial neoplasia: 4-year end-of-study analysis of the randomised, double-blind PATRICIA trial. *Lancet Oncol* 2012 Jan; 13(1): 89–99.

49. Available at http://healthypeople.gov/2020/.

50. Darden PM, Thompson DM, Roberts JR, et al. Reasons for not vaccinating adolescents: National Immunization Survey of Teens, 2008–2010. *Pediatrics* 2013 Apr; 131(4): 645–51. doi:10.1542/peds.2012–2384. Epub Mar 18, 2013.

51. Fagan JJ. Developing World ENT: a global responsibility. *J Laryngol Otol* 2012 Jun; 126(6): 544–47.

52. Pfister DG, Laurie SA, Weinstein GS, et al. American Society of Clinical Oncology clinical practice guideline for the use of larynx-preservation strategies

in the treatment of laryngeal cancer. American Society of Clinical Oncology. *J Clin Oncol* 2006 Aug 1; 24(22): 3693–704.

53. Brizel DM, Albers ME, Fisher SR, et al. Hyperfractionated irradiation with or without concurrent chemotherapy for locally advanced head and neck cancer. *N Engl J Med* 1998 Jun 18; 338(25): 1798–804.

54. Staar S, Rudat V, Stuetzer H, et al. Intensified hyperfractionated accelerated radiotherapy limits the additional benefit of simultaneous chemotherapy—results of a multicentric randomized German trial in advanced head-and-neck cancer. *Int J Radiat Oncol Biol Phys* 2001 Aug 1; 50(5): 1161–71.

55. Denis F, Garaud P, Bardet E, et al. Final results of the 94–01 French Head and Neck Oncology and Radiotherapy Group randomized trial comparing radiotherapy alone with concomitant radiochemotherapy in advanced-stage oropharynx carcinoma. *J Clin Oncol* 2004 Jan 1; 22(1): 69–76.

56. Vermorken JB, Mesia R, Rivera F, et al. Platinum-based chemotherapy plus cetuximab in head and neck cancer. *N Engl J Med* 2008 Sep 11; 359(11): 1116–27. doi:10.1056/NEJMoa0802656.

57. Bernier J, Domenge C, Ozsahin M, et al. Postoperative irradiation with or without concomitant chemotherapy for locally advanced head and neck cancer. *N Engl J Med* 2004 May 6; 350(19): 1945–52.

58. Cooper JS, Pajak TF, Forastiere AA, et al. Postoperative concurrent radiotherapy and chemotherapy for high-risk squamous-cell carcinoma of the head and neck. *N Engl J Med* 2004 May 6; 350(19): 1937–44.

59. Barton MB, Frommer M, Shafiq J. Role of radiotherapy in cancer control in low-income and middle-income countries. *Lancet Oncol* 2006 Jul; 7(7): 584–95.

# 2

# Global Breast Cancer Care: Disparities and Challenges

*Kenneth D. Miller, Tamna Wangjam,
Cara Miller, and Bella Nadler*

## TWO CASE HISTORIES

*United States:* Michelle is a 56-year-old postmenopausal woman, who on a yearly screening mammogram was found to have a new 0.7-cm indeterminate lesion in her right breast which could not be identified by a breast ultrasound that was performed at the same time. An MRI-guided biopsy was performed 2 days later, and it revealed a Grade II infiltrating ductal breast cancer that was estrogen and progesterone receptor positive and negative for Her2-Neu. Gene expression profiling indicated a low recurrence score. She was seen by a multidisciplinary team and 5 days later underwent a lumpectomy and sentinel node biopsy. Three weeks later she started radiation, and after completing radiation, she began a 5-year course of treatment with an aromatase inhibitor.

*East Africa:* Rachel is a 38-year-old woman who lives in northern Ethiopia. Two years ago she noted a lump in her right breast that was the size of a marble, which she thought was a scar. One year ago, it had increased to the size of an egg, and she saw a local healer who recommended herbal medication which she took for 6 months. Progressively, her breast became hard, the nipple became inverted, and she began to bleed. She was seen at a local clinic, referred to a regional hospital, and underwent a mastectomy which confirmed the diagnosis of breast cancer with multiple positive nodes. Two months later she traveled 12 hours by bus to the cancer institute. Treatment with six cycles of cyclophosphamide, Adriamycin, and 5-fluorouracil was recommended as well as radiation for the chest wall and axilla. She waited 2 months and with funds donated from her village and from selling her property she was able to receive two cycles of adjuvant chemotherapy but then decided to not receive additional chemotherapy because of the cost. She did not return to receive radiation therapy to the chest wall.

## INTRODUCTION

Breast cancer contributes greatly to the global burden of disease but more personally is the cause of deep suffering for women, their families, and communities. It is one of the most common cancers in high-income countries (HICs), and the incidence rates are increasing rapidly in low- and middle-income countries (LMICs), which has been attributed to an increasingly Westernized lifestyle. At the same time, divergent trends for the incidence of breast cancer within and between countries in the same region (e.g., Venezuela and Colombia or Thailand and Singapore) are a reminder that the known, major risk factors, such as reproductive history, obesity, and diet, account for some but not all recognized incidence patterns.[1,2] It is likely that the interaction between genetics and individual risk factors, and environmental factors may together explain these divergent trends.[3] The complexity of the changing incidence of breast cancer focuses on the importance of building better surveillance systems to inform the development of national cancer control strategies.[3]

## BREAST CANCER ETIOLOGY

International variation in breast cancer incidence has provided important clues to understanding the role of hormonal carcinogenesis. A woman living up to age 80 in North America has a one in nine chance of developing breast cancer, but Asian women in Asia (who have substantially lower concentrations of estrogens and progesterone than women in North America) have one-fifth or less of the risk of developing breast cancer. In contrast, Asian women who immigrate to westernized nations and more notably their daughters have sex steroid hormone concentrations and risks identical to those of their Western counterparts.[5–7]

The length of menstrual life (particularly the fraction occurring before first full-term pregnancy) is a substantial contributor to the total lifetime risk of breast cancer. Similarly, the duration of maternal nursing also correlates with substantial risk reduction, which is independent of either parity or age at first full-term pregnancy.[8–10] Three dates in a woman's life have a major impact on breast cancer incidence, including age at menarche, age at first full-term pregnancy, and age at menopause. Together, these three factors account for up to 70% to 80% of the variation in breast cancer frequency in different countries. More specifically,

1. women with menarche at age 16 or above have only 50% to 60% of the breast cancer risk of a woman with menarche at age 12 and the lower risk persists throughout life;

2. women with menopause occurring 10 years before the median age of menopause (52 years), whether natural or surgically induced, have a 35% reduction in lifetime breast cancer risk; and

3. in addition, women who have a first full-term pregnancy by age 18 have a 30% to 40% lower risk of breast cancer compared with nulliparous women.

The role of diet and environmental exposures in breast cancer etiology is more controversial. Although there are associative links between total caloric and fat intake and breast cancer risk, the exact role of dietary fat is unproven.[11,12] Increased caloric intake contributes to breast cancer risk in multiple ways: earlier menarche, later age at menopause, and increased postmenopausal estrogen concentrations reflect enhanced aromatase activities in fatty tissues. Moderate alcohol intake also increases the risk, and radiation exposure is a risk factor in younger women. Women who have been exposed before age 30 to radiation in the form of multiple fluoroscopies (200 to 300 cGy) or treatment for Hodgkin's disease (>3,600 cGy) have a substantial increase in risk of breast cancer, whereas radiation exposure after age 30 poses less risk for the development of a subsequent breast cancer.[13,14]

## GLOBAL BREAST CANCER EPIDEMIOLOGY

### Breast Cancer Incidence

Breast cancer is the most common cancer among women both in developed and in developing countries with an estimated 1.38 million new cancer cases diagnosed in 2008 (23% of all cancers).[3] Global breast cancer incidence increased from 641,000 (95% certainty interval 610,000 to 750,000) cases in 1980 to 1,643,000 (1,421,000 to 1,782,000) cases in 2010, for an annual rate of increase of 3.1%.[1–3] Incidence rates vary greatly from 19.3 per 100,000 women in eastern Africa to 89.7 per 100,000 women in Western Europe. The incidence is particularly high (greater than 80 per 100,000) in HIC (except Japan) and low (less than 40 per 100,000) in LMICs (Figure 2.1). There has been an increasing incidence of breast cancer in most regions during the past three decades, but this increase is more prominent in the Middle East, South Asia, Southeast Asia, and Latin America (Figure 2.2). In 2010, a little more than two-thirds of cases of breast cancer were seen in women aged 50 years and older, the majority of whom were in developed countries (39%) (Figure 2.3).[3] For younger women aged 15 to 49 years, there were twice as many breast cancer cases in developing countries (23%) than that in developed countries (10%).[3,17,18]

## Breast Cancer Mortality

Breast cancer is the fifth leading cause of death from cancer overall (458,000 deaths); however, in women, it is still the most frequent cause of cancer death in both developing (269,000 deaths) and developed regions (189,000 deaths). The mortality rates range from approximately 6 to 19 per 100,000.[3,16–18] This is a treatable cancer, and so mortality rates are lower than the incidence of developing the disease. Despite vast differences

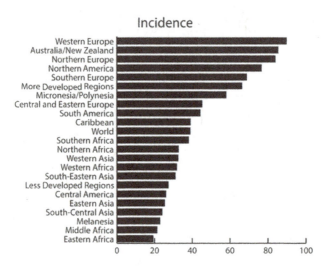

**FIGURE 2.1** Estimated age-standardized incidence rates for breast cancer (adapted from reference 2).

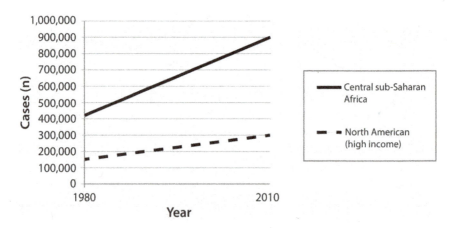

**FIGURE 2.2** Trends in the incidence of breast cancer in individuals aged 15 years and older, 1980 to 2010 (adapted from references 3,16).

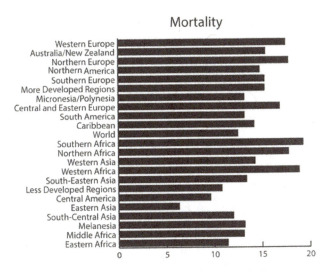

**FIGURE 2.3** Estimated age-standardized mortality rates for breast cancer (adapted from reference 2).

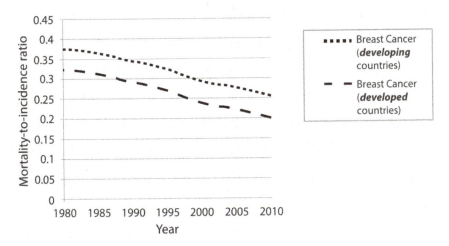

**FIGURE 2.4** Age-standardized mortality-to-incidence ratio for breast and cervical cancer in developed and developing countries in women aged 15 years or older, 1980 to 2010 (adapted from references 3,16).

in the mortality-to-incidence (M/I) ratios for breast cancer between developed and developing regions, the M/I ratios for both have decreased since the mid-1980s. Increased availability of screening, decreased use of hormone replacement therapy, and improved treatment may be contributing to this improvement in outcomes (Figure 2.4).

## REGIONAL BREAST CANCER STATISTICS: A BRIEF REVIEW

### United States: Incidence Related to Age and Race

SEER Cancer Statistics in 2006 to 2010 from 18 SEER geographic areas indicate that the age-adjusted breast cancer incidence rate was 123.8 per 100,000 women/year and the age-adjusted death rate was 23/100,000 women/year.[19] In 2013 it was estimated that 232,340 women and 2,240 men in the United States would be diagnosed with breast cancer. Breast cancer mortality in the United States varied with age and of those who died 0.9% were between 20 and 34 years, 5.3% between 35 and 44 years, 14.6% between 45 and 54 years, 21.6% between 55 and 64 years, 20.2% between 65 and 74 years, 21.5% between 75 and 84 years, and 15.9% for 85+ years. The breast cancer incidence and mortality in the United States also varied with race/ethnicity. The incidence rate was highest for white women, whereas breast cancer mortality rates were highest in black women (Table 2.1).

### Europe: Significant Regional Differences Seen in Rates and Trends

Breast cancer was a very common cancer in all European countries in 2012 (13.5% of all cancer cases in all populations) and the most common cancer in women (28.8% of cancer diagnoses). It is estimated that in 2012 there were 464,000 new cases of breast cancer, which was also the leading cause of death in women (131,000 cases) followed by colorectal and lung cancer.[20,21]

Within Europe, there are geographical variations in the incidence rates, ranging from 49 to 148 per 100,000.[20,21] The highest incidence rates were noted in Western European countries, including Belgium (147/100,000), France (137), the Netherlands (131), and Northern Europe, (particularly the United Kingdom [129], the Nordic countries [143], and Iceland [131]). In contrast, incidence rates in Eastern European countries were much lower,

TABLE 2.1 Breast Cancer Incidence and Mortality by Race (adapted from SEER Data[19])

| Incidence Rates by Race | Death Rates by Race |
|---|---|
| Race/Ethnicity | Race/Ethnicity |
| Female | Female |
| All Races | All Races |
| 123.8 per 100,000 women | 22.6 per 100,000 women |
| White | White |
| 127.4 per 100,000 women | 22.1 per 100,000 women |
| Black | Black |
| 121.4 per 100,000 women | 30.8 per 100,000 women |

including in the Ukraine (54) and Moldova (53) (Figure 2.5). Incidence rates are increasing across all age groups in each European country, except in Scotland, Slovenia, and Switzerland.[16] Breast cancer mortality rates varied in Europe from 15 to 36 per 100,000. Highest breast cancer mortality rates were observed in Northern Europe (e.g., Belgium, 29, and Denmark, 28) and in Southern Europe (e.g., Serbia, 31, and Macedonia, 36).

## Africa: Incidence Rising to Equal HICs

There are few cancer registries in Africa, and incidence and mortality rates can be extrapolated only from data available from two cancer registries in Africa, including the Zimbabwe National Cancer Registry and the Kampala

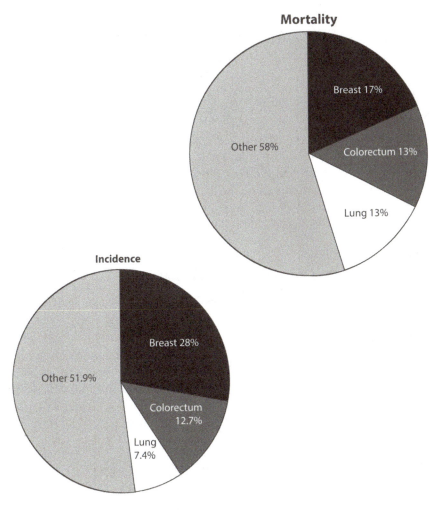

**FIGURE 2.5** Distribution of the expected cases and deaths for the most common cancers in Europe in females, 2012 (adapted from reference 16).

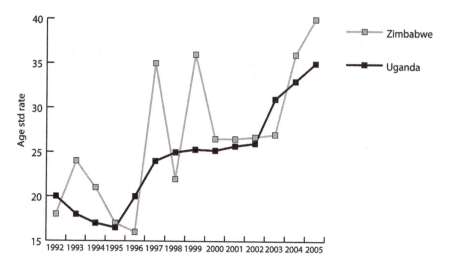

**FIGURE 2.6** Trends in age-standardized incidence rates of breast cancer in Uganda and Zimbabwe 1992 to 2005 (adapted from reference 22).

Cancer Registry in Uganda.[22,23] There has been a steady increase in the incidence of cancer in both sexes, which for women in Kampala is now similar to that of HICs.[22,23] From 1991 to 2010, breast cancer in Zimbabwe was the third most common cancer in women (10.4% of cases) after cancer of the cervix (24.6% of cases) and Kaposi sarcoma (17.4%). Unfortunately, breast cancer incidence has increased markedly at an average annual rate of 3.3% (95% CI 2.0 to 4.6%) over a 20-year period so that the age-specific rate in 2006 to 2010 was 103.8 per 100,000 (Figure 2.6).

## Asia: Changing Urban to Rural Case Ratio

China:[24,25] In 2008, breast cancer was the second most common cancer in China (incidence 21.6/100,000) and the sixth leading cause of cancer mortality (mortality rate 5.7/100,000). This increase in the incidence and mortality rate of breast cancer was noted in both urban and rural settings. In urban areas of Beijing, incidence and mortality rates rose from 2004 to 2008 from 55.43/100,000 and 10.65/100,000 to 70.70/100,000 and 15.01/100,000, respectively. In rural areas, these rates rose from 30.60/100,000 and 5.54/100 000 in 2004 to 44.78/100 000 and 7.49/100,000 in 2008.

## BREAST CANCER SURVIVAL: SIGNIFICANT GLOBAL VARIATION

The National Comprehensive Cancer Network has published extensive guidelines for the diagnosis and treatment of breast cancer, and guidelines have also been developed by the Breast Health Global Initiative on treatment of breast cancer, including the 2012 guidelines for the treatment of advanced breast cancer.[26,27] Unfortunately, these excellent guidelines are juxtaposed with the reality of the limited availability and affordability of comprehensive breast cancer care as well as the late stage of diagnosis. Broadly viewed, the 5-year survival ranges from 12% in parts of Africa to almost 90% in the United States.[28] The 5-year survival rate from breast cancer was 89% in the United States, 82% in Switzerland, and 80% in Spain, 38.8% in Algeria, 36.6% in Brazil, and 12% in the Gambia.[29] These differences in survival are noted between continents but also exist within regions. In the Nordic countries, 5- and 10-year relative survival increased by 20% to 30% but 5-year survival was 79% for 1999 to 2003 in Denmark but 83% to 87% in the other Nordic countries.[30] Finally, as might be expected, breast cancer survival differences are also seen when comparing the same ethnic or cultural groups who are living in different geographic settings. A study of age-adjusted 5-year relative survival of incident cases from 1993 to 2002 compared Filipinos, Filipino-Americans, and Caucasians in the SEER 13 database.[31] The 5-year relative survival rates of Manila residents, Filipino-Americans, and Caucasians were 58.6%, 89.6%, and 88.3%, respectively. Multiple factors contribute to prognosis for women with breast cancer, including delay in diagnosis, stage at the time of diagnosis, compliance with care, and the availability, affordability, and accessibility of comprehensive breast cancer care.[32]

## DELAY OF DIAGNOSIS AND BREAST CANCER STAGE

In the United States and other developed countries, breast cancer is typically diagnosed at an early stage. In contrast, in moderate- and low-income countries, women often present as locally advanced or metastatic breast cancer, treatment options are limited, and outcomes are poor. A survey of articles on breast cancer care in low- and medium-income countries, including Nigeria, Malaysia, Pakistan, Libya, and Indonesia, demonstrates a different situation:

*Nigeria:* In a series of 179 new cases of breast cancer presenting from 1998–2005 in Nigeria the majority of women were young, (mean of 46.85 years [SD 12.98]) with peak age ranges 30–39 and 40–49.[32–35] There was commonly a significant delay from initial symptoms to hospital presentation with 47% presenting after 6–12 months, 17% between 12 and 24 months, and 9% at more than 24 months. These investigators noted a decrease in the incidence of presentation with advanced breast cancer compared to 1960 but clinical staging in their cohort was; Stage I -3%, Stage II -25%, Stage III -68%, Stage IV -4%. Axillary lymph node were clinical positive in >70%. The investigators

hypothesize that some of the reasons for late diagnosis include, "ignorance, superstition, self-denial, fear of mastectomy and unavailability of
treatment facilities."[36]

http://www.ncbi.nlm.nih.gov/pmc/articles/PMC2486264/figure/F4/

*Malaysia:* In a study of 774 women with breast cancer at Hospital
Kuala Lumpur in Malaysia from 1998–2001 50% to 60% presented in
late stages (Stages 3 and 4).[40] During the same period, at the University
Malaya Medical Centre, 752 new cases of breast cancer were diagnosed
and 30% to 40% had advanced disease. They attributed the delay in
presentation to, "a strong belief in traditional medicine, the negative
perception of the disease, poverty and poor education, coupled with
fear and denial."

In a related study of 328 Malaysian women with breast cancer data
was collected on the delay in diagnosis.[41] The median time to consultation with a general practitioner was 2 months, which is shorter than in
other reported series. A delay in diagnosis (the time between the general practitioner and obtaining a histologic diagnosis) of more than 3
months was 72.6% and delay of more than 6 months occurred in 45.5%
of the cases. The factors associated with delay in diagnosis included the
use of alternative therapy, a false-negative diagnostic test, and a negative attitude toward treatment. In this group, the stage of breast cancer
was Stage I -5%, Stage II -39%, Stage III -45%, Stage IV -11%.

*Pakistan:* From 2004–2008 60 women were admitted to a hospital
in Nawabshah, Pakistan for treatment of breast cancer.[42] In this group,
the mean age is 43.5 +/– 10.4 years (age range 28–80 years) and in
95% of patients the first visit was more than 6 months of the start of
any breast cancer related symptoms or findings. The investigators noted
that, "Most cases of breast cancer presented in advanced stage due to
poor economic status, illiteracy and negligence by patients or their family members and general practitioners." Staging in this group was Stage
I -5%, Stage II -25%, Stage III -38%, Stage IV -19%.

*Libya:* 200 women, aged 22 to 75 years were diagnosed with breast
cancer during 2008–2009.[42] Only 30.0% of patients were diagnosed
within 3 months after symptoms while 14% of patients were diagnosed
within 3–6 months and 56% within a period longer than 6 months. The
investigators site a number of reasons for the delay in diagnosis including;
Symptoms were not considered serious in 27% of patients, alternative
therapy was initiated in 13.0% of the patients, fear and shame prevented
the visit to the doctor in 10% and 4.5% of patients respectively. Staging
was; Stage I -9%, Stage II -25%, Stage III -54%, Stage IV -12%.

*Jakarta, Indonesia:* 637 consecutive patients who were diagnosed at
the Dharmais Cancer Centre in 2010.[43] In this group clinical staging
was; Stage I -5%, Stage II -32%, Stage III -41%, Stage IV -22%. These

investigators also noted that some of the barriers to care include financial problems but also fatalism and belief in alternative medicine.

## Barriers to Care: Affordability

There are many barriers to breast cancer care in low- and medium-income countries regarding treatment. Cost is a major problem for many women with breast cancer, particularly in the absence of health insurance or public subsidy of cancer care. A study in central Vietnam estimated that the average cost of breast cancer care was $975 per patient (range $11.7 to $3,955) and the cost of initial treatment including chemotherapy accounted for 65% of the total cost. The authors note that "patients at later stages of breast cancer did not differ significantly in their total costs from those at earlier stages but their survival time was much shorter. Absence of health insurance was the main factor limiting service uptake."[44,45] In the United States, the estimated cost of breast cancer treatment per patient per month was $2,896 or approximately $34,752 per year.[46] The estimated 4-year cost for patients with stage III breast cancer was more than $60,000, but lower (though still substantial at $21,000) in patients with Stage I disease. The investigators note that affordability needs to be interpreted within the context of family income. The calculated costs of breast cancer treatment per month would take 5.4 days of salary for a middle-income country such as Pakistan and 18.4 days for a low-income country such as Malawi.[47,48]

## REGIONAL DIFFERENCES IN BREAST CANCER TREATMENT

Breast cancer surgery differs significantly between and within HICs and LMICs. In a large study of 9,779 women from 566 sites in nine countries (Belgium, France, Germany, Greece, Japan, the Netherlands, the United Kingdom/Ireland, and the United States), 58% of the women had T1 tumors (less than 2 cm), 37% had T2 tumors (2 to 5 cm), and 5% had larger/more advanced (T3/T4) tumors.[49] The overall mastectomy rate was 44%, with the lowest rate in France (19%) and the highest rate in Greece (56%).[49,50] In a similar study, the rates of mastectomy varied greatly. In contrast, in the Filipino study described earlier, during 1991, 1994, and 1997, 97% of incident cases of early breast cancer underwent modified radical mastectomy.[32] Similarly, in a study of 145 women treated at three referral hospitals from 2007 to 2011 in a low-income country, Rwanda, many women presented with metastatic cancer and 48% underwent mastectomy, 20% lumpectomy, and 3% mastectomy and chemotherapy.[51] Mastectomy rates vary significantly, as noted in Table 2.2.

**TABLE 2.2  Mastectomy Rates in Different Countries**

| France | 28% | Italy | 41% | Netherlands | 48% |
|---|---|---|---|---|---|
| United Kingdom | 31% | Germany | 43% | Greece | 56% |
| Belgium | 37% | Switzerland | 47% | | |

## Breast Cancer Radiation

The use of radiation therapy for women with breast cancer varies significantly. France and Belgium were the only countries to report essentially 100% radiation treatment rates after breast-conserving surgery (BCS), whereas the percentages of cases who did not receive radiation after BCS were Japan (14%), the United Kingdom and Ireland (13%), and the United States (14%). *Radiation therapy* is often not available for women with breast cancer.[52-56] In a study published in 1999, only 22 of 56 African nations had radiation facilities; these were concentrated in the southern and northern extremes of the continent and the population served by each unit ranged from 0.6 million to 70 million. In a later study in 2013, radiation therapy was still only available in 23 of 52 African nations. A third study notes that "many departments were found to treat patients without simulators or treatment planning systems."

The status of radiation oncology facilities in Latin America is different and 18 of 19 nations have radiation therapy centers. The authors of this study reported that 470 treatment centers were identified in 18 countries and were staffed with 933 radiation oncologists, 357 physicists, and 2,326 radiation therapy technologists. Availability of equipment and personnel was related to economic status of the country. They also noted that the major restriction to patient service is an insufficient number of specialists in 16 of the 18 countries.

A study in Korea provided quantitative data on the change in the availability of radiation oncology care over a decade. It found that radiation oncology facilities have steadily increased for 10 years and reached 60 sites in 2006 (see Figure 2.7) but that "radiation therapy equipment and human resources per population are relatively low compared with advanced countries."

## Systemic Therapy for Breast Cancer

*Systemic therapy after breast cancer surgery* also varies significantly.[52-56] The affordability and availability of hormone receptor testing are limited in many settings. In a randomized clinical trial conducted in Vietnam and China, adjuvant treatment with oophorectomy and tamoxifen was compared to observation alone. "5-year disease-free survival rates were 75% and 58% (P = .0003 unadjusted; P = .0075 adjusted) for the adjuvant and observation groups,

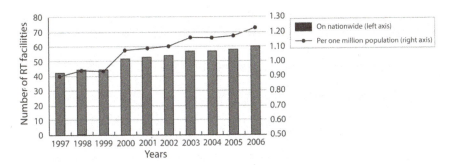

**FIGURE 2.7** Radiation oncology facilities in North Korea.

respectively," though as might be expected the only benefit was in women who were later found to have hormone receptor positive breast cancer. This study also found that oophorectomy and tamoxifen costs $350 per year of life saved in Vietnam. Where testing has been done, the results have been heterogeneous. In a study in Kenya[57] ER/PR was tested in 120 breast cancer specimens; 24% were ER-positive, 10% were ER-negative but PR-positive, and 66% were negative for ER and PR. ER/PR was not associated with age, stage, or node metastases; 26.5% over-expressed Her2. In a study in the Philippines, hormone receptor was positive in 65% of mastectomy specimens.

## TREATMENT WITH SYSTEMIC CHEMOTHERAPY

Adjuvant chemotherapy and treatment with chemotherapy for advanced breast cancer are available globally but with great variability.[59–61]

1. In a large study of over 4,000 patients seen in Singapore–Malaysia, 70% had mastectomy while 30% had BCS. Chemotherapy was then administered to 56% of patients and hormonal treatment to 60%.
2. In a study of 1,165 women with breast cancer in Singapore, mastectomy was the most common surgical therapy, and about 90% of patients received adjuvant therapy. At a median follow-up of 81 months, the median 5-year survival was as follows: stage I, 97%, stage II, 78%, stage III, 52%, and stage IV, 13%.
3. In Morocco, 152 women with triple-negative breast cancer were studied.[60] Clinical staging was stage I, 8%, stage II, 60%, and stage III, 28%; 72% underwent a radical mastectomy with axillary lymph nodes dissection; 131 patients received adjuvant chemotherapy and in 76% this contained an anthracycline. Overall survival at 5 years for all patients was 76.5%.

More common issues in low-income settings may be the low percentage of women who actually receive treatment and also compliance issues for those who do receive therapy. For example, in the study reported earlier in Rwanda, only 3% of patients underwent mastectomy followed by chemotherapy. Compliance with completing treatment may also be incomplete, even in countries with higher uptake of adjuvant and neoadjuvant therapy. In a study of 44 patients treated with neoadjuvant chemotherapy in Nigeria, 17 patients (32%) did not complete the planned course of chemotherapy. Ten patients had inadequate funds to purchase chemotherapy, three patients insisted on immediate mastectomy, and four patients refused mastectomy after achieving a complete clinical response. Twenty patients had treatment delays.

## CONCLUSIONS

In the United States over 12,000 medical oncologists care for approximately 320 million people. In contrast, Ethiopia has a population of 90 million people, one cancer center, four oncologists, and two radiation vaults, and Uganda has a population of 30 million people, one cancer center, seven oncologists, and two radiation vaults. In LMICs, the incidence of breast cancer is increasing, but many women need to travel long distances and then join long waiting lists that delay treatment for weeks or months. Often, receptor testing cannot be performed, tamoxifen is not affordable, and chemotherapy is not available or affordable. In HICs, many breast cancers are detected by mammography as small microcalcifications and then breast ultrasound and MRI may follow. Hormone receptor and Her2-Neu testing is uniform and often gene expression is studied to even better define prognosis and treatment options. Frequently, definitive treatment is provided almost immediately.

As noted at the beginning of this chapter, breast cancer is a major part of the global burden of disease but more personally also a major source of human suffering for women, their families, and communities. Progress in HICs needs to be transferred, translated, affordable, and available for women globally.

## REFERENCES

1. Ferlay J, Shin HR, Bray F, Forman D, Mathers C, Parkin DM. *GLOBOCAN 2008 v1.2, Cancer Incidence and Mortality Worldwide: IARC CancerBase No. 10 [Internet]*. Lyon, France: International Agency for Research on Cancer, 2010. Available at http://globocan.iarc.fr. Accessed July 2012.
2. Ferlay J, Shin HR, Bray F, Forman D, Mathers C, Parkin DM. Estimates of worldwide burden of cancer in 2008: GLOBOCAN 2008. *Int J Cancer* 2010; 127(12): 2893–917.
3. Forouzanfar MH, Foreman KJ, Delossantos AM, et al. Breast and cervical cancer in 187 countries between 1980 and 2010: a systematic analysis. *Lancet* 2011; 378(9801): 1461–84.
4. Setiawan VW, Haiman CA, Stanczyk FZ, Le Marchand L, Henderson BE. Racial/ethnic differences in postmenopausal endogenous hormones: the Multiethnic

Cohort Study. *Cancer Epidemiol Biomarkers Prev* 2006; 15: 1849–55. doi:10.11 58/1055–9965.EPI-06–0307.

5. Boyapati SM, Shu XO, Gao YT, et al. Correlation of blood sex steroid hormones with body size, body fat distribution, and other known risk factors for breast cancer in post-menopausal Chinese women. *Cancer Causes Control* 2004; 15: 305–11. doi:10.1023/B:CACO.0000024256.48104.50.

6. Lukanova A, Lundin E, Zeleniuch-Jacquotte A, et al. Body mass index, circulating levels of sex-steroid hormones, IGF-I and IGF-binding protein-3: a cross-sectional study in healthy women. *Eur J Endocrinol* 2004; 150: 161–71. doi:10.1530/eje.0.1500161.

7. Chan MF, Dowsett M, Folkerd E, et al. Usual physical activity and endogenous sex hormones in postmenopausal women: the European prospective investigation into cancer-Norfolk population study. *Cancer Epidemiol Biomarkers Prev* 2007; 16: 900–905. doi:10.1158/1055–9965.EPI-06–0745.

8. MacMahon B, Cole P, Lin TM, et al. Age at first birth and breast cancer risk. *Bull World Health Organ* 1970; 43(2): 209–21.

9. Woods KL, Smith SR, Morrison JM. Parity and breast cancer: evidence of a dual effect. *Br Med J* 1980; 281(6237): 419–21. doi:10.1136/bmj.281.6237.419.

10. Lord SJ, Bernstein L, Johnson KA, et al. Breast cancer risk and hormone receptor status in older women by parity, age of first birth, and breastfeeding: a case–control study. *Cancer Epidemiol Biomarkers Prev* 2008; 17(7): 1723–30. doi:10.1158/1055–9965.EPI-07–2824.

11. Holmes MD, Willett WC. Does diet affect breast cancer risk? *Breast Cancer Res* 2004; 6(4): 170–78.

12. Hopkins Tanne J. Diets high in animal fats increase risk of breast cancer, while painkillers lower risk. *Br Med J* 2003 July 26; 327(7408): 181.

13. Ibrahim E. Risk of second breast cancer in female Hodgkin's lymphoma survivors: a meta-analysis. *BMC Cancer* 2012; 12: 197.

14. Schneider U, Sumila M, Robotka J, Gruber G, Mack A, Besserer J. Dose–response relationship for breast cancer induction at radiotherapy dose. *Radiat Oncol* 2011; 6: 67.

15. Parkin DM, Bray F, McCarron P. The changing global patterns of female breast cancer incidence and mortality. *Breast Cancer Res* 2004; 6(6): 229–39.

16. GlobalCan 2012: Estimated Global Incidence, Mortality, and Prevalence Worldwide in 2012. IARC 2014. Available at http://globocan.iarc.fr/.

17. Tfayli A, Temraz S, Abou Mrad R, and Shamseddine A. Breast cancer in low- and middle-income countries: an emerging and challenging epidemic. *J Oncol* 2010, Article ID 490631: 5 pages. doi:10.1155/2010/490631.

18. Bray F. The changing global patterns of female breast cancer incidence and mortality. *Breast Cancer Res* 2004; 6(6): 229–39.

19. SEER Cancer Statistics Review, 1975–2010, National Cancer Institute. Bethesda, MD. Available at http://seer.cancer.gov/csr/1975_2010/, based on November 2012 SEER data submission, posted to the SEER website, 2013.

20. Ferlay J, Steliarova-Foucher E, Lortet-Tieulent J. Cancer incidence and mortality patterns in Europe: estimates for 40 countries in 2012. *Eur J Cancer* 2013 Apr; 49(6): 1374–403.

21. Botha JL, Bray F, Sankila R, Parkin DM. Breast cancer incidence and mortality trends in 16 European countries. *Eur J Cancer* 2003; 39: 1718–29.

22. Parkin DM, Nambooze S, Wabwire-Mangen F, Wabinga HR. Changing cancer incidence in Kampala, Uganda, 1991–2006. *Int J Cancer* 2010 Mar 1; 126(5): 1187–95.

23. Chokunonga E. Trends in the incidence of cancer in the black population of Harare, Zimbabwe 1991–2010. *Int J Cancer* 2013 Aug 1; 133(3): 721–29.

24. Zhang ML, Huang ZZ, Zheng Y. Estimates and prediction on incidence, mortality and prevalence of breast cancer in China, 2008. *Zhonghua Liu Xing Bing Xue Za Zhi* 2012 Oct; 33(10): 1049–51. [Article in Chinese.]

25. Yang L, Sun TT, Wang N. The incidence and mortality trends of female breast cancer in Beijing, China: between 2004 and 2008. *Zhonghua Yu Fang Yi Xue Za Zhi* 2012 Nov; 46(11): 1009–14. [Article in Chinese].

26. Cardoso F, Costa A. 1st International consensus guidelines for advanced breast cancer (ABC 1). *Breast* 2012; 21(3): 242–52.

27. Anderson BO. Cancer Guideline implementation for breast healthcare in low-income and middle-income countries: overview of the Breast Health Global Initiative Global Summit 2007 Supplement: Guidelines for International Breast Health and Cancer Control–Implementation. *Cancer* 2008 Oct 15; 113(Suppl 8): 2221–43.

28. Mettlin C. Global breast cancer mortality statistics. *CA Cancer J Clin* 1999 May/June; 49(3): 138–44.

29. Youlden DR, Cramb SM, Dunn NA, Muller JM, Pyke CM, Baade PD. The descriptive epidemiology of female breast cancer: an international comparison of screening, incidence, survival and mortality. *Cancer Epidemiol* 2012 Jun; 36(3): 237–48. Epub Mar 27, 2012.

30. Tryggvadóttir L, Gislum M, Bray F, et al. Trends in the survival of patients diagnosed with breast cancer in the Nordic countries 1964–2003 followed up to the end of 2006. *Acta Oncol* 2010 Jun; 49(5): 624–31.

31. Redaniel MT, Laudico A, Mirasol-Lumague MR, et al. Breast cancer survival in different country settings: comparisons between a Filipino resident population, Filipino-Americans and Caucasians. *Breast* 2010 Apr; 19(2): 109–14.

32. Anyanwu SNC. Breast cancer in Eastern Nigeria: a ten year review. *West Afr J Med* 2000; 19(2): 120–125.

33. Pearson JB. Carcinoma of the breast in Nigeria. A review of 100 patients. *Br J Cancer* 1963; 17: 559–65.

34. Atoyebi OA, Atimomo CE, Adesanya AA, Berdugo BK, da Rocha-Afodu JT. An appraisal of 100 patients with breast cancer seen at the Lagos University Teaching Hospital, Lagos, Nigeria. *Nig Quart J Hosp Med* 1997; 7(2): 104–8.

35. Chiedozi LC. Breast cancer in Nigeria. *Cancer* 1985; 55: 563–67.

36. Lannin DR, Mathews HF, Mitchell J, Swanson MS. Impacting cultural attitudes in African-American women to decrease breast cancer. *Am J Surg* 2002; 184(5): 418–23.

37. Velanovich V, Yood MU, Bawle U, et al. Racial differences in the presentation and surgical management of breast cancer. *Surgery* 1999; 125(4): 375–79.

38. Smith RA, Caleffi M, Albert US, et al. Breast cancer in limited-resource countries: early detection and access to care. *Breast J* 2006; 12(Suppl 1): S16–S26.

39. Shavers VL, Harlan LC, Stevens JL. Racial/ethnic variation in clinical presentation, treatment, and survival among breast cancer patients under age 35. *Cancer* 2003; 97(1): 134–47.

40. Hisham AN, Yip CH. Overview of breast cancer in Malaysian women: a problem with late diagnosis. *Asian J Surg* 2004 Apr; 27(2): 130–33.

41. Norsa'adah B, Rampal KG, Rahmah MA, Naing NN, Biswal BM. Diagnosis delay of breast cancer and its associated factors in Malaysian women. *BMC Cancer* 2011 Apr 17; 11: 141. doi:10.1186/1471–2407–11–141.

42. Talpur AA, Surahio AR, Ansari A, Ghumro AA. Late presentation of breast cancer: a dilemma. *J Pak Med Assoc* 2011 Jul; 61(7): 662–66.

43. Ermiah E, Abdalla F, Buhmeida A, Larbesh E, Pyrhönen S, Collan Y. Diagnosis delay in Libyan female breast cancer. *BMC Res Notes* 2012 Aug 21; 5: 452. doi:10.1186/1756–0500–5-452.

44. Ng CH, Pathy NB, Taib NA, et al. Comparison of breast cancer in Indonesia and Malaysia—a clinico-pathological study between Dharmais Cancer Centre Jakarta and University Malaya Medical Centre, Kuala Lumpur. *Asian Pac J Cancer Prev* 2011; 12(11): 2943–46.

45. Hoang Lan N, Laohasiriwong W, Stewart JF, Tung ND, Coyte PC. Cost of treatment for Breast Cancer in Central Vietnam. *Glob Health Action* 2013 Feb 4; 6: 18872.

46. Chu PC, Hwang JS, Wang JD, Chang YY. Estimation of the financial burden to the national health insurance for patients with major cancers in Taiwan [abstract]. *J Formos Med Assoc* 2008; 107: 54–63.

47. Mendis S, Fukino K, Cameron A, et al. The availability and affordability of selected essential medicines for chronic diseases in six low and middle income countries. *Bull World Health Organ* 2007; 85: 279–88. doi:10.2471/BLT.06.033647.

48. Steinbrook R. Closing the affordability gap for drugs in low income countries. *N Engl J Med* 2007; 357: 1996–1999.

49. Van Nes JG, Seynaeve C, Jones S, et al. Variations in locoregional therapy in postmenopausal patients with early breast cancer treated in different countries. *Br J Surg* 2010 May; 97(5): 671–79).

50. Pain SJ, Miles D, Harnett A. Variations in treatment and survival in breast cancer. *Lancet Oncol* 2001 Dec; 2(12): 719–25.

51. Mody GN, Nduaguba A, Ntirenganya F, Riviello R. Characteristics and presentation of patients with breast cancer in Rwanda. *Am J Surg* 2013 Apr; 205(4): 409–11.

52. Levin CV, El Gueddari B, Meghzifene A. Radiation therapy in Africa: distribution and equipment. *Radiother Oncol* 1999 Jul; 52(1): 79–84.

53. Abdel-Wahab M, Bourque JM, Pynda Y, et al. Status of radiotherapy resources in Africa: an International Atomic Energy Agency analysis. *Lancet Oncol* 2013 Apr; 14(4): e168–75.

54. Zubizarreta EH, Poitevin A, Levin CV. Overview of radiotherapy resources in Latin America: a survey by the International Atomic Energy Agency (IAEA). *Radiother Oncol* 2004 Oct; 73(1): 97–100.

55. Tatsuzaki H, Levin CV. Quantitative status of resources for radiation therapy in Asia and Pacific region. *Radiother Oncol* 2001 Jul; 60(1): 81–89.

56. Ji YH, Jung H, Yang K, et al. Trends for the past 10 years and international comparisons of the structure of Korean radiation oncology. *Jpn J Clin Oncol* 2010 May; 40(5): 470–75. Epub Feb 5, 2010.

57. Bird PA, Hill AG, Houssami N. Poor hormone receptor expression in East African breast cancer: evidence of a biologically different disease? *Ann Surg Oncol* 2008 Jul; 15(7): 1983–88.

58. Pathy NB, Yip CH, Taib NA, et al. Breast cancer in a multi-ethnic Asian set-
    ting: results from the Singapore-Malaysia hospital-based breast cancer registry.
    *Breast* 2011 Apr; 20(Suppl 2): S75–S80.
59. Lim SE, Back M, Quek E, Iau P, Putti T, Wong JE. Clinical observations from a
    breast cancer registry in Asian women. *World J Surg* 2007 Jul; 31(7): 1387–92.
60. Rais G, Raissouni S, Aitelhaj M, et al. Triple negative breast cancer in Moroccan
    women: clinicopathological and therapeutic study at the National Institute of
    Oncology. BMC *Womens Health* 2012 Oct 7; 12: 35.
61. Egwuonwu OA, Anyanwu SN, Nwofor AM. Default from neoadjuvant che-
    motherapy in premenopausal female breast cancer patients: what is to blame?
    *Niger J Clin Pract* 2012 Jul–Sep; 15(3): 265–69.

# 3

# Lung Cancer: Challenges and Progress

*Christopher S. Lathan, Kenneth D. Miller,*
*Harleen Chahil, Rahul Gosain,*
*and Amitoj S. Gill*

## SECTION I: OVERVIEW OF GLOBAL LUNG CANCER

Leading both global incidence and mortality rates, lung cancer is the most common form of cancer in the world today and has been since 1985.[1-6] As mortality rates decrease (in men) or plateau (in women) in the more developed world, they are increasing across the less developed world.[7] The most significant progress in addressing this burden has been the efforts to curb the intake of tobacco through research, public action, and government policy related to tobacco control and elimination.[8-10] Recent advances in diagnosis and treatment have not yet been implemented uniformly enough to result in any real change in international mortality trends. The more developed countries continue to struggle with the financial and human cost of lung cancer, a future that awaits less developed countries if their patterns of health behavior and health system development follow current trends.

By 2030 the global burden of cancer is expected to increase by 8.1 million cases/year according to demographic changes alone, a result that will disproportionately impact the developing world.[6]

### Tobacco

Since the early 20th century there has been strong evidence supporting tobacco use as a dominant risk factor for developing lung cancer.[11] The U.S. Surgeon General publicly recognized the link in 1964, years after case–control studies had been conducted in the 1930s in Germany and further studies had been performed in the 1950s in the United Kingdom and the United States.[11] A 2012 Lee et al.[11] comprehensive systematic review and meta-analysis, of

studies conducted in the 20th century relating smoking to all major pheno-
types of lung cancer, clarified the causal relationship through confirmation of
the increased risk by people who do or have ever smoked; that risk increases
despite sex, age, and geographic location; and that risk increases as amount
and duration of smoking increase.

The International Agency for Research on Cancer (IARC), an entity of
the World Health Organization (WHO), published the most comprehensive
global data on cancer in 2008. Lung cancer accounted for 12% of the total
incidence of all cancers, except for non-melanoma skin cancer, and 18.2%
of the total mortality of 7.6 million people in 2008. Taking into account a
lag of 20 to 30 years[12] (increasing lung cancer incidence among Israelis) for
tobacco use to translate into lung cancer, one can see the close relationship between trends in tobacco consumption and lung cancer incidence and
mortality.[5,13]

## RESEARCH, PUBLIC ACTION, GOVERNMENT POLICY

Recognizing that lung cancer has been a common form of cancer since
the mid-1980s, the irrefutably poor survival rates, and taking into account
the relative risk of increase with tobacco use, participants of the 49th World
Health Assembly (WHA) in 1996 spurred the director-general to take action. Seven years later, the WHA adopted the Framework Convention on
Tobacco Control (FCTC). By May 2011, there were 173 parties to the first
international treaty generated by the WHO, covering 87% of the world's
population.[9] In a 1994 article, Lopez et al. described a four-stage model of
the cigarette epidemic. Formed from information from the more developed
world, this four-stage description is a model still pertinent today and can
be observed through country-specific data generated through stipulations in
the FCTC.

Stage I is identified as the beginning of the epidemic, when cigarette
consumption is still low (less than 500 cigarettes per adult) and predominantly among men, tobacco control measures are minimally or not present,
and health consequences due to tobacco use are not yet prominent. Stage
II is identified when smoking rates reach a range of 1,000 to 3,000 per person per year, both sexes see a rapid increase in consumption, tobacco control
measures are not well developed or do not have political and public support, and a rapid increase in seen in lung cancer rates in men but not yet in
women. Stage III sees the start of a shift away from smoking being socially
acceptable, rates of ex-smokers increasing, prevalence of smoking declines
for men and declines minimally or plateaus in women, public support for
tobacco control measures increases as education of negative consequences of
smoking increase, some smoke-free environments are established, and there

is a rapid rise in incidence of tobacco-related mortality of men while the incidence for women remains relatively low. Stage IV is characterized by a continued decline in smoking rates, a significant increase in public advocacy for smoke-free environments and tobacco control policies put in place along with appropriate support measures, and an early peak and then a decline in male mortality rates while female rates continue to increase rapidly and see a much later peak consistent with the smoking rates of 20 to 30 years earlier.[9,14]

On a global scale, the WHO FCTC provides international, political, and judicial backing for scientifically proven and measurable initiatives to push local educational and political agendas to be ahead of the curve of smoking trends and mortality rates of the four-stage model mentioned earlier. The application of this model to present-day circumstances can be seen in the countries and regions explored in Section II: Country and Regional Perspectives of Lung Cancer.

## Other Causes

The strong emphasis on tobacco avoidance and cessation is due to the link between its use and risk of lung cancer and also an underestimation of the number of users worldwide and the full extent of its addictiveness and harm. Lung cancer in those who have never smoked, defined as less than 100 cigarettes in a lifetime, ranks seventh in mortality of global cancer.[15,16] The IARC published a 2012 update to its listing of known human lung carcinogens. The most prominent environmental and occupational causes of lung cancer are radon, asbestos, polycyclic aromatic hydrocarbons, arsenic, silica, and secondhand smoke.[14,15]

Occupationally, miners, smelters, metal workers, railroad workers, mechanics, dock workers, and those in construction are the most at risk for constant exposure,[15,17] with an estimated 1.6 million disability-adjusted life years due to occupational exposure. Environmentally, women in developing countries who cook in homes with poor ventilation and urban dwellers are at substantially higher risks for developing lung cancer.[18] Cooking and heating with coal is the cause for 1.5% of all lung cancer deaths (http://www .who.int/cancer/prevention/en/). Women nonsmokers in Asia especially have high rates of lung cancer, particularly adenocarcinoma, possibility attributable to cooking oil vapors and using coal, wood, or other biomass for cooking and heating.[3] The increase in particulate matter and other factors in urban areas raises the rates of lung cancer by 10% to 40%. Other risk factors related to increased incidence of lung cancer include HIV, diet, age, history of lung disease, and inherited genetic mutations.[17,19,20] Other risk factors related to increase mortality of lung cancer include socioeconomic status, age, and comorbidities.[21]

## Lung Cancer Histology and Stage

The International Association for the Study of Lung Cancer (IASLC) and the Union for International Cancer Control released a revised staging standard in 2010, the seventh edition of TNM classification. Appropriate staging is vital as over 70% of lung cancers are diagnosed as stage III or IV when surgical resection is no longer possible and survival rates are significantly reduced.[22] The 2004 WHO classifications of lung cancer are currently augmented by multidisciplinary classification published in 2011 by the IASLC in conjunction with the American Thoracic Society and the European Respiratory Society.[22] The biggest changes in the 2004 classification system is the incorporation of genetics along with traditional, histological, and clinical factors in diagnosis.

Although overall incidence of lung cancer has decreased in men and reached a plateau in women in developed countries, including Australia, Canada, the United Kingdom, and the United States,[3,13] it masks a major shift in the incidence of different histology manifestations.[5,22] The evidence of the relationship between smoking and lung cancer is overwhelming, and a 2012 systematic review by Lee et al.[11] showed the strongest correlation between smoking and squamous and small cell carcinoma. Global trends of the different forms of lung cancer show an increase in adenocarcinoma, predominantly manifesting in peripheral lung tissue, closely matched by a decrease in squamous cell carcinoma, historically presenting as central lung tumors, occurring around the time filtered cigarettes were introduced. The years 1950 to 1990 saw the U.S. industry shift toward filtered cigarettes, with coverage of 97% by the end of the 1990s (Worldwide trends). Globally there is also an increase in adenocarcinomas, the most common phenotype of lung carcinomas since 1987.[23] There is a prominent increase among nonsmoking women in developing countries, with the highest burden in Asia.[24,25] This trend is bringing increased attention to the need to focus on tobacco primarily but also environmental risk factors related to lung cancer.

## Burden

The burden of lung cancer on more developed countries has been constantly increasing. At 31% in 1980, by 2002 less developed countries accounted for 50% of lung cancer cases, and this is expected to increase to 60% by 2030.[6] Tobacco consumption in the less developed world accounted for 71% of total consumption in 2010.[6,17] This puts the population of those countries at a clearly elevated risk and should be a major call to action for development of cost-effective screening, treatment, and palliative care measures.

In addition to the differing burden of lung cancer between countries, there are also significant disparities within individual countries.[5,26] The cause for these disparities is multifaceted and ranges from cultural issues to a lack of services available to people of low socioeconomic status (SES). Despite these differences, research shows that after controlling for race and SES, the outcomes for lung cancer patients with similar-stage presentation are equal. This information is extremely important when reviewing data of outcomes and survival rates for different populations, as people of low SES and minorities in the more developed world are more likely to be smokers and be exposed to environmental risk factors for developing lung cancer. In the more developed world, even in countries where a national health system exists, persons of low SES have less access to care and receive less treatment interventions than people of higher SES.[6,21,27] This disparity is present in practically all societies and is especially pronounced in less developed countries where the sheer presence of screening, prevention, treatment, and palliative measures is lacking, not to mention trained men and women to provide those services.

## SECTION II: COUNTRY AND REGIONAL PERSPECTIVES OF LUNG CANCER

### More Developed Countries

The more developed world is experiencing a general decline in the lung cancer epidemic, especially in relation to the influence of tobacco. There is an overall decline in the mortality trends in men, with slight variation in the rate of change. Women in some countries, such as Australia, Japan, and the United States, are seeing a plateau in incidence, whereas many countries in places like Western Europe are still seeing an increase in mortality rates. At the same time, the average 5-year survival rate is still poor. Trends in tobacco use, incidence and mortality of lung cancer, and policy status regarding tobacco control and cessation measures place most countries of the more developed world in stage IV of the model, characterized by a continued decline in smoking rates, increase in public advocacy for smoke-free environments, an early peak and then a decline in male mortality rates, while female rates continue to increase rapidly and see a much later peak consistent with the smoking rates of 20 to 30 years earlier.[9,14]

### A Global Survey of Lung Cancer

#### United States

Lung cancer incidence and mortality in the United States have been concordant with the historical gender difference in the uptake and then the reduction in tobacco use. In the United States, the incidence of lung cancer for men has been declining at approximately 2.8% per year, but among women, this decline is newer and less dramatic at 1% per year.[28] Lung cancer incidence rates in men decreased from 1996 through 2005 in 24 of 28 states that were studied. In contrast, during the same time period, lung cancer incidence rates in women increased in eight states (Pennsylvania, Illinois, Iowa, Michigan, Minnesota, Nebraska, Kentucky, and Idaho).

Lung cancer mortality has also been declining for men since 1991 and for women since 2003. The mortality rates however differ with race. Between 2001 and 2005 lung cancer mortality rate for white men was 71.3/100,000 and for blacks 93.1/100,000, though declining trends were seen in both.[28] In a comprehensive study of lung cancer incidence and mortality from 1996 to 2005, Jemal et al. noted that lung cancer mortality decreased during 1996 to 2005 in 43 of the 50 states for men.[13] "The decrease in the lung cancer death rate began first and has been largest in California, where the male death rate is approaching that in Utah." During the same period, lung cancer mortality for women decreased only in three states and increased in 13 states.

Due to medical advancements in surgical techniques and the combination of therapies, the survival rate for lung cancer has improved. The 1-year survival rate for patients with non–small cell lung cancer (NSCLC) increased from 37% in 1975 to 1979 to 44% in 2005 to 2008, but 5-year survival rate for all stages of lung cancer is 16% and for the localized stage is 52%. Five-year survival is 52% for patients with localized disease, but only 15% of cases are detected at this stage. In general, NSCLC has a higher 5-year survival rate of 18% compared to the rate of 6% for small cell lung cancer.[58] The economic cost of caring for patients with lung cancer is very large. In a study of 4,068 patients with metastatic NSCLC, followed for a mean of 334 days, cumulative total health-care costs were $125,849 ($120,228, $131,231).[29]

### Australia

Lung cancer is the leading cause of cancer death. From 1982 to 2007 the incidence in men decreased by 32% whereas for women it increased by 72% in Australia. The mortality rate over the same period decreased 46% in men while increasing 56% among women. Almost 90% and 65% of lung cancer incidence was attributed to smoking.[30]

As with other more developed countries, Australia's main burden of lung cancer is highest among those geographically and economically challenged. The indigenous population is more likely to live in rural areas, have low SES, and is twice as likely to be current smokers. Although these risk factors also apply to the nonindigenous population, there is evidence that the survival rate among the indigenous population is worse than that among the nonindigenous population. This occurred even after controlling for histologic phenotype, stage at presentation, and comorbidities, suggesting a disparity in treatment in men and women, respectively.

### Role of Tobacco

The 2012 WHO FCTC report for Australia recorded an overall smoking prevalence of 15.1% for daily smokers aged 14 years and older. Separated by sex, the daily smoker prevalence is 16.5% in males and 13.9% in females, a significant decrease from their peaks when approximately 58% of men smoked (1964) and 33% of women smoked (mid-1970s).[31] Analyzed within the parameters of the Lopez et al. four-stage model, Australia is categorized as being in stage IV, a continued decline in smoking rates and changes in mortality rates corresponding to smoking rates from approximately two to three decades earlier.

A 2011 survey in the state of Western Australia found that a majority of citizens do not see smoking as socially acceptable and 92% live in smoke-free homes. This public support has led to a gradual increase in political action and measures of support: in 1992 the government banned tobacco advertising; in 1996 the government declared lung cancer as a National Health Priority Area; and most recently, in 2012, a law went into effect mandating packaging with updated and expanded graphic health warnings for all tobacco products manufactured or processed in Australia (Australia FCTC report). In addition to favorable demographic shifting, strong political support for tobacco elimination programs will continue to benefit the campaign against lung cancer.

### *Europe*

In Europe, approximately 90% of lung cancer in men and 66% of lung cancer in women[1,2,32,33] are associated with tobacco use. A number of studies have examined the incidence and mortality of lung cancer in Europe. A large study of 36 European nations concluded that tobacco accounts for one-fifth of the cancer-related deaths.[1] Lung cancer mortality in men has been decreasing during the past 20 years, but in women it is still increasing in many countries. The authors conclude, "Men and women are clearly in very different phases of the smoking epidemic" and that there is an "urgent need for national and European prevention strategies that target tobacco cessation and prevention among European women."

In Eastern Europe, the trends were essentially the same in demonstrating a declining incidence and lung cancer mortality in men but not in women.[2]

A large study of 15 European Union countries also reported that lung cancer incidence in men was typically leveling or declining.[32] In contrast, in women in the United Kingdom and Ireland, the incidence was declining, but for women in other European countries, "there are unambiguous upsurges in rates seen in younger and older women . . . and little sign that the epidemic has or will soon reach a peak." This group divided the lung cancer risk and trends for men and for women in EU countries into six groups for women, including

Groups I (Denmark) The risk for women is high and rising rapidly.

Group II (United Kingdom) In both populations, risk is declining.

Group III countries (the Netherlands, Luxembourg, Sweden, Austria) represent females at intermediate risk but increasing rapidly.

Group IV (Ireland) where risk in women is moderate and declining rapidly for a decade.

Group V contains a large group of countries (Germany, Belgium, Italy, Finland, Greece, France) with moderate to low risk but increasing. In older women, rates are increasing quite rapidly.

Group VI (Portugal and Spain) low risk but increasing.

These authors conclude that reducing tobacco smoking in youth is of the "most important ways to reduce the future lung cancer burden in current and new EU member states."

## Asia

Asia collectively is the home of a large percentage of the world citizenry. China has the distinction of being the largest producer and consumer of tobacco worldwide. It is estimated that 34.7 million cartons of cigarettes are sold annually and that there are over 320 million Chinese smokers. These numbers have risen because of the rapid increase in cigarette smoking by teenagers; 53.5% of citizens are exposed to passive smoking.[34] In this setting, 21.7% of incident cancers were lung cancer in men and 14.3% in women.[35]

In another study in the Western Pacific and Southeast Asia, the prevalence of smoking in Asia is up to 65% in men and 50% in women, and the fraction of lung cancer deaths attributable to smoking was up to 40% in Asian women and 49% in Asian men.[36] Several articles conclude that "the peak of smoking-induced diseases is still to come and therefore, it is very important to strengthen anti-smoking measures so as to have a far-reaching effects."

Lung cancer is also a major problem in India and accounts for 9.4% of all cancers in males and 2.7% of those in females in Greater Mumbai.[37] There has been a significant decreasing incidence in men and increasing incidence among women. One out of every 74 men and 1 out of every 242 women will contract lung cancer at some time in their whole life in the absence of other causes of death, assuming that the current trends prevail over the time period. Most of them will acquire the disease after the age of 40 years, after which risk increases with time.

### Africa

Cancer is a common disease in Africa with an estimated incidence of 650,000 people each year, but unlike other regions, lung cancer is not the most common cause of cancer death. The cancers with the highest incidence are cervical, breast, and now HIV-associated Kaposi's sarcoma.[38–40]

Data on lung cancer incidence and mortality is difficult to obtain because of the limited number of tumor registries, but one study estimated the lung cancer mortality at 4 to 5 times what was reported by GLOBOCAN. It estimates that up to 2030, lung cancer deaths are expected to increase in general and by over 100% in Benin and Niger.[39] A similar report estimates that in sub-Saharan Africa there were 44,076 lung cancer deaths in 2005, which was 2.6 times the 2003 WHO estimate of 17,000 deaths. A similar ratio when comparing 2005 to 2003 was also found in Ethiopia.[40]

## GLOBAL LUNG CANCER CARE DISPARITIES IN THE ERA OF PERSONALIZED MEDICINE

Differential outcomes medicated by access to care and infrastructure are an important and timely issue in the study of lung cancer.[40–56] Not only do treatment differences affect survival in early-stage disease, but it is likely they will also impact the quality of life of patients with advanced disease, especially as advances continue in the areas of personalized medicine and adjuvant and maintenance therapy.[32,54–72]

The idea that equal treatment can lead to equal outcomes is the central tenet of treatment equity. In the United States, in a review of clinical trial data from the Southwest Oncology Group, Albain and colleagues found that for patients in clinical trials, there were no survival differences for lung cancer related to race after adjusting for confounders.[57] This work can be extrapolated to region and SES. These studies suggest that equal treatment can lead to equal outcomes, even when patients present with advanced lung cancer and comorbid diseases.

Lung cancer treatment is moving beyond basic treatment with surgery, radiation, and chemotherapy and into the era of personalized medicine. Treatment for lung cancer today is best guided by a combination of the histologic and molecular characteristics of the tumor and the adequacy of tumor samples is extremely important, and the absence is detrimental to therapy. The access to personalized medicine approaches in lung cancer is rare in less developed countries that lack the infrastructure or economic means to evaluate tissue and obtain targeted therapies exacerbating already existing treatment disparities, morbidity, and mortality. Certainly, we cannot make great strides in the treatment of lung cancer if we continue to leave the most vulnerable patients behind.

Targeted therapy is now an option for a sizable number of lung cancer patients, but there has been little research on racial disparities or regional disparities in the use of targeted agents for lung cancer.[1,2,28,32–38] Given the disparities seen in every other treatment modality, however, it seems likely that targeted therapy will also be a source of treatment disparities related to race and class, and region. At this time, few publications have evaluated the frequency of the somatic mutations outside of American/European patients and patients of East Asian descent. As targeted therapies become more widely used, it is important to ensure that all lung cancer patient populations benefit from these treatment advances. Otherwise, the very patients who are most affected by lung cancer will continue to have inferior access to the most effective therapies.

## REFERENCES

1. Bray FI, Weiderpass E. Lung cancer mortality trends in 36 European countries: secular trends and birth cohort patterns by sex and region 1970–2007. *Int J Cancer* 2010; 126(6): 1454–66.
2. Tyczynski JE, Bray F, Aareleid T, et al. Lung cancer mortality patterns in selected Central, Eastern and Southern European countries. *Int J Cancer* 2004; 109(4): 598–610.
3. Katanoda K, Yako-Suketomo H. Trends in lung cancer mortality rates in Japan, USA, UK, France and Korea based on the WHO mortality database. *Jpn J Clin Oncol* 2012; 42(3): 239–40.
4. Janssen-Heijnen ML, Coebergh JW. The changing epidemiology of lung cancer in Europe. *Lung Cancer* 2003; 41(3): 245–58.
5. Toh CK. The changing epidemiology of lung cancer. *Methods Mol Biol* 2009; 472: 397–411.
6. Kanavos P. The rising burden of cancer in the developing world. *Ann Oncol* 2006; 17(Suppl 8): viii15–viii23.
7. Novello S, Vavala T. Lung cancer and women. *Future Oncol* 2008; 4(5): 705–16.
8. Powell HA, Iyen-Omofoman B, Hubbard RB, Baldwin DR, Tata LJ. The association between smoking quantity and lung cancer in men and women. *Chest* 2013; 143(1): 123–29.

9. Sinha DN, Narain JP, Kyaing NN, Rinchen S. WHO framework convention on tobacco control and its implementation in South-East Asia region. *Indian J Public Health* 2011; 55(3): 184–91.

10. Jayalekshmy PA, Akiba S, Nair MK, et al. Bidi smoking and lung cancer incidence among males in Karunagappally cohort in Kerala, India. *Int J Cancer* 2008; 123(6): 1390–97.

11. Lee PN, Forey BA, Coombs KJ. Systematic review with meta-analysis of the epidemiological evidence in the 1900s relating smoking to lung cancer. *BMC Cancer* 2012; 12: 385.

12. Tarabeia J, Green MS, Barchana M, et al. Increasing lung cancer incidence among Israeli Arab men reflects a change in the earlier paradox of low incidence and high smoking prevalence. *Eur J Cancer Prev* 2008; 17(4): 291–96.

13. Jemal A, Thun MJ, Ries LA, et al. Annual report to the nation on the status of cancer, 1975–2005, featuring trends in lung cancer, tobacco use, and tobacco control. *J Natl Cancer Inst* 2008; 100(23): 1672–94.

14. Hoggart C, Brennan P, Tjonneland A, et al. A risk model for lung cancer incidence. *Cancer Prev Res* (Phila) 2012; 5(6): 834–46.

15. Field RW, Withers BL. Occupational and environmental causes of lung cancer. *Clin Chest Med* 2012; 33(4): 681–703.

16. Wakelee HA, Chang ET, Gomez SL, et al. Lung cancer incidence in never smokers. *J Clin Oncol* 2007; 25(5): 472–78.

17. Lam WK, White NW, Chan-Yeung MM. Lung cancer epidemiology and risk factors in Asia and Africa. *Int J Tuberc Lung Dis* 2004; 8(9): 1045–57.

18. Pauk N, Kubík A, Zatloukal P, Krepela E. Lung cancer in women. *Lung Cancer* 2005; 48(1): 1–9.

19. Sigel K, Wisnivesky J, Gordon K. HIV as an independent risk factor for incident lung cancer. *AIDS* 2012; 26(8): 1017–25.

20. Shiels MS, Cole SR, Mehta SH, Kirk GD. Lung cancer incidence and mortality among HIV-infected and HIV-uninfected injection drug users. *J Acquir Immune Defic Syndr* 2010; 55(4): 510–15.

21. Kutikova L, Bowman L, Chang S, Long SR, Obasaju C, Crown WH. The economic burden of lung cancer and the associated costs of treatment failure in the United States. *Lung Cancer* 2005; 50(2): 143–54.

22. Travis WD. Pathology of lung cancer. *Clin Chest Med* 2011; 32(4): 669–92.

23. Travis WD, Brambilla E, Noguchi M. International Association for the Study of Lung Cancer/American Thoracic Society/European Respiratory Society: international multidisciplinary classification of lung adenocarcinoma: executive summary. *Proc Am Thorac Soc* 2011; 8(5): 381–85.

24. Moore MA, Ariyaratne Y, Badar F, et al. Cancer epidemiology in South Asia—past, present and future. *Asian Pac J Cancer Prev* 2010; 11(Suppl 2): 49–66.

25. Moore MA, Attasara P, Khuhaprema T, et al. Cancer epidemiology in mainland South-East Asia—past, present and future. *Asian Pac J Cancer Prev* 2010; 11(Suppl 2): 67–80.

26. Lozano R, Naghavi M, Foreman K, et al. Global and regional mortality from 235 causes of death for 20 age groups in 1990 and 2010: a systematic analysis for the Global Burden of Disease Study 2010. *Lancet* 2012; 380(9859): 2095–128.

27. LaPar DJ, Bhamidipati CM, Harris DA, et al. Gender, race, and socioeconomic status affects outcomes after lung cancer resections in the United States. *Ann Thorac Surg* 2011; 92(2): 434–39.

28. American Cancer Society. *Cancer Facts and Figures 2013*. Atlanta, GA: American Cancer Society, 2013.

29. Vera-Llonch M, Weycker D, Glass A, et al. Healthcare costs in patients with metastatic lung cancer receiving chemotherapy. *BMC Health Serv Res* 2011 Nov 10; 11: 305.

30. Anikeeva O, Bi P, Hiller JE, Ryan P, Roder D, Han GS. Trends in cancer mortality rates among migrants in Australia: 1981–2007. *Cancer Epidemiol* 2012 Apr; 36(2): e74–e82. doi:10.1016/j.canep.2011.10.011. Epub Nov 21, 2011.

31. Progress Report on Implementation of the WHO Framework Convention on Tobacco Control, 2012. Available at http://www.who.int/fctc/reporting/2012_global_progress_report_en.pdf.

32. Bray F, Tyczynski JE, Parkin DM. Going up or coming down? The changing phases of the lung cancer epidemic from 1967 to 1999 in the 15 European Union countries. *Eur J Cancer* 2004; 40: 96–125.

33. Brennan P, Bray I. Recent trends and future directions for lung cancer mortality in Europe. *Br J Cancer* 2002 July 1; 87(1): 43–48.

34. Zhang H, Cai B. The impact of tobacco on lung health in China. *Respirology* 2003 Mar; 8(1): 17–21.

35. Globocan database. The Global Cancer Atlas. http://globocan.iarc.fr.

36. Martiniuk A, Lee CM, Woodward M, Huxley R. Burden of lung cancer deaths due to smoking for men and women in the WHO Western Pacific and South East Asian regions. *Asian Pac J Cancer Prev* 2010; 11(1): 672.

37. Agarwal N, Yeole BB, Ram U. Lifetime risk and trends in lung cancer incidence in greater Mumbai. *Asian Pac J Cancer Prev* 2009 Jan–Mar; 10(1): 75–82.

38. Parkin DM, Sitas F, Chirenje M, Stein L, Abratt R, Wabinga H. Part I: cancer in indigenous Africans—burden, distribution, and trends. *Lancet Oncol* 2008 Jul; 9(7): 683–92.

39. Winkler V, Ott JJ, Cowan M, Becher H. Smoking prevalence and its impacts on lung cancer mortality in Sub-Saharan Africa: an epidemiological study. *Prev Med* 2013 Nov; 57(5): 634–40, Epub Sep 5, 2013.

40. Ng N, Winkler V, Van Minh H, Tesfaye F, Wall S, Becher H. Predicting lung cancer death in Africa and Asia: differences with WHO estimates. *Cancer Causes Control* 2009 Jul; 20(5): 721–30.

41. Paez JG, Jänne PA, Lee JC, et al. EGFR mutations in lung cancer: correlation with clinical response to gefitinib therapy. *Science* 2004; 304(5676): 1497–500.

42. Gandhi L, Janne PA. Crizotinib for ALK-rearranged non-small cell lung cancer: a new targeted therapy for a new target. *Clin Cancer Res* 2012; 18(14): 3737–42.

43. Janne PA, Meyerson M. ROS1 rearrangements in lung cancer: a new genomic subset of lung adenocarcinoma. *J Clin Oncol* 2012; 30(8): 878–79.

44. Oxnard GR, Janne PA. KRAS wild-type lung cancer: a moving target in an era of genotype migration. *J Clin Oncol* 2012 Sep 20; 30(27): 3322–24.

45. Sequist LV, Heist RS, Shaw AT, et al. Implementing multiplexed genotyping of non-small-cell lung cancers into routine clinical practice. *Ann Oncol* 2011; 22(12): 2616–24.

46. Lynch TJ, Bell DW, Sordella R, et al. Activating mutations in the epidermal growth factor receptor underlying responsiveness of non-small-cell lung cancer to gefitinib. *N Engl J Med* 2004; 350(21): 2129–39.

47. Yang SH, Mechanic LE, Yang P, et al. Mutations in the tyrosine kinase domain of the epidermal growth factor receptor in non-small cell lung cancer. *Clin Cancer Res* 2005; 11(6): 2106–10.

48. Krishnaswamy S, Kanteti R, Duke-Cohan JS, et al. Ethnic differences and functional analysis of MET mutations in lung cancer. *Clin Cancer Res* 2009; 15(18): 5714–23.

49. Leidner RS, Fu P, Clifford B, et al. Genetic abnormalities of the EGFR pathway in African American patients with non-small-cell lung cancer. *J Clin Oncol* 2009; 27(33): 5620–26.

50. Cote ML, Haddad R, Edwards DJ, et al. Frequency and type of epidermal growth factor receptor mutations in African Americans with non-small cell lung cancer. *J Thorac Oncol* 2011; 6(3): 627–30.

51. Janku F, Garrido-Laguna I, Petruzelka LB, Stewart DJ, Kurzrock R. Novel therapeutic targets in non-small cell lung cancer. *J Thorac Oncol* 2011; 6(9): 1601–12.

52. Mok TS. Personalized medicine in lung cancer: what we need to know. *Nat Rev Clin Oncol* 2011; 8(11): 661–68.

53. Paik PK, Arcila ME, Fara M, et al. Clinical characteristics of patients with lung adenocarcinomas harboring BRAF mutations. *J Clin Oncol* 2011; 29(15): 2046–51.

54. Reinersman JM, Johnson ML, Riely GJ, et al. Frequency of EGFR and KRAS mutations in lung adenocarcinomas in African Americans. *J Thorac Oncol* 2011; 6(1): 28–31.

55. Earle C, Venditti LN, Nuemann, PJ, et al. Who gets chemotherapy for metastatic lung cancer? *Chest* 2000; 117(5): 1239–46.

56. Sitas F. Part II: cancer in indigenous Africans—causes and control. *Lancet Oncol* 2008 Aug; 9(8): 786–95.

57. Esnaola NF, Gebregziabher M, Knott K, et al. Underuse of surgical resection for localized, non-small cell lung cancer among whites and African Americans in South Carolina. *Ann Thorac Surg* 2008; 86(1): 220–26; discussion 227.

58. Gadgeel SM, Kalemkerian GP. Racial differences in lung cancer. *Cancer Metastasis Rev* 2003; 22: 39–46.

59. Haiman CA, Stram DO, Wilkens LR, et al. Ethnic and racial differences in the smoking-related risk of lung cancer. *N Engl J Med* 2006; 354(4): 333–42.

60. Hardy D, Liu CC, Xia R, et al. Racial disparities and treatment trends in a large cohort of elderly black and white patients with nonsmall cell lung cancer. *Cancer* 2009; 115(10): 2199–211.

61. Lathan CS, Neville BA, Earle CC. Racial composition of hospitals: effects on surgery for early-stage non-small-cell lung cancer. *J Clin Oncol* 2008; 26(26): 4347–52.

62. Lathan CS, Neville BA, Earle CC. The effect of race on invasive staging and surgery in non-small-cell lung cancer. *J Clin Oncol* 2006; 24(3): 413–18.

63. Margolis M, Christie JD, Silvestri G, Kaiser L, Santiago S. Racial differences pertaining to a belief about lung cancer surgery. *Ann Intern Med* 2003; 139(7): 558–63.

64. Menvielle G, Boshuizen H, Kunst AE, et al. The role of smoking and diet in explaining educational inequalities in lung cancer incidence. *J Natl Cancer Inst* 2009; 101(5): 321–30.

65. Molina JR, Yang P, Cassivi SD, Schild SE, Adjei AA. Non-small cell lung cancer: epidemiology, risk factors, treatment, and survivorship. *Mayo Clin Proc* 2008; 83(5): 584–94.

66. Neighbors CJ, Rogers ML, Shenassa ED, Sciamanna CN, Clark MA, Novak SP. Ethnic/racial disparities in hospital procedure volume for lung resection for lung cancer. *Med Care* 2007; 45(7): 655–63.

67. Potosky AL, Saxman S, Wallace RB, Lynch CF. Population variations in the initial treatment of non-small cell lung cancer. *J Clin Oncol* 2004; 22(16): 3261–68.

68. Stewart J. Lung cancer in African Americans. *Cancer* 2001; 91(12): 2476–81.

69. Arriagada R, Bergman B, Dunant A, et al. Cisplatin-based adjuvant chemotherapy in patients with completely resected non-small-cell lung cancer. *N Engl J Med* 2004; 350(4): 351–60.

70. Pirker R, Pereira JR, Szczesna A, et al. Cetuximab plus chemotherapy in patients with advanced non-small-cell lung cancer (FLEX): an open-label randomised phase III trial. *Lancet* 2009; 373(9674): 1525–31.

71. Sandler A, Gray R, Perry MC, et al. Paclitaxel-carboplatin alone or with bevacizumab for non-small-cell lung cancer. *N Engl J Med* 2006; 355(24): 2542–50.

72. Albain KS, Unger JM, Crowley JJ, Coltman CA Jr, Hershman DL. Racial disparities in cancer survival among randomized clinical trials patients of the Southwest Oncology Group. *J Natl Cancer Inst* 2009; 101(14): 984–92.

# 4

# Mesothelioma: Increasing Incidence

## Jonathan Daniel

## BACKGROUND AND HISTORICAL CONTEXT

A patient enters the office complaining of shortness of breath and cough, two chief complaints that are ubiquitous from clinic to clinic throughout the world. The majority of time this likely represents benign disease such as pneumonia or upper respiratory illness. Occasionally, the clinician will auscultate a paucity of breath sounds and perhaps even use percussion to determine if a fluid interface exists. If chest x-ray is readily available and performed, a pleural effusion can be confirmed.

Pleural effusions from lung and all other primary sites are considered stage IV disease. Primary pleural malignancy or mesothelioma is routinely associated with a pleural effusion; however, metastatic disease exists only if there is involvement outside the ipsilateral hemithorax.

Unfortunately, few malignancies are as aggressive and poorly responsive to treatment as mesothelioma irrespective of stage. Despite advances in multidisciplinary evaluation and treatment, the 5-year survival remains approximately 5%, including countries with excellent access to diagnosis and treatment. Currently, no effective screening tool is available for patients at high risk. The typical patient presents with progressive shortness of breath with cough due to increasing pleural effusion and resulting atelectasis. Thoracentesis is usually the first maneuver performed; however, the ability to make a firm diagnosis is limited due to the poor sensitivity of cytology in detecting malignant cells (30% to 40%). This leads to a significant delay in eventual diagnosis and treatment. Once a diagnosis is made, median survival is generally 9 to 12 months without any treatment. Therapy is generally focused on palliation with possible life extension, and curative intent is rare.

An estimated 43,000 people worldwide die from mesothelioma each year.[1] The increasing incidence of the disease is continually reported in multiple countries, both industrialized and developing. However, the true incidence is probably much higher due to failure of diagnosis and poor reporting in many nonindustrialized countries.[2]

As with most cancers, the greatest hope relies on effective prevention, particularly in countries that do not have comprehensive health care available. Mesothelioma is known to be associated with asbestos exposure in 80% of cases. The remaining cases are likely also linked to asbestos, but a clear exposure cannot always be identified. Spontaneous cases of mesothelioma are considered to be extremely rare. As a result, the incidence of this cancer and other related disease could be effectively controlled or even stopped with total cessation of asbestos use. The World Health Organization (WHO) position statement on dangerous chemicals recognized asbestos as responsible for over half of all occupational carcinogen-related cancers and called for a worldwide ban.[3] This report estimated 125 million people are occupationally exposed to asbestos each year.

Asbestos is a naturally occurring mineral composed of small-diameter fibers classified as serpentine (chrysotile) and amphibole (crocidolite). Its use has been documented over 4,000 years ago, and during the first half of the 21st century, it was mined in large scale due to its widespread applications. Durable, cost-effective, and easily found, the material was thought to be a magical element for industrial countries developing infrastructure and buildings. Asbestos was used to help with pipe production, insulation, reinforcing softer materials, and even came in a spray application. As the automotive industry grew, asbestos was also instrumental in outfitting brakes, clutch, and engine parts.

In England and the eastern United States, areas of high ship building activity were linked to mesothelioma cases where vessels were insulated with asbestos. At one point the material was so commonly used and easily applied that even school playgrounds were being sprayed with asbestos. People known to be at high risk for asbestos exposure included metal plate workers, automotive builders, plumbers, carpenters, and military personnel. At its peak in 1977, almost 5 million metric tons was produced and 85 countries were involved in some manufacture of the compound.

All types of fibers from asbestos are thought to produce malignancy. Why the cancer has a predilection for pleural disease is unclear. The particle size may be small enough to be filtered to the pleura via macrophages. The macrophages then potentially cause malignant transformation through initiation of an inflammatory cascade or mutagenic behavior. Asbestos plaques will often form along the parietal pleura and are a marker of asbestos exposure but interestingly do not have the capability to undergo malignant transformation. The fact that these plaques do occur however lends credence to the theory that repetitive exposure or injury of the pleural is occurring. In addition, benign forms of mesothelioma do exist, and again, it is unclear what prevents this form from undergoing malignant transformation.

Primary mesothelioma can also occur in the peritoneum and pericardium though less common. How inhaled asbestos fibers can cause malignancy within these sites is even more uncertain, but the strong causal relationship is now undeniable. A potential relationship with lung cancer has also been documented. The risk is thought to increase when combined with tobacco use. Additional solid organ tumors, including ovarian, laryngeal, and testicular cancers, have been linked to asbestos exposure.

A causal relationship between asbestos exposure and mesothelioma was difficult to initially determine due to the latency period between exposure and development of malignancy. A 1960 report in the *British Journal of Industry* was one of the first to highlight a correlation between asbestos exposure and pleural mesothelioma.[4] Nicknamed the "asbestos belt," the Northwestern Cape Province of Africa represented a concentrated region of land available for blue asbestos mining. A number of workers were developing asbestos-related disease, and at autopsy, a hard, pleural malignancy was being identified. It was reports such as this that slowly uncovered asbestos as the occupational carcinogen it is now known to represent. Challenges occurred when explaining the significant latency period seen with onset of malignancy as the majority of patients who were affected presented in the seventh and eighth decades of life. With time, however, various cohorts and series came to fruition and confirmed the strong link between exposure and development of mesothelioma.

Recent notable examples from various nations include the following.

## United States

Follow-up through 1986 of 17,800 asbestos insulation applicators found 458 mesotheliomas in this cohort.[5]

## Australia

A crocidolite mine in Wittenoom with workers exposed between 1943 and 1966, includes data on 6,358 men with 222 deaths from mesothelioma and 302 deaths from lung cancer.[6]

## Canada

A Quebec cohort of 11,000 workers in asbestos mines and mills, with 38 deaths identified from mesothelioma. In a study of women residing near asbestos mining communities, there was a 7-fold increase in the mortality rate from mesothelioma.[7]

## Turkey

Three villages in areas where erionite asbestos is mined coupled with a possible genetic link were responsible for a mesothelioma-related mortality of 50% among this population.[8]

## Britain

The United Kingdom is the ideal example of an industrialized country initially at the forefront of asbestos use with subsequent high numbers of disease prevalence. The British mesothelioma rate is currently the highest in the world. The projected lifetime risk of the disease in British men born in the 1940s is 0.59% or 1 in 170 of all deaths.[9] This is in large part due to Britain's rapid growth of industry and reliance on high-volume asbestos mining in the first half of the 20th century. Asbestos supply and consumption at its peak are followed by a bimodal effect, with sharp rises in mesothelioma cases after the known 20- to 30-year latency period is reached.

## Japan

In June 2005 Japanese media reported on 51 asbestos-related deaths of employees at a machinery company known for asbestos products, eventually becoming known as the "Kubota Shock."[10] As word spread, the number of victims including residents near the factory began to grow. As far back as 1971, asbestos risk was recognized by Japan and measures for asbestos handling and also medical evaluations of workers were instituted. In 1995 the use of certain forms of asbestos including crocidolite was prohibited. However, it was not until the 2005 report that Japan eventually ratified the Asbestos Convention and imposed a total ban. The importation of raw asbestos has ceased since 2005. Before this ban, the first maneuver was to try and regulate the controlled use and handling of asbestos, which then subsequently changed to limiting the types of items allowed. The total ban was thus an evolutionary process over many decades that eventually culminated in media frenzy, leading to essentially a national panic. This similar process is what was seen with a number of additional industrialized countries, before total bans taking effect. Only in 1986 was asbestos even declared a proven human carcinogen by the U.S. Environmental Protection Agency. To date there is no agreement on what should be considered a safe amount of exposure or if a safe amount even exists.

## DIAGNOSIS AND TREATMENT

Malignant mesothelioma also presents in varied histological forms. Epithelioid, sarcomatoid, and biphasic (combined) elements are used to classify this tumor. The epithelioid form has some response to treatment and can be considered for surgery in early stages; however, the purely sarcomatoid form is resistant to all forms of treatment and surgery should not be considered for those patients. Diagnosis of specific histological type can only be made with surgical pleural biopsy (via open or thoracoscopic technique) and therefore is not widely used in many areas without access to this type of intervention.

The initial experimentation with surgery for this disease was started in Britain. The roots of surgery for mesothelioma were built on intervention for infectious disease, namely tuberculosis.[11] For advanced cases with destroyed lung, the extrapleural pneumonectomy was performed and was a rigorous surgery requiring removal of the entire pleura, lung, pericardium and diaphragm in the ipsilateral hemithorax. The surgery was extrapolated to use with mesothelioma due to the widespread disease seen and the hope of complete tumor removal via complete extirpation of the thoracic organs exposed to malignant cells. Dr. Eric Butchart was the first to attempt a series of this

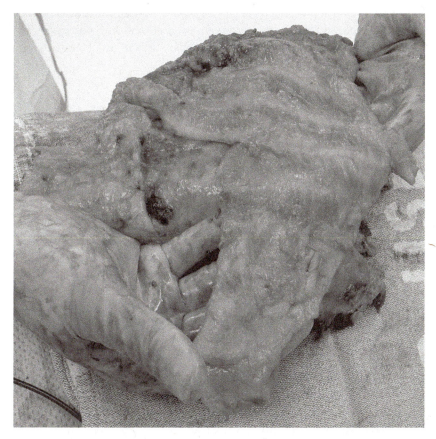

**FIGURE 4.1** Pleural tumor debulking from the lung—radical pleurectomy.

operation, and the operative mortality of greater than 30% eventually called into question aggressive treatments for a disease that was incurable.[12] In his series of 29 patients, the median survival was only 10 months. It was not until the late 1980s that the surgery was revitalized and reconsidered for this patient population. A landmark report by Sugarbaker and colleagues in 1999 established that the operation could be performed with acceptable mortality (3.2%) in experienced centers; however, the utility of this operation is still controversial due to the poor long-term survival rate seen.[13] A paradigm shift to tumor debulking alone with radical pleurectomy (Figure 4.1) is now the favored approach at many centers, but definitive data to suggest this is preferred is lacking, mostly because of the failure to achieve statistical power in studies based on the rarity of this disease. Nonetheless, operations of this magnitude remain an option only in developed countries, with tertiary medical centers capable of providing the intensive support required to run a successful program. When multidisciplinary approach is not feasible, standard chemotherapy is an option in medically fit patients for possible life extension. Cisplatin and Alimta are considered first-line agents and can be administered safely in a wide range of scenarios with a limited side effect profile. Early consideration for palliative intervention is critical with pleurodesis for recurrent effusions and pain management for chest wall involvement often required.

## COMPETING INTERESTS

So despite the known carcinogenic effect of asbestos, why does its use persist? An analysis by the International Consortium of Investigative Journalists has tracked nearly $100 million in public and private money spent by these groups since the mid-1980s in three countries alone—Canada, India, and Brazil—to keep asbestos in commerce. Their strategy, critics say, is one borrowed from the tobacco industry: create doubt, contest litigation, and delay regulation.

Lobbyist groups such as the Chrysotile Institute (representing the Quebec Mining Industry) continue to promote the false notion that asbestos can be handled safely. Canada has campaigned vigorously to protect its $97 million asbestos exportation industry. In 1997, when France banned all forms and uses of asbestos, including chrysotile, the move set off an international dispute with Canada. Canada subsequently petitioned the World Trade Organization, claiming that safe practice for handling asbestos was available and a ban would unjustly cause economic devastation. After 3 years of debate, the World Trade Organization ruled that chrysotile was indeed dangerous, that claims about the safety of controlled use could not be supported, and that the French ban was legal to protect public health.[14]

Companies and countries with economic incentive to develop or sell asbestos have shifted from countries with bans to developing countries that are still reliant on growth in the construction sector and led by leaders who are willing to disregard potential for widespread health risks due to the overall benefits to their gross national product. These countries continue to cite studies that contest asbestos as a carcinogen despite the poor science contained within them. Product defense via industry-sponsored studies that are less rigorously monitored by scientific methods is responsible for attempting to conflict the known causal relationships of asbestos and mesothelioma. GM, Ford, and Chrysler, for instance, have paid $37 million between 2001 and 2008 to scientist consultant companies for presentation of these studies at national meetings.[15]

## NECESSITY FOR A UNIVERSAL BAN

Japanese researchers found that the adoption of an asbestos ban doubled the pace of reduction in asbestos use and observed that changes in asbestos use during 1970 to 1985 correlated with changes in the age-adjusted mortality rates of pleural mesothelioma during 1996 to 2005.[16] The current ban is fairly complete in industrialized nations, but the shift has now been made to developing countries where asbestos mining and use are still high. Based on the latency period and bimodal distribution of prevalence seen, these countries should expect a sharp rise in cases similar to their industrial predecessors.

Asia accounts for 64% of the world's current asbestos use but only 13% of the recent asbestos-related deaths in the WHO mortality data.[17] But a significant disclaimer is the likely failure of these developing countries to effectively capture mesothelioma-related deaths due to poor health-care access and lack of mandatory reporting. The malignant mesothelioma latency period has not yet achieved peak saturation in these countries and should be expected over the next 20 to 40 years. The proportion of global asbestos use attributed to Asia has been steadily increasing over the years from 14% (1920 to 1970) to 33% (1971 to 2000) to 64% (2001 to 2007).[18] Russia remains the leading producer of asbestos worldwide, followed by China, Kazakhstan, Brazil, Canada, Zimbabwe, and Colombia. These six countries accounted for 96% of the world production of asbestos in 2007.[19] Most of the asbestos mined in Russia is exported, whereas China is the number one consumer of asbestos in the world followed by Russia, India, Kazakhstan, and Brazil. These countries lack any meaningful data on mesothelioma.[20]

Only 3% of Asian countries have ratified the International Labour Organization (ILO) Asbestos Convention (an agreement for safe practices regarding asbestos) compared with 17.8% of countries worldwide.[18] The hope is that all Asian countries will not only ban asbestos use immediately but also ratify the ILO and reduce exposure concurrently.

India no longer produces asbestos but remains one of the leading importers from Canada. Essentially the government is balancing the low cost of this mineral versus the long-term risks of exposure and disease development. In 2011 there was a promising turn when Indian officials made a move toward a complete ban. However, India reversed its stand on asbestos at the recent Rotterdam Convention (May 2013), citing discredited studies on chrysotile promoted by industry lobbyists who continue to benefit from the billion-dollar domestic asbestos industry. The handling of imported asbestos remains poorly regulated, and low-income workers are being exposed to a high toxic burden of fibers.

Continued cases of mesothelioma should be expected even in industrialized countries due to ongoing dust contamination related to previous construction and use of asbestos. In Australia over one-third of homes built between 1945 and 1980 used asbestos cement materials. Massive exposure to asbestos likely occurred during the fall of the World Trade Center. Natural deposits within many states have been cited in places like New York City's Central Park, and U.S. Environmental Protection Agency workers have measured increased airborne asbestos levels in California playgrounds.

Iceland was the first nation to ban asbestos in 1983. Since then over 50 countries have acknowledged this dangerous carcinogen and instituted complete bans on the importation or exportation of asbestos. Unlike most solid organ cancers, mesothelioma can be made virtually extinct if a uniform ban is adopted. This represents a unique area for intervention not normally seen in the oncological world. In the meantime, the disease will continue to devastate and hurt its hosts—the majority of whom have little hope for any potentially effective therapy.

## REFERENCES

1. Driscoll T, Nelson, D, Steenland K, et al. The global burden of disease due to occupational carcinogens. *Am J Ind Med* 2005; 48: 397–408.
2. Delgermaa V, Takahasi K, Park E, Le GV, Hara T, Sorahan T. Global mesothelioma deaths reported to the World Health Organization between 1994–2008. *Bull World Health Organ* 2011; 89: 716–24.
3. *Elimination of Asbestos-Related Diseases.* Geneva: World Health Organization, 2006.
4. Wagner JC, Sleggs CA, Marcand P. Diffuse pleural mesothelioma and asbestos exposure in Northwestern Cape Province. *Br Ind Med* 1960; 17: 260–71.
5. Selikoff IJ, Seidman H. Asbestos associated deaths among insulation workers in the United States and Canada, 1967–1987. *Ann N Y Acad Sci* 1991; 643: 1–14.
6. Berry G, Reid A, Aboagye-Sarfo P, et al. Malignant mesotheliomas in former miners and millers of crocidolite at Wittenoom (Western Australia) after more than 50 years follow-up. *Br J Cancer* 2012 Feb 28; 106(5): 1016–20.

7. Camus M, Siemiatycki J, Meek B. Nonoccupational exposure to chrysotile asbestos and the risk of lung cancer. *N Engl J Med* 1998: 1565–71.

8. Roushdy-Hammady I, Siegal J, Emri S, Testa JR, Carbone M. Genetic susceptibility factor and malignant mesothelioma in the Cappadocian region of Turkey. *Lancet* 2001: 357: 444–45.

9. Hodgson JT, McElvenny DM, Darnton AJ, Price MJ, Peto J. The expected burden of mesothelioma mortality in Great Britain from 2002–2050. *Br J Cancer* 2005; 92: 583–93.

10. Takahashi Y, Miyaki K, Nakayama T. Analysis of news of the Japanese asbestos panic: a supposedly resolved issue that turned out to be a time bomb. *J Public Health* 2007; 29: 62–9.

11. Sarot IA. Extrapleural pneumonectomy and pleurectomy in pulmonary tuberculosis. *Thorax* 1949; 4: 173.

12. Butchart EG, Ashcroft T, Barnsley WC, Holden MP. Pleuropneumonectomy in the management of diffuse malignant mesothelioma of the pleura. *Thorax* 1976; 31: 15–24.

13. Sugarbaker DJ, Flores RM, Jaklitsch MT, et al. Resection margins, extrapleural nodal status, and cell type determine postoperative long-term survival in trimodality therapy of malignant pleural mesothelioma: results in 183 patients. *J Thorac Cardiovasc Surg* 1999; 117: 54–63.

14. Castleman B. WTO confidential: the case of asbestos. *Int J Health Serv* 2002; 32(3): 489–501.

15. Dietz et al. *v.* ACandS Inc., et al. Supplemental Responses to Plaintiff's Interrogatories and Document Requests Directed to Defendant Ford Motor Company. Superior Court for Baltimore City; Baltimore, MD: 2009. Mar 20, Mesothelioma Trial Cluster (M-102) Consolidated Case No 2408000004.

16. Nishikawa K, Takahashi K, Karjalainen A, et al. Recent mortality from pleural mesothelioma, historical patterns of asbestos use, and adoption of bans: a global assessment. *Environ Health Perspect* 2008; 116: 1675–80.

17. Le GV, Takahashi K, Park EK, et al. Asbestos use and asbestos-related diseases in Asia: past, present and future. *Respirology* 2011; 16: 767–75.

18. Giang V, Takahashi K, Park EK, et al. Asbestos use and asbestos-related diseases in Asia: past, present and future. *Respirology* 2011: 767–75.

19. Virta R. *Worldwide Asbestos Supply and Consumption Trends from 1900 through 2003*. Reston, VA: U.S. Geological Survey, 2006.

20. Bianchi C, Bianchi T. Malignant mesothelioma: global incidence and relationship with asbestos. *Ind Health* 2007; 45: 379–387.

# 5

# Colorectal Cancer

## *James J. Lee, Tae W. Kim, and Edward Chu*

### EPIDEMIOLOGY

Colorectal cancer (CRC) remains a major public health problem in the United States and worldwide. In the United States, it is the third most common cancer in both men and women and the second leading cause of cancer-related deaths.[1] Nearly 145,000 new CRC cases and 50,000 deaths from CRC are expected to occur in the United States in 2014.[1] Globally, CRC is the third most common cancer after lung cancer and breast cancer, and it is estimated that over 1 million new cases will be diagnosed. Each year, more than 500,000 cancer deaths are associated with this disease worldwide.[2] Of note, the incidence of CRC varies over 10-fold throughout the world. The incidence rates are highest in North America, Europe, Australia, and New Zealand, whereas the lowest rates are seen in Africa and South-Central Asia.

Over the past 15 years, the incidence of CRC in the United States has declined by approximately 2% to 3% per year, and there has been a corresponding 2.7% per year decline in the cancer death rate from CRC during the 1980s and 1990s in the United States.[3] In contrast, there has been a rapid increase in CRC incidence in several areas around the world, which have typically been at low risk, and these include Spain, Eastern Europe, and eastern Asia.[4]

The incidence of CRC is estimated to be about 4-fold higher in more highly developed countries than that in less developed countries.[2] These increased rates in highly developed countries are felt to result from increased exposure to risk factors such as obesity, physical inactivity, and smoking, as well as an increased exposure to an unhealthy, Western-style diet.[4] Between the 1970s and the 1990s, the incidence of CRC had increased in most parts of the world except in the United States.[2] In addition, individuals of low socioeconomic status are at an increased risk for developing CRC. The same modifiable elements that are responsible for the increased risk in highly developed regions of the world account for the socioeconomic disparity in CRC incidence.

Overall, CRC mortality rates have declined in the more highly developed countries, whereas they continue to rise in the less developed countries of South America and Eastern Europe. The steady decline of CRC mortality rate in these countries is attributed, in large part, to improved screening and early detection strategies as well as more effective treatments for early-stage disease, in the form of adjuvant chemotherapy, and for advanced, metastatic disease. The mortality-to-incidence rate ratios (MR:IR) are lowest in North America (0.34 to 0.35) and highest in Africa (0.88 to 0.89), suggesting significant global disparities of cancer care, which span the entire continuum from screening and early detection practices to multidisciplinary care and to treatment of early-stage and advanced disease.[2]

## ETIOLOGY

Sporadic CRC accounts for approximately 80% to 85% of the CRC cases diagnosed. The most important risk factor for sporadic CRC is age, with >90% of the cases being diagnosed in patients older than 50 years. Personal or family history of sporadic CRC, in the absence of a well-defined familial genetic syndrome, is also an important risk factor for CRC. Metachronous primary CRC occurs in 3% of patients in the first 5 years after resection of primary CRC. A personal history of large adenomatous polyps (>1 cm) or polyps of villous or tubulovillous histology increases the risk of CRC.[5] A family history of one first-degree relative with CRC increases the risk of CRC by about 2-fold.

Approximately 10% to 15% of CRC can be attributed to well-defined hereditary CRC syndromes, including familial adenomatous polyposis (FAP) and hereditary non-polyposis colorectal cancer (HNPCC).[6] FAP is caused by germ-line mutations in the adenomatous polyposis coli (APC) gene and accounts for less than 1% of CRC cases. Ninety percent of untreated individuals carrying these mutations develop CRC by age 45.[6] HNPCC is caused by defects in one of the mismatch repair genes, most commonly hMLH1, hMSH2, hMSH6, or PMS2,[7] and this is an autosomal dominant syndrome. HNPCC accounts for approximately 3% to 5% of CRC cases.[8] The mean age of initial CRC diagnosis in these HNPCC patients is 48 years, with some patients presenting in their early twenties. In addition to CRC, extra-colonic cancers can develop, including endometrial, ovarian, breast, stomach, small bowel, hepatobiliary, brain, and genitourinary cancer.

There is a well-established association between inflammatory bowel disease and CRC. Specifically, the extent and duration of disease are the two main factors that determine the potential development of CRC in patients with ulcerative colitis (UC). In fact, it has been shown that UC involving the entire colon for more than 10 years increases the risk of CRC by 5- to 15-fold.[9] The incidence of CRC is usually about 0.5% per year during the first 10 to 20 years after the diagnosis of UC and then 1% per year thereafter. The pancolitis of Crohn's disease carries a similar risk of CRC as UC involving the entire colon.

Several studies have shown that diabetes mellitus and insulin resistance increase the risk of CRC.[10-16] A meta-analysis of prior studies estimated that the risk of CRC is 20% to 38% higher among diabetics than non-diabetics.[16]

Moderate to heavy consumption of alcohol increases the risk of CRC.[17-19] Multiple studies show that cigarette smoking increases the risk of CRC.[20]

Obesity has become a significant health-care issue responsible for steadily increasing incidence of several major medical conditions. Prospective trials have shown that high body mass index (BMI) increases the risk of CRC in both men and women.[21,22] Waist circumference and waist-to-hip ratio are strong risk factors for colon cancer.[22] A meta-analysis showed that 5 kg/m$^2$ increase in BMI was associated with increased risk of CRC in men with a relative risk (RR) of 1.24.[23]

Several factors that appear to protect against the occurrence of CRC have been identified. Perhaps the most important factor is physical activity where prospective trials have shown a reduction in CRC risk.[21,22] The Nurses' Health Study (NHS) showed that women who expended more than 21 MET-hours per week on leisure-time physical activity had an RR of CRC of 0.54 compared with women who expended less than 2 MET-hours per week.[21] Another prospective cohort study conducted in the United States showed that physical activity was inversely associated with risk for CRC with an RR of 0.53 in male health professionals with high quintiles of average energy expenditure on leisure-time activities compared with those with low quintiles.[22] A meta-analysis of 52 published studies through June 2008 (24 case–control studies and 28 cohort studies) demonstrated that increased physical activity was able to reduce the risk of CRC with an overall RR of 0.76.[24]

The effect of diet on CRC risk remains somewhat controversial. The current general consensus is that there is a relatively marginal benefit of reducing the risk of CRC by increasing the consumption of fruits and vegetables beyond the levels associated with a reasonably balanced diet.[25-27] The protective benefit of dietary fiber is also controversial.[28-36]

Increased calcium intake has been associated with a significant reduction of CRC risk.[37-39] A combined analysis of two prospective studies, the NHS and the Health Professionals Follow-up Study (HPFS), showed that higher calcium intake (>1,250 mg/day vs. ≤500 mg/day) was associated with a reduced risk of distal CRC (RR of 0.58 in men and 0.73 in women).[37] The NIH-AARP Diet and Health Study revealed that the intake of dairy food and calcium was inversely associated with the risk of cancers of the digestive system, especially CRC. This study also showed that the use of supplemental calcium was inversely associated with the risk of CRC.[39]

Aspirin has been actively investigated for its protective benefit against CRC. Long-term follow-up of several randomized aspirin trials (Thrombosis Prevention Trial, British Doctors Aspirin Trial, Swedish Aspirin Low Dose Trial, UK-TIA Aspirin Trial, Dutch TIA Aspirin Trial) showed that daily aspirin intake reduced the 20-year risk of colon cancer by 24% (incidence hazard ratio [HR], 0.76). With respect to the optimal dose of aspirin, there was no further increased benefit at doses of aspirin greater than 75 mg daily, with an absolute reduction of 1.76% in 20-year risk of CRC after 5-year scheduled treatment with 75 to 300 mg daily.[40] The CAPP2 randomized controlled trial (n = 861) showed that daily intake of 600 mg aspirin significantly reduced the risk of CRC in carriers of Lynch syndrome (HR, 0.63).[41] The molecular pathologic epidemiology study (n = 964) of NHS and HPFS recently showed that the regular use of aspirin among CRC patients with mutated-PIK3CA was associated with superior CRC-specific survival (HR for cancer-related death, 0.18) and overall survival (HR for death from any cause, 0.54).[42]

## SCREENING

The current model for CRC screening is based on the well-established adenoma–carcinoma sequence. In this model, CRC arises from adenomatous polyps where adenomas progress from small to large polyps (>1 cm), and then to dysplasia and cancer.[43] This progression results from both inherited and acquired genetic defects,[43] and the process from adenomatous polyp to true cancer takes, on average, at least 8 to 12 years.[44]

Most colorectal polyps are either adenomatous or hyperplastic in nature. In general, hyperplastic polyps usually do not progress to cancer. Two-thirds of colonic polyps are adenomatous. Adenomatous polyps are found in about 25% of men and 15% of women, and the prevalence increases with age.[45] The risk of CRC increases with histology (villous adenoma), polyp size (≥1 cm), degree of atypia (high-grade dysplasia), and number of adenomas (≥3).[46]

Now, there are two different categories of CRC screening methods: stool-based tests and structural-based strategies. Stool tests include guaiac-based fecal occult blood test (gFOBT) and immunochemical-based fecal occult blood test (iFOBT). The potential advantage of stool tests is that they are noninvasive and relatively inexpensive, with fecal immunochemical testing being more expensive than FOBT. Both of these tests require annual testing with colonoscopy for follow-up of positive results. Randomized studies have shown that CRC screening with gFOBT significantly reduced mortality from CRC.[47–50] Although these stool-based tests are noninvasive and inexpensive, they require patient compliance with annual testing and colonoscopic follow-up for positive results. One other disadvantage of gFOBT is that it has relatively low sensitivity for polyps and relatively low specificity for cancer.[51] These diagnostic strategies are used predominantly in Europe and Australia.

Structural-based tests include double-contrast barium enema (DCBE), flexible sigmoidoscopy, colonoscopy, and computed tomographic colonography, also known as virtual colonoscopy. DCBE was one of the first radiologic imaging techniques used for CRC screening, and it can visualize the colon in its entirety. While it is a relatively safe procedure, the main limitations of this method are its reduced sensitivity to detect polyps <1 cm when compared with endoscopic techniques and the operator dependence on the radiologist in performing and interpreting the examination. In addition, abnormal findings must be followed by colonoscopy.[51]

Randomized trials have shown that flexible sigmoidoscopy screening reduced the incidence of CRC by 18% to 23% and CRC mortality by 22% to 31% over 10 to 12 years follow-up period.[52,53] Flexible sigmoidoscopy identifies lesions in the distal 60 cm of the large intestine, and it can be performed with minimal patient preparation and does not require sedation. However, this method cannot visualize the proximal part of the colon, and abnormal findings by flexible sigmoidoscopy require follow-up colonoscopy to visualize the entire colon.

Colonoscopy is the predominant method of CRC screening in the United States, and it is felt to be the gold standard for screening and early detection. However, it should be noted that the current recommendation of colonoscopy as a screening test in the United States is based only on indirect data and observational studies due to lack of data from randomized studies evaluating the effect of colonoscopy on CRC mortality. The National Polyp Study showed that removal of adenomatous polyps was effective in preventing the development of CRC.[54] Six-year follow-up of 1,418 patients after colonoscopic removal of one or more polyps revealed that the incidence of CRC was 90% lower in these patients when compared to patients reported in other studies who had polyps that were not removed and 76% lower than in the general population.[54] The prevalence of left-sided CRC was strongly reduced within a 10-year period after colonoscopy (prevalence ratio of 0.33).[55] A population-based case–control study showed that colonoscopy in the preceding 10 years was associated with 77% lower risk for both left-sided and right-sided CRC.[56]

The advantages of colonoscopy is that it can remove polyps, which are known to be the major cause of CRC, as well as identify CRC at its earliest stage. However, the potential downsides of this screening approach are that it requires conscious sedation and a vigorous bowel regimen before the procedure.[51] Moreover, there is a low, albeit real, risk of bowel perforation and bleeding.

CT colonography (CTC, virtual colonoscopy) is an imaging examination of the entire colon and rectum using CT to acquire images and advanced 2-D and 3-D image display methods for subsequent interpretation. This procedure does not require sedation, it typically takes only 10 to 15 minutes, and no recovery time is needed. As with colonoscopy, this procedure requires aggressive bowel preparation, and patients with one or more polyps ≥1 cm or 3 or more polyps ≥0.6 cm should be referred for colonoscopy.[51] CTC should be especially considered in those individuals with significant comorbidities for whom colonoscopy may be contraindicated.

A joint guideline from the American Cancer Society, the United States Multi-Society Task Force on Colorectal Cancer, and the American College of Radiology was published in 2008 for screening and surveillance for the early detection of CRC and adenomatous polyps.[51] The recommended tests for detection of adenomatous polyps and cancer in asymptomatic adults aged 50 years and older include flexible sigmoidoscopy every 5 years, colonoscopy every 10 years, DCBE every 5 years, or computed tomographic colonography every 5 years. The recommended tests that primarily detect cancer are annual gFOBT with high sensitivity for cancer, annual fecal immunochemical test with high sensitivity for cancer, or stool DNA test with high sensitivity for cancer annually. For individuals with a family history of either CRC or adenomatous polyps in one first-degree relative before age 60 years or in two or more first-degree relatives at any age, the recommendation is to have colonoscopy at age 40 years or 10 years before the youngest case in the immediate family.

One important issue relates to screening in African American individuals. There is now strong evidence in the literature that CRC is diagnosed at an earlier age in African Americans than in whites, with higher mortality rates in the African American population. In the United States, the screening rates are generally lower for African Americans by approximately 10%. Based on these various factors, the recommendation in the United States is to begin CRC screening in African Americans at the age of 45, which is 5 years earlier than screening for average-risk individuals.

On a global level, it is noteworthy that different screening strategies are being considered based on the incidence of CRC, availability of health-care resources, and economic development of a given country. In the United States and in some European countries, nationwide CRC screening programs with colonoscopy have been implemented. In contrast, CRC screening rates are low in most Asian countries. Despite the implementation of a nationwide CRC screening program in Korea in 2004 and an increased use of FOBT and endoscopy testing over a 4-year period, still less than 50% of Korean adults are undergoing CRC screening.[57] In most Asian countries with national health-care systems in place, screening colonoscopy is performed only in patients with positive FOBT.[58]

## DIAGNOSIS

The definitive diagnosis of CRC is usually made by colonoscopic biopsy of a mass lesion visualized in the gastrointestinal (GI) tract with histological confirmation of tumor cells. Cancer staging provides the extent of disease with three main components: primary tumor (T), status of regional nodes (N), and distant metastasis (M). These three components are combined to form a stage grouping, from I to IV. Stage groupings permit the stratification of prognosis, which is useful for the selection of treatment. The most important indicator of long-term clinical outcome following resection of primary colon cancer is the pathologic stage at the time of surgery.[59]

At the time of initial presentation, clinical staging of colon cancer is best accomplished by physical examination and radiologic imaging including CT scans of the chest, abdomen, and pelvis, which can identify locoregional tumor involvement, regional lymph node and distant metastases, and tumor-related complications such as obstruction, perforation, or fistula formation. The initial staging of primary rectal cancer requires a complete analysis of the extent of the disease including the depth of tumor invasion through the rectal wall and regional lymph node involvement. Rectal MRI and/or rectal ultrasound are the best modalities for evaluating the extent of localized disease.

Serum carcinoembryonic antigen (CEA) levels are usually obtained preoperatively in patients with newly diagnosed CRC. This serum marker is particularly useful in the postsurgical follow-up of patients to identify those who may be presenting with possible recurrent disease. Elevated preoperative CEA levels that do not normalize after surgical resection suggest the presence of persistent disease.

## SURGERY

Approximately 80% of CRCs are localized to the colon and/or regional nodes, and surgery remains the only curative modality for localized disease. The goal of surgical resection of early-stage CRC is complete removal of the tumor, the major vascular pedicle, and the lymphatic drainage basin of the affected segment of the colon.

With respect to rectal cancer, total mesorectal excision has become the standard surgical treatment around the world. This technique, however, does not treat lateral lymph node involvement. Among the lateral lymph nodes, the middle rectal, obturator, and internal iliac lymph nodes are important from the viewpoint of both the incidence of metastasis and treatment effects. As a result, the extent of lymph node dissection may differ according to the specific country. In Japan and some other Asian countries, a more involved D3 lateral lymph node dissection is usually performed in patients with T3 rectal cancer.[60]

Local recurrence is a major concern after surgical resection of locally advanced rectal cancer, and several studies have shown that pelvic radiation with concurrent chemotherapy reduces the incidence of local recurrence.[61,62] Based on the pivotal study conducted by Sauer et al. in Germany, preoperative pelvic radiation with concurrent fluoropyrimidine chemotherapy results in a higher sphincter preservation rate and is much better tolerated than postoperative combined modality therapy.[62] Therefore, this approach of giving preoperative radiotherapy and fluoropyrimidine chemotherapy, with either infusional 5-fluorouracil or oral capecitabine, has become standard of care in the United States, Europe, and throughout the world.

Surgical resection provides a potentially curative option for selected patients with site-limited metastatic disease, predominantly in liver and lung. Long-term survival can be achieved with metastasectomy in a significant number of cases, and an aggressive surgical approach to both the primary and the metastatic sites is warranted, in conjunction with systemic chemotherapy.

There is a greater than 50% to 70% chance of CRC recurrence after initial definitive surgical resection of the primary tumor in localized CRC, and postoperative surveillance is warranted. Consensus groups including National Comprehensive Cancer Network (NCCN) recommend close surveillance after surgical resection of primary tumor for stage II or III CRC: history and physical examination every 3 to 6 months for the first 2 years, and then every 6 months for a total of 5 years; CT scan of chest/abdomen/pelvis annually for up to 5 years for patients at high risk of recurrence; colonoscopy in 1 year from surgery, then repeat in 1 year if advanced adenoma found, or repeat in 3 years if no advanced adenoma found; and CEA level every 3 to 6 months for 2 years, and then every 6 months for a total of 5 years.

## ADJUVANT THERAPY

For patients who have undergone potentially curative surgical resection, disease recurrence is thought to arise from clinically occult micrometastases that are present at the time of surgery. The goal of postoperative adjuvant therapy is to eradicate these micrometastases, thereby increasing the chance of cure.

During the past four decades, 5-FU has been the major backbone of combination chemotherapy for the treatment of CRC in both the adjuvant and metastatic disease settings. Several agents have been approved by the U.S. Food and Drug Administration (US FDA) for the treatment of CRC over the past decade, including three cytotoxic agents and five biologics: irinotecan (CPT-11), a topoisomerase I inhibitor; oxaliplatin, the third-generation platinum analog; and capecitabine, an oral fluoropyrimidine; bevacizumab, a monoclonal antibody against vascular endothelial growth factor (VEGF);

cetuximab and panitumumab, monoclonal antibodies against epidermal growth factor receptor (EGFR); aflibercept, an anti-VEGF recombinant fusion protein; most recently, regorafenib, a multikinase small molecule inhibitor.

The combination of 5-FU and the reduced folate leucovorin (LV) represents the backbone of adjuvant chemotherapy for CRC over the past 30 years.[63] Several major randomized trials in the United States established the role of bolus 5-FU/LV as a standard adjuvant regimen for patients with stage III CRC following surgical resection.[64–66] GERCOR C96.1 trial was a randomized phase III randomized trial conducted in Europe to compare infusional 5-FU/LV (LV5FU2, de Gramont regimen) versus bolus 5-FU/LV (Mayo Clinic regimen).[67,68] This trial showed that LV5FU2 was much better tolerated than bolus 5-FU/LV with similar efficacy in 6-year disease-free survival (DFS) and overall survival (OS),[67,68] and based on the results of this study, infusional LV5FU2 was adopted as the new backbone for all subsequent adjuvant combination trials.[68]

The oral fluoropyrimidines like capecitabine offer increased convenience and potentially improved therapeutic benefit when compared to intravenous 5-FU-based chemotherapy.[69] The X-ACT study showed that oral capecitabine therapy for 6 months is at least as effective and much better tolerated as bolus 5-FU/LV for adjuvant treatment of resected stage III CRC.[70] UFT is another oral fluoropyrimidine, which is a combination of tegafur and uracil, combined at a molar ratio of 1:4.[71] Uracil competitively inhibits the degradation of 5-FU, thereby resulting in sustained concentrations in both plasma and tumor. The NSABP C-06 trial compared UFT with IV bolus 5-FU/LV in patients with stage II/III colon cancer. This study showed UFT to be at least equivalent, in terms of clinical efficacy, to that of IV bolus 5-FU/LV.[71] Unfortunately, UFT was not granted approval by the US FDA, and as a result, it is not available as a treatment option for adjuvant therapy in the United States. However, UFT is widely available throughout other regions of the world, such as Asia, Australia, Europe, and South America for patients who have undergone surgical resection and require adjuvant chemotherapy.

Oxaliplatin is a diaminocyclohexane, third-generation platinum compound that has been studied in the setting of adjuvant therapy of surgically resected early-stage CRC. MOSAIC was the pivotal randomized phase III trial (n = 2246) conducted in Europe to evaluate the benefit of LV5FU2 in combination with oxaliplatin (FOLFOX4) versus LV5FU2 monotherapy in patients with resected Stages II and III CRC.[72,73] This trial showed that FOLFOX4 significantly improved 5-year DFS and 6-year OS in patients with stage III CRC when compared to LV5FU2 alone. A subsequent subset analysis revealed that patients with high-risk stage II disease also derived the same level of clinical benefit as those with stage III disease. However, there was not benefit for those with average-risk stage II disease. Based largely on the results of this trial, FOLFOX4 was approved for adjuvant therapy of completely re-sected stage III CRC in the United States, Europe, and throughout the world. Although FOLFOX4 is viewed as the regulatory standard that was approved for use in the United States, most U.S. oncologists prefer to use either modified FOLFOX6 or FOLFOX7 due to an improved safety profile with reduced myelosuppression and GI toxicity. The combination of the oral fluoropyrimidine capecitabine plus oxaliplatin (XELOX) has also been investigated in the adjuvant setting, and when compared to bolus 5-FU/LV, the XELOX regimen showed improved clinical efficacy along with an improved safety profile.[74] As a result, XELOX is considered a standard treatment option in patients with stage III CRC.

As will be discussed in the next section, irinotecan-based chemotherapy has documented clinical efficacy in the treatment of metastatic CRC (mCRC). Unfortunately, none of the irinotecan-based regimens showed clinical benefit as adjuvant therapy.[75-77] Several randomized phase III trials have investigated the potential role of combining oxaliplatin-based chemotherapy with one of the active biologic agents, including bevacizumab, cetuximab, and panitumumab, in the adjuvant setting given the clinical activity of these combination regimens in mCRC. To date, all of the studies combining these antibody therapies with FOLFOX chemotherapy in the adjuvant setting have not demonstrated any clinical benefit.[75-81]

The role of adjuvant therapy in resected stage II CRC remains a subject of much debate.[82-86] In general, the majority of randomized clinical trials have not documented clinical benefit in treating stage II patients with adjuvant chemotherapy. However, the QUASAR study conducted in the United Kingdom and the pooled analysis conducted by Sargent et al. of individual patient data from nearly 21,000 patients treated on 18 randomized trials suggest that adjuvant therapy with 5-FU/LV confers a small but real clinical benefit in terms of OS, somewhere in the range 3% to 5%.[87,88]

There are several clinicopathologic features associated with poor prognosis in patients with stage II disease, which include T4 primary;[59,89] poorly differentiated histology (including signet ring and mucinous tumors);[90] lymphovascular invasion (LVI);[89,91-93] perineural invasion;[89,94,95] bowel obstruction or perforation at presentation;[96-98] and inadequately sampled lymph nodes in the surgical resection specimens (<12 lymph nodes in the surgical specimen).[99] Presently, the ASCO guidelines recommend that adjuvant therapy be carefully discussed with medically fit patients with high-risk clinicopathologic features:[100] inadequately sampled lymph nodes (<13 lymph nodes); T4 lesions; tumor perforation; LVI; poorly differentiated histology; or neural invasion.

The gold standard to define benefit from adjuvant therapy has been improvement in OS. However, DFS at 2 or 3 years has become an acceptable surrogate end point for 5-year OS.[87,101] Significant improvements in 3-year

DFS formed the basis for the approval of adjuvant FOLFOX and XELOX in the United States.

Adjuvant chemotherapy is typically initiated within 6 to 8 weeks of surgical resection to allow sufficient time for the surgical wound to heal and to allow the patient's performance status to return to normal baseline. There is now growing data suggesting an adverse impact of delaying adjuvant chemotherapy beyond 8 weeks.[102,103] Moreover, there is recent clinical data suggesting improved clinical outcomes with early initiation of adjuvant chemotherapy within 2 to 4 weeks of surgery.

## SYSTEMIC CHEMOTHERAPY FOR METASTATIC CRC

Approximately 20% of newly diagnosed CRCs are metastatic at the time of initial presentation. Unfortunately, in patients who initially present with early-stage disease, up to 50% of these patients will develop recurrent, metastatic disease. The most common sites of metastatic spread are liver, lungs, and peritoneum. Recent major advances in systemic chemotherapy have improved median survival of patients with mCRC from 8–12 months to 24 months or longer. However, mCRC is still associated with poor prognosis with 5-year OS in the range 5% to 8%. While systemic cytotoxic chemotherapy has been the primary modality for the treatment of patients with mCRC, new developments in biological and targeted agents have also contributed to the improvement of the survival of patients with metastatic disease, especially in those with site-limited involvement.

Capecitabine is an oral fluoropyrimidine with the main advantage over infusional 5-FU as it does not require a central venous catheter and ambulatory infusion pump. Two phase III trials compared capecitabine monotherapy to the Mayo Clinic regimen of bolus 5-FU/LV in patients with mCRC and showed similar clinical efficacy with improved safety profile.[104,105] Patients have also expressed a strong preference for oral medication over the IV form. Moreover, there is growing evidence suggesting a potential pharmacoeconomic advantage of oral capecitabine over IV 5-FU whether the economic analyses have been conducted in the United States, France, Spain, Italy, and Asia.

Despite the potential advantages of oral capecitabine, there is significant geographical difference in tolerability of this agent. Capecitabine at a dose of 1,250 mg/m$^2$ twice daily is often poorly tolerated by U.S. patients, whereas patients in Europe and Asia seem to be better able to tolerate this same dose.[106] This difference in tolerability might be attributed, in part, to population-specific pharmacogenomic variability as well as dietary and lifestyle differences. For example, the diet in the United States is much more heavily fortified with folic acid than it is in other countries and there is probably a greater focus placed on folic acid supplementation in the United States than in other countries around the world.

Capecitabine is the only oral fluoropyrimidine approved for use in the United States. However, two other oral fluoropyrimidines are widely used in Asian countries to treat mCRC, and they are UFT and S-1. As noted previously, UFT is composed of tegafur and uracil, whereas S-1 (TS-1) is an orally active combination of tegafur, gimeracil (an inhibitor of dihydropyrimidine dehydrogenase), and oteracil (an inhibitor of orotate phosphoribosyltransferase) in a molar ratio of 1:0.4:1. Phase II and III studies have shown UFT/LV to have comparable clinical efficacy and improved safety when compared to 5-FU/LV. In the frontline setting, UFT in combination with oxaliplatin (TEGAFOX) or irinotecan (TEGAFIRI) have similar efficacy and tolerability when compared to the corresponding 5-FU and capecitabine-based regimens. As with UFT, S-1 has similar clinical activity to infusional 5-FU when combined with either oxaliplatin or irinotecan. However, in contrast to UFT, which appears to be well tolerated in European patients, S-1 would not be presently recommended for use outside of Asia given the increased GI toxicity observed in European and other non-Asian patient population.[107–109]

FOLFOX4 has become the most commonly used first-line chemotherapy backbone for mCRC in the United States largely based on the NCCTG and INT N9741 trials.[110,111] Two European trials, GERCOR[112] and GOIM trials,[113] showed that FOLFIRI is as efficacious as FOLFOX in the first-line setting. FOLFOX and FOLFIRI are considered acceptable and equivalent treatment options for the first-line treatment of mCRC. Capecitabine plus oxaliplatin (XELOX) was compared to FOLFOX in the first-line setting in several randomized phase III trials in the United States and Europe, and these studies have shown that the clinical efficacy of XELOX, with respect to RR, PFS, and OS, is nearly identical to FOLFOX,[114–116] along with an improved safety profile.

The main side effects of irinotecan-containing regimens are diarrhea and marrow toxicity. However, the GI toxicity is usually not cumulative, and it can be administered until disease progression. Oxaliplatin-containing regimens are less likely to cause diarrhea and alopecia, and they are generally safe in patients with hepatic or renal dysfunction with no need for dose modification.[117,118] The dose-limiting side effect of oxaliplatin is a cumulative dose-dependent neuropathy, and with prolonged therapy, neuropathy can adversely affect quality of life.

Several biologic agents are approved by the regulatory authorities for the treatment of patients with mCRC. One class targets the VEGF signaling pathway. Bevacizumab is the first in this category to be approved in the United States for the treatment of mCRC. Bevacizumab is a humanized monoclonal antibody that targets all forms of VEGF-A. The benefit of adding bevacizumab to a variety of irinotecan and oxaliplatin-containing combination chemotherapy regimens has been confirmed in the first-line treatment of mCRC.[119–122] Immediately following the approval of bevacizumab in 2004, FOLFOX plus bevacizumab emerged as the most commonly used combination regimen for palliative first-line treatment of mCRC despite the absence of phase II or phase III data confirming the superiority of this regimen over any other regimen. Since 2004, the vast majority of patients with mCRC in the United States have received bevacizumab as a component of first-line therapy regardless of the specific regimen chosen for the chemotherapy backbone. In contrast, the situation differs sharply in other parts of the world, where fewer than 50% of patients are treated with bevacizumab in the first-line setting.

Ziv-aflibercept (VEGF Trap) is a recombinant fusion protein, composed of the VEGF binding portions from key domains of human VEGF receptors 1 and 2 fused to the Fc portion of human immunoglobulin G1. This molecule acts as a soluble "decoy" receptor that binds to human VEGF-A, VEGF-B, and placental growth factor. Ziv-aflibercept inhibits the binding of these ligands and activation of their respective receptors. VELOUR trial was a phase III randomized study to evaluate the benefit of ziv-aflibercept in combination with FOLFIRI in patients with oxaliplatin-refractory mCRC. This study showed that the addition of ziv-aflibercept to FOLFIRI significantly prolonged median OS (13.5 months vs. 12.1 months).[123] Based on this study, ziv-aflibercept was approved in the United States and in Europe for use in combination with FOLFIRI for the second-line treatment of patients with mCRC that is resistant to or has progressed following an oxaliplatin-containing regimen.

Antibodies targeting EGFR represent another important class of biologic agents presently available for the treatment of mCRC. There are two such antibodies, and they include the chimeric IgG1 antibody cetuximab and the fully human IgG2 antibody panitumumab. Cetuximab has significant activity against mCRC as a single agent[124–126] and in combination with irinotecan-containing chemotherapy regimens.[127] The randomized phase III CRYSTAL trial showed that cetuximab in combination with FOLFIRI has significant clinical efficacy in the first-line treatment of patients with mCRC.[127] Panitumumab was first shown to have clinical activity as a single agent in refractory mCRC. Subsequent studies have documented its clinical activity in combination with FOLFOX4 in the first-line treatment of mCRC[128] as well as activity in combination with FOLFIRI in the second-line treatment of mCRC. Currently, both cetuximab and panitumumab are indicated for mCRC with wild-type KRAS in the frontline setting where surgical resection is being considered for site-limited metastatic disease or in the second- or third-line setting either as monotherapy or in combination with irinotecan-based chemotherapy. However, there are some subtle differences in the recommendations put forth by NCCN and the ESMO guidelines. For example, only the combination of cetuximab and FOLFIRI is recommended by NCCN in the United States in the frontline setting, whereas the combination of cetuximab and FOLFIRI as well as cetuximab and FOLFOX is recommended by ESMO in Europe.

Regorafenib is an oral small molecule inhibitor of several key multikinases, including angiogenic (VEGFR1–3, TIE2), stromal (PDGRF-β, FGFR), and oncogenic kinases (KIT, RET, and B-RAF).[129] The randomized phase III CORRECT trial was the pivotal trial documenting the clinical benefit of regorafenib in patients with chemo-refractory mCRC.[130] Significant improvement of median OS was observed in the regorafenib arm when compared to placebo (median OS, 6.4 months vs. 5.0 months; one-sided p-value = 0.0052). Regorafenib also significantly improved PFS compared to placebo (median PFS, 1.9 months vs. 1.7 months; one-sided p-value < 0.000001). This study led to the recent approval of regorafenib in the US FDA for the treatment of patients with mCRC who have been previously treated with fluoropyrimidine-, oxaliplatin- and irinotecan-based chemotherapy, an anti-VEGF therapy, and, if KRAS wild type, an anti-EGFR therapy.[130,131]

It should be noted that significant differences exist with respect to access and availability of these novel targeted agents for treating mCRC in different countries around the world. In fact, these targeted agents are either significantly under-reimbursed or not reimbursed at all in most Asian countries, which then represents a huge barrier for access to effective therapy.

## CONCLUSION

There is a significant disparity of CRC-specific incidence and mortality among different regions globally. The disparity of CRC-specific incidence is attributed, at least in part, to different levels of exposure to risk factors of CRC, such as unhealthy Western diet, physical inactivity, and obesity. The significant part of the known risk factors of CRC is related with lifestyle and modifiable with education and preventive measures.

The global disparity of CRC-specific mortality is directly linked with the availability and/or accessibility of health-care resources for CRC screening and timely treatment of diagnosed CRC in adjuvant and/or metastatic settings. This disparity depends on several important societal and political factors, including health-care policy in each region or country. However, some of this disparity, especially between developed countries and underdeveloped countries, requires close collaboration among nations on a global scale.

Significant advances have been made in the systemic treatment of patients with CRC over the past 15 years. However, these results continue to be far too short of our goal for curative treatment as well prevention of cancer recurrence in patients with CRC, and there remains a significant unmet need for new agents and/or treatment regimens.

## CASE 1

Mr. H is a 52-year-old gentleman, who was in good health without any unusual symptoms until 3 weeks ago when he underwent a colonoscopy for CRC screening, which revealed a sessile mass in the sigmoid region of the colon. Biopsy of this mass revealed a moderately differentiated adenocarcinoma. He also underwent esophagogastroduodenoscopy on the same day, which revealed six hyperplastic gastric polyps without any evidence of invasive cancer. His past medical history is unremarkable except for a seizure disorder for which he takes valproic acid and clonazepam. In terms of family history, his father was diagnosed with pancreatic cancer at the age of 71. He did not have any other significant risk factor for CRC.

He underwent surgical resection of the sigmoid colon mass. Surgical pathology revealed a moderately differentiated, invasive adenocarcinoma reaching the muscularis propria without penetration. Two of eight lymph nodes were positive for adenocarcinoma. All surgical margins were free of cancer. Pathological staging was T2 N1Mx. He had an uneventful postoperative course and recovered fully from surgery.

Medical oncology was consulted for consideration of adjuvant chemotherapy. A pre-op CEA level had not been obtained, and a post-op CEA level was within normal range. CT evaluation of chest/abdomen/pelvis did not reveal any evidence of metastatic disease. The final diagnosis was stage III (T2N1M0) colon cancer, and the decision was made to treat him with 6 months of FOLFOX adjuvant chemotherapy.

## CASE 2

Mr. S is a 69-year-old gentleman with a history of stage II colon cancer. He has a significant history of hypertension and coronary artery disease (CAD) for which he had coronary stent placement in December 2008.

In May 2010, he was found to have a mass lesion in the transverse colon for which he underwent right hemicolectomy. Surgical pathology revealed a 3-cm moderately differentiated adenocarcinoma arising in a background of tubulovillous adenoma. The tumor invaded the muscularis propria into the pericolic fat, and the surgical margins were free of cancer. Angiolymphatic invasion was identified. Nineteen lymph nodes were identified in the surgical resection specimen, and 0 of 19 were positive for tumor involvement. The final pathologic stage was pT3N0M0, stage II cancer CRC. Molecular analysis revealed a high level of microsatellite instability in the tumor specimen.

He had a discussion with his medical oncologist about adjuvant chemotherapy and opted not to have adjuvant chemotherapy due to concerns about potential complications of the chemotherapy although his cancer had features of high risk. He had a follow-up colonoscopy in November 2011, which did not reveal any evidence of polyps or recurrent disease.

He had annual CT scan evaluation for surveillance. A recent CT scan of chest/abdomen/pelvis revealed a new 2-cm nodule in the left lobe of the liver without evidence of any other metastatic disease. CT scan of the chest/abdomen/pelvis performed 1 year earlier did not reveal any abnormal findings except multiple cystic lesions in the liver, which had been stable and not related with the new nodule.

He underwent a CT-guided biopsy of the liver lesion in July 2012, which showed malignant cells positive for CAM5.2, AE1, CDX2, CK7, and CK20, consistent with metastatic adenocarcinoma of the colon. Molecular evaluation of this metastatic lesion did not show the presence of KRAS or BRAF mutations.

He has no significant history of cancer in his family, and he does not have any significant risk factors for CRC. He takes lipitor, aspirin, and metoprolol for his known CAD and hypertension. His pre-op CEA was within normal limit. He underwent wedge resection of the liver nodule in August 2012 and had an uneventful postoperative course. Medical oncology was consulted, and FOLFOX chemotherapy was recommended after a long discussion about the potential risks and benefits of systemic chemotherapy.

## REFERENCES

1. Siegel R, Naishadham D, Jemal A. Cancer statistics, 2012. CA *Cancer J Clin* 2012; 62(1): 10–29.
2. Kamangar F, Dores GM, Anderson WF. Patterns of cancer incidence, mortality, and prevalence across five continents: defining priorities to reduce cancer disparities in different geographic regions of the world. *J Clin Oncol* 2006; 24(14): 2137–50.
3. Kohler BA, Ward E, McCarthy BJ, et al. Annual report to the nation on the status of cancer, 1975–2007, featuring tumors of the brain and other nervous system. *J Natl Cancer Inst* 2011; 103(9): 714–36.
4. Center MM, Jemal A, Smith RA, Ward E. Worldwide variations in colorectal cancer. CA *Cancer J Clin* 2009; 59(6): 366–78.
5. Atkin WS, Morson BC, Cuzick J. Long-term risk of colorectal cancer after excision of rectosigmoid adenomas. *N Engl J Med* 1992; 326(10): 658–62.
6. Burt RW, DiSario JA, Cannon-Albright L. Genetics of colon cancer: impact of inheritance on colon cancer risk. *Annu Rev Med* 1995; 46(7598472): 371–79.
7. Spirio L, Olschwang S, Groden J, et al. Alleles of the APC gene: an attenuated form of familial polyposis. *Cell* 1993; 75(5): 951–57.
8. Lynch HT, Smyrk TC, Watson P, et al. Genetics, natural history, tumor spectrum, and pathology of hereditary nonpolyposis colorectal cancer: an updated review. *Gastroenterology* 1993; 104(5): 1535–49.
9. Ekbom A, Helmick C, Zack M, Adami HO. Ulcerative colitis and colorectal cancer. A population-based study. *N Engl J Med* 1990; 323(18): 1228–33.

10. Inoue M, Iwasaki M, Otani T, Sasazuki S, Noda M, Tsugane S. Diabetes mellitus and the risk of cancer: results from a large-scale population-based cohort study in Japan. *Arch Intern Med* 2006; 166(17): 1871–77.

11. Hu FB, Manson JE, Liu S, et al. Prospective study of adult onset diabetes mellitus (type 2) and risk of colorectal cancer in women. *J Natl Cancer Inst* 1999; 91(6): 542–47.

12. Jee SH, Ohrr H, Sull JW, Yun JE, Ji M, Samet JM. Fasting serum glucose level and cancer risk in Korean men and women. *JAMA* 2005; 293(2): 194–202.

13. Nilsen TI, Vatten LJ. Prospective study of colorectal cancer risk and physical activity, diabetes, blood glucose and BMI: exploring the hyperinsulinaemia hypothesis. *Br J Cancer* 2001; 84(3): 417–22.

14. He J, Stram DO, Kolonel LN, et al. The association of diabetes with colorectal cancer risk: the Multiethnic Cohort. *Br J Cancer* 2010; 103(1): 120–26.

15. Larsson SC, Orsini N, Wolk A. Diabetes mellitus and risk of colorectal cancer: a meta-analysis. *J Natl Cancer Inst* 2005; 97(22): 1679–87.

16. Yuhara H, Steinmaus C, Cohen SE, Corley DA, Tei Y, Buffler PA. Is diabetes mellitus an independent risk factor for colon cancer and rectal cancer? *Am J Gastroenterol* 2011; 106(11): 1911–21.

17. Fedirko V, Tramacere I, Bagnardi V, et al. Alcohol drinking and colorectal cancer risk: an overall and dose-response meta-analysis of published studies. *Ann Oncol* 2011; 22(9): 1958–72.

18. Cho E, Smith-Warner SA, Ritz J, et al. Alcohol intake and colorectal cancer: a pooled analysis of 8 cohort studies. *Ann Intern Med* 2004; 140(8): 603–13.

19. Giovannucci E, Rimm EB, Ascherio A, Stampfer MJ, Colditz GA, Willett WC. Alcohol, low-methionine—low-folate diets, and risk of colon cancer in men. *J Natl Cancer Inst* 1995; 87(4): 265–73.

20. Botteri E, Iodice S, Bagnardi V, Raimondi S, Lowenfels AB, Maisonneuve P. Smoking and colorectal cancer: a meta-analysis. *JAMA* 2008; 300(23): 2765–78.

21. Martinez ME, Giovannucci E, Spiegelman D, Hunter DJ, Willett WC, Colditz GA. Leisure-time physical activity, body size, and colon cancer in women. Nurses' Health Study Research Group. *J Natl Cancer Inst* 1997; 89(13): 948–55.

22. Giovannucci E, Ascherio A, Rimm EB, Colditz GA, Stampfer MJ, Willett WC. Physical activity, obesity, and risk for colon cancer and adenoma in men. *Ann Intern Med* 1995; 122(5): 327–34.

23. Renehan AG, Tyson M, Egger M, Heller RF, Zwahlen M. Body-mass index and incidence of cancer: a systematic review and meta-analysis of prospective observational studies. *Lancet* 2008; 371(9612): 569–78.

24. Wolin KY, Yan Y, Colditz GA, Lee IM. Physical activity and colon cancer prevention: a meta-analysis. *Br J Cancer* 2009; 100(4): 611–16.

25. Terry P, Giovannucci E, Michels KB, et al. Fruit, vegetables, dietary fiber, and risk of colorectal cancer. *J Natl Cancer Inst* 2001; 93(7): 525–33.

26. Michels KB, Edward Giovannucci, Joshipura KJ, et al. Prospective study of fruit and vegetable consumption and incidence of colon and rectal cancers. *J Natl Cancer Inst* 2000; 92(21): 1740–52.

27. Koushik A, Hunter DJ, Spiegelman D, et al. Fruits, vegetables, and colon cancer risk in a pooled analysis of 14 cohort studies. *J Natl Cancer Inst* 2007; 99(19): 1471–83.

28. Peters U, Sinha R, Chatterjee N, et al. Dietary fibre and colorectal adenoma in a colorectal cancer early detection programme. *Lancet* 2003; 361(9368): 1491–95.

29. Bingham SA, Day NE, Luben R, et al. Dietary fibre in food and protection against colorectal cancer in the European Prospective Investigation into Cancer and Nutrition (EPIC): an observational study. *Lancet* 2003; 361(9368): 1496–501.

30. Larsson SC, Giovannucci E, Bergkvist L, Wolk A. Whole grain consumption and risk of colorectal cancer: a population-based cohort of 60,000 women. *Br J Cancer* 2005; 92(9): 1803–7.

31. Dahm CC, Keogh RH, Spencer EA, et al. Dietary fiber and colorectal cancer risk: a nested case-control study using food diaries. *J Natl Cancer Inst* 2010; 102(9): 614–26.

32. Fuchs CS, Giovannucci EL, Colditz GA, et al. Dietary fiber and the risk of colorectal cancer and adenoma in women. *N Engl J Med* 1999; 340(3): 169–76.

33. Beresford SA, Johnson KC, Ritenbaugh C, et al. Low-fat dietary pattern and risk of colorectal cancer: the Women's Health Initiative Randomized Controlled Dietary Modification Trial. *JAMA* 2006; 295(6): 643–54.

34. Park Y, Hunter DJ, Spiegelman D, et al. Dietary fiber intake and risk of colorectal cancer: a pooled analysis of prospective cohort studies. *JAMA* 2005; 294(22): 2849–57.

35. Schatzkin A, Lanza E, Corle D, et al. Lack of effect of a low-fat, high-fiber diet on the recurrence of colorectal adenomas. Polyp Prevention Trial Study Group. *N Engl J Med* 2000; 342(16): 1149–55.

36. Alberts DS, Martínez ME, Roe DJ, et al. Lack of effect of a high-fiber cereal supplement on the recurrence of colorectal adenomas. Phoenix Colon Cancer Prevention Physicians' Network. *N Engl J Med* 2000; 342(16): 1156–62.

37. Wu K, Willett WC, Fuchs CS, Colditz GA, Giovannucci EL. Calcium intake and risk of colon cancer in women and men. *J Natl Cancer Inst* 2002; 94(6): 437–46.

38. Cho E, Smith-Warner SA, Spiegelman D, et al. Dairy foods, calcium, and colorectal cancer: a pooled analysis of 10 cohort studies. *J Natl Cancer Inst* 2004; 96(13): 1015–22.

39. Park Y, Leitzmann MF, Subar AF, Hollenbeck A, Schatzkin A. Dairy food, calcium, and risk of cancer in the NIH-AARP Diet and Health Study. *Arch Intern Med* 2009; 169(4): 391–401.

40. Rothwell PM, Wilson M, Elwin, et al. Long-term effect of aspirin on colorectal cancer incidence and mortality: 20-year follow-up of five randomised trials. *Lancet* 2010; 376(9754): 1741–50.

41. Burn J, Gerdes AM, Macrae F, et al. Long-term effect of aspirin on cancer risk in carriers of hereditary colorectal cancer: an analysis from the CAPP2 randomised controlled trial. *Lancet* 2011; 378(9809): 2081–87.

42. Liao X, Lochhead P, Nishihara R, et al. Aspirin use, tumor PIK3CA mutation, and colorectal-cancer survival. *N Engl J Med* 2012; 367(17): 1596–606.

43. Fearon ER, Vogelstein B. A genetic model for colorectal tumorigenesis. *Cell* 1990; 61(5): 759–67.

44. Winawer SJ, Fletcher R, Rex D, et al. Colorectal cancer screening: clinical guidelines and rationale. *Gastroenterology* 1997; 112(2): 594–642.

45. Ferlitsch M, Reinhart K, Pramhas S, et al. Sex-specific prevalence of adenomas, advanced adenomas, and colorectal cancer in individuals undergoing screening colonoscopy. JAMA 2011; 306(12): 1352–58.

46. Laiyemo AO, Murphy G, Albert PS, et al. Postpolypectomy colonoscopy surveillance guidelines: predictive accuracy for advanced adenoma at 4 years. Ann Intern Med 2008; 148(6): 419–26.

47. Mandel JS, Church TR, Ederer F, Bond JH. Colorectal cancer mortality: effectiveness of biennial screening for fecal occult blood. J Natl Cancer Inst 1999; 91(5): 434–37.

48. Hardcastle JD, Chamberlain JO, Robinson MH, et al. Randomised controlled trial of faecal-occult-blood screening for colorectal cancer. Lancet 1996; 348(9040): 1472–77.

49. Kronborg O, Fenger C, Olsen J, Jørgensen OD, Søndergaard O. Randomised study of screening for colorectal cancer with faecal-occult-blood test. Lancet 1996; 348(9040): 1467–71.

50. Faivre J, Dancourt V, Lejeune C, et al. Reduction in colorectal cancer mortality by fecal occult blood screening in a French controlled study. Gastroenterology 2004; 126(7): 1674–80.

51. Levin B, Lieberman DA, McFarland B, et al. Screening and surveillance for the early detection of colorectal cancer and adenomatous polyps, 2008: a joint guideline from the American Cancer Society, the US Multi-Society Task Force on Colorectal Cancer, and the American College of Radiology. CA Cancer J Clin 2008; 58(3): 130–60.

52. Atkin WS, Edwards R, Kralj-Hans I, et al. Once-only flexible sigmoidoscopy screening in prevention of colorectal cancer: a multicentre randomised controlled trial. Lancet 2010; 375(9726): 1624–33.

53. Segnan N, Armaroli P, Bonelli L, et al. Once-only sigmoidoscopy in colorectal cancer screening: follow-up findings of the Italian Randomized Controlled Trial—SCORE. J Natl Cancer Inst 2011; 103(17): 1310–22.

54. Winawer SJ, Zauber AG, Ho MN, et al. Prevention of colorectal cancer by colonoscopic polypectomy. The National Polyp Study Workgroup. N Engl J Med 1993; 329(27): 1977–81.

55. Brenner H, Hoffmeister M, Arndt V, Stegmaier C, Altenhofen L, Haug U. Protection from right- and left-sided colorectal neoplasms after colonoscopy: population-based study. J Natl Cancer Inst 2010; 102(2): 89–95.

56. Brenner H, Chang-Claude J, Seiler CM, Rickert A, Hoffmeister M. Protection from colorectal cancer after colonoscopy: a population-based, case-control study. Ann Intern Med 2011; 154(1): 22–30.

57. Choi KS, Jun JK, Lee HY, Hahm MI, Oh JH, Park EC. Increasing uptake of colorectal cancer screening in Korea: a population-based study. BMC Public Health 2010; 10: 265.

58. Ku G, Tan IB, Yau T, et al. Management of colon cancer: resource-stratified guidelines from the Asian Oncology Summit 2012; Lancet Oncol 2012; 13(11): e470–81.

59. O'Connell JB, Maggard MA, Ko CY. Colon cancer survival rates with the new American Joint Committee on Cancer sixth edition staging. J Natl Cancer Inst 2004; 96(19): 1420–25.

60. Watanabe T, Itabashi M, Shimada Y, et al. Japanese Society for Cancer of the Colon and Rectum (JSCCR) guidelines 2010 for the treatment of colorectal cancer. *Int J Clin Oncol* 2012; 17(1): 1–29.

61. Bosset JF, Collette L, Calais G, et al. Chemotherapy with preoperative radiotherapy in rectal cancer. *N Engl J Med* 2006; 355(11): 1114–23.

62. Sauer R, Becker H, Hohenberge W, et al. Preoperative versus postoperative chemoradiotherapy for rectal cancer. *N Engl J Med* 2004; 351(17): 1731–40.

63. Pinedo HM, Peters GF. Fluorouracil: biochemistry and pharmacology. *J Clin Oncol* 1988; 6(10): 1653–64.

64. Wolmark N, Rockette H, Fisher B, et al. The benefit of leucovorin-modulated fluorouracil as postoperative adjuvant therapy for primary colon cancer: results from National Surgical Adjuvant Breast and Bowel Project protocol C-03. *J Clin Oncol* 1993; 11(10): 1879–87.

65. Moertel CG, Fleming TR, Macdonald JS, et al. Fluorouracil plus levamisole as effective adjuvant therapy after resection of stage III colon carcinoma: a final report. *Ann Intern Med* 1995; 122(5): 321–26.

66. Wolmark N, Rockette H, Mamounas E, et al. Clinical trial to assess the relative efficacy of fluorouracil and leucovorin, fluorouracil and levamisole, and fluorouracil, leucovorin, and levamisole in patients with Dukes' B and C carcinoma of the colon: results from National Surgical Adjuvant Breast and Bowel Project C-04. *J Clin Oncol* 1999; 17(11): 3553–59.

67. Andre T, Quinaux E, Louvet C, et al. Phase III study comparing a semimonthly with a monthly regimen of fluorouracil and leucovorin as adjuvant treatment for stage II and III colon cancer patients: final results of GERCOR C96.1. *J Clin Oncol* 2007; 25(24): 3732–38.

68. Andre T, Colin P, Louvet C, et al. Semimonthly versus monthly regimen of fluorouracil and leucovorin administered for 24 or 36 weeks as adjuvant therapy in stage II and III colon cancer: results of a randomized trial. *J Clin Oncol* 2003; 21(15): 2896–903.

69. Cassidy J, Douillard JY, Twelves C, et al. Pharmacoeconomic analysis of adjuvant oral capecitabine vs intravenous 5-FU/LV in Dukes' C colon cancer: the X-ACT trial. *Br J Cancer* 2006; 94(8): 1122–29.

70. Twelves C, Wong A, Nowacki MP, et al. Capecitabine as adjuvant treatment for stage III colon cancer. *N Engl J Med* 2005; 352(26): 2696–704.

71. Lembersky BC, Wieand HS, Petrelli NJ, et al. Oral uracil and tegafur plus leucovorin compared with intravenous fluorouracil and leucovorin in stage II and III carcinoma of the colon: results from National Surgical Adjuvant Breast and Bowel Project Protocol C-06. *J Clin Oncol* 2006; 24(13): 2059–64.

72. Andre T, Boni C, Mounedji-Boudiaf L, et al. Oxaliplatin, fluorouracil, and leucovorin as adjuvant treatment for colon cancer. *N Engl J Med* 2004; 350(23): 2343–51.

73. Andre T, Boni C, Navarro M, et al. Improved overall survival with oxaliplatin, fluorouracil, and leucovorin as adjuvant treatment in stage II or III colon cancer in the MOSAIC trial. *J Clin Oncol* 2009; 27(19): 3109–16.

74. Haller DG, Tabernero J, Maroun J, et al. Capecitabine plus oxaliplatin compared with fluorouracil and folinic acid as adjuvant therapy for stage III colon cancer. *J Clin Oncol* 2011; 29(11): 1465–71.

75. Saltz LB, Niedzwiecki D, Hollis D, et al. Irinotecan fluorouracil plus leucovorin is not superior to fluorouracil plus leucovorin alone as adjuvant treatment for stage III colon cancer: results of CALGB 89803. *J Clin Oncol* 2007; 25(23): 3456–61.

76. Van Cutsem E, Labianca R, Bodoky G, et al. Randomized phase III trial comparing biweekly infusional fluorouracil/leucovorin alone or with irinotecan in the adjuvant treatment of stage III colon cancer: PETACC-3. *J Clin Oncol* 2009; 27(19): 3117–25.

77. Ychou M, Raoul JL, Douillard JY, et al. A phase III randomised trial of LV5FU2 + irinotecan versus LV5FU2 alone in adjuvant high-risk colon cancer (FNCLCC Accord02/FFCD9802). *Ann Oncol* 2009; 20(4): 674–80.

78. Allegra CJ, Yothers G, O'Connell MJ, et al. Phase III trial assessing bevacizumab in stages II and III carcinoma of the colon: results of NSABP protocol C-08. *J Clin Oncol* 2011; 29(1): 11–16.

79. Allegra CJ, Yothers G, O'Connell MJ, et al. Initial safety report of NSABP C-08: a randomized phase III study of modified FOLFOX6 with or without bevacizumab for the adjuvant treatment of patients with stage II or III colon cancer. *J Clin Oncol* 2009; 27(20): 3385–90.

80. De Gramont A, Van Cutsem E, Tabernero J, et al. AVANT: results from a randomized, three-arm multinational phase III study to investigate bevacizumab with either XELOX or FOLFOX4 versus FOLFOX4 alone as adjuvant treatment for colon cancer. ASCO Meeting Abstracts. *J Clin Oncol* 2011; 29(Suppl 4): 362.

81. Alberts SR, Sargent DJ, Nair S, et al. Effect of oxaliplatin, fluorouracil, and leucovorin with or without cetuximab on survival among patients with resected stage III colon cancer: a randomized trial. *JAMA* 2012; 307(13): 1383–93.

82. Efficacy of adjuvant fluorouracil and folinic acid in colon cancer. International Multicentre Pooled Analysis of Colon Cancer Trials (IMPACT) investigators. *Lancet* 1995; 345(8955): 939–44.

83. Moertel CG, Fleming TR, Macdonald JS, et al. Intergroup study of fluorouracil plus levamisole as adjuvant therapy for stage II/Dukes' B2 colon cancer. *J Clin Oncol* 1995; 13(12): 2936–43.

84. Moore HC, Haller DG. Adjuvant therapy of colon cancer. *Semin Oncol* 1999; 26(5): 545–55.

85. Gray R, Barnwell J, McConkey C, et al. Adjuvant chemotherapy versus observation in patients with colorectal cancer: a randomised study. *Lancet* 2007; 370(9604): 2020–29.

86. Schippinger W, Samonigg H, Schaberl-Moser R, et al. A prospective randomised phase III trial of adjuvant chemotherapy with 5-fluorouracil and leucovorin in patients with stage II colon cancer. *Br J Cancer* 2007; 97(8): 1021–27.

87. Sargent DJ, Patiyil S, Yothers G, et al. End points for colon cancer adjuvant trials: observations and recommendations based on individual patient data from 20,898 patients enrolled onto 18 randomized trials from the ACCENT Group. *J Clin Oncol* 2007; 25(29): 4569–74.

88. Comparison of fluorouracil with additional levamisole, higher-dose folinic acid, or both, as adjuvant chemotherapy for colorectal cancer: a randomised trial. QUASAR Collaborative Group. *Lancet* 2000; 355(9215): 1588–96.

89. Quah HM, Chou JF, Gonen M, et al. Identification of patients with high-risk stage II colon cancer for adjuvant therapy. *Dis Colon Rectum* 2008; 51(5): 503–7.

90. Gill S, Loprinzi CL, Sargent DJ, et al. Pooled analysis of fluorouracil-based adjuvant therapy for stage II and III colon cancer: who benefits and by how much? *J Clin Oncol* 2004; 22(10): 1797–806.

91. Michelassi F, Ayala JJ, Balestracci T, Goldberg R, Chappell R, Block GE. Verification of a new clinicopathologic staging system for colorectal adenocarcinoma. *Ann Surg* 1991; 214(1): 11–18.

92. Sternberg A, Sibirsky O, Cohen D, Blumenson LE, Petrelli NJ. Validation of a new classification system for curatively resected colorectal adenocarcinoma. *Cancer* 1999; 86(5): 782–92.

93. Betge J, Pollheimer MJ, Lindtner RA, et al. Intramural and extramural vascular invasion in colorectal cancer: prognostic significance and quality of pathology reporting. *Cancer* 2012; 118(3): 628–38.

94. Liebig C, Ayala G, Wilks J, et al. Perineural invasion is an independent predictor of outcome in colorectal cancer. *J Clin Oncol* 2009; 27(31): 5131–37.

95. Huh JW, Kim HR, Kim YJ. Prognostic value of perineural invasion in patients with stage II colorectal cancer. *Ann Surg Oncol* 2010; 17(8): 2066–72.

96. Faivre-Finn C, Bouvier-Benhamiche AM, Phelip JM, Manfredi S, Dancourt V, Faivre J. Colon cancer in France: evidence for improvement in management and survival. *Gut* 2002; 51(1): 60–64.

97. Petersen VC, Baxter KJ, Love SB, Shepherd NA. Identification of objective pathological prognostic determinants and models of prognosis in Dukes' B colon cancer. *Gut* 2002; 51(1): 65–69.

98. Chen HS, Sheen-Chen SM. Obstruction and perforation in colorectal adenocarcinoma: an analysis of prognosis and current trends. *Surgery* 2000; 127(4): 370–76.

99. Chang GJ, Rodriguez-Bigas MA, Skibber JM, Moyer VA. Lymph node evaluation and survival after curative resection of colon cancer: systematic review. *J Natl Cancer Inst* 2007; 99(6): 433–41.

100. Benson AB 3rd, Schrag D, Somerfield MR, et al. American Society of Clinical Oncology recommendations on adjuvant chemotherapy for stage II colon cancer. *J Clin Oncol* 2004; 22(16): 3408–19.

101. Punt CJ, Buyse M, Köhne CH, et al. Endpoints in adjuvant treatment trials: a systematic review of the literature in colon cancer and proposed definitions for future trials. *J Natl Cancer Inst* 2007; 99(13): 998–1003.

102. Biagi JJ, Raphael MJ, Mackillop WJ, Kong W, King WD, Booth CM. Association between time to initiation of adjuvant chemotherapy and survival in colorectal cancer: a Systematic review and meta-analysis. *JAMA* 2011; 305(22): 2335–42.

103. Des Guetz G, Nicolas P, Perret GY, Morere JF, Uzzan B. Does delaying adjuvant chemotherapy after curative surgery for colorectal cancer impair survival? A meta-analysis. *Eur J Cancer* 2010; 46(6): 1049–55.

104. Hoff PM, Ansari R, Batist G, et al. Comparison of oral capecitabine versus intravenous fluorouracil plus leucovorin as first-line treatment in 605 patients

with metastatic colorectal cancer: results of a randomized phase III study. *J Clin Oncol* 2001; 19(8): 2282–92.

105. Van Cutsem E, Twelves C, Cassidy J, et al. Oral capecitabine compared with intravenous fluorouracil plus leucovorin in patients with metastatic colorectal cancer: results of a large phase III study. *J Clin Oncol* 2001; 19(21): 4097–106.

106. Haller DG, Cassidy J, Clarke SJ, et al. Potential regional differences for the tolerability profiles of fluoropyrimidines. *J Clin Oncol* 2008; 26(13): 2118–23.

107. Bennouna J, Saunders M, Douillard JY. The role of UFT in metastatic colorectal cancer. *Oncology* 2009; 76(5): 301–10.

108. Hong YS, Park YS, Lim HY, et al. S-1 plus oxaliplatin versus capecitabine plus oxaliplatin for first-line treatment of patients with metastatic colorectal cancer: a randomised, non-inferiority phase 3 trial. *Lancet Oncol* 2012; 13(11): 1125–32.

109. Muro K, Boku N, Shimada Y, et al. Irinotecan plus S-1 (IRIS) versus fluorouracil and folinic acid plus irinotecan (FOLFIRI) as second-line chemotherapy for metastatic colorectal cancer: a randomised phase 2/3 non-inferiority study (FIRIS study). *Lancet Oncol* 2010; 11(9): 853–60.

110. Goldberg RM, Sargent DJ, Morton RF, et al. A randomized controlled trial of fluorouracil plus leucovorin, irinotecan, and oxaliplatin combinations in patients with previously untreated metastatic colorectal cancer. *J Clin Oncol* 2004; 22(1): 23–30.

111. Goldberg RM, Sargent DJ, Morton RF, et al. Randomized controlled trial of reduced-dose bolus fluorouracil plus leucovorin and irinotecan or infused fluorouracil plus leucovorin and oxaliplatin in patients with previously untreated metastatic colorectal cancer: a North American Intergroup Trial. *J Clin Oncol* 2006; 24(21): 3347–53.

112. Tournigand C, André T, Achille E, et al. FOLFIRI followed by FOLFOX6 or the reverse sequence in advanced colorectal cancer: a randomized GERCOR study. *J Clin Oncol* 2004; 22(2): 229–37.

113. Colucci G, Gebbia V, Paoletti G, et al. Phase III randomized trial of FOLFIRI versus FOLFOX4 in the treatment of advanced colorectal cancer: a multicenter study of the Gruppo Oncologico Dell'Italia Meridionale. *J Clin Oncol* 2005; 23(22): 4866–75.

114. Cassidy J, Clarke S, Díaz-Rubio E, et al. Randomized phase III study of capecitabine plus oxaliplatin compared with fluorouracil/folinic acid plus oxaliplatin as first-line therapy for metastatic colorectal cancer. *J Clin Oncol* 2008; 26(12): 2006–12.

115. Porschen R, Arkenau HT, Kubicka S, et al. Phase III study of capecitabine plus oxaliplatin compared with fluorouracil and leucovorin plus oxaliplatin in metastatic colorectal cancer: a final report of the AIO Colorectal Study Group. *J Clin Oncol* 2007; 25(27): 4217–23.

116. Diaz-Rubio E, Tabernero J, Gómez-España A, et al. Phase III study of capecitabine plus oxaliplatin compared with continuous-infusion fluorouracil plus oxaliplatin as first-line therapy in metastatic colorectal cancer: final report of the Spanish Cooperative Group for the Treatment of Digestive Tumors Trial. *J Clin Oncol* 2007; 25(27): 4224–30.

117. Takimoto CH, Remick SC, Sharma S, et al. Dose-escalating and pharmacological study of oxaliplatin in adult cancer patients with impaired renal function: a National Cancer Institute Organ Dysfunction Working Group Study. *J Clin Oncol* 2003; 21(14): 2664–72.

118. Doroshow JH, Synold TW, Gandara D, et al. Pharmacology of oxaliplatin in solid tumor patients with hepatic dysfunction: a preliminary report of the National Cancer Institute Organ Dysfunction Working Group. *Semin Oncol* 2003; 30(4 Suppl 15): 14–19.

119. Fuchs CS, Marshall J, Mitchell E, et al. Randomized, controlled trial of irinotecan plus infusional, bolus, or oral fluoropyrimidines in first-line treatment of metastatic colorectal cancer: results from the BICC-C Study. *J Clin Oncol* 2007; 25(30): 4779–86.

120. Hochster HS, Hart LL, Ramanathan R, et al. Safety and efficacy of oxaliplatin and fluoropyrimidine regimens with or without bevacizumab as first-line treatment of metastatic colorectal cancer: results of the TREE Study. *J Clin Oncol* 2008; 26(21): 3523–29.

121. Saltz LB, Clarke S, Díaz-Rubio E, et al. Bevacizumab in combination with oxaliplatin-based chemotherapy as first-line therapy in metastatic colorectal cancer: a randomized phase III study. *J Clin Oncol* 2008; 26(12): 2013–19.

122. Fuchs CS, Marshall J, Barrueco J. Randomized, controlled trial of irinotecan plus infusional, bolus, or oral fluoropyrimidines in first-line treatment of metastatic colorectal cancer: updated results from the BICC-C study. *J Clin Oncol* 2008; 26(4): 689–90.

123. Van Cutsem E, Tabernero J, Lakomy R, et al. Addition of aflibercept to fluorouracil, leucovorin, and irinotecan improves survival in a phase III randomized trial in patients with metastatic colorectal cancer previously treated with an oxaliplatin-based regimen. *J Clin Oncol* 2012; 30(28): 3499–506.

124. Cunningham D, Humblet Y, Siena S, et al. Cetuximab monotherapy and cetuximab plus irinotecan in irinotecan-refractory metastatic colorectal cancer. *N Engl J Med* 2004; 351(4): 337–45.

125. Karapetis CS, Khambata-Ford S, Jonker DJ, et al. K-ras mutations and benefit from cetuximab in advanced colorectal cancer. *N Engl J Med* 2008; 359(17): 1757–65.

126. Pessino A, Artale S, Sciallero S, et al. First-line single-agent cetuximab in patients with advanced colorectal cancer. *Ann Oncol* 2008; 19(4): 711–16.

127. Van Cutsem E, Köhne CH, Hitre E, et al. Cetuximab and chemotherapy as initial treatment for metastatic colorectal cancer. *N Engl J Med* 2009; 360(14): 1408–17.

128. Douillard JY, Siena S, Cassidy J, et al. Randomized, phase III trial of panitumumab with infusional fluorouracil, leucovorin, and oxaliplatin (FOLFOX4) versus FOLFOX4 alone as first-line treatment in patients with previously untreated metastatic colorectal cancer: the PRIME study. *J Clin Oncol* 2010; 28(31): 4697–705.

129. Wilhelm SM, Dumas J, Adnane L, et al. Regorafenib (BAY 73-4506): a new oral multikinase inhibitor of angiogenic, stromal and oncogenic receptor tyrosine

kinases with potent preclinical antitumor activity. *Int J Cancer* 2011; 129(1): 245–55.

130. Van Cutsem E, Sobrero AF, Siena S, et al. Phase III CORRECT trial of rego-rafenib in metastatic colorectal cancer (mCRC). ASCO Meeting Abstracts. *J Clin Oncol* 2012; 30(15 Suppl): 3502.

131. Stivarga [package insert]. Wayne, NJ: Bayer HealthCare Pharmaceuticals Inc, 2012.

# 6

# Esophageal Cancer

## Radu Pescarus and Christy M. Dunst

### EPIDEMIOLOGY

Esophageal cancer is the eighth most common cancer worldwide.[1] In the United States, esophageal cancer ranks third among cancers of the gastrointestinal tract, behind colorectal and gastric cancers.[2] It is estimated that there will be around 18,000 new cases of esophageal cancer in 2014 in the United States alone and will be responsible for 4% of cancer-related deaths in the male population this year.[2] Together, adenocarcinoma (AC) and squamous cell cancer subtypes account for more than 90% of all esophageal cancers.[3] The remainder 10% is composed of esophageal lymphoma, gastrointestinal stromal tumor or other mesenchymal tumors, carcinoid and other endocrine tumors, melanoma, metastatic lesions, and other rare pathologies.

Esophageal cancer is known for its markedly aggressive course, with an overall mortality rate of approximately 85% due to the advanced stage at which most esophageal cancers are diagnosed. According to the most recent statistics, there were approximately 480,000 new esophageal cancer cases and 405,000 deaths secondary to esophageal tumors worldwide in 2008.[4] Overall, there is a 3- to 4-fold higher incidence in men than women.[4] The highest rates of esophageal cancer are found in southern and eastern Africa as well as eastern Asia. The lowest rates are seen in western and northern Africa as well as Central America. There is therefore up to a 16-fold difference in the prevalence of this condition internationally when all subtypes are pooled together.[4]

However, there are important differences in the biology of the subtypes of esophageal cancer that impact its prevalence. Squamous cell carcinoma (SCC) of the esophagus is thought to arise as a result of direct, repeated contact with carcinogens that are ingested, such as tobacco and alcohol. On the other hand, gastroesophageal reflux (GER) is strongly associated with esophageal AC. The presence of weekly reflux symptoms equates with a 5-fold increased risk for esophageal AC, while having daily reflux symptoms increases the risk 7-fold.[5] Furthermore, the strongest risk factor for AC is the presence of intestinal metaplasia in the esophagus (Barrett's esophagus). The link between Barrett's esophagus and GER disease is well established. Therefore, the incidence of certain subtypes of esophageal cancer is directly linked to the underlying risk factors prevalent in the region. Changes in personal habits have had a direct impact on the incidence of esophageal cancer. For example, historically, the incidence of SCC of the esophagus far exceeded that of AC until the mid-1990s. This is partly due to a sharp decrease in SCC

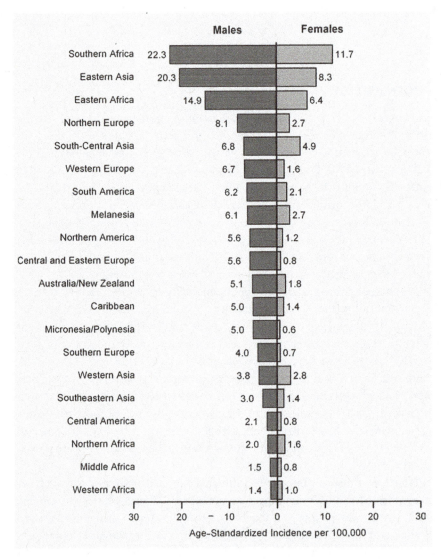

**FIGURE 6.1** Age-standardized incidence of esophageal cancer per 100,000 in males (left) and females (right) in various world areas. (Reference 4. Permission for use obtained from John Wiley and Sons.)

beginning in the 1980s likely attributed to the rise in awareness of the association between smoking and cancer, which in turn led to declining cigarette use over the same time period. Meanwhile, the incidence of esophageal AC is increasing at an alarming rate and has become the most frequent histological subtype of esophageal cancer in the developed world.[6] This change is most evident in the white male U.S. population,[6] whereas the incidence of SCC of the esophagus is stable or decreasing in the same population.[7] Interestingly, this parallels the worsening obesity epidemic in the same population,[4] but the exact cause is unknown.

Indeed, fewer than 30% of newly diagnosed esophageal cancers in the United States and Western Europe are SCC.[8] Conversely, the prevalence of SCC is much greater than that of AC in the African population.[9] Indeed SCC accounted for up to 78% of esophageal cancer cases in a series from Ghana.[10] Other published series from Kenya and southern India report over 90% of cases as being SCC.[11] In Asia, Mongolia, northwestern China, the Central Asian Republics, and the countries bordering the Caspian Sea have been collectively named the Central Asian Esophageal Cancer Belt (Figures 6.1 and 6.2) due to the high incidence of esophageal cancer that is almost

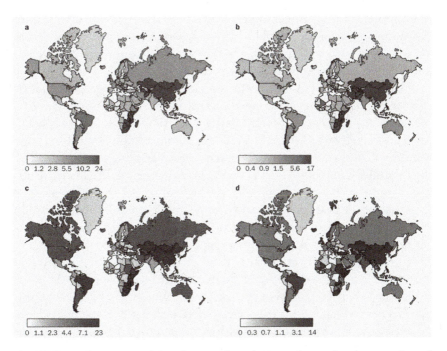

**FIGURE 6.2** International distribution of incidence and mortality from esophageal cancer based on the most recent estimates (2008). The age-standardized incidence per 100,000 in males (A) and females (B). Below, age-standardized mortality per 100,000 in males (C) and females (D). (Reference 13. Permission for use obtained from Nature Publishing Group.)

exclusively SCC.[12] In addition, southeastern Africa is also noted to have a particularly high incidence of SCC (Figure 6.2).[13]


## ETIOLOGY

As with other tumors, the etiology of esophageal cancer is multifactorial. It is thought that during one's life esophageal mucosa is exposed to toxic stimuli triggering a sequence of dysplastic events in predisposed individuals eventually leading to cancer. Various DNA mutations confer a genetic susceptibility and at least seven susceptibility loci have been identified in the esophageal cancer sequence.[14] It is thought that up to 13% of esophageal AC cases have an underlying genetic predisposition.[15] The predisposing mutations seem to be affecting macrophage function and inflammatory pathways.[15]

Smoking and alcohol consumption significantly increase the risk of SCC.[3] Other risk factors are the consumption of nitrites found in processed meats and preserved vegetables, drinking hot beverages, achalasia (stasis), history of previous caustic injury, previous thoracic radiotherapy, history of head and neck neoplasia, malnutrition, micronutrient deficiencies, palmar tylosis, and low economic status.[16-19] The common theme among most of these risk factors is repeated squamous cell injury, which likely leads to a susceptibility of the epithelium to topical exposure by carcinogens. Squamous cell tumors are more likely to be located more proximal in the esophagus where the concentration of injury and exposure is at its peak.

Tobacco smoking has also been associated with esophageal AC, albeit its relative causative impact is less than that for SCC.[6] For esophageal AC, the presence of Barrett's esophagus is arguably the most important risk factor. Barrett's esophagus occurs as a result of chronic exposure to gastric juice seen in reflux disease. Up to 15% of patients undergoing screening endoscopy for GER symptoms and 1% to 2% of asymptomatic American adults have Barrett's.[20] Barrett's esophagus can be defined as the displacement of the squamocolumnar junction proximal to the gastroesophageal junction with a biopsy positive for intestinal metaplasia.[21] In other words, the normal human esophagus is lined with squamous epithelium to the level of the gastroesophageal junction. With years of damaging reflux, the esophageal mucosa undergoes a well-documented metaplastic event whereby the squamous lining changes to a columnar-type epithelium. By itself, this change is not thought to confer an increased risk of cancer, but in some individuals, the change is more sinister, marked by the presence of goblet cells. This so-called specialized epithelium defines intestinal metaplasia, otherwise known as Barrett's esophagus. The reflux-metaplasia-dysplasia sequence is well known and explains why ACs are more likely to occur in the distal esophagus where, theoretically, the exposure to carcinogens in gastric juice is more concentrated. Exactly what is the ultimate carcinogen, or carcinogens, responsible for the progression from benign Barrett's esophagus to cancer is unknown. The incidence of progression from Barrett's esophagus to AC is approximately 0.5% per year.[21] The rates of AC have continued to skyrocket in the Western world despite the introduction of potent antacid medications, implying that acid alone is unlikely the ultimate carcinogen. Given the fact that the rising incidence of Barrett's esophagus and AC actually correlates with the introduction of proton pump inhibitors, some wonder if the altered chemistry in susceptible individuals could be of influence. The varying activity of molecules such as bile acids and digestive enzymes in acidic (natural) and neutral or basic (medicated) environments is an area of active research around the world.[22]

Another theory gaining popularity regarding the development of esophageal AC is the link to obesity. It is well known that obesity along with GER increases the risk of distal esophageal AC.[3,23] The association between increasing body mass index (BMI) and the presence of esophageal AC is stronger than the association of any other cancer with obesity.[24] As an example, a BMI over 30 confers a relative risk of 2.7,[25] whereas a BMI above 40 confers a 4.8 relative risk of developing esophageal AC.[26] The most simplistic explanation for the link between obesity and esophageal AC is that chronic overeating causes prolonged gastric distention and weakening of the antireflux barrier with unfolding of the lower esophageal sphincter and secondary reflux. Furthermore, increased abdominal pressure promotes the flow of gastric juice into the esophagus and leads to hiatal herniation of the gastroesophageal junction. However, data is fast accumulating regarding the risk of all cancers in obese patients due to chronic inflammation and altered metabolism—a mechanism far more complex than merely overeating.[27] Insulin resistance and elevated serum leptin, a regulator of appetite and secreted by adipose tissue, have been recently linked to increased risk of progression from Barrett's to AC.[28] Dietary composition itself seems to play a role as esophageal AC is more common in people with low intake of fruits and vegetables.[6] It is likely that the association between obesity and esophageal AC is a complex interplay between mechanical and biochemical factors.

## PREVENTION

### Modification of Risk Factors

Unfortunately, most esophageal cancers are already in an advanced stage upon diagnosis, which highlights the importance of prevention and early detection. General public education to increase awareness of the associations between changeable personal habits and cancer is vital to the success of widespread risk factor modification. Four primary factors, obesity, GER, smoking, and a diet low in fruit and vegetables, account for 76% to 79% of esophageal AC cases in population studies from the United States and Australia.[29,30] Smoking and alcohol consumption are the main risk factors for esophageal SCC in China and Japan.[31] Therefore, both esophageal AC and SCC appear to be at least partially preventable through risk factor modifications. Increasing dietary fruits and vegetables and decreasing tobacco and alcohol use represent the easiest of these measures to implement. Impacting GER and obesity is a little more complicated. At the very least, improved awareness of the association between these factors and cancer should lead to improved screening for at-risk individuals. Furthermore, weight loss strategies including bariatric surgery may have a role to play in the prevention of esophageal cancer.[6] Theoretically, effective reflux therapy should influence the development of esophageal AC. However, no definitive controlled studies have demonstrated a protective effect of neither antacid medical therapy nor antireflux surgery. Although there is evidence suggesting a favorable effect of antireflux surgery on the prevention of esophageal cancer, the data is reported only in uncontrolled studies.[32] If the theory that the carcinogen responsible for the development of esophageal AC is contained in gastric juice is correct, then a fundoplication should halt the progression to cancer as it prevents the reflux of all materials into the esophagus regardless of pH or composition. Unfortunately, recurrent reflux occurs in approximately 15% of fundoplications. A recent study found that patients who developed AC after a fundoplication were 3 times more likely to have recurrent reflux compared to those who did not.[33] Proton pump inhibition has also been shown to have a preventive effect on the progression of Barrett's esophagus to AC in a few uncontrolled studies.[34,35] To date, the relationship of proton pump inhibition to the progression of esophageal AC remains unclear, but potential protective effects may be related to anti-inflammatory properties.[36] Three recent meta-analyses have described a protective effect of nonsteroidal anti-inflammatory (NSAIDs) medication and aspirin with a 32% to 36% decrease in the risk of esophageal cancer.[6] Along with their positive effect, NSAIDs also have multiple side effects, and it is unclear at this point whether the protective effect outweighs the possible side effects. The answer might come from a European randomized chemoprevention study that is currently under way, assessing the role of aspirin in the prevention of cancer progression in patients with Barrett's esophagitis.[37]

## Early Detection and Screening

Endoscopic screening is the gold standard procedure through which esophageal cancer and dysplastic lesions are diagnosed.[13] However, the ideal goal of screening is to identify high-risk individuals before they have developed invasive cancer. Once diagnosed, the presence of Barrett's esophagus provides an excellent method of risk stratification and identified patients can be enrolled in established surveillance protocols. Currently, the recommended endoscopic surveillance protocol consists of random four-quadrant biopsies every 1 to 2 cm throughout the entire length of metaplasia at 3-year intervals.[38] Unfortunately, there is no consensus regarding which patients should undergo routine screening. The American College of Gastroenterology has stated that the highest yield for primary screening would be in the Caucasian overweight male aged 50 years and older with long-standing GER symptoms.[39] Still, many experts argue that more liberal indications for screening endoscopy should be considered to increase the sensitivity of diagnosing Barrett's esophagus. The debate inevitably involves economic concerns regarding appropriate stewardship of medical resources. Accordingly, decreasing the cost of widespread screening is a topic of great interest. Newer technologies such as the ultrathin endoscope are designed for in-office use without the need for sedation, monitoring, and other expenses that come with routine endoscopy. Although they provide adequate visualization, their capability for biopsy remains limited. Non-endoscopic screening techniques are also under development, such as esophageal sponges or inflatable balloons. Although conceptually attractive and demonstrating good specificity, their very poor sensitivity makes them difficult to use on a large scale in their current state.[13]

## Removal of High-Risk Lesions

Despite the fact that the presence of Barrett's esophagus increases the risk of developing esophageal AC, the risk is still quite low (0.5% per year). However, the 5-year risk of cancer becomes significantly increased with the development of low-grade dysplasia (LGD) (4%) and high-grade dysplasia (HGD) (59%) in the setting of Barrett's esophagus.[20,40] Identification of dysplastic Barrett's provides an opportunity for intervention and prevention of invasive cancer. Historically, esophagectomy was the general recommendation for patients diagnosed with HGD to prevent progression. Although esophageal resection is an effective treatment for HGD, its high morbidity is well documented. Today, a variety of effective endoscopic modalities are currently available as acceptable alternatives to esophagectomy for dysplasia. The first option is to increase endoscopic surveillance. Current recommendations for those who chose this option are 1-year intervals for an LGD and 3-month interval surveillance until definitive therapy in HGD.[38] The second option is eradication of the epithelium at risk. In the absence of visible nodules, the entire Barrett's mucosa can be removed. The most popular and best-studied method is endoscopic radiofrequency ablation (RFA). Complete eradication of dysplasia has been demonstrated in 90.5% of LGD and 81% of HGD after a mean of 3.5 treatments with RFA.[41] In a subsequent report, long-term eradication was demonstrated in 98% of LGD and 93% of HGD at 3-year follow-up.[42] Surveillance for patients following successful ablation therapy should be annually for life.

## TREATMENT

Over the past 20 years there have been major changes in our approach to esophageal cancer. Traditionally, surgical resection, esophagectomy, was the only acceptable treatment for all stages of local–regional disease. Today, many early lesions can be treated with endoscopic therapy, preserving the esophagus. More advanced tumors can be stratified to receive neoadjuvant chemoradiation therapy before esophagectomy to improve the likelihood of complete resection.[3] Some tumors, particularly SCC, can often be treated with definitive chemoradiotherapy.

## STAGING

Locally invasive cancers, those extending beyond the muscularis mucosa, require a complete staging evaluation to identify involved lymph nodes and rule out metastatic disease. Initially staged and treated differently, the AC and SCC are now staged with the same algorithm.[3] In the United States, staging includes computed tomography (CT) of the chest and abdomen, PET-CT, endoscopic ultrasound (EUS), and bronchoscopy (for lesions above the carina).[43] Endoscopic mucosal resection (EMR) can be used to help differentiate the depth of early tumors beyond the sensitivity of EUS.

### Endoscopic Therapy for Early Esophageal Cancer

Multiple endoscopic therapies are now available for patients with cancers limited to the superficial mucosa of the esophagus or intramucosal AC.[6] Endoscopic therapy for early esophageal cancer has increased from 3% in 1998 to 29% in 2009, with cure rates similar to surgical resection.[44] Various ablative techniques such as RFA, argon plasma coagulation, and photodynamic therapy are all part of the armamentarium of the interventional endoscopist.[21] One disadvantage of these ablative techniques is the absence of a pathological specimen. The experienced endoscopist can recognize subtle abnormalities in the mucosa, such as a nodule, that may signify a deeper lesion. When a nodule is found, it can be removed using targeted endoscopic techniques. EMR or endoscopic submucosal dissection (ESD) can be used to completely excise superficial tumors avoiding the high morbidity and mortality associated with an esophagectomy.[45,46] The EMR procedure utilizes an endoscopic cap and snare technique to remove small lesions to the level of the submucosa. This produces a much larger and deeper pathologic specimen that can be evaluated microscopically for depth and margins. The ESD technique is more technically demanding but allows the en bloc removal of more extensive, superficial lesions. If isolated mucosal involvement is confirmed with EMR or ESD, the patient is placed on a more aggressive endoscopic surveillance program for life to monitor for recurrence or new tumors. If the lesion is found to extend into the submucosa, esophagectomy with lymph node removal is recommended due to the high risk of lymph node involvement associated with this depth of invasion. Risk stratification of submucosal lesions based on tumor characteristics is an area of active research that aspires to further spare low-risk patients an unnecessary esophagectomy. The expertise required for successful use of these newer technologies has limited widespread use mostly to specialized centers. From a global perspective, these techniques are most commonly used in Asian countries, where they were developed. However, their use is expanding as supportive data accrues and interventional endoscopists are becoming facile with endoscopic resection.

## SURGICAL RESECTION: ESOPHAGECTOMY

Surgical resection remains the cornerstone of treatment for locally advanced esophageal cancers. Esophagectomy is regarded as a technically demanding operation associated with high morbidity rates. Given the level of complexity, esophagectomy should be performed by experienced teams in dedicated foregut centers. Indeed, it has clearly been shown that short-term mortality is significantly lower in the hands of high-volume esophageal surgeons and in high-volume centers.[47,48] Esophagectomy is most commonly performed using one of two approaches: trans-thoracic or trans-hiatal. The trans-thoracic approach allows for direct visualization of the thoracic esophagus and its surrounding structures. This facilitates resection of tumors in the middle to upper esophagus, including regional thoracic lymph nodes. The distal esophagus and abdominal lymph nodes are then accessed through the abdomen separately to complete the resection. The trans-hiatal operation, or esophagectomy without thoracotomy, uses a relative blind approach to the thoracic esophagus through the esophageal hiatus of the diaphragm while focusing direct visual dissection on the distal esophagus and surrounding lower mediastinal and celiac lymph nodes. Both operations use similar techniques for the restoration of gastrointestinal continuity using a suitable replacement organ, most commonly the stomach (gastric pull-up procedure). Each approach has its advantages and possible complications, and both can be done using minimally invasive techniques. Up to 30% to 50% of patients have significant complications after an esophagectomy, with more than 5%

mortality.[6] No difference in survival has been clearly demonstrated between these two approaches.[49]

## CHEMORADIOTHERAPY

Older studies comparing neoadjuvant chemoradiation followed by surgery with surgery alone obtained nonsignificant results.[17] However, improvements in chemotherapeutic regimens and radiotherapeutic technology have identified protocols that are now a routine adjunct to surgery in most parts of the world. In the MAGIC trial, 503 patients with resectable esophagogastric cancer were randomized to surgery alone or perioperative chemotherapy consisting of three cycles of intravenous epirubicin-cisplatin-fluorouracil given before and after surgery. This study found a significant improvement in disease-free 5-year survival in the chemotherapy group (36%) compared to the surgery-alone group (23%) without an increase in surgical complications.[50] While these results are encouraging, generalizations beyond gastric cancer are criticized as only 26% of the patients in each group had esophageal cancer. Another recent multicenter study, the CROSS Trial, demonstrated better results with neoadjuvant treatment.[51] In this trial, 366 patients were randomized to receive either preoperative carboplatin-paclitaxel-based chemotherapy with 41.4 Gy external beam radiation or surgery alone. The 5-year survival was 47% versus 34% favoring neoadjuvant chemoradiation.[51] These two studies have had a major impact on the treatment of esophageal cancer.

## SURVIVAL

The overall 5-year survival of esophageal AC amounts to 15% in the Western world, including those presenting with metastatic disease or inoperable tumors.[52] With neoadjuvant chemotherapy and a better selection of operative candidates, the 5-year survival of patients after curatively intended therapy is 30% to 55% overall.[6,53] Importantly, survival is significantly improved for early invasive cancer, with 5-year survival rates of 76% for stage I disease.[54] Unfortunately, in the developing countries, the 5-year survival rate is less than 10%.[13]

## PALLIATION

Patients in both developing countries and Western nations often present with advanced esophageal disease. It has been estimated that approximately 79% of patients presenting with esophageal AC are not candidates to curative treatment.[55] For patients with metastatic or recurrent disease, palliative chemotherapy and/or radiotherapy can be used to prolong survival and relieve symptoms such as dysphagia and pain from bone metastasis. Endoscopic therapies such as endoluminal stenting or brachytherapy are also used to relieve the esophageal obstruction.[17] Unfortunately, as effective endoscopic palliation requires expensive technology, most patients in developing countries have no access to this type of treatment. The unavailability of stents leads to the use of morbid palliative operations such as colonic bypasses in cases of metastatic esophageal disease, as described in one retrospective review from Ghana.[10] Though surgical palliative techniques, such as esophageal bypass, are durable and can improve quality of life, the morbidity and mortality rates are too high to justify their regular use worldwide.

## INTERNATIONAL PERSPECTIVE

Esophageal cancer in the developing world not only is a different disease as illustrated by the SCC histology but also more importantly affects different populations with diverse socioeconomic statuses and cultural beliefs. In the absence of adequate screening capabilities, a high percentage of patients in developing countries present with advanced incurable disease. Along with the efforts in public education and improvement in sanitation and diet as well as other primary prevention strategies, the importance of delivering effective palliative treatments has to be highlighted.

One great example of innovation in the field of palliative esophageal cancer in the developing countries is the story of Professor Pankaj Jani. Looking for an effective and affordable idea, Professor Jani from the University of Nairobi, Kenya, has pioneered the use of plastic stents for incurable esophageal cancer. These stents eliminate the constant vomiting secondary to the esophageal obstruction and allow the patients to hydrate themselves. Ultimately, they can return to their homes and die in dignity (A. Park, personal communication, 2013).

As our understanding at a molecular level of this aggressive disease progresses, the use of molecularly targeted chemotherapeutic agents will hopefully improve the prognosis of at least certain groups of patients. Nonetheless, primary prevention through general public education to modify risk factors is essential in reducing exposure to the main risk factors described earlier. Finally, establishing good screening programs in high-risk populations and developing more affordable and less invasive non-endoscopic screening modalities might contribute to better outcomes in the future for this highly lethal disease.

## REFERENCES

1. Kamangar F, Dores GM, Anderson WF. Patterns of cancer incidence, mortality, and prevalence across five continents: defining priorities to reduce cancer

disparities in different geographic regions of the world. *J Clin Oncol* 2006; 24: 2137–50.

2. Siegel R, Naishadham D, Jemal A. Cancer statistics, 2013. *CA Cancer J Clin* 2013; 63: 11–30.

3. Shridhar R, Imani-Shikhabadi R, Davis B, Streeter OA, Thomas CR Jr. Curative treatment of esophageal cancer: an evidenced based review. *J Gastrointest cancer* 2013; 44(4): 375–84.

4. Jemal A, Bray F, Center MM, Ferlay J, Ward E, Forman D. Global cancer statistics. *CA Cancer J Clin* 2011; 61:69–90.

5. Rubenstein JH, Taylor JB. Meta-analysis: the association of oesophageal adenocarcinoma with symptoms of gastro-oesophageal reflux. *Aliment Pharmacol Ther* 2010; 32: 1222–27.

6. Lagergren J, Lagergren P. Recent developments in esophageal adenocarcinoma. *CA Cancer J Clin* 2013; 63: 232–48.

7. Cook MB, Chow WH, Devesa SS. Oesophageal cancer incidence in the United States by race, sex, and histologic type, 1977–2005. *Br J Cancer* 2009; 101:855–59.

8. Trivers KF, Sabatino SA, Stewart SL. Trends in esophageal cancer incidence by histology, United States, 1998–2003. *Int J Cancer* 2008; 123:1422–28.

9. Pickens A, Orringer MB. Geographical distribution and racial disparity in esophageal cancer. *Ann Thorac Surg* 2003; 76: S1367–69.

10. Tettey M, Edwin F, Aniteye E, et al. The changing epidemiology of esophageal cancer in sub-Saharan Africa—the case of Ghana. *Pan Afr Med J* 2012; 13:6.

11. Cherian JV, Sivaraman R, Muthusamy AK, Jayanthi V. Carcinoma of the esophagus in Tamil Nadu (South India): 16-year trends from a tertiary center. *J Gastrointest Liver Dis* 2007; 16: 245–49.

12. Melhado R. The changing face of esophageal cancer. *Cancers* 2010; 2: 1379–404.

13. Lao-Sirieix P, Fitzgerald RC. Screening for oesophageal cancer. *Nat Rev Clin Oncol* 2012; 9: 278–87.

14. Wu C, Hu Z, He Z, et al. Genome-wide association study identifies three new susceptibility loci for esophageal squamous-cell carcinoma in Chinese populations. *Nat Genet* 2011; 43: 679–84.

15. Orloff M, Peterson C, He X, et al. Germline mutations in MSR1, ASCC1, and CTHRC1 in patients with Barrett esophagus and esophageal adenocarcinoma. *JAMA* 2011; 306: 410–19.

16. Palladino-Davis AG, Mendez BM, Fisichella PM, Davis CS. Dietary habits and esophageal cancer. *Dis Esophagus* 2013.

17. Pennathur A, Gibson MK, Jobe BA, Luketich JD. Oesophageal carcinoma. *Lancet* 2013; 381: 400–12.

18. Jakszyn P, Gonzalez CA. Nitrosamine and related food intake and gastric and oesophageal cancer risk: a systematic review of the epidemiological evidence. *World J Gastroenterol* 2006; 12: 4296–303.

19. Andreollo NA, Tercioti V Jr, Lopes LR, Coelho-Neto Jde S. Neoadjuvant chemoradiotherapy and surgery compared with surgery alone in squamous cell carcinoma of the esophagus. *Arq Gastroenterol* 2013; 50: 101–6.

20. Cossentino MJ, Wong RK. Barrett's esophagus and risk of esophageal adenocarcinoma. *Semin Gastrointest Dis* 2003; 14: 128–35.

21. Rajendra S, Sharma P. Management of Barrett's oesophagus and intramucosal oesophageal cancer: a review of recent development. *Therap Adv Gastroenterol* 2012; 5: 285–99.

22. Ghatak S, Reveiller M, Toia L, Ivanov A, Godfrey TE, Peters JH. Bile acid at low pH reduces squamous differentiation and activates EGFR signaling in esophageal squamous cells in 3-D culture. *J Gastrointest Surg* 2013; 17(10): 1723–31.

23. Lagergren J, Bergstrom R, Lindgren A, Nyren O. Symptomatic gastroesophageal reflux as a risk factor for esophageal adenocarcinoma. *N Engl J Med* 1999; 340: 825–31.

24. Renehan AG, Tyson M, Egger M, Heller RF, Zwahlen M. Body-mass index and incidence of cancer: a systematic review and meta-analysis of prospective observational studies. *Lancet* 2008; 371: 569–78.

25. Turati F, Tramacere I, La Vecchia C, Negri E. A meta-analysis of body mass index and esophageal and gastric cardia adenocarcinoma. *Ann Oncol* 2013; 24: 609–17.

26. Hoyo C, Cook MB, Kamangar F, et al. Body mass index in relation to oesophageal and oesophagogastric junction adenocarcinomas: a pooled analysis from the International BEACON Consortium. *Int J Epidemiol* 2012; 41: 1706–18.

27. Calle EE, Kaaks R. Overweight, obesity and cancer: epidemiological evidence and proposed mechanisms. *Nat Rev Cancer* 2004; 4:5 79–91.

28. Duggan C, Onstad L, Hardikar S, Blount PL, Reid BJ, Vaughan TL. Association between markers of obesity and progression from Barrett's esophagus to esophageal adenocarcinoma. *Clin Gastroenterol Hepatol* 2013; 11: 934–43.

29. Engel LS, Chow WH, Vaughan TL, et al. Population attributable risks of esophageal and gastric cancers. *J Natl Cancer Inst* 2003; 95: 1404–13.

30. Olsen CM, Pandeya N, Green AC, Webb PM, Whiteman DC, Australian Cancer Study. Population attributable fractions of adenocarcinoma of the esophagus and gastroesophageal junction. *Am J Epidemiol* 2011; 174: 582–90.

31. Lin Y, Totsuka Y, He Y, et al. Epidemiology of esophageal cancer in Japan and China. *J Epidemiol*/Japan Epidemiological Association 2013; 23: 233–42.

32. Chang EY, Morris CD, Seltman AK, et al. The effect of antireflux surgery on esophageal carcinogenesis in patients with barrett esophagus: a systematic review. *Ann Surg* 2007; 246: 11–21.

33. Lofdahl HE, Lu Y, Lagergren P, Lagergren J. Risk factors for esophageal adenocarcinoma after antireflux surgery. *Ann Surg* 2013; 257: 579–82.

34. Kastelein F, Spaander MC, Steyerberg EW, et al. Proton pump inhibitors reduce the risk of neoplastic progression in patients with Barrett's esophagus. *Clin Gastroenterol Hepatol* 2013; 11: 382–88.

35. El-Serag HB, Aguirre TV, Davis S, Kuebeler M, Bhattacharyya A, Sampliner RE. Proton pump inhibitors are associated with reduced incidence of dysplasia in Barrett's esophagus. *Am J Gastroenterol* 2004; 99: 1877–83.

36. Miyashita T, Shah FA, Harmon JW, et al. Do proton pump inhibitors protect against cancer progression in GERD? *Surg Today* 2013; 43: 831–37.

37. Das D, Chilton AP, Jankowski JA. Chemoprevention of oesophageal cancer and the AspECT trial. *Recent Results Cancer Res* 2009; 181: 161–69.

38. Wang KK, Sampliner RE, Practice Parameters Committee of the American College of Gastroenterology. Updated guidelines 2008 for the diagnosis,

surveillance and therapy of Barrett's esophagus. *Am J Gastroenterol* 2008; 103: 788–97.

39. Katz PO, Gerson LB, Vela MF. Guidelines for the diagnosis and management of gastroesophageal reflux disease. *Am J Gastroenterol* 2013; 108: 308–28; quiz 29.

40. Reid BJ, Levine DS, Longton G, Blount PL, Rabinovitch PS. Predictors of progression to cancer in Barrett's esophagus: baseline histology and flow cytometry identify low- and high-risk patient subsets. *Am J Gastroenterol* 2000; 95: 1669–76.

41. Shaheen NJ, Sharma P, Overholt BF, et al. Radiofrequency ablation in Barrett's esophagus with dysplasia. *N Engl J Med* 2009; 360: 2277–88.

42. Shaheen NJ, Overholt BF, Sampliner RE, et al. Durability of radiofrequency ablation in Barrett's esophagus with dysplasia. *Gastroenterology* 2011; 141: 460–68.

43. Esophageal and Esophagogastric Junction Cancers. Version 2.2013.

44. Ngamruengphong S, Wolfsen HC, Wallace MB. Survival of patients with superficial esophageal adenocarcinoma after endoscopic treatment vs surgery. *Clin Gastroenterol Hepatol* 2013; 11(11):1424–29.

45. Kato H, Nakajima M. Treatments for esophageal cancer: a review. *Gen Thorac Cardiovasc Surg* 2013; 61: 330–35.

46. Chennat J, Waxman I. Endoscopic treatment of Barrett's esophagus: from metaplasia to intramucosal carcinoma. *World J Gastroenterol* 2010; 16: 3780–85.

47. Birkmeyer JD, Stukel TA, Siewers AE, Goodney PP, Wennberg DE, Lucas FL. Surgeon volume and operative mortality in the United States. *N Engl J Med* 2003; 349: 2117–27.

48. Ghaferi AA, Birkmeyer JD, Dimick JB. Variation in hospital mortality associated with inpatient surgery. *N Engl J Med* 2009; 361: 1368–75.

49. Omloo JM, Lagarde SM, Hulscher JB, et al. Extended transthoracic resection compared with limited transhiatal resection for adenocarcinoma of the mid/distal esophagus: five-year survival of a randomized clinical trial. *Ann Surg* 2007; 246: 992–1000; discussion 1.

50. Cunningham D, Allum WH, Stenning SP, et al. Perioperative chemotherapy versus surgery alone for resectable gastroesophageal cancer. *N Engl J Med* 2006; 355: 11–20.

51. van Hagen P, Hulshof MC, van Lanschot JJ, et al. Preoperative chemoradiotherapy for esophageal or junctional cancer. *N Engl J Med* 2012; 366: 2074–84.

52. Ferlay J, Shin HR, Bray F, Forman D, Mathers C, Parkin DM. Estimates of worldwide burden of cancer in 2008: GLOBOCAN 2008. *Int J Cancer* 2010; 127: 2893–917.

53. Hong JC MJ, Wang SJ, Koong AC, Chang DT. Chemoradiotherapy before and after surgery for locally advanced esophageal cancer: a SEER-Medicare analysis. *Ann Surg Oncol* 2013; 20(12): 3999–4007.

54. Peyre CG, Hagen JA, DeMeester SR, et al. The number of lymph nodes removed predicts survival in esophageal cancer: an international study on the impact of extent of surgical resection. *Ann Surg* 2008; 248: 549–56.

55. Coupland VH, Lagergren J, Luchtenborg M, et al. Hospital volume, proportion resected and mortality from oesophageal and gastric cancer: a population-based study in England, 2004–2008. *Gut* 2013; 62: 961–66.

# 7

# Gastric Cancer

## Han-Kwang Yang, *Erin Gilbert, and John G. Hunter*

## INCIDENCE AND MORTALITY

The world incidence of gastric adenocarcinoma is currently estimated at al-most 1,000,000 people per year with a mortality of 700,000 deaths per year. It is the fourth most common cancer in the world, and it is the second leading cause of cancer deaths in both men and women. It had been documented as the leading cause of cancer deaths from the very first formal cancer stud-ies conducted in Verona, Italy (1760 to 1839), by Rigoni Stern up until the 1980s when lung cancer became the number one cause. Five-year prevalence data available in the GLOBOCAN database of the World Health Organiza-tion International Agency for Research on Cancer is estimated at 1.6 mil-lion cases[1] and is higher in less developed as compared to more developed countries.[2]

Both incidence and age-related mortality vary widely depending on geo-graphical location. The highest incidence rates can be found in East Asia and Eastern Europe as well as in South America, with much lower rates in North America, Australia, and parts of Africa (Figure 7.1).[1] Intermediate risk countries include Malaysia, Singapore, and Taiwan. Age-adjusted mor-tality is highest in South Korea at 30.7 per 100,000 person-years in males and 11.3 per 100,000 person-years in females and lowest in the United States at 3.2 per 100,000 person-years in males and 1.6 per 100,000 person-years in females (Figures 7.2A and B).[3] The difference between Eastern and Western mortality rates is almost 10-fold, and it highlights the worldwide variation of many aspects of this disease. It suggests that cultural differences in diet, ethnicity, and environment all play a vital role in the incidence of this disease.

According to the National Cancer Institute, the estimated number of new cases of gastric cancer in 2013 in the United States is 21,600, with 10,990

## Stomach: Both Sexes, All Ages

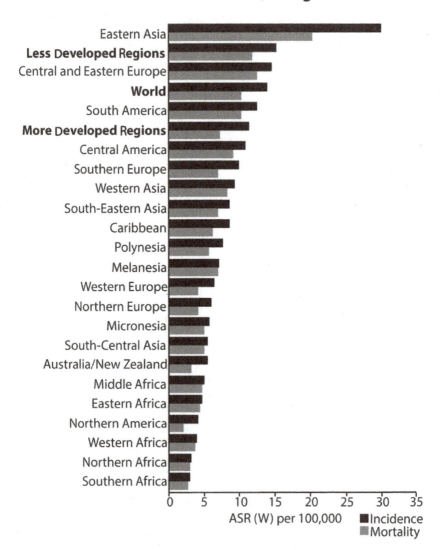

**FIGURE 7.1** Estimated age-adjusted incidence and mortality rates per 100,000 (reference 1).

associated deaths.[4] Nearly 80% of all gastric cancers occur in Asia and only 2.2% of all cases worldwide are seen in North America. A more specific example of how dramatic this geographical variation is the difference in incidence of gastric cancer in Japan as compared to the United States. In Japan it is the number one most common cancer diagnosed in men, whereas in the

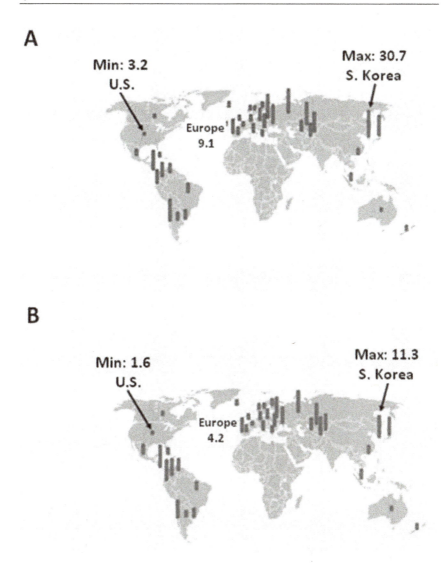

**FIGURE 7.2A** Age-adjusted incidence and mortality per 100,000 person-years, male for Japan.

**FIGURE 7.2B** Age-adjusted incidence and mortality per 100,000 person-years, male for the United States.

United States it is ranked only 12th (Figure 7.3).[1] Moreover, the "fatality-to-case ratio" of gastric cancer is also significantly different among countries. For example, the estimated number of new cases and deaths were 21,320 and 10,540 in the United States in 2012; however, in Korea the new cases and deaths were 29,727 and 10,135 in 2009.[5] The fatality-to-case ratio in

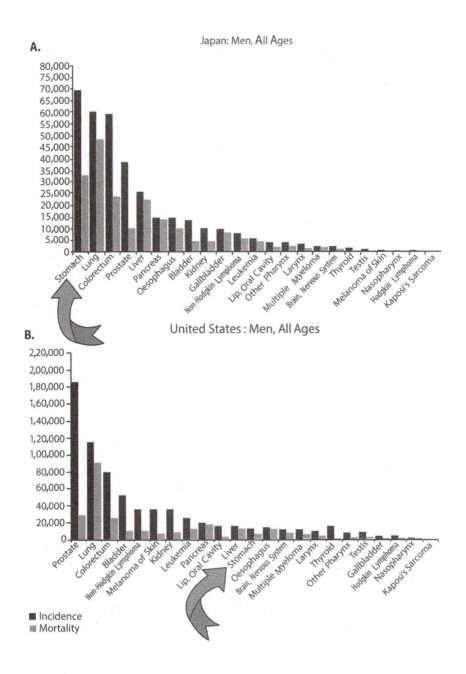

**FIGURE 7.3** Incidence and mortality in men of cancer in Japan (A) and the United States (B) (Reference 1).

the United States was 49.4%, but in Korea, it was only 34.1%. Globally, a fatality-to-case ratio of gastric cancer is estimated at 70%. This is significantly higher than other common malignancies such as prostate and breast cancers that have a ratio of 30% and 33%.[6] This regional disparity of fatality-to-case ratios can be explained by two factors: early detection and extent of lymph node dissection in surgery, both of which are quite different in Western and Eastern countries.

## Temporal Trends in Incidence and Mortality

Gastric cancer was the leading cause of cancer deaths worldwide until the 1980s when lung cancer exceeded it. Since the mid-1960s the incidence of gastric cancer has markedly declined across the globe.[7–9] Reasons for this decline are not completely understood, but almost certainly include factors such as a more varied diet with better food conservation, including refrigeration, a decreasing prevalence of *Helicobacter pylori* (*H. pylori*) infection, a decrease in smoking prevalence, and the implementation of screening measures in high-risk areas.[10] This decline in incidence is less pronounced in developing countries for reasons that are not altogether known.[11] Cancers of the gastric body and antrum are decreasing in incidence, whereas the incidence of tumors of the cardia and upper third of the stomach have been stable or even increasing over time.[12] Notable increases in purely non-cardia gastric cancers have been seen in the United States in Caucasians aged 25 to 39 years and also in the very young and very old Chinese populations. The absolute number of new cases continues to rise, however, mainly as a function of the world's enlarging aging population. In South Korea, the absolute number of gastric cancer cases increased from 26,000 in 2005 to 30,000 in 2010 and, at the same time, peak age shifted from the fifties to the sixties, suggesting that this increase in the absolute number of gastric cancer patients is indeed due to an aging population. On the other hand, the proportion of gastric cardia cancer patients has not increased in Korea in the last 20 years.

## The Migration Effect

First-generation international migrants from high-incidence to lower-incidence countries sustain the risk rate of their native country.[13] In a study of Japanese-born residents of Sao Paulo, Brazil, gastric cancer had the highest incidence of all cancers (69.3% male and 32.0% female); however, ethnic Japanese living several generations in Brazil have a significantly lower incidence of gastric cancer.[14] More recent studies have confirmed that Japanese who migrate to the United States have a decrease in incidence and mortality

from gastric cancer. The incidence declines further in subsequent generations.[15] This suggests the etiology may rest more heavily on environmental
rather than ethnic or genetic factors.

## ETIOLOGY

There are two distinct types of gastric adenocarcinoma, intestinal-type
(well-differentiated) and diffuse-type (undifferentiated) carcinoma. These
disease entities have a very different pathogenesis, epidemiology, and genetic
profile. The main carcinogenic-inciting event in the formation of diffuse-type
gastric adenocarcinoma is loss of expression of E-cadherin (CDH1), a surface
protein responsible for maintaining the structural organization of the epithelial tissues.

The pathophysiological progression of normal gastric mucosa to
intestinal-type cancer is not as systematic, although it is almost always initiated by infection with H. pylori bacteria coupled with increased salt intake.[16] The progression of intestinal-type gastric cancer to frank malignancy
begins with chronic superficial gastritis as caused by one or more of the commonly known risk factors for gastric cancer. With time, damage to the mucosal layer is manifest as atrophic gastritis followed by intestinal metaplasia.
The transformation from metaplasia to low-grade and high-grade dysplasia
is the last step before frank malignancy is apparent (Figure 7.4). Because the
intestinal-type gastric cancer is far and away the most prevalent accounting
for >90% of all cases, it will be the focus of our chapter.

The risk of gastric cancer that is attributable to H. pylori infection is at
least 6- to 20-fold higher than that of unaffected individuals.[17] The causality
between H. pylori infection and gastric cancer is so strong that the World
Health Organization's International Agency for Research on Cancer classified it as a definite carcinogen in 1994. It is the risk factor for gastric cancer
best linked to scientific evidence of biological plausibility and increasing risk
of non-cardia gastric cancer. In early studies, this relative risk was estimated
at a 3-fold increase, but better controlled studies with strong statistical meth-
odologies estimate the relative risk of H. pylori infection to be 20-fold or even
greater than noninfected controls.

Other well-known risk factors that increase the probability of developing
gastric cancer include smoking,[18] a high salt diet,[19] and a body mass index

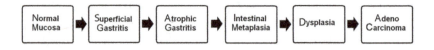

**FIGURE 7.4** Pathophysiology of the development of intestinal-type gastric cancer.

> 25.[20] Throughout the world there is a strong and consistent correlation between amount of salt consumption and gastric cancer incidence. This association is biologically sound as salt can lead to mucosal inflammation and injury. A number of studies have addressed this association and found a 2-fold increase in cancer risk with high salt diets.[19,21] In addition, a diet high in allium vegetables reduces the risk of intestinal-type gastric cancer. Allium vegetables include garlic, onion, leeks, chives, and scallions. A recent meta-analysis combined 21 studies which analyzed the effect of high versus low allium vegetable consumption. The authors found that by eating the equivalent of one garlic bulb daily the risk of developing gastric cancer was reduced by 50%.

## PREVENTION AND SCREENING

H. pylori infection is the strongest and most consistent risk factor for gastric cancer. There is strong evidence that its eradication may reduce the risk of gastric cancer development. Therefore, prevention of this infection and its early eradication once infection is established are two of the most promising strategies for decreasing the incidence of gastric cancer. Prevention and eradication of H. pylori has been confirmed to reduce the incidence of gastric cancer in a number of randomized controlled trials and cohort studies.[22–24] It is thought that H. pylori infection begins in infancy or early childhood, and after a long latency period, cancers are generally diagnosed four or five decades later. Early detection with a urea breath test or blood or stool antibody test is often employed as a way to focus eradication efforts. Once H. pylori has been eradicated, there is a significant durable regression of intestinal metaplasia and gastric atrophy.[25] The prevalence of H. pylori in Western countries ranges from approximately 10% to 60%,[26] whereas in developing countries, it may be as high as 90%.[27] Eradication studies performed in high-risk geographical areas such as Taiwan have demonstrated a significant reduction in H. pylori infection (78.7% reduction, 95% CI 76.8%-80.7%) corresponding to a significant decrease in the incidence of atrophic gastritis (77.2% reduction, 95% CI 72.3%-81.2%) at a cost of a 6% increase in esophagitis following treatment.[28] The hypothesis of increasing esophagitis following H. pylori eradication is that restoration of normal gastric acid secretion with resolving gastritis will lead to more erosive esophagitis in those with a defective lower esophageal sphincter. A commonly employed adjunct to primary prevention of gastric cancer is the prophylactic treatment of H. pylori infection in first-degree relatives of patients with gastric cancer as they are at twice the risk of having not only H. pylori but also atrophic gastritis and intestinal metaplasia.

One obstacle of H. pylori eradication is that its treatment requires a multidrug regimen, and there is known drug resistance, especially with the more commonly used antibiotics such as amoxicillin, erythromycin, and clarithro-mycin.[29] It is believed that prevention of H. pylori infection together with a childhood vaccine may reduce the incidence of gastric cancer by 40%. Therefore, another promising intervention for the prevention of gastric cancer that avoids these difficulties is the prevention rather than eradication of H. pylori infection via the use of a vaccine. This would also be a cost-saving intervention, as the cost of testing all patients with dyspepsia and treating all of those patients with infection is expensive and inherently misses identifying many infected individuals who are not symptomatic. Vaccination against H. pylori is difficult as the H. pylori bacterium colonizes the gastric mucosa with-out crossing it where it would be susceptible to the body's immune system.[30] Vaccines with three antigens, vacuolating cytotoxin A, cytotoxin-associated antigen, and neutrophil-activating protein, alone or in combination, have been shown to be safe and effective in animals.[31,32] Phase I trials in humans have been completed. These studies show the vaccines are well tolerated and have a high percentage of seroconversion, reflecting a strong immunogenic T-cell-mediated response.[33,34]

Secondary prevention in the form of screening is ubiquitous in East Asia and virtually absent in Western countries. The objective of any screening program is to detect disease in asymptomatic populations at an early and potentially curable stage. This approach is cost effective for gastric cancer, but only in high-incidence regions such as Japan, China, and South Korea. In North America and Western Europe, no formal screening programs are in place for the general population because the low incidence precludes the cost benefit of such an approach.[13] In fact, endoscopic screening studies per-formed in 50-year-old asymptomatic patients in the United States estimate that the incidence of gastric cancer would have to increase more than 300% to justify their use.[35] The American Society for Gastrointestinal Endoscopy points out in its guidelines that endoscopic surveillance for gastric intestinal metaplasia and other premalignant conditions has not been extensively stud-ied in the United States and therefore cannot be uniformly recommended. Therefore, it only recommends endoscopic screening and surveillance of as-ymptomatic patients for high-risk individuals with familial adenopolyposis syndrome, hereditary non-polyposis colon cancer, Peutz–Jeghers syndrome, and Ménétrier's disease.[36] Considering the ethnic disparity in gastric cancer incidence even in the United States, a person of a high-incidence ethnic group such as Asian (a Korean immigrant has a 5 times higher incidence than a native Caucasian) with a risk factor like H. pylori infection may be con-sidered a candidate for screening in the United States.[37] Prospective studies on screening in high-incidence geographical locations, however, have essen-tially proven a beneficial effect on both the development of pre-neoplastic conditions, such as atrophic gastritis, and the prevention of gastric cancer itself as well as in a reduction in mortality from gastric cancer.[38,39]

Mass screening appears to be most effective in decreasing gastric cancer incidence in patients without any evidence of pre-neoplastic lesions or with only mild atrophic gastritis[40] and in those with the highest pretest probability.[41] Currently, population-based screening at the national level is performed only in East Asia. In China and Japan the screening approach is a combination of barium radiography and serum pepsinogen testing, which is 88% sensitive at cancer detection. In South Korea, the population-based endoscopic or upper gastrointestinal series screening of people over 40 years every year (National Cancer Screening Program for Medical Aid Program Recipients) has been in place since 1999 and has a rate of pre-neoplastic or cancer detection of 75%. Considering other screening methods such as opportunistic screening and the organized screening program conducted by the National Institutes of Health, the overall screening rate for gastric cancer in Korea is reported as 53.5%.[42]

Early detection ensures that a higher proportion of gastric cancer can be treated in its earlier stage, and consequently, treatment outcomes improve. The Korean Gastric Cancer Association has reported a 5-year-interval nationwide survey regularly, which shows that the proportion of early (T1) gastric cancer that is detected has rapidly increased from 28.6% in 1995 to 32.8% in 1999, 47.4% in 2004, and finally reached 57.7% in 2009.[43] In addition, the 5-year survival rate of gastric cancer in Korea, reported by Korean Central Cancer Registry, has increased from 42.8% in 1993–1995 to 65.3% in 2005–2009. However, in Western countries where the incidence of gastric cancer is low and the cost of endoscopy is higher, a different approach to reduce gastric cancer mortality through screening is required. Due to the rarity of cancer-specific antigens and their low expression, only several multi-panel approaches have been reported in serum or stool in gastric or other gastrointestinal cancer until now.[44] Recent achievements in genomics, proteomics, and sequencing technology may lead us into the new era of gastric cancer screening in the near future.

## TREATMENT

### Surgery

Once a diagnosis of gastric cancer has been made, the next step is to complete clinical staging. According to the most recent National Comprehensive Center Network (NCCN) guidelines,[45] staging should consist of a computed tomography (CT) scan of the chest, abdomen, and pelvis, with consideration for an endoscopic ultrasound (EUS) assessment. It also includes a recommendation for diagnostic laparoscopy for tumor stage III or clinical evidence of lymph node involvement, as positive peritoneal washings would indicate stage IV disease precluding a possible curative surgical resection. Other criteria of unresectablilty include level 4 lymph node involvement, invasion or encasement of major vessels, or distant metastasis. Barring evidence of unresectable disease surgery is warranted to achieve a possible curative resection.

Although the NCCN does not mandate EUS evaluation in the United States, worldwide it has become indispensable in the preoperative tumor staging of gastric cancer. Compared to CT, EUS is superior in accurately determining tumor stage with a sensitivity of approximately 83% (65% to 90%) and a tendency toward over-staging rather than under-staging. It is also sensitive at determining nodal involvement with sensitivities of 50% to 90%. It loses sensitivity when trying to identify T1m (mucosa) disease (77% sensitivity) and Tism (submucosa) disease (46% sensitivity) because the anatomical distinction between these two stages is difficult to discern with EUS.

Once clinical staging is complete, the method of resection varies with location, depth, and size of tumor. For in situ tumors (Tis or T1a) that have no sign of submucosal extension, endoscopic mucosal resection (EMR) or endoscopic submucosal resection (ESD) may be employed. The rationale behind the use of EMR for early tumors arises from the knowledge that small well-differentiated intramucosal tumors have a small risk of lymph node involvement, a risk that is lower than the risk of mortality from gastric surgery. The tumor should also possess pathologic grade 1 or 2 and be intramucosal in location. Any elevated lesion should be ≤2 cm and a depressed lesion can be no more than 1 cm in diameter. Also, any sign of ulceration precludes the use of EMR as an adequate treatment for an intramucosal lesion. Indications for ESD include any intramucosal lesions without ulceration, intramucosal ulcerated lesions that are ≤3 cm in diameter and well-differentiated tumors ≤3 cm without submucosal infiltration and without lymphatic or vascular invasion. A recent study comparing EMR and ESD found that ESD outperforms EMR with lesions >1 cm because it allows for the thorough removal of these larger lesions with complete excision rates of >95% for lesions up to 2 cm and 79% to 97% for lesions >2 cm.[46] After ESD, if tumor cells invade the submucosa, a radical gastrectomy should be performed due to possibility of regional lymph node metastasis.

For any ulcerated lesion >3 cm or T1b staged or higher, an adequate resection with at least 5-cm margins should be performed. The standard operation is a radical subtotal gastrectomy. In general, tumors confined to the proximal one-third of the stomach are treated with total gastrectomy to ensure adequate margins and a good functional result. Proximal gastrectomy for cardia cancers should rarely be performed, as a large South Korean study demonstrated a significant increase in the complication rate when proximal gastrectomy was performed, as compared to total gastrectomy without any improvement in survival.[47] For cancers in the body and antrum of the stomach, total gastrectomy adds no additional survival benefit to partial gastrectomy and has higher postoperative morbidity and mortality.[48,49] Patients undergoing sub-total gastrectomies have shorter hospital stays and a better long-term nutritional status. T4 lesions require en bloc resection with involved structures.

In the past, lymph nodes were classified according to their distance from the primary tumor; however, the topographic definition of D1 D2 lymph nodes by the Japanese Gastric Cancer Association (JGCA) is widely accepted and used for the description of lymph node dissection. Recently, the JGCA has simplified the definition of D1 and D2 depending on distal, subtotal gastrectomy, and total gastrectomy.

The extended D2 lymphadenectomy, initially championed by Japanese surgeons, has been shown to confer survival benefits in many Asian studies. When examined in Western countries, however, patients undergoing D2 dissections had equivalent survival as those having D1 dissections but an increased morbidity. The discrepancies in findings between East and West studies evaluating the benefits of extended lymphadenectomies have been theorized to stem from a difference in operative experience as the surgeons lacked previous training in extended (D2) lymphadenectomy and the rate of pancreatectomy/splenectomy was much higher, which may explain the survival differences. Even in a large Dutch randomized controlled trial proctored by Japanese surgeons here was an increase in complications (D1 25%, D2 43%) and mortality (D1 4%, D2 10%) without any improvement in 5-year survival (D1 45%, D2 47%).[50] One consideration is that even in this Dutch trial, the number of enrolled cases for each investigator was very low. In long-term follow-up, however, there was a significant improvement in survival for patients who underwent D2 in terms of death due to gastric cancer.

There is strong evidence even in the United States that the higher the number of lymph nodes removed, the better the survival. Using Surveillance, Epidemiology, and End Results (SEER) data from 1973 to 1999, the relationship between number of lymph nodes examined and overall survival was analyzed and for the subgroups of patients with T1-3 and N1 disease, the more lymph nodes that were resected, the better the postgastrectomy survival. Interestingly, there was no cutoff point for the number of nodes examined, but the trend toward superior outcome could be followed to numbers greater than 40 without signs of plateauing.[51] The number of nodes harvested is directly related to the type of nodal dissection employed. In only 40% of D1 dissections are 15 or more lymph nodes resected. This is in comparison to D2 dissections where 15 or more lymph nodes are resected in approximately 95% of cases.[52]

Regardless of the results of large Western European and North American trials where there is no overall survival benefit to a D2 dissection,[53] the current standard of care in submucosal and more advanced gastric cancers is that at least 15 lymph nodes are necessary to accurately stage the tumor. There is a tendency toward noncompliance in the United States, with studies conducted within the past 10 to 15 years showing a minority of surgeons follow guidelines for precise lymph node staging (10% to 44%) and as few as 20% have ≥15 lymph nodes analyzed.[54] For proper treatment and prognostication of gastric cancer, an extended lymph node dissection (D1, D2) is crucial, but ex vivo dissection of lymph node stations is also important for proper pathologic evaluation. In a recent publication from a high-volume center in the United States adopting ex vivo dissection of the stomach specimen, lymph node harvest was increased significantly.[55]

For a long time, D2 lymphadenectomy has been regarded as a procedure of high complication rate for gastric cancer treatment in Western countries; therefore, D1 lymphadenectomy plus adjuvant chemoradiotherapy was considered the treatment of choice for advanced gastric cancer. However, studies show that a D2 lymphadenectomy can be performed safely not only in Asia but also in United States and Europe, with acceptable morbidity and mortality rates of 15% to 20% and less than 3%.[56]

Laparoscopic surgery is now increasingly applied in many oncologic surgeries, including gastric cancer surgery. Several randomized controlled trials have been conducted, comparing laparoscopic with open gastric cancer surgery in Korea, Japan, and China including KLASS-01, 02, 03 trials and the JCOG-0912 trial. In addition to the known benefits of laparoscopic surgery such as less postoperative pain, improved cosmesis, and improved quality of life, a lower postoperative complication rate was also reported following laparoscopic surgery, compared to open surgery.[57] Laparoscopic surgery may have an additional benefit of fine and meticulous lymph node dissection from the magnified, clear image of the laparoscope. One limitation of current laparoscopic surgery technology is the limited degree of freedom in motion. Robotic instrumentation can be an alternative approach to overcome this limitation. On the other hand, the cost of robotic instruments is very expensive; therefore, the benefit of robotic surgery should be proven before its clinical application.

## Adjuvant and Neoadjuvant Therapy

The poor survival rates of patients with stage II and greater gastric cancers stem from the fact that the majority of patients develop a locoregional recurrence. Efforts to improve survival in these patients have focused on finding effective perioperative systemic therapies to enhance the benefits of surgery or even to achieve down-staging, providing some patients an opportunity to undergo a surgical procedure that was not initially possible. Early efforts at survival improvement with systemic therapies were initially mixed, but have become more positive with time. Three Western studies have molded current Western clinical practice: the U.S. Intergroup 0116 and CALGB 80101 trials and the British MAGIC (Medical Research Council) trial. INT0116 was a large U.S. trial comparing adjuvant chemoradiotherapy (5-FU and leucovorin) following surgery to surgery alone for the treatment of resectable gastric cancer. Overall survival was significantly improved with combined modality therapy (50% vs. 41%).[58] With longer follow-up, these benefits were maintained with 5-year overall survival rates of 43% versus 28% (HR 1.32, CI 1.10, 1.60). The CALGB 80101 trial compared the regimen used in INT0116 with postoperative epirubicin cisplatin and 5-fluorouracil (ECF). Patients receiving ECF had lower rates of drug-related toxicities and similar overall survival (52% vs. 50% for ECF and 5-FU/leucovorin, respectively), although the study was not powered for non-inferiority comparison of the two regimens.

The MAGIC trial was the largest Western randomized trial of neoadjuvant treatment of gastric cancer, with over 500 patients, almost 75% of whom had gastric rather than distal esophageal or esophagogastric junction cancer. The trial compared perioperative epirubicin, cisplatin and 5-fluorouracil (ECF) with surgery alone. Members of the group who received ECF were more likely to have a curative resection and were more likely to have T1 or T2 lesions. Although the majority of patients receiving perioperative ECF were unable to complete the full chemotherapeutic course, there was still a significant improvement in overall survival in this group. In other words, there was an absolute 5-year survival benefit of 13% and in a 10% higher resectability rate with perioperative ECF.[59] Building on the positive results of the MAGIC trial, an ongoing Dutch trial "CRITICS" trial will demonstrate whether the addition of radiotherapy to perioperative chemotherapy (epirubicin, cisplatin, and capecitabine) will further improve clinical outcomes.[60]

The Japanese S-1 trial (ACTS-GC trial) investigated the efficacy of S-1, an oral fluoropyrimidine, in over 1,000 patients with stage II or III gastric cancer following curative resection with D2 dissection. The patients were randomly assigned to 1 year of S1 postoperatively or no adjuvant therapy. Five-year overall survival was improved in both groups over results from Western trials but with superior survival in the experimental group (72% vs. 61%).[61] This has led to the implementation of a 1-year course of S1 following gastric resection as the standard approach for all East Asian patients as well as patients in Europe. These two Asian trials in effect ended the controversy surrounding the role of adjuvant chemotherapy after curative dissection in Japan and Korea.

In Japan and Korea, radiation therapy is not considered after curative resection of advanced gastric cancer. The viewpoint is that in Western countries, the reason for improvement of locoregional recurrence after chemoradiotherapy in Western trials is due to inadequate surgical resection (only 10% was D2 surgery in INT0116). The improved locoregional recurrence rate in this Western study was higher than the locoregional recurrence rate after surgery alone in Japan or Korea. This emphasizes that inadequate lymph node dissection can be benefited by radiotherapy but radiotherapy cannot replace an adequate lymph node dissection.

Another large Asian trial conducted in Taiwan, South Korea, and China called the CLASSIC trial reinforced the benefit of adjuvant chemotherapy. The regimen used (capecitabine and oxaliplatin) was difficult to tolerate and led to dose modifications in 90%, but despite the fact that only 56% were able to complete the full regimen, 3-year survival was improved with adjuvant therapy (74% vs. 59%).[62] Many other clinical trials compare adjuvant systemic therapies with surgery alone that have produced negative results, showing no survival advantage for those receiving adjuvant chemotherapy. Given this variability, several meta-analyses have been completed, all of which support the use of adjuvant chemotherapy even when results from Asian countries are excluded. The survival benefit conferred by the addition of adjuvant chemotherapy is estimated at as much as 18% and has cemented the use of multimodal therapy over surgery alone as the standard of care both in the East and in the West.[63]

## SURVIVAL

Around the world, death from gastric cancer is decreasing. The annual percentage change in mortality over the past 10 years ranges from –4.3% in Korea, –4% in Europe, –3.6% in the United States, and –3.5% in Japan to –1.6% in Latin America.[11] This geographical disparity is reflected in survival rates as well. Five-year survival rates are only about 25%[64,65] compared to rates of over 60% in Japan and other East Asian countries.[66] The improved survival in Japan and South Korea is attributable at least in part to the higher proportion of early-stage disease at the time of diagnosis largely as a result of aggressive screening programs. From 1993 to 2005, over 50% of gastric cancers diagnosed in Japan were localized as compared to only 27% in the United States during the same time frame according to SEER data (Figure 7.5).[67]

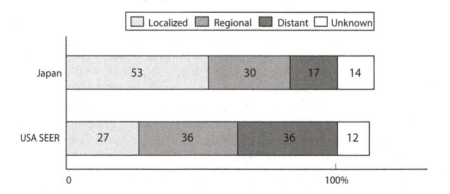

**FIGURE 7.5** Stage distribution of gastric cancer in Japan and the United States from 1995 to 2000. (Reference 9. Used by permission of BMJ Publishing Group Ltd.)

When gastric cancer is diagnosed early, 5-year survival of 90% and more is achieved in Eastern countries compared to lower rates of just over 60% in the United States [64,68,69] A similar low rate of localized cancer at diagnosis is suspected in other Western countries. When survival is examined over time, it is seen to improve stage by stage at a similar level to the percentage that localized disease has increased, whereas there has been no survival improvement over time for stage IV disease, indicating that proportion of cases detected at earlier stages may have strongly contributed to improvements in overall survival.

## A PATIENT'S STORY

Patient D is a 26-year-old woman who was referred to a gastroenterologist by her primary-care physician for a sensation of occasional dysphagia at the suprasternal notch coupled with a family history positive for gastric cancer. Her father died at age 40 after he presented with ascites and endoscopy revealed a 10-cm soft villous tumor with polypoid lesions throughout the stomach sparing the distal half of the stomach. Although, biopsies of the polyps and cytology of the ascitic fluid failed to reveal a definitive pathology, the impression was that this was a gastric cancer. He died shortly after presentation and no autopsy was performed to confirm his doctors' suspicions. Her paternal aunt died of adenocarcinoma of unknown primary, which was also felt to be gastric in origin. A complete four-generation pedigree was completed during a consultation with a geneticist (Figure 7.6). Based on this unique family history, D and her siblings underwent screening endoscopy. One of her brothers had hyperplastic polyps in the fundus of his stomach on endoscopy without evidence of dysplasia. Her other two brothers had no polyps on endoscopy. In contrast, D was found to have hundreds of 1- to 10-mm polyps carpeting the proximal portion of her stomach, three of which were adenomatous on biopsy. In addition, her duodenum and ampulla were normal. Despite the fact that no juvenile polyps were identified on D's screening endoscopy, only three polyps were biopsied and therefore one could not conclude definitively that it was a representative biopsy. D subsequently underwent colonoscopy to further rule out familial adenomatous polyposis (FAP) or juvenile polyposis syndrome. No polyps or lesions were identified on colonoscopy. D has no family history of Crohn's disease, colon cancer, or liver disease. She herself has no past medical or surgical history. She has never taken a proton pump inhibitor or any other acid suppression medication, and her *H. pylori* testing was negative.

An increased incidence of familial gastric cancers has been recognized as a component of several inherited cancer syndromes, including FAP, hereditary diffuse gastric cancer (HDGC), Lynch syndrome, Li–Fraumeni syndrome

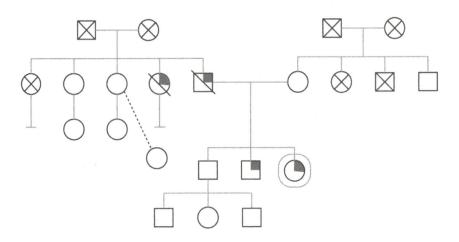

**FIGURE 7.6** Patient D's family pedigree.

Peutz–Jeghers syndrome, juvenile polyposis syndrome, and gastric adenocarcinoma and proximal polyposis of the stomach (GAPPS). Although most gastric cancers are adenocarcinomas, it is still important to distinguish between HDGC caused by mutations in CDH1 and other familial gastric cancers. The finding of multiple polyps on M's endoscopy argued against HDGC and points more toward FAP or juvenile polyposis syndrome. Juvenile polyposis was ruled out in D as she had negative genetic testing for BMPR1A and SMAD4 deletions or duplications. As her colonoscopy was normal, based on the pattern of disease incidence in her family and the findings on endoscopy, D was suspected to have GAPPS, an autosomal dominant syndrome. She displayed the key features of GAPPS syndrome: multiple fundic gland polyps of the proximal stomach with sparing of the antrum. This is a newly described syndrome based on the study of a large family in Australia as well as two families in the United States.[70] The estimated patient risk for cancer of the stomach with this syndrome is at least 25%, with malignant deterioration usually occurring in the fourth decade of life. The polyposis found in GAPPS is restricted to oxyntic mucosa explaining the geography of the polyps' location, as the antral mucosa, lacking oxyntic cells, may extend along the lesser curve.

D had an increased risk of gastric cancer based on endoscopic findings and her family history as she was nearing the age at which cancer develops. She underwent laparoscopic total gastrectomy, esophagojejunostomy, jejunostomy feeding tube placement, and upper endoscopy. Surgical pathology revealed a villous adenoma with high-grade dysplasia, multiple fundic polyps, and adenomatous polyps with low-grade dysplasia localized in the proximal stomach. Even though a formal D2 was not undertaken as she did not have a diagnosis of cancer, 45 lymph nodes were found in the surgical specimen and all were negative for invasive adenocarcinoma.

D had an uneventful recovery from surgery and was discharged home on hospital day eight. She used her feeding tube for supplemental nutrition for approximately 5 weeks following the operation. It was removed after a stable weight was confirmed for 2 weeks off of tube feeding. D met the criteria suggested in the literature for a diagnosis of GAPPS with >100 polyps of the proximal stomach, no evidence of colorectal or duodenal polyps, and a predominance of fundic gastric polyps some with dysplasia. GAPPS is a new syndrome already found worldwide. Affected families have been identified in North America, Japan,[71] and Australia. It is unclear if this syndrome will represent a significant minority of familial gastric cancers or what its geographical extent and distribution will be. In our current global medical community where the ease of communication aids the characterization of new clinical entities such as GAPSS, we are likely to have the answers soon.

## REFERENCES

1. Ferlay J, Shin HR, Bray F, Forman D, Mathers C, Parkin DM. *GLOBOCAN 2008 v2.0, Cancer Incidence and Mortality Worldwide*. IARC CancerBase No. 10 [Internet]. Lyon, France: International Agency for Research on Cancer, 2010. Available at http://globocan.iarc.fr.

2. Bray F, Ren JS, Masuyer E, Ferlay J. Global estimates of cancer prevalence for 27 sites in the adult population in 2008. *Int J Cancer* 2013; 132(5): 1133–45.

3. de Manzoni G, Roviello F, Siquini W (Eds). *Surgery in the Multimodal Management of Gastric Cancer*. 1st ed. Milan, Italy: Springer-Verlag Italia, 2012.

4. National Cancer Institute at the National Institutes of Health: Stomach (gastric) Cancer. Available at http://www.cancer.gov/cancertopics/types/stomach. Accessed July 11, 2013.

5. Siegel R, Naishadham D, Jemal A. Cancer statistics, 2012. *CA Cancer J Clin* 2012; 62(1): 10–29.

6. Guggenheim DE, Shah MA. Gastric cancer epidemiology and risk factors. *J Surg Oncol* 2013; 107(3): 230–36.

7. Klint A, Engholm G, Storm HH, et al. Trends in survival of patients diagnosed with cancer of the digestive organs in the Nordic countries 1964–2003 followed up to the end of 2006. *Acta Oncol* 2010; 49(5): 578–607.

8. Dassen AE, Lemmens VE, van de Poll-Franse LV, et al. Trends in incidence, treatment and survival of gastric adenocarcinoma between 1990 and 2007: a population-based study in the Netherlands. *Eur J Cancer* 2010; 46(6): 1101–10.

9. Inoue M, Tsugane S. Epidemiology of gastric cancer in Japan. *Postgrad Med J* 2005; 81(957): 419–24.

10. Levi F, Lucchini F, Gonzalez JR, Fernandez E, Negri E, La Vecchia C. Monitoring falls in gastric cancer mortality in Europe. *Ann Oncol* 2004; 15(2): 338–45.

11. Bertuccio P, Chatenoud L, Levi F, et al. Recent patterns in gastric cancer: a global overview. *Int J Cancer* 2009; 125(3): 666–73.

12. Steevens J, Botterweck AA, Dirx MJ, van den Brandt PA, Schouten LJ. Trends in incidence of oesophageal and stomach cancer subtypes in Europe. *Eur J Gastroenterol Hepatol* 2010; 22(6): 669–78.

13. Gore RM. Gastric cancer: clinical and pathologic features. *Radiol Clin North Am* 1997; 35(2): 295–310.

14. Tsugane S, de Souza JM, Costa ML Jr, et al. Cancer incidence rates among Japanese immigrants in the city of Sao Paulo, Brazil, 1969–78. *Cancer Causes Control* 1990; 1(2): 189–93.

15. Haenszel W, Kurihara M, Segi M, Lee RK. Stomach cancer among Japanese in Hawaii. *J Natl Cancer Inst* 1972; 49(4): 969–88.

16. Correa P. Human gastric carcinogenesis: a multistep and multifactorial process—first American Cancer Society Award Lecture on Cancer Epidemiology and Prevention. *Cancer Res* 1992; 52(24): 6735–40.

17. Brenner H, Arndt V, Stegmaier C, Ziegler H, Rothenbacher D. Is *Helicobacter pylori* infection a necessary condition for noncardia gastric cancer? *Am J Epidemiol* 2004; 159(3): 252–58.

18. Ladeiras-Lopes R, Pereira AK, Nogueira A, et al. Smoking and gastric cancer: systematic review and meta-analysis of cohort studies. *Cancer Causes Control* 2008; 19(7): 689–701.

19. D'Elia L, Rossi G, Ippolito R, Cappuccio FP, Strazzullo P. Habitual salt intake and risk of gastric cancer: a meta-analysis of prospective studies. *Clin Nutr* 2012; 31(4): 489–98.

20. Yang P, Zhou Y, Chen B, et al. Overweight, obesity and gastric cancer risk: results from a meta-analysis of cohort studies. *Eur J Cancer* 2009; 45(16): 2867–73.

21. Zhong C, Li KN, Bi JW, Wang BC. Sodium intake, salt taste and gastric cancer risk according to Helicobacter pylori infection, smoking, histological type and tumor site in China. *Asian Pac J Cancer Prev* 2012; 13(6): 2481–84.

22. Yanaoka K, Oka M, Ohata H, et al. Eradication of Helicobacter pylori prevents cancer development in subjects with mild gastric atrophy identified by serum pepsinogen levels. *Int J Cancer* 2009; 125(11): 2697–703.

23. Uemura N, Okamoto S, Yamamoto S, et al. Helicobacter pylori infection and the development of gastric cancer. *N Engl J Med* 2001; 345(11): 784–89.

24. Take S, Mizuno M, Ishiki K, et al. The effect of eradicating Helicobacter pylori on the development of gastric cancer in patients with peptic ulcer disease. *Am J Gastroenterol* 2005; 100(5): 1037–42.

25. Mera R, Fontham ET, Bravo LE, et al. Long term follow up of patients treated for Helicobacter pylori infection. *Gut* 2005; 54(11): 1536–40.

26. Graham DY, Malaty HM, Evans DG, Evans DJ Jr, Klein PD, Adam E. Epidemiology of *Helicobacter pylori* in an asymptomatic population in the united states. Effect of age, race, and socioeconomic status. *Gastroenterology* 1991; 100(6): 1495–501.

27. Frenck RW Jr, Clemens J. Helicobacter in the developing world. *Microbes Infect* 2003; 5(8): 705–713.

28. Lee YC, Chen TH, Chiu HM, et al. The benefit of mass eradication of helicobacter pylori infection: a community-based study of gastric cancer prevention. *Gut* 2013; 62(5): 676–682. doi:10.1136/gutjnl-2012-302240. Epub Jun 14, 2012.

29. Graham DY, Fischbach L. Helicobacter pylori treatment in the era of increasing antibiotic resistance. *Gut* 2010; 59(8): 1143–53.

30. Agarwal K, Agarwal S. Helicobacter pylori vaccine: from past to future. *Mayo Clin Proc* 2008; 83(2): 169–75.

31. Del Giudice G, Covacci A, Telford JL, Montecucco C, Rappuoli R. The design of vaccines against Helicobacter pylori and their development. *Annu Rev Immunol* 2001; 19: 523–63.

32. Ihan A, Pinchuk IV, Beswick EJ. Inflammation, immunity, and vaccines for Helicobacter pylori infection. *Helicobacter* 2012; 17(Suppl 1): 16–21.

33. Malfertheiner P, Megraud F, O'Morain CA, et al. Management of helicobacter pylori infection—the Maastricht IV/Florence Consensus Report. *Gut* 2012; 61(5): 646–64.

34. Malfertheiner P, Schultze V, Rosenkranz B, et al. Safety and immunogenicity of an intramuscular Helicobacter pylori vaccine in noninfected volunteers: a phase I study. *Gastroenterology* 2008; 135(3): 787–95.

35. Gupta N, Bansal A, Wani SB, Gaddam S, Rastogi A, Sharma P. Endoscopy for upper GI cancer screening in the general population: a cost-utility analysis. *Gastrointest Endosc* 2011; 74(3): 610–24.e2.

36. Hirota WK, Zuckerman MJ, Adler DG, et al. Standards of Practice Committee, American Society for Gastrointestinal Endoscopy. ASGE guideline: the role of endoscopy in the surveillance of premalignant conditions of the upper GI tract. *Gastrointest Endosc* 2006; 63(4): 570–80.

37. Cho NH, Moy CS, Davis F, Haenszel W, Ahn YO, Kim H. Ethnic variation in the incidence of stomach cancer in Illinois, 1986–1988. *Am J Epidemiol* 1996; 144(7): 661–64.

38. Fukao A, Tsubono Y, Tsuji I, HIsamichi S, Sugahara N, Takano A. The evaluation of screening for gastric cancer in Miyagi prefecture, Japan: a population-based case-control study. *Int J Cancer* 1995; 60(1): 45–48.

39. Arisue T, Tamura K, Tebayashi A. [End results of gastric cancer detected by mass survey: analysis using the relative survival rate curve]. *Gan To Kagaku Ryoho* 1988; 15(4 Pt 2–1): 929–36.

40. Fuccio L, Zagari RM, Eusebi LH, et al. Meta-analysis: can Helicobacter pylori eradication treatment reduce the risk for gastric cancer? *Ann Intern Med* 2009; 151(2): 121–28.

41. Watabe H, Mitsushima T, Yamaji Y, et al. Predicting the development of gastric cancer from combining Helicobacter pylori antibodies and serum pepsinogen status: a prospective endoscopic cohort study. *Gut* 2005; 54(6): 764–68.

42. Lee YY, Oh DK, Choi KS, Jung KW, Lee HY, Jun JK. The current status of gastric cancer screening in Korea: report on the national cancer screening programme, 2009. *Asian Pac J Cancer Prev* 2011; 12(12): 3495–500.

43. Ahn HS, Lee HJ, Yoo MW, et al. Changes in clinicopathological features and survival after gastrectomy for gastric cancer over a 20-year period. *Br J Surg* 2011; 98(2): 255–60.

44. Ahlquist DA, Zou H, Domanico M, et al. Next-generation stool DNA test accurately detects colorectal cancer and large adenomas. *Gastroenterology* 2012; 142(2): 248–56.

45. Jaffer AA. NCCN clinical practice guidelines in oncology: gastric cancer version 2.2012. Available at http://www.nccn.org/professionals/physician_gls/f_guidelines.asp. Accessed August 14, 2013.

46. Nakamoto S, Sakai Y, Kasanuki J, et al. Indications for the use of endoscopic mucosal resection for early gastric cancer in Japan: a comparative study with endoscopic submucosal dissection. *Endoscopy* 2009; 41(9): 746–50.

47. An JY, Youn HG, Choi MG, Noh JH, Sohn TS, Kim S. The difficult choice between total and proximal gastrectomy in proximal early gastric cancer. *Am J Surg* 2008; 196(4): 587–91.

48. Bozzetti F, Marubini E, Bonfanti G, Miceli R, Piano C, Gennari L. Subtotal versus total gastrectomy for gastric cancer: five-year survival rates in a multicenter randomized Italian trial. Italian Gastrointestinal Tumor Study Group. *Ann Surg* 1999; 230(2): 170–78.

49. Gouzi JL, Huguier M, Fagniez PL, et al. Total versus subtotal gastrectomy for adenocarcinoma of the gastric antrum. A French prospective controlled study. *Ann Surg* 1989; 209(2): 162–66.

50. Bonenkamp JJ, Hermans J, Sasako M, et al. Extended lymph-node dissection for gastric cancer. *N Engl J Med* 1999; 340 (12): 908–14.

51. Smith DD, Schwarz RR, Schwarz RE. Impact of total lymph node count on staging and survival after gastrectomy for gastric cancer: data from a large US-population database. *J Clin Oncol* 2005; 23(28): 7114–24.

52. Verlato G, Roviello F, Marchet A, et al. Indexes of surgical quality in gastric cancer surgery: experience of an Italian network. *Ann Surg Oncol* 2009; 16(3): 594–602.

53. Yang SH, Zhang YC, Yang KH, et al. An evidence-based medicine review of lymphadenectomy extent for gastric cancer. *Am J Surg* 2009; 197(2): 246–51.

54. Mullaney PJ, Wadley MS, Hyde C, et al. Appraisal of compliance with the UICC/AJCC staging system in the staging of gastric cancer. Union Internacional Contra la Cancrum/American Joint Committee on Cancer. *Br J Surg* 2002; 89(11): 1405–8.

55. Schmidt CM, Powell ES, Yiannoutsos CT, et al. Pancreaticoduodenectomy: a 20-year experience in 516 patients. *Arch Surg* 2004; 139(7): 718–25.

56. Sasako M, Sano T, Yamamoto S, et al. D2 lymphadenectomy alone or with para-aortic nodal dissection for gastric cancer. *N Engl J Med* 2008; 359(5): 453–62.

57. Vinuela EF, Gonen M, Brennan MF, Coit DG, Strong VE. Laparoscopic versus open distal gastrectomy for gastric cancer: a meta-analysis of randomized controlled trials and high-quality nonrandomized studies. *Ann Surg* 2012; 255(3): 446–56.

58. Smalley SR, Benedetti JK, Haller DG, et al. Updated analysis of SWOG-directed intergroup study 0116: a phase III trial of adjuvant radiochemotherapy versus

observation after curative gastric cancer resection. *J Clin Oncol* 2012; 30(19): 2327–33.

59. Cunningham D, Allum WH, Stenning SP, et al. Perioperative chemotherapy versus surgery alone for resectable gastroesophageal cancer. *N Engl J Med* 2006; 355(1): 11–20.

60. Dikken JL, van Sandick JW, Maurits Swellengrebel HA, et al. Neo-adjuvant chemotherapy followed by surgery and chemotherapy or by surgery and chemoradiotherapy for patients with resectable gastric cancer (CRITICS). *BMC Cancer* 2011; 11: 329.

61. Sasako M, Sakuramoto S, Katai H, et al. Five-year outcomes of a randomized phase III trial comparing adjuvant chemotherapy with S-1 versus surgery alone in stage II or III gastric cancer. *J Clin Oncol* 2011; 29(33): 4387–93.

62. Bang YJ, Kim YW, Yang HK, et al. Adjuvant capecitabine and oxaliplatin for gastric cancer after D2 gastrectomy (CLASSIC): a phase 3 open-label, randomised controlled trial. *Lancet* 2012; 379(9813): 315–21.

63. GASTRIC (Global Advanced/Adjuvant Stomach Tumor Research International Collaboration) Group, Paoletti X, Oba K, et al. Benefit of adjuvant chemotherapy for resectable gastric cancer: a meta-analysis. *JAMA* 2010; 303(17): 1729–37.

64. Howlader N, Noone AM, Krapcho M, et al. SEER Cancer Statistics Review, 1975–2010, National Cancer Institute, Bethesda, MD. Available at http://seer.cancer.gov/csr/1975_2010/. Accessed July 2, 2013.

65. Verdecchia A, Corazziari I, Gatta G, et al. Explaining gastric cancer survival differences among European countries. *Int J Cancer* 2004; 109(5): 737–41.

66. Nashimoto A, Akazawa K, Isobe Y, et al. Gastric cancer treated in 2002 in Japan: 2009 annual report of the JGCA nationwide registry. *Gastric Cancer* 2013; 16(1): 1–27.

67. Matsuda T, Ajiki W, Marugame T, et al. Population-based survival of cancer patients diagnosed between 1993 and 1999 in Japan: a chronological and international comparative study. *Jpn J Clin Oncol* 2011; 41(1): 40–51.

68. Onodera H, Tokunaga A, Yoshiyuki T, et al. Surgical outcome of 483 patients with early gastric cancer: prognosis, postoperative morbidity and mortality, and gastric remnant-cancer. *Hepatogastroenterology* 2004; 51(55): 82–85.

69. Kikuchi S, Katada N, Sakuramoto S, et al. Survival after surgical treatment of early gastric cancer: surgical techniques and long-term survival. *Langenbecks Arch Surg* 2004; 389(2): 69–74.

70. Worthley DL, Phillips KD, Wayte N, et al. Gastric adenocarcinoma and proximal polyposis of the stomach (GAPPS): a new autosomal dominant syndrome. *Gut* 2012; 61(5): 774–79.

71. Yanaru-Fujisawa R, Nakamura S, Moriyama T, et al. Familial fundic gland polyposis with gastric cancer. *Gut* 2012; 61(7): 1103–4.

# 8

# Liver Cancer

## Kinsey A. McCormick, Manoj P. Menon, and William P. Harris

### GLOBAL EPIDEMIOLOGY

Hepatocellular carcinoma (HCC), which disproportionately affects resource-poor countries, represents nearly 90% of the total burden of all primary liver cancers. The burden HCC exerts worldwide is enormous, representing the seventh most common cause of all cancers globally and the third leading cause of death.[1] Annually, approximately 750,000 incident cases are diagnosed and almost 700,000 deaths are attributed to HCC.[1] A recent systematic analysis of the leading causes of death corroborated these findings and noted that between 1990 and 2010, the number of deaths attributed to liver cancer is estimated to have increased by over 60%, from 463,000 to 752,100.[2] Nearly 85% of both cases and death secondary to HCC occur in the less developed world, defined as all regions of Africa, Asia (excluding Japan), Latin America and the Caribbean, Melanesia, Micronesia, and Polynesia. These resource-limited areas are often characterized by an inadequate health-care infrastructure, which may result in a lack of primary preventive efforts, delayed diagnoses, and inadequate treatment options. The toll of HCC in China is particularly taxing, accounting for over half of the global burden of disease.[3]

The incidence and prevalence of HCC parallels the geographic distribution and epidemiology of hepatitis B (HBV) and hepatitis C (HCV) infection (Figure 8.1). Accordingly, the burden of HCC in endemic countries is expectedly high. Eastern Asia (i.e., China, Chinese Taipei, Japan, Democratic People's Republic of Korea, Republic of Korea, and Mongolia) maintains the highest incidence and mortality from HCC, with an age-standardized incidence and mortality (age-standardized) of 24.0 cases and 21.6 deaths per 100,000 people, respectively.[1] Similarly, the incidence and mortality rates in less developed regions were 13.0 and 12.1 per 100,000 people—nearly 3 times

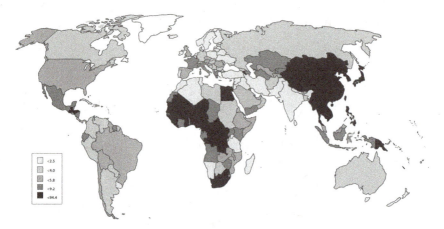

**FIGURE 8.1** GLOBOCAN map of worldwide age-standardized incidence from primary liver cancer, 2008 estimates. Rates per 100,000 person-years. (Ferlay J, Shin HR, Bray F, Forman D, Mathers C, Parkin DM. GLOBOCAN 2008 v2.0, Cancer Incidence and Mortality Worldwide: IARC CancerBase No. 10 [Internet]. Lyon, France: International Agency for Research on Cancer, 2010. Available at http://glo bocan.iarc.fr. Accessed July 7, 2013.)

the rates of 5.2 and 4.6 per 100,000 people seen in more developed regions (i.e., all regions of Europe and Northern America, Australia/New Zealand).[1]

Although the relative burden of HCC in the United States is low, the age-adjusted incidence tripled from 1.6 per 100,000 to 4.9 per 100,000 between 1975 and 2005 as calculated from Surveillance, Epidemiology, and End Results registry data.[4] This increase is thought to be secondary to sequelae from chronic HCV and an increased prevalence of HBV among recent immigrants to the United States from Southeast Asia. Although the prevalence of chronic infectious hepatitis may be decreasing in the United States, other factors including a rise in nonalcoholic steatohepatitis (NASH) may result in a continued upward trend.[5,6] Conversely, despite China having the highest prevalence of HCC in the world, the incidence of HCC in urban Shanghai decreased from 33.9 to 25.8 per 100,000 among men and 11.4 to 8.5 per 100,000 among women, attributed in part to widespread hepatitis B vaccination, during a similar time period using an age-period-cohort model for the time period between 1976 and 2005.[7]

## Age and Gender

The incidence of HCC typically increases with age, a trend seen in both low-prevalence regions, including the United States, where infection is typically acquired in adulthood, and the very highly prevalent regions in East

Asia, where acquisition frequently occurs via perinatal transmission.[8] However, despite a relatively high prevalence of disease, the incidence of HCC in sub-Saharan Africa, for unclear reasons, remains relatively stable between the ages of 55 and 75.[9]

The age of acquisition of an etiologic risk factor, most commonly HCV or HBV is particularly relevant, due to both the temporal relationship between virus acquisition and carcinogenesis and the risk of developing chronic disease. The majority of oncogenic viral-mediated cases of HCC occur a number of years after infection, given the role of chronic inflammation in the pathogenesis of HCC. In addition, acquisition of HBV via perinatal transmission dramatically increases the risk of developing chronic infection when compared to infection acquisition in adulthood.[10,11]

The global incidence of HCC among men is approximately twice that of women, with distinct geographic variation.[1] Although the reason for this sex discrepancy is not fully understood, potential explanations are related to sex-specific variations in exposure to known risk factors (e.g., alcohol consumption, viral infections), and a hormonal influence.

### Race

There are observed ethnic/racial differences in the incidence of HCC. In part secondary to differences in exposure to risk factors, Asian Americans have nearly twice the rate of HCC compared to African Americans and 4 times the rate when compared to white persons.[4] Interestingly, approximately 90% of HCC among whites is associated with HCV, whereas nearly 75% of HCC among Asians living in the United States was associated with HBV.[12] Similar ethnic variation in the incidence of HCC has been documented in other countries as well.[13]

## ETIOLOGY

### Hepatitis B

The majority of all cases of HCC worldwide are secondary to HBV, a double-stranded DNA virus that can lead to chronic infection.[14,15] The attributable fraction of HCC secondary to HBV infection is even greater in endemic countries, accounting for up to 80% of the burden of HCC.[13]

Although the exact mechanism of HBV oncogenesis has not been fully elucidated, one explanation is that the hepatitis B viral DNA is inserted proximal to tumor suppressor genes and upregulates expression of tumorigenicity and blocks the function of tumor suppressor genes.[16,17] Up to 90% of HBV-associated cases develop in the setting of underlying chronic liver disease, typically 25 to 30 years after initial infection, and a minority of hepatitis B–associated HCC occurs in the absence of cirrhosis.[3] Indeed, the lifetime risk of HCC is up to 25% among patients with chronic HBV infection.[13] Multiple cohort studies have described the direct relationship with HBV DNA levels and risk of HCC.[18,19] Although the risk is higher among patients with active chronic HBV, carriers with inactive chronic HBV are also at elevated risk.[20] In a prospective cohort study of Alaskan natives, the incidence of HCC was significantly lower among patients who had cleared the antigen compared to their counterparts (36.8 per 100,000 per year vs. 195.7 cases per 100,000 person-years; $p < 0.001$).[21] Although HBeAg seroconversion is associated with a better prognosis, the incidence of HCC after clearing HBsAg remains elevated and ongoing surveillance is recommended.[21] The role of chronic infection is particularly relevant in highly endemic regions where transmission is typically vertical, allowing for a longer exposure period.

In addition to the adverse risk of cirrhosis among patients with HBV, demographic factors (sex, age, ethnicity), exposures (alcohol, tobacco, aflatoxin), and viral factors, including viral load and genotype, are each associated with an additive risk of HCC among this population.[10] In addition, a meta-analysis revealed the profound negative synergistic effect of coinfection with HCV and HBV.[22]

## Hepatitis C

Although the mechanism is not yet clear, the carcinogenic potential of HCV, via chronic inflammation leading to cirrhosis, has been well documented, with an annual incidence in patients with cirrhosis between 2% and 5%.[23] While the majority of HCC globally is secondary to HBV, HCV is responsible for the majority of HCC cases in resource-abundant areas, including the United States.[24] Surveillance data from the U.S. Centers for Disease Control and Prevention reveals a greater than 90% decline in incidence of HCV between 1989 when an estimated 47,800 cases were reported and 2010 in which only 2,800 cases were estimated in the United States;[25] however, the prevalence of HCV globally remains high and continues to rise with an estimated incidence of approximately 3%, with highest prevalence documented in Central/East Asia, northern Africa, and the Middle East.[26]

The risk of HCV-associated HCC, although elevated, varies globally.[3] In a large community-based prospective study of over 12,000 men in Taiwan, researchers noted that the risk of HCC among anti-HCV-positive patients was 20 times greater than patients who were anti-HCV negative.[27] A case–control study (164 cases, 250 controls) in three countries in North Africa revealed that 60% of HCC patients were anti-HCV positive, with an odds ratio (OR) of 32 for anti-HCV.[28]

## Aflatoxin

Aflatoxin B1, characterized as a group 1 carcinogen by the International Agency for Research on Cancer in 1994, is produced by *Aspergillus* fungi. Largely due to improper storage, it is a relatively common contaminant among foods in Asia and sub-Saharan Africa.[28] Consequently, an estimated 4.5 billion people live in areas exposed to this toxin.[29] Aflatoxin is thought to induce carcinogenesis via mutations in the p53 tumor suppressor gene, resulting in chronic hepatitis or cirrhosis.[30,31] A systematic review of 17 studies in China, Taiwan, or sub-Saharan Africa revealed that the population-attributable risk of aflatoxin was 17%, with an OR of 6.37 for the development of HCC. Notably, the effect of aflatoxin and HBV was synergistic with a combined OR of 73.0.[32]

## Nonalcoholic Fatty Liver Disease (NAFLD)

The prevalence of NAFLD, defined as macrovesicular steatosis in greater than 5% of hepatocytes, and NASH, which requires the addition of hepatocyte swelling and lobular inflammation, has paralleled the increasing prevalence of obesity.[37,38] Globally, the estimated prevalence of NAFLD ranges between 6% and 35%.[39] In the United States, the prevalence is even higher, with noted variation by ethnicity, presence of diabetes, and obesity.[40,41] Indeed, in a review of medical claims between 2002 and 2008, NAFLD/NASH was the most common risk factor for HCC in the United States.[42]

## Alcohol and Other Etiologies

Although the mechanism by which alcohol leads to HCC has not been fully elucidated, the role of alcohol in promoting cirrhosis is clear. In areas of relatively low HCC prevalence, including the United States, the role of alcohol as a risk factor for HCC is particularly prominent.[33] However, the association between alcohol and HCC is less strong in regions of high prevalence. Recently, a large cohort study of over 11,000 Taiwanese men, which examined the multiple risk factors associated with HCC, failed to document an independent effect of alcohol. However, an interaction effect was demonstrated between alcohol intake and HbsAg positivity.[34] Multiple other studies have also previously documented the synergistic effect of alcohol and viral hepatitis on the risk of HCC.[35,36]

In addition to the factors mentioned earlier, rarer etiologies correlate with risk of developing HCC, including autoimmune hepatitis, primary biliary cirrhosis, hemochromatosis, and alpha-1-antitrypsin deficiency.. Regardless, upon development of cirrhosis, all patients harbor a risk of developing HCC with approximate risk of greater than 1.5% annual incidence and should be screened accordingly. In addition, HIV coinfection with hepatitis B or C may lead to more rapidly progressive liver disease and consequently HCC.[43]

## PREVENTION

### Hepatitis B

Primary prevention, which involves exposure reduction to carcinogens, includes vaccination against hepatitis B. The hepatitis B vaccine, which first became available nearly 30 years ago, was recommended to be implemented globally in 1992 by the World Health Assembly.[44] Since that time, the utilization of the vaccine has dramatically increased, and as of 2010, the hepatitis B vaccine is included in the national infant immunization program in over 90% of the countries in the world.[45] This increase is in large part due to the various studies that show the protective effect of hepatitis B vaccination in reducing both horizontal and vertical transmission and the incidence of HCC.[46-49] In Taiwan, widespread implementation of the hepatitis B vaccine began in 1984. Researchers reviewed data from the National Cancer Registry and from the country's major medical facilities and found that the average annual incidence of HCC declined from 0.70 per 100,000 children 6 to 14 years for the interval between 1981 and 1986 to 0.36 per 100,000 between 1990 and 1994 ($p < 0.01$).[47]

The incidence of transfusion-transmitted HBV (and HCV) in resource-abundant areas has dramatically decreased, yielding an estimated risk of 1 in 280,000 and 1 in 1,100,000 units, respectively.[50,51] However, the role of blood supply surveillance in resource-poor settings is limited. As such, improved hemovigilance in resource-poor settings will also prevent the transmission of both hepatitis B and C.

In addition to preventing the acquisition of HBV, cancer prevention efforts also are aimed toward treating patients with hepatitis B before the development of HCC. Based on preclinical and clinical data suggesting that patients with persistent HBe antigenemia have an increased risk of liver failure and HCC, multiple researchers have evaluated the effectiveness of antiviral therapy in preventing disease progression.[52-54] In a randomly controlled prospective study, over 600 patients with chronic hepatitis B with histologically confirmed cirrhosis or advanced fibrosis were randomized to receive continuous treatment with either the antiviral drug lamivudine or placebo. The incidence of HCC was significantly greater (HR 0.49; $p = 0.047$) in the placebo group (7.4%) than the treatment group (3.9%).[55] A more recent meta-analysis also observed a treatment benefit, with either interferon, nucleoside, or nucleotide analogue in reducing the risk of HCC.[56] More recently, algorithms integrating multiple variables, including age, gender, ALT levels, HBeAg status, and HBV DNA levels, show promise in identifying which non-cirrhotic chronic HBV-infected patients derive benefit from treatment with antiviral therapy.[57]

## Hepatitis C

Currently, no vaccine is available for HCV. Therefore, prevention efforts revolve around risk reduction strategies, including improved hemovigilance and the use of single-use medical supplies to prevent nosocomial transmission. Multiple meta-analyses have documented the protective effect of interferon in reducing the incidence of HCC in patients with HCV-associated cirrhosis; however, prospective data indicates that the benefit is primarily limited to those patients who achieve a sustained virologic response.[58-61] Regardless, the clinical utility of interferon therapy in resource-poor areas is limited. Newer treatment strategies for genotype 1 HCV, including protease inhibitors alone or in combination with peginterferon-ribavirin, demonstrate promise in obtaining sustained virologic responses in over 60% of patients, but the high cost of such therapies serves as a current barrier to widespread global implementation.[62,63]

## Aflatoxin

As contamination of food by aflatoxin can occur both preharvest and postharvest, prevention measures must target both crop growth and postharvest storage conditions. Although certain crops are more susceptible to contamination than others, altering crop selection may be logistically difficult. One potential preventive option, under study, is to reduce exposure to aflatoxin in the development of *Aspergillus*-resistant crops.[64,65]

In order to assess the impact of postharvest interventions, researchers conducted a community-based study involving 20 villages. Ten villages received a package of interventions, consisting of both education (e.g., how to identify contaminated or damaged groundnuts, how to properly sun-dry ground nuts) and commodities (e.g., fiber mats for drying, fiber jute bags for storage, insecticide); the other 10 villages implemented their standard practice. After 5 months, villagers living in the treatment villages had significantly lower concentrations of blood aflatoxin-albumin adducts than those villagers living in the control village (8.0 pg/mg vs. 18.7 pg/mg; $p < 0.0001$), suggesting that such interventions can reduce exposure to aflatoxin in a resource-poor setting.[66] The role of trapping agents, such as sodium calcium aluminosilicate, and chlorophyllin, which is thought to sequester aflatoxin, is under study.[67-69]

## Nonalcoholic Fatty Liver Disease

Various studies have documented the effect of lifestyle modification, including diet, exercise, and behavioral therapy, in improving NAFLD.[70-73] The role of pharmacotherapy, including vitamin E and insulin-sensitizing agents, as disease-modifying agents is less certain. In a recent randomized controlled trial, patients with NASH without diabetes were randomized to receive vitamin E, pioglitazone, or placebo to assess the improvements in histology as the primary outcome measure. When compared to placebo, the patients receiving vitamin E did have improved histologic features; however, there was not a statistically significant difference among the group receiving the insulin-sensitizing agent.[42]

## Screening for Hepatocellular Carcinoma in High-Risk Populations

Screening protocols for HCC in high-risk populations can identify patients with early-stage tumors potentially amenable to curative therapy. Individuals deemed high risk include cirrhotic patients from any etiology with Child–Pugh stage A or B, non-cirrhotic HBV carriers with active hepatitis or family history of HCC, non-cirrhotic chronic HCV patients with advanced fibrosis, or any cirrhotic patient awaiting liver transplantation according to recent European Association for the Study of the Liver (EASL)/EORTC recommendations.[74] Evidence from several studies suggests that screening confers a survival advantage, earlier stage migration, and cost-efficacy in the Western world.[43] Zhang et al. in a large randomized controlled trial from China demonstrated that semiannual ultrasound was associated with a statistically significant 37% reduction in mortality, and this study remains the highest quality evidence to date on the topic.[75]

Ultrasound represents the most common method of surveillance due to the noninvasiveness of the procedure, moderate cost, and feasibility. Ultrasound identifies the majority of tumors before onset of clinical symptoms and carries a sensitivity of approximately 60% to 90% and a specificity of >90%.[74,76] This method is highly operator dependent, and specialized training for the ultrasonographer is critical. Semiannual ultrasound is associated with improved sensitivity (70% vs. 50%) and improved clinical outcomes in some studies and remains the schedule of choice when compared to annual ultrasound surveillance.[77,78] The benefit of concurrent alpha-fetoprotein (AFP) testing is controversial and provides minimal additional benefit in the surveillance setting to ultrasound, detecting 6% to 8% of cases not identified by this modality.[79] Although many experts argue against integration of AFP into screening guidelines due to the added expense of evaluating false-positive findings, its use in screening remains country dependent. However, in the absence of ultrasound availability, AFP levels may aid in diagnosis if persistently elevated above 400 ng/mL or increasing rapidly. Research efforts targeting validation of new serologic biomarkers for identification of HCC are an area of intense investigation, and improvement upon AFP accuracy in the screening setting represents a clear clinical need.

## Diagnosis and Staging of Hepatocellular Carcinoma

Upon identification of a suspicious lesion greater than 1 cm on ultrasound, confirmation is required by either diagnostic contrast-enhanced cross-sectional imaging or biopsy. Smaller lesions can be followed by ultrasound at 3- to 6-month intervals, with a return to standard surveillance after 2 years of stability. For lesions greater than 1 cm, cross-sectional dynamic imaging with either multiphase CT or MRI is indicated for staging and potentially diagnosis. Diagnosis can be achieved with imaging alone in the majority of cases, avoiding the 2% to 3% risk of tumor seeding along the needle biopsy tract and up to 0.5% risk of hemorrhagic complications.[43] High-quality contrast-enhanced imaging or biopsy confirmation is required to differentiate HCC from dysplastic nodules, intrahepatic cholangiocarcinoma, metastatic disease from other sites, or other entities.

Noninvasive imaging guidelines regarding interpretation of CT/MRI vary among international organizations, and further standardization among these organizations is required. The broadly implemented EASL/EORTC guidelines consider multiphase CT or MRI imaging demonstrating arterial phase enhancement and portal venous washout in delayed phases, if performed at centers of expertise with optimal equipment, diagnostic of HCC in cirrhotic patients.[74] Confirmatory cross-sectional imaging with a second modality should be considered for lesions 1 to 2 cm in settings lacking optimal equipment or radiology expertise. Additional imaging features that may favor the radiographic diagnosis of HCC include evidence of venous tumor thrombus, presence of surrounding enhancing capsule, T2 mild-moderate hyperintensity on MRI, interval growth on interim imaging, or fat deposition within the lesion.[80] In patients without underlying cirrhosis, patients with indeterminate enhancement patterns, or if adequate cross-sectional imaging is not possible, percutaneous needle biopsy is recommended. In regard to alternative imaging methods, contrast-enhanced ultrasound and PET imaging are not recommended, whereas gadoxetate-enhanced MRI (hepatobiliary-enhanced MRI) for smaller and indeterminate lesions may prove useful in differentiating dysplastic nodules from HCC when available.[81]

Numerous staging systems, the Barcelona Clinic Liver Cancer (BCLC), Okuda, Japanese Integrated Staging (JIS) score, and Cancer of the Liver Italian Program (CLIP), have been described and validated. In general terms, integrations of estimates of disease burden, underlying hepatic function, and the patients' overall functional status provide critical information regarding prognosis and treatment options. For general practice in the Western world, the EASL and American Association for the Study of Liver Diseases (AASLD) endorse the BCLC system, and this is a commonly employed standard in Western clinical practice and research settings. In this system, tumor stage is linked with specific prognosis and correlated with general treatment guidelines.

Regional preferences regarding prognostic staging systems and subsequent treatment algorithms exist. For example, the modified JIS system has been promoted in Japan as a superior determinate of predicting outcome in Japanese surgical candidates who are often identified at an early stage due to existence of robust early detection programs.[82] In contrast, the CLIP score may provide good prognostic stratification in lower-resource settings without routine access to early detection programs and higher-cost medical imaging.[82] The Asian Pacific Association for the Study of the Liver (APASL) provides general treatment guidelines commonly used in China and Southeast Asia which differ from Western guidelines, as discussed in the subsequent section.[83]

## TREATMENT AND ASSOCIATED SURVIVAL OUTCOMES

Optimal therapy for HCC varies from potentially definitive local therapies (surgery, radiofrequency or ethanol ablation, and liver transplant) to palliative therapies (catheter-based therapy, sorafenib) based on extent of disease, underlying hepatic reserve, and the patient's functional status. Variability

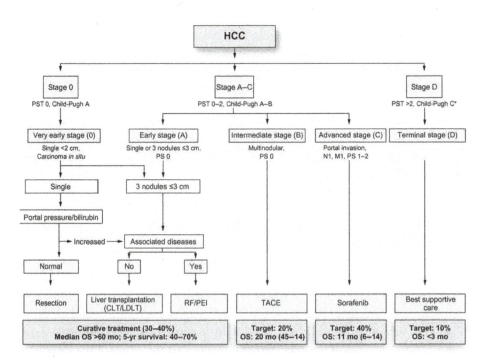

**FIGURE 8.2** BCLC treatment algorithm. (Figure reprinted from *Journal of Hepatology* 56(4): 908–43. European Association for the Study of the Liver, European Organization for Research and Treatment of Cancer. EASL-EORTC Clinical Practice Guidelines: Management of hepatocellular carcinoma. April 2012.)

in international guidelines between Asia and the Western world suggests a trend toward more aggressive local intervention in Asia. Regional discrepancies (e.g., surgical candidacy of Child Turcotte Pugh [CTP]-B patients, administration of chemoembolization in patients with focal vascular invasion) highlight the need for ongoing clinical research and robust cost-efficacy analyses. The BCLC treatment algorithm, often used in the Western world, is provided in Figure 8.2. A more nuanced discussion of commonly employed interventions for HCC is detailed in this section.

## Surgical Resection (SR)

SR provides significant curative potential in well-selected patients, with 5-year survivals of 60% to 80% in optimal candidates. This remains the recommended first-line intervention in patients with solitary HCC and adequate hepatic reserve.[74,84] Critical factors considered in determining resectability include tumor biology (size and number of lesions, absence of vascular invasion, grade), technical considerations for resection (extent of resection and future liver remnant estimates, medical comorbidities to surgery), and current hepatic function (CTP score, evidence of portal hypertension).

In non-cirrhotic patients, extensive resections can be performed with acceptable morbidity and outcomes (30% to 50% 5-year survival), and surgery remains the standard of care in potentially resectable disease. In cirrhotic patients, optimal candidates are selected based on CTP-A hepatic function and absence of portal hypertension to minimize operative mortality. A careful assessment of underlying hepatic function, critical in determining surgical risk, can be refined beyond the CTP score with evaluation of portal hypertension as defined by hepatic venous pressure >10 mm Hg, platelet count <100,000 with associated splenomegaly, or using the indocyanine green retention rate at 15 minutes (ICGR 15%, often employed in Asia).[85] Current Western surgical standards in cirrhotic patients target 60% 5-year overall survival (OS) rates with perioperative mortality of 2% to 3%.[74]

Controversial topics include whether surgical resection (SR) should be performed in the setting of factors predicting poorer surgical outcomes and disease recurrence. While increased tumor size corresponds to microscopic vascular invasion and poorer survival rates, this is not typically considered a contraindication to surgery as an isolated factor.[86] Tumor multifocality (greater than three lesions), portal hypertension, limited vascular invasion, prior tumor rupture, and even CTP-B hepatic function suggest likelihood of poorer outcomes but may not represent absolute contraindications to surgery based on surgical series involving experienced surgeons at high-volume centers.[87] In many regions of Asia, the APASL guidelines are commonly employed, which promote more routine resection of multifocal disease if technically amenable and allow more clinical judgment in determining adequate hepatic reserve than the Western EASL/AASLD guidelines (often integrating information from ICGR 15% to predict hepatic reserve).[83,88] Regardless, in such high-risk populations, careful discussion in a multidisciplinary group setting remains critical in determining surgical candidacy.

Careful preoperative staging, including contrast-enhanced abdominal CT or MRI, chest CT, and bone scan, if clinically indicated, should be performed. If surgery is undertaken, anatomic resections are preferred with a goal of 2-cm margins if future liver remnant volumes allow. The role of preoperative portal vein embolization and minimally invasive techniques remains under investigation but show promise.[74] Despite surgical intervention, the majority of patients (approximately 50% to 70%) will unfortunately recur.[89] No definitive data exists to support adjuvant therapy after resection at this time.

## Percutaneous Ethanol Injection (PEI)

PEI involves insertion of a needle, typically under ultrasound guidance, into a liver lesion with subsequent injection of ethanol, leading to cellular dehydration, protein denaturation, chemical occlusion of tumor-feeding vessels, and ultimately coagulation necrosis of the tumor.[90]

This procedure is effective for treating small tumors (<2 cm) in patients who are not candidates for liver transplant or SR, and when more definitive local therapies such as radiofrequency ablation (RFA) are not possible. Among those with early-stage disease, treatment with PEI achieves complete tumor necrosis in 66% to 100% of cases and yields 3-year survival rates of 59% to 81%.[91–95] PEI is well tolerated, inexpensive, and relatively easy to perform and does not require general anesthesia.

Multiple limitations to PEI exist. This procedure is suboptimal for treating larger tumors, as its efficacy has been shown to decrease with increasing tumor size.[96] PEI is associated with relatively high rates of local recurrence; at 2 years, the local recurrence rate is up to 44% for tumors >3 cm and up to 27% for tumors <3 cm.[97,98] Finally, in order to achieve complete tumor necrosis, PEI may require multiple treatment sessions in contrast to radiofrequency ablation or other modalities.

## Radiofrequency Ablation (RFA)

RFA involves the placement of electrodes within a tumor to generate high-frequency alternating electric current, which subjects the target tissue to cytotoxic temperatures. RFA is typically performed via a percutaneous approach under ultrasound guidance, but may be performed intraoperatively. As thermal power decreases with increasing distance from the electrode, larger lesions (>3 cm) may be inadequately treated. Tumor location is critical, as RFA is less effective for tumors located near large vessels due to heat loss from perfusion-mediated tissue cooling.[99] The risk of incomplete ablation and of major complications increases when treating tumors near the gallbladder or in subcapsular locations.[99]

RFA is superior to PEI in the treatment of early-stage HCC, having replaced PEI in high-resource settings. Five randomized controlled trials (RCTs) comparing PEI to RFA in patients with early-stage HCC have all shown that RFA is associated with a higher rate of complete tumor necrosis and improved local disease control.[91–95] Three of the five studies documented a survival advantage with RFA, a finding that has been confirmed by three independent meta-analyses.[100–102] PEI, on the other hand, costs less than RFA (despite requiring more treatment sessions) and is associated with fewer major complications.[92,94]

SR and RFA likely yield similar long-term outcomes for patients with early-stage HCC. Shiina et al. conducted a prospective cohort study of 1,170 patients with HCC meeting Milan criteria who were either ineligible for or had declined SR and/or transplant and were instead treated with RFA.[89] In this study, 5- and 10-year OS rates were 60.2% and 27.3%, respectively, and the corresponding local tumor progression rates were both remarkably low at 3.2%. For those meeting criteria for SR, as per the BCLC classification system, the 5-year survival rate was even higher, at 76%.[103] Importantly, these outcomes are comparable to the 5- and 10-year survival rates reported for patients treated with resection alone, which have ranged from 34.4% to 70% and 10.5% to 52%, respectively.[89]

In addition to these observational data, RFA has been directly compared to SR in patients with early-stage HCC. Two randomized trials, including patients with HCC within Milan criteria, demonstrated that RFA and SR were equivalent with regard to disease-free and overall survival.[104,105] In the study by Chen et al., the 1- and 4-year disease-free survival rates were 87% and 52% versus 86% and 46% for SR and RFA, respectively. The corresponding 1- and 4-year survival rates were 93% and 64% versus 96% and 68%. Another randomized trial, however, found SR to be superior to RFA with regard to recurrence-free and overall survival.[106] Multiple non-randomized studies have also compared SR to RFA; Whereas some have found no difference in survival between these two treatment approaches,[107–110] others have demonstrated improved survival with SR.[111–113] Notably, in comparison to SR, RFA is associated with shorter treatment times, decreased length of hospital stay, fewer blood transfusions, and a lower complication rate, all of which contribute to its lower cost.[104–107,109,111–113]

Whether RFA can replace SR for patients with a solitary tumor and no significant liver disease remains an open question. In high-resource settings,

RFA is recommended as first-line treatment for patients with very early-stage HCC (single tumor <2 cm) who are not candidates for liver transplant, as well as for those with early-stage disease (single or three nodules <3 cm, CPT-A or B, PS 0) who are not candidates for SR or transplant.[103] In practice, however, RFA is increasingly being used in patients with small tumors, who are also suitable surgical candidates.

## Liver Transplantation for Hepatocellular Carcinoma

Orthotopic liver transplantation, when available, offers the possibility of curing malignancy and underlying cirrhosis. For patients within the classic Milan criteria (single tumor <5 cm or less than three tumors <3 cm without vascular invasion or extrahepatic disease), deceased donor liver transplantation is associated with 5-year survival rates of 65% to 78%, with reported 10-year survival rates of approximately 50%. Surgical series of patients within Milan criteria who instead underwent resection describe 5-year survival rates of up to 60% in comparison.[114,115] Disadvantages to transplantation include lack of donor livers leading to dropout from the waiting lists, requirement for long-term immunosuppression, cost, and perioperative mortality rates of approximately 3%.[116]

Areas of controversy in liver transplantation include whether patients with increased tumor volume or number might achieve similar survival benefit, one example being the UCSF criteria demonstrating promising outcomes despite less stringent criteria (single tumor <6.5 cm or two to three nodules <4.5 cm with cumulative volume <8 cm).[116,117] Whether expansion beyond the Milan criteria improves outcomes in an intention-to-treat analysis remains unclear and an area of intense research. Similarly, outcomes of patients downstaged to within Milan criteria require further study. Finally, living donor transplantation has been assessed as an alternative to deceased donor transplantation. While use of this technique continues in some regions, concerns have been raised in Western countries over the early reports of morbidity (2% life-threatening complications) and mortality (0.3%) to healthy donors,[118] although more recent Chinese experience is more encouraging.[118,119] This method remains an area of investigation, but use of living donors for patients outside of Milan criteria appears to be associated with poorer outcomes and uncertainty exists regarding how best to integrate this option into clinical care.[120]

## Conventional Transarterial Chemoembolization (cTACE) and Transarterial Embolization (TAE)

cTACE is a palliative technique widely used for patients with intermediate-stage HCC. In this procedure, a chemotherapy agent (typically doxorubicin or cisplatin in a lipid-based emulsion) is injected into the hepatic arterial vessels supplying the tumor. This is followed by injection of an embolic agent to obstruct arterial flow, thereby combining ischemic necrosis with the cytotoxic activity of a chemotherapeutic agent. cTACE is typically performed on more than one occasion, but the optimal treatment schedule has not been defined. TAE involves the injection of an embolic agent without chemotherapy. Although the definitive survival advantage of cTACE over embolization alone remains unclear, cTACE has been widely adopted around the world.

Two RCTs have shown that cTACE, as compared to conservative management, improves survival in selected patients with unresectable HCC.[90,121] In these two positive trials, the relative risk of death was 0.47[90] and 0.49,[121] favoring cTACE, with 2-year OS rates increasing 10% to 36%. Although several other RCTs have failed to demonstrate a survival advantage, all of the trials conducted to date have included different patient populations and have used different embolization techniques, treatment schedules, chemotherapy drugs and doses, and embolic particles, which likely account for the disparate results.[90,122–125] In a meta-analysis that included all but one of the earlier-referenced RCTs, cTACE was associated with a significant improvement in 2-year survival as compared to conservative management or suboptimal treatment (OR, 0.53).[126] In one recent prospective observational cohort from Japan, the median survival of 8,507 patients treated with cTACE was noted to be 2.74 years, suggesting survival estimates may be improving in comparison to older studies.[122]

Not all patients with localized, unresectable HCC benefit equally from cTACE, and careful patient selection is important.[123] Currently, cTACE is recommended for patients with intermediate-stage disease, as defined by the BCLC staging system (i.e., patients with large and/or multinodular tumors, CTP-A or B cirrhosis, and ECOG PS 0).[103] Patients with intermediate-stage disease, however, represent a heterogeneous group with varying degrees of tumor burden and liver dysfunction. Per expert consensus, absolute contraindications to cTACE include decompensated cirrhosis, extensive tumor burden with replacement of both lobes of the liver, severely reduced portal vein flow, technical contraindications (e.g., arteriovenous fistula), and significant renal insufficiency.[123] Optimal cTACE candidates include patients with CPT-A cirrhosis and multifocal HCC without vascular invasion, and initial radiographic response to therapy predicts survival benefit. Notably, catheter-based therapies such as cTACE are commonly employed in Asia despite focal vascular tumor invasion as evidenced by the APASL treatment guidelines, but definitive data to support this consensus recommendation is lacking. Factors associated with worse outcomes among patients undergoing cTACE include ascites, elevated AFP (>400 ng/mL), poor performance status (WHO PS 1–4), age >60, *greater than or equal to three* liver lesions, tumor size >10 cm, and diffusely infiltrative tumor.[123]

cTACE is associated with known toxicities, with post-embolization syndrome (usually self-limited episode of fever, abdominal pain, and nausea) being the most common, occurring in 35% to 100% of patients.[123] In one meta-analysis, the mean rate of severe adverse events (AEs) was 5.6% (range 0% to 50%), and death within 30 days of cTACE occurred in 0% to 10% of cases.[124] Other potential complications include transient deterioration in liver function, development of ascites, and gastrointestinal bleeding. Liver failure following cTACE is relatively rare, but is more likely in patients with baseline elevation in total bilirubin, prolonged prothrombin time, and more advanced cirrhosis.[125]

## Drug Eluting Bead TACE (DEB-TACE)

DEBs are biocompatible, nonresorbable hydrogel beads impregnated with doxorubicin, which are injected into the arterial vessels supplying a tumor. In addition to obstructing flow, these beads release doxorubicin in a slow, sustained fashion, achieving high intra-tumoral concentration of drug, while minimizing systemic exposure.[127,128]

DEB-TACE has been compared to cTACE, with promising trends toward improved tolerance and efficacy. In a randomized trial conducted in Europe, which included patients with CPT-A or B cirrhosis and large and/or multinodular, unresectable HCC, there was a nonsignificant trend toward improved response with DEB-TACE (52% vs. 44% for DEB-TACE vs. cTACE, respectively; p = 0.11).[129] In the subgroup of patients with more advanced disease (CPT-B, ECOG 1, bilobar, or recurrent disease), however, DEB-TACE achieved significantly better objective response and disease control rates. DEB-TACE was also associated with less liver toxicity and fewer doxorubicin-related AEs. In another large, case–control study performed in Asia, patients who received DEB-TACE had a higher rate of complete response, as well as improved time to disease progression and OS compared to those who underwent cTACE.[130] One registry from Barcelona, including mainly CTP-A patients with BCLC stage A/B disease, noted an encouraging median OS of 48 months.[131] Based on these and other studies, DEB-TACE is increasingly used as the first-line transcatheter approach for selected patients with unresectable HCC.

## Transarterial Radioembolization (TARE)

TARE utilizes micron-sized embolic particles loaded with a radioisotope, most commonly Yttrium-90 ($^{90}$Y). These particles are injected into the arterial vessels supplying a tumor, exposing the tumor to high doses of radiation, while mostly sparing normal liver parenchyma, which receives most of its blood supply from the portal vein.

TARE appears to be safe and well tolerated in patients with unresectable HCC, including those with portal vein thrombosis.[132–136] A mild post-embolization syndrome, characterized by fatigue, fever, and abdominal discomfort occurs in 20% to 55% of patients.[137] Transient hyperbilirubinemia and lymphopenia are also common. Severe complications, such as gastrointestinal ulceration, radiation pneumonitis and radiation-induced liver disease, are rare.[137]

Multiple retrospective and prospective studies have demonstrated good antitumor efficacy with TARE.[134–136,138] Some have even suggested that TARE may be superior[139] or at least equivalent[140,141] to TACE, but randomized studies are lacking. The role of TARE in the treatment of patients with focal vascular invasion, large and/or multifocal HCC not amenable to curative therapy, remains to be defined through ongoing randomized phase 3 trials.

## Systemic Therapy

The majority of patients present with advanced HCC not amenable to any potentially curative approach. Of those who are initially candidates for locoregional treatment, the majority will relapse. Systemic therapy plays a palliative role in appropriately selected patients with metastatic disease or in those patients refractory to locoregional therapeutic interventions.

Many cytotoxic chemotherapy agents have been studied in patients with advanced HCC, the most promising of which has been doxorubicin. Response rates to doxorubicin, however, are relatively low, in the 10% to 20% range.[142–145] Moreover, when compared to best supportive care, doxorubicin has been shown to improve survival in only one study, and the benefit, though statistically significant, was minimal (10.6 vs. 7.5 weeks; p = 0.036).[142] Combination regimens, including FOLFOX (5-FU and oxaliplatin) and PIAF (cisplatin, interferon, doxorubicin, and 5-FU) have also been studied, and although they may increase response rates, they are also associated with significant toxicity and have not been shown to confer a definitive survival advantage over single-agent chemotherapy.[103,146] Multiple noncytotoxic agents, including tamoxifen, octreotide, and antiandrogens, have also failed to improve outcomes.[74]

As our understanding of the genetic and molecular alterations driving HCC has improved, attention has turned to targeted therapies. Sorafenib is an oral multikinase inhibitor, which inhibits Raf-1, BRAF, vascular endothelial growth factor receptor (VEGFR), and platelet-derived growth factor receptor-$\beta$ (PDGFR-$\beta$). Signaling through the Raf-1 and VEGF pathways appears to play a role in HCC carcinogenesis, making sorafenib a potentially useful agent.[147]

The Sorafenib HCC Assessment Randomized Protocol (SHARP) was a large randomized, double-blind, placebo-controlled trial designed to evaluate the safety and efficacy of sorafenib in patients with advanced HCC who had not previously received systemic therapy.[147] To be eligible, patients were also required to have CPT-A cirrhosis and a good performance status (ECOG PS 0–2). In this population, sorafenib was associated with statistically improved time to disease progression (5.5 vs. 2.8 months) and OS (10.7 vs. 7.9 months) despite response rates of 2%. Grade 3 hand-foot skin reactions (HFSRs) and diarrhea did occur significantly more often in the sorafenib arm. While the SHARP trial included mostly North American and European patients with HCV- or alcohol-related cirrhosis, the efficacy and safety of sorafenib have also been established in an Asian, HBV-infected population, where median OS was extended from 4.2 to 6.5 months with sorafenib therapy.[148] In addition, in an economic evaluation of sorafenib, this drug was found to be cost-effective when compared to best supportive care in a high-resource setting.[149] For patients with advanced-stage HCC, sorafenib is now considered the standard of care. It is worth noting that the benefit of sorafenib in patients with more advanced liver disease has not been established, and use in CPT-B patients represents an extrapolation of existing data.

Experimental agents and new combinations are being rigorously assessed given the substantial clinical need. The combination of sorafenib and doxorubicin is currently under evaluation in randomized phase 3 trials against a sorafenib control group based on promising initial randomized phase 2 data comparing the combination to doxorubicin alone.[150] In this phase 2 study, the combination arm was associated with a significant improvement in both time to progression (TTP) (6.4 vs. 2.8 months) and OS (13.7 vs. 6.5 months) as compared to doxorubicin. These results, while encouraging, came at the cost of moderate toxicity, with almost 50% of patients developing grade 3 or 4 hematologic AEs and 19% experiencing a decline in left ventricular systolic function.

Newer targeted agents in development have shown promise in early-phase studies. In a randomized, placebo-controlled phase 2 trial including patients with unresectable HCC, treatment with an oral c-met inhibitor was associated with improved survival compared to placebo among the approximately 60% of patients with MET-high tumors (7.2 vs. 3.8 months, respectively; HR 0.38; p = 0.01).[151] Notably, the median OS of patients with low MET expression randomized to placebo was 9 months. Thus, in addition to confirming the poor survival of patients with high as compared to low MET expression, this study suggests that the negative prognostic impact of MET over-expression could largely be reversed with a targeted inhibitor. Subsequent trials exploring c-met inhibition are under way and may eventually lead to biomarker-driven selection of systemic therapy in time. Additional areas of clinical research include optimization of anti-angiogenic therapy and early assessment of immune modulators such as CTLA-4 and PD1 inhibitors.

Finally, there is growing interest in the use of targeted therapies in conjunction with locoregional treatments to prevent or delay recurrence in patients with earlier-stage HCC. In one recent study, 307 patients with intermediate-stage HCC (BCLC B) were randomized to DEB-TACE in combination with sorafenib versus placebo.[152] The sorafenib arm was associated with a trend toward improved TTP (HR 0.80; 95% CI 0.588 to 1.080; p = 0.072), but the combination increased toxicity as expected without preliminary evidence of improved OS. Additional investigation is required before this strategy can be adopted into routine clinical practice; the results of ongoing phase 3 studies are eagerly awaited. The benefit of sorafenib after SR or RFA is also being evaluated in a phase 3 trial, with initial results pending. Thus, although theoretically promising, the role of sorafenib in combination with localized therapies or in the adjuvant setting remains unclear at this time.

## Palliative Care and Symptom Management

The majority of patients present with advanced HCC, which is not curable. The median survival for these patients is 2 to 4 years for those receiving palliative catheter-based therapy and 6 to 11 months for those with vascular invasion and/or metastatic disease. In addition, symptoms related to tumor burden, underlying cirrhosis, and/or treatment are common among patients with HCC. Thus, effective palliation of symptoms is critical in the management of patients with HCC.

Pain is common among patients with HCC. In a cohort of patients with advanced HCC admitted to a hospice ward in Taiwan, 76% reported pain at the time of presentation.[153] The majority described abdominal pain, characterized as a dull visceral discomfort. Bony pain was also relatively common in this cohort, reflecting the tendency of HCC to metastasize to bone.

Opioids represent the mainstay of treatment for pain due to HCC, but careful attention to drug selection and dosing is required. In the setting of hepatic impairment, fentanyl and methadone can be safely used, and oxycodone can be used with caution. Drugs with significant hepatic metabolism that should be avoided, if possible, include morphine, codeine, meperidine, and propoxyphene. Patients should also be cautioned against taking acetaminophen-containing regimens and should use nonsteroidal anti-inflammatory medications with care. When starting an opioid in a patient with severe liver dysfunction, the usual dose of the drug should be reduced by 50% and the dosing interval increased. For those with pain related to bony metastases, single dose or abbreviated radiation schedules can provide effective palliation of pain in approximately 80% of patients, as HCC has proven to be an exquisitely radiosensitive disease.[154]

Other symptoms commonly associated with advanced HCC include fatigue, anorexia, vomiting, cachexia, and symptoms related to hepatic decompensation such as ascites, variceal bleeding, peripheral edema, and hepatic encephalopathy.[153] These symptoms should be managed with usual supportive care measures, including lactulose and diuretic therapies. In the setting of hepatic decompensation, the possibility of spontaneous bacterial peritonitis should be considered and pursued.

In addition to cancer- and cirrhosis-related symptoms, patients with advanced HCC must also contend with the side effects of treatment. In the landmark study that established sorafenib as the standard of care for patients with advanced HCC, HFSR was one of the most common sorafenib-related AEs, occurring in 21% of patients.[147] Other common side effects included fatigue, diarrhea, nausea, anorexia, and weight loss. Based on recent randomized data from China, patients beginning sorafenib should be counseled to use a urea-based cream twice daily to minimize HFSR.[155] In addition, antidiarrheals and antiemetics, to be used on an as-needed basis, should be provided in conjunction with sorafenib. Finally, dose reductions and/or interruptions with subsequent reintroduction are often required to manage sorafenib-related toxicities.

## GLOBAL STRATEGIES TO OPTIMIZE TREATMENT

HCC is a global epidemic, with the majority of global cases affecting low- to moderate-resource regions. Despite multiple advances in early diagnosis and treatment, the majority of cases arise in regions of limited resources. Such patients, who often present symptomatically with vascular invasion or metastatic disease, harbor the least favorable prognosis, and therapy is palliative in nature with a median survival of 6 to 11 months. Introduction of rigorous screening programs for high-risk individuals can identify those patients amenable to more definitive therapy such as SR, ablative therapy, or transplant, where 5-year survival rates may reach 50% to 80% in early-stage patients. For those patients with multifocal HCC not amenable to definitive therapy, treatment with catheter-based therapy prolongs survival, with median OS in the range 24 to 48 months.

Current guidelines apply to high-resource settings, but implementation in the low- to moderate-resource settings where most patients are diagnosed remains a substantial challenge. General recommendations based on available resources have been developed by the World Gastroenterology Organization, which define minimal-resource settings as those in which treatment options are extremely limited and medium-resource settings as those in which both resection and ablation are available, but liver transplantation is not. High-resource settings are defined by the availability of liver transplantation.[156]

In minimal-resource settings, where adequate cross-sectional imaging and definitive local therapy are not routinely available, the morbidity and mortality associated with HCC can be addressed in a cost-effective manner by implementing primary prevention–oriented public health measures, including hepatitis B vaccination programs such as newborn vaccination programs, food storage programs for aflatoxin control, and health education and health-care programs to minimize the spread of viral hepatitis. Treatment of HBV infection should be considered, if indicated, although costs of therapy remain prohibitive in many regions. Even if the medical expertise and imaging technology required for HCC surveillance are available, mass screening is recommended only in areas where resection or ablation could be offered to those diagnosed with early-stage disease. With regard to management of patients diagnosed with HCC in minimal-resource settings, the focus is on supportive care. Sorafenib, reportedly available in generic form in some regions for $600/year, remains costly and of modest benefit.

While primary HCC prevention strategies remain critical, surveillance programs represent a dominant shift in strategy toward early intervention in medium-resource settings where curative treatments are available. For those diagnosed with HCC, SR, ablation, TACE, and systemic therapy should be considered. Development of regional centers of excellence in such settings can minimize equipment costs while facilitating better patient selection for appropriate interventions. Infrastructure development, including ultrasound screening programs and the associated interventions, comes with a predictable increase in expenditure for the associated medical gains. One illustrative example by Taiwanese researchers evaluated medical resource consumption by patients with HCC undergoing RFA. This analysis demonstrated a striking increase in the use of RFA over the time period studied, with 238 procedures performed in 2002 compared to 1,941 in 2006. The mean cost of hospitalization for a patient undergoing RFA was $1,403, and annual expenditures rose 900% over a 4-year period. The authors concluded that although there is an important role for RFA in the management of HCC, the cost of this procedure is placing a major strain on the Taiwanese health-care budget.[157]

In the high-resource setting, careful attention to appropriate regional guidelines such as EASL/EORTC or APASL is warranted.[74,83] Comprehensive programs aimed at early identification and treatment of individuals who may benefit from antiviral therapy should be supported, and efforts to increase participation in HCC screening should be a priority. A critical need to transition infrastructure and training to regions of the world most affected by HCC remains. Providing tools for primary prevention and interventional therapy to minimal-resource regions at acceptable cost remains a global health imperative and should be a primary goal of future clinical research endeavors in the field.

## REFERENCES

1. Ferlay J, Shin HR, Bray F, Forman D, Mathers C, Parkin DM. GLOBOCAN 2008 v2.0, Cancer Incidence and Mortality Worldwide: IARC CancerBase No. 102010, May 30, 2013.

2. Lozano R, Naghavi M, Foreman K, et al. Global and regional mortality from 235 causes of death for 20 age groups in 1990 and 2010: a systematic analysis for the Global Burden of Disease Study 2010. *Lancet* 2012 Dec 15; 380(9859): 2095–128.

3. El-Serag HB, Rudolph KL. Hepatocellular carcinoma: epidemiology and molecular carcinogenesis. *Gastroenterology* 2007 Jun; 132(7): 2557–76.

4. Altekruse SF, McGlynn KA, Reichman ME. Hepatocellular carcinoma incidence, mortality, and survival trends in the United States from 1975 to 2005. *J Clin Oncol* 2009 Mar 20; 27(9): 1485–91.

5. El-Serag HB. Hepatocellular carcinoma: recent trends in the United States. *Gastroenterology* 2004 Nov; 127(5 Suppl 1): S27–S34.

6. El-Serag HB. Epidemiology of hepatocellular carcinoma in USA. *Hepatol Res* 2007 Sep; 37(Suppl 2): S88–S94.

7. Gao S, Yang WS, Bray F, et al. Declining rates of hepatocellular carcinoma in urban Shanghai: incidence trends in 1976–2005. *Eur J Epidemiol* 2012 Jan; 27(1): 39–46.

8. Evans AA, O'Connell AP, Pugh JC, et al. Geographic variation in viral load among hepatitis B carriers with differing risks of hepatocellular carcinoma. *Cancer Epidemiol Biomarkers Prev* 1998 Jul; 7(7): 559–65.

9. Yang JD, Roberts LR. Hepatocellular carcinoma: a global view. *Nat Rev Gastroenterol Hepatol* 2010 Aug; 7(8): 448–58.

10. El-Serag HB. Epidemiology of viral hepatitis and hepatocellular carcinoma. *Gastroenterology* 2012 May; 142(6): 1264–73 e1.

11. Edmunds WJ, Medley GF, Nokes DJ, Hall AJ, Whittle HC. The influence of age on the development of the hepatitis B carrier state. *Proc Biol Sci* 1993 Aug 23; 253(1337): 197–201.

12. Barazani Y, Hiatt JR, Tong MJ, Busuttil RW. Chronic viral hepatitis and hepatocellular carcinoma. *World J Surg* 2007 Jun; 31(6): 1243–48.

13. McGlynn KA, London WT. The global epidemiology of hepatocellular carcinoma: present and future. *Clin Liver Dis* 2011 May; 15(2): 223–43, vii-x.

14. Bosch FX, Ribes J, Diaz M, Cleries R. Primary liver cancer: worldwide incidence and trends. *Gastroenterology* 2004 Nov; 127(5 Suppl 1): S5–S16.

15. Parkin DM. The global health burden of infection-associated cancers in the year 2002. *Int J Cancer* 2006 Jun 15; 118(12): 3030–44.

16. Arzumanyan A, Reis HM, Feitelson MA. Pathogenic mechanisms in HBV- and HCV-associated hepatocellular carcinoma. *Nat Rev Cancer* 2013 Feb; 13(2): 123–35.

17. Feitelson MA. Hepatitis B virus in hepatocarcinogenesis. *J Cell Physiol* 1999 Nov; 181(2): 188–202.

18. Beasley RP, Hwang LY, Lin CC, Chien CS. Hepatocellular carcinoma and hepatitis B virus. A prospective study of 22 707 men in Taiwan. *Lancet* 1981 Nov 21; 2(8256): 1129–33.

19. Evans AA, Chen G, Ross EA, Shen FM, Lin WY, London WT. Eight-year follow-up of the 90,000-person Haimen City cohort: I. Hepatocellular carcinoma

mortality, risk factors, and gender differences. *Cancer Epidemiol Biomarkers Prev* 2002 Apr; 11(4): 369–76.

20. Chen JD, Yang HI, Iloeje UH, et al. Carriers of inactive hepatitis B virus are still at risk for hepatocellular carcinoma and liver-related death. *Gastroenterology* 2010 May; 138(5): 1747–54.

21. Simonetti J, Bulkow L, McMahon BJ, et al. Clearance of hepatitis B surface antigen and risk of hepatocellular carcinoma in a cohort chronically infected with hepatitis B virus. *Hepatology* 2010 May; 51(5): 1531–37.

22. Donato F, Boffetta P, Puoti M. A meta-analysis of epidemiological studies on the combined effect of hepatitis B and C virus infections in causing hepatocellular carcinoma. *Int J Cancer.* 1998 Jan 30; 75(3): 347–54.

23. Leone N, Rizzetto M. Natural history of hepatitis C virus infection: from chronic hepatitis to cirrhosis, to hepatocellular carcinoma. *Minerva Gastroenterol Dietol* 2005 Mar; 51(1): 31–46.

24. Di Bisceglie AM, Lyra AC, Schwartz M, et al. Hepatitis C-related hepatocellular carcinoma in the United States: influence of ethnic status. *Am J Gastroenterol* 2003 Sep; 98(9): 2060–63.

25. Control CfD. CDC. Viral Hepatitis Statistics and Surveillance, United States, 2009–2011, 2013 [cited July 4, 2013]. Available at http://www.cdc.gov/hepatitis/Statistics/index.htm.

26. Mohd Hanafiah K, Groeger J, Flaxman AD, Wiersma ST. Global epidemiology of hepatitis C virus infection: new estimates of age-specific antibody to HCV seroprevalence. *Hepatology* 2013 Apr; 57(4): 1333–42.

27. Sun CA, Wu DM, Lin CC, et al. Incidence and cofactors of hepatitis C virus-related hepatocellular carcinoma: a prospective study of 12,008 men in Taiwan. *Am J Epidemiol* 2003 Apr 15; 157(8): 674–82.

28. Bahri O, Ezzikouri S, Alaya-Bouafif NB, et al. First multicenter study for risk factors for hepatocellular carcinoma development in North Africa. *World J Hepatol* 2011 Jan 27; 3(1): 24–30.

29. Williams JH, Phillips TD, Jolly PE, Stiles JK, Jolly CM, Aggarwal D. Human aflatoxicosis in developing countries: a review of toxicology, exposure, potential health consequences, and interventions. *Am J Clin Nutr* 2004 Nov; 80(5): 1106–22.

30. Gursoy-Yuzugullu O, Yuzugullu H, Yilmaz M, Ozturk M. Aflatoxin genotoxicity is associated with a defective DNA damage response bypassing p53 activation. *Liver Int* 2011 Apr; 31 (4): 561–71.

31. Ozturk M. p53 mutation in hepatocellular carcinoma after aflatoxin exposure. *Lancet* 1991 Nov 30; 338(8779): 1356–59.

32. Liu Y, Chang C-CH, Marsh GM, Wu F. Population attributable risk of aflatoxin-related liver cancer: systematic review and meta-analysis. *Eur J Cancer* 2012 Sep; 48(14): 2125–36.

33. El-Serag HB, Mason AC. Risk factors for the rising rates of primary liver cancer in the United States. *Arch Intern Med* 2000 Nov 27; 160(21): 3227–30.

34. Liao SF, Yang HI, Lee MH, Chen CJ, Lee WC. Fifteen-year population attributable fractions and causal pies of risk factors for newly developed hepatocellular carcinomas in 11,801 men in Taiwan. *PloS One* 2012; 7(4): e34779.

35. Donato F, Tagger A, Gelatti U, et al. Alcohol and hepatocellular carcinoma: the effect of lifetime intake and hepatitis virus infections in men and women. *Am J Epidemiol* 2002 Feb 15; 155(4): 323–31.

36. Yuan JM, Govindarajan S, Arakawa K, Yu MC. Synergism of alcohol, diabetes, and viral hepatitis on the risk of hepatocellular carcinoma in blacks and whites in the U.S. *Cancer* 2004 Sep 1; 101(5): 1009–17.

37. Brunt EM. Nonalcoholic steatohepatitis: definition and pathology. *Semin Liver Dis* 2001; 21(1): 3–16.

38. Matteoni CA, Younossi ZM, Gramlich T, Boparai N, Liu YC, McCullough AJ. Nonalcoholic fatty liver disease: a spectrum of clinical and pathological severity. *Gastroenterology* 1999 Jun; 116(6): 1413–19.

39. Vernon G, Baranova A, Younossi ZM. Systematic review: the epidemiology and natural history of non-alcoholic fatty liver disease and non-alcoholic steato-hepatitis in adults. *Aliment Pharmacol Ther* 2011 Aug; 34(3): 274–85.

40. Browning JD, Szczepaniak LS, Dobbins R, et al. Prevalence of hepatic steatosis in an urban population in the United States: impact of ethnicity. *Hepatology* 2004 Dec; 40(6): 1387–95.

41. Williams CD, Stengel J, Asike MI, et al. Prevalence of nonalcoholic fatty liver disease and nonalcoholic steatohepatitis among a largely middle-aged population utilizing ultrasound and liver biopsy: a prospective study. *Gastroenterology* 2011 Jan; 140(1): 124–31.

42. Sanyal A, Poklepovic A, Moyneur E, Barghout V. Population-based risk factors and resource utilization for HCC: US perspective. *Curr Med Res Opin* 2010 Sep; 26(9): 2183–91.

43. Sherman M, Bruix J, Porayko M, Tran T, AASLD Practice Guidelines Committee. Screening for hepatocellular carcinoma: the rationale for the American Association for the Study of Liver Diseases recommendations. *Hepatology* 2012; 56(3): 793–96.

44. Kane M. Global programme for control of hepatitis B infection. *Vaccine* 1995; 13(Suppl 1): S47–S49.

45. Kane MA. Preventing cancer with vaccines: progress in the global control of cancer. *Cancer Prev Res* (Philadelphia, Pa) 2012 Jan; 5(1): 24–29.

46. Chang MH, Chen CJ, Lai MS, et al. Universal hepatitis B vaccination in Taiwan and the incidence of hepatocellular carcinoma in children. Taiwan Childhood Hepatoma Study Group. *N Engl J Med* 1997 Jun 26; 336(26): 1855–59.

47. Chang MH, You SL, Chen CJ, et al. Decreased incidence of hepatocellular carcinoma in hepatitis B vaccinees: a 20-year follow-up study. *J Natl Cancer Inst* 2009 Oct 7; 101(19): 1348–55.

48. Hsu HM, Chen DS, Chuang CH, et al. Efficacy of a mass hepatitis B vaccination program in Taiwan. Studies on 3464 infants of hepatitis B surface antigen-carrier mothers. *JAMA* 1988 Oct 21; 260(15): 2231–35.

49. Ni YH, Chang MH, Wu JF, Hsu HY, Chen HL, Chen DS. Minimization of hepatitis B infection by a 25-year universal vaccination program. *J Hepatol* 2012 Oct; 57(4): 730–35.

50. Zou S, Stramer SL, Dodd RY. Donor testing and risk: current prevalence, incidence, and residual risk of transfusion-transmissible agents in US allogeneic donations. *Transfus Med Rev* 2012 Apr; 26(2): 119–28.

51. Zou S, Stramer SL, Notari EP, et al. Current incidence and residual risk of hepatitis B infection among blood donors in the United States. *Transfusion* 2009 Aug; 49(8): 1609–20.

52. Fattovich G, Giustina G, Realdi G, Corrocher R, Schalm SW. Long-term outcome of hepatitis B e antigen-positive patients with compensated cirrhosis treated with interferon alfa. European Concerted Action on Viral Hepatitis (EUROHEP). *Hepatology* 1997 Nov; 26(5): 1338–42.

53. Lin SM, Sheen IS, Chien RN, Chu CM, Liaw YF. Long-term beneficial effect of interferon therapy in patients with chronic hepatitis B virus infection. *Hepatology* 1999 Mar; 29(3): 971–75.

54. Tangkijvanich P, Thong-ngam D, Mahachai V, Kladchareon N, Suwangool P, Kullavanijaya P. Long-term effect of interferon therapy on incidence of cirrhosis and hepatocellular carcinoma in Thai patients with chronic hepatitis B. *Southeast Asian J Trop Med Public Health* 2001 Sep; 32(3): 452–58.

55. Liaw Y-F, Sung JJY, Chow WC, et al. Lamivudine for patients with chronic hepatitis B and advanced liver disease. *N Engl J Med* 2004; 351(15): 1521–31.

56. Sung JJ, Tsoi KK, Wong VW, Li KC, Chan HL. Meta-analysis: treatment of hepatitis B infection reduces risk of hepatocellular carcinoma. *Aliment Pharmacol Ther* 2008 Nov 1; 28(9): 1067–77.

57. Chen TM, Chang CC, Huang PT, Wen CF, Lin CC. Performance of Risk Estimation for Hepatocellular Carcinoma in Chronic Hepatitis B (REACH-B) score in classifying treatment eligibility under 2012 Asian Pacific Association for the Study of the Liver (APASL) guideline for chronic hepatitis B patients. *Aliment Pharmacol Ther* 2013; 37(2): 243–51.

58. Camma C, Giunta M, Andreone P, Craxi A. Interferon and prevention of hepatocellular carcinoma in viral cirrhosis: an evidence-based approach. *J Hepatol* 2001 Apr; 34(4): 593–602.

59. Papatheodoridis GV, Papadimitropoulos VC, Hadziyannis SJ. Effect of interferon therapy on the development of hepatocellular carcinoma in patients with hepatitis C virus-related cirrhosis: a meta-analysis. *Aliment Pharmacol Ther* 2001 May; 15(5): 689–98.

60. Singal AK, Singh A, Jaganmohan S, et al. Antiviral therapy reduces risk of hepatocellular carcinoma in patients with hepatitis C virus-related cirrhosis. *Clinical Gastroenterol Hepatol* 2010 Feb; 8(2): 192–99.

61. Shiratori Y, Ito Y, Yokosuka O, et al. Antiviral therapy for cirrhotic hepatitis C: association with reduced hepatocellular carcinoma development and improved survival. *Ann Intern Med* 2005 Jan 18; 142(2): 105–14.

62. Jacobson IM, McHutchison JG, Dusheiko G, et al. Telaprevir for previously untreated chronic hepatitis C virus infection. *N Engl J Med* 2011 Jun 23; 364(25): 2405–16.

63. Poordad F, McCone J Jr, Bacon BR, et al. Boceprevir for untreated chronic HCV genotype 1 infection. *N Engl J Med* 2011 Mar 31; 364(13): 1195–206.

64. Brown RL, Chen ZY, Warburton M, et al. Discovery and characterization of proteins associated with aflatoxin-resistance: evaluating their potential as breeding markers. *Toxins* 2010 Apr; 2(4): 919–33.

65. Menkir A, Brown RL, Bandyopadhyay R, Chen ZY, Cleveland TE. A USA-Africa collaborative strategy for identifying, characterizing, and developing maize germplasm with resistance to aflatoxin contamination. *Mycopathologia* 2006 Sep; 162(3): 225–32.

66. Turner PC, Sylla A, Gong YY, et al. Reduction in exposure to carcinogenic afla-toxins by postharvest intervention measures in west Africa: a community-based intervention study. *Lancet* 2005 Jun 4–10; 365(9475): 1950–56.

67. Kabak B, Dobson AD. Biological strategies to counteract the effects of mycotox-ins. *J Food Prot* 2009 Sep; 72 (9): 2006–16.

68. Kabak B, Dobson AD, Var I. Strategies to prevent mycotoxin contamination of food and animal feed: a review. *Crit Rev Food Sci Nutr* 2006; 46(8): 593–619.

69. Kumar M, Verma V, Nagpal R, et al. Effect of probiotic fermented milk and chlo-rophyllin on gene expressions and genotoxicity during AFB(1)-induced hepa-tocellular carcinoma. *Gene* 2011 Dec 15; 490(1–2): 54–59.

70. Bhat G, Baba CS, Pandey A, Kumari N, Choudhuri G. Life style modification improves insulin resistance and liver histology in patients with non-alcoholic fatty liver disease. *World J Hepatol* 2012 Jul 27; 4(7): 209–17.

71. Keating SE, Hackett DA, George J, Johnson NA. Exercise and non-alcoholic fatty liver disease: a systematic review and meta-analysis. *J Hepatol* 2012 Jul; 57(1): 157–66.

72. Rodriguez B, Torres DM, Harrison SA. Physical activity: an essential component of lifestyle modification in NAFLD. *Nat Rev Gastroenterol Hepatol* 2012 Dec; 9(12): 726–31.

73. Thoma C, Day CP, Trenell MI. Lifestyle interventions for the treatment of non-alcoholic fatty liver disease in adults: a systematic review. *J Hepatol* 2012 Jan; 56(1): 255–66.

74. European Association for the Study of the Liver, European Organisation for Re-search and Treatment of Cancer. EASL–EORTC Clinical Practice Guidelines: management of hepatocellular carcinoma. *J Hepatol* 2012 Apr; 56(4): 908–43.

75. Zhang B-H, Yang B-H, Tang Z-Y. Randomized controlled trial of screening for hepatocellular carcinoma. *J Cancer Res Clin Oncol* 2004 Jul; 130(7): 417–22. English.

76. Bolondi L. Screening for hepatocellular carcinoma in cirrhosis. *J Hepatol* 2003 Dec; 39(6): 1076–84.

77. Singal A, Volk ML, Waljee A, et al. Meta-analysis: surveillance with ultrasound for early-stage hepatocellular carcinoma in patients with cirrhosis. *Aliment Pharmacol Ther* 2009; 30(1): 37–47.

78. Santi V, Trevisani F, Gramenzi A, et al. Semiannual surveillance is superior to annual surveillance for the detection of early hepatocellular carcinoma and patient survival. *J Hepatol* 2010 Aug/; 53(2): 291–97.

79. Zhang B, Yang B. Combined α fetoprotein testing and ultrasonography as a screening test for primary liver cancer. *J Med Screen* 1999 June 1, 1999; 6(2): 108–10.

80. Radiology ACo. Liver Imaging Reporting and Data System (LI-RADS) version 2013.1, 2013. Available at www.acr.org/Quality-Safety/Resources/LIRADS/Archive/.

81. Tang A, Cruite I, Sirlin CB. Toward a standardized system for hepatocellular carcinoma diagnosis using computed tomography and MRI. *Expert Rev Gastro-enterol Hepatol* 2013 Mar; 7(3): 269–79.

82. Kudo M, Izumi N, Kokudo N, et al. Management of Hepatocellular Carcinoma in Japan: Consensus-Based Clinical Practice Guidelines proposed by the Japan

Society of Hepatology (JSH) 2010 updated version. *Dig Dis* 2011; 29(3): 339–64.

83. Omata M, Lesmana LA, Tateishi R, et al. Asian Pacific Association for the Study of the Liver consensus recommendations on hepatocellular carcinoma. *Hepatol Int* 2010; 4(2): 439–74.

84. Poon RT, Ng IO, Fan ST, et al. Clinicopathologic features of long-term survivors and disease-free survivors after resection of hepatocellular carcinoma: a study of a prospective cohort. *J Clin Oncol* 2001 Jun 15; 19(12): 3037–44.

85. Rahbari NN, Mehrabi A, Mollberg NM, et al. Hepatocellular carcinoma: current management and perspectives for the future. *Ann Surg* 2011 Mar; 253(3): 453–69.

86. Ikai I, Arii S, Kojiro M, et al. Reevaluation of prognostic factors for survival after liver resection in patients with hepatocellular carcinoma in a Japanese nationwide survey. *Cancer* 2004 Aug 15; 101(4): 796–802.

87. Ishizawa T, Hasegawa K, Aoki T, et al. Neither multiple tumors nor portal hypertension are surgical contraindications for hepatocellular carcinoma. *Gastroenterology* 2008 Jun; 134(7): 1908–16.

88. Chow PK-H. Resection for hepatocellular carcinoma: is it justifiable to restrict this to the American Association for the Study of the Liver/Barcelona Clinic for Liver Cancer criteria? *J Gastroenterol Hepatol* 2012; 27(3): 452–57.

89. Shiina S, Tateishi R, Arano T, et al. Radiofrequency ablation for hepatocellular carcinoma: 10-year outcome and prognostic factors. *Am J Gastroenterol* 2012 Apr; 107(4): 569–77; quiz 78.

90. Llovet JM, Real MI, Montana X, et al. Arterial embolisation or chemoembolisation versus symptomatic treatment in patients with unresectable hepatocellular carcinoma: a randomised controlled trial. *Lancet* 2002 May 18; 359(9319): 1734–39.

91. Lencioni RA, Allgaier HP, Cioni D, et al. Small hepatocellular carcinoma in cirrhosis: randomized comparison of radio-frequency thermal ablation versus percutaneous ethanol injection. *Radiology* 2003 Jul; 228(1): 235–40.

92. Lin SM, Lin CJ, Lin CC, Hsu CW, Chen YC. Radiofrequency ablation improves prognosis compared with ethanol injection for hepatocellular carcinoma < or =4 cm. *Gastroenterology* 2004 Dec; 127(6): 1714–23.

93. Shiina S, Teratani T, Obi S, et al. A randomized controlled trial of radiofrequency ablation with ethanol injection for small hepatocellular carcinoma. *Gastroenterology* 2005 Jul; 129(1): 122–30.

94. Lin SM, Lin CJ, Lin CC, Hsu CW, Chen YC. Randomised controlled trial comparing percutaneous radiofrequency thermal ablation, percutaneous ethanol injection, and percutaneous acetic acid injection to treat hepatocellular carcinoma of 3 cm or less. *Gut* 2005 Aug; 54(8): 1151–56. Pubmed Central PMCID: 1774888.

95. Brunello F, Veltri A, Carucci P, et al. Radiofrequency ablation versus ethanol injection for early hepatocellular carcinoma: a randomized controlled trial. *Scand J Gastroenterol* 2008; 43(6): 727–35.

96. Vilana R, Bruix J, Bru C, Ayuso C, Sole M, Rodes J. Tumor size determines the efficacy of percutaneous ethanol injection for the treatment of small hepatocellular carcinoma. *Hepatology* 1992 Aug; 16(2): 353–57.

97. Khan KN, Yatsuhashi H, Yamasaki K, et al. Prospective analysis of risk factors for early intrahepatic recurrence of hepatocellular carcinoma following ethanol injection. *J Hepatol* 2000 Feb; 32(2): 269–78.

98. Koda M, Murawaki Y, Mitsuda A, et al. Predictive factors for intrahepatic recurrence after percutaneous ethanol injection therapy for small hepatocellular carcinoma. *Cancer* 2000 Feb 1; 88(3): 529–37.

99. Lencioni R. Loco-regional treatment of hepatocellular carcinoma. *Hepatology* 2010 Aug; 52(2): 762–73.

100. Orlando A, Leandro G, Olivo M, Andriulli A, Cottone M. Radiofrequency thermal ablation vs. percutaneous ethanol injection for small hepatocellular carcinoma in cirrhosis: meta-analysis of randomized controlled trials. *Am J Gastroenterol* 2009 Feb; 104(2): 514–24.

101. Germani G, Pleguezuelo M, Gurusamy K, Meyer T, Isgro G, Burroughs AK. Clinical outcomes of radiofrequency ablation, percutaneous alcohol and acetic acid injection for hepatocelullar carcinoma: a meta-analysis. *J Hepatol* 2010 Mar; 52(3): 380–88.

102. Cho YK, Kim JK, Kim MY, Rhim H, Han JK. Systematic review of randomized trials for hepatocellular carcinoma treated with percutaneous ablation therapies. *Hepatology* 2009 Feb; 49(2): 453–59.

103. Bruix J, Sherman M, American Association for the Study of Liver Diseases. Management of hepatocellular carcinoma: an update. *Hepatology* 2011 Mar; 53(3): 1020–22. Pubmed Central PMCID: 3084991.

104. Chen MS, Li JQ, Zheng Y, et al. A prospective randomized trial comparing percutaneous local ablative therapy and partial hepatectomy for small hepatocellular carcinoma. *Ann Surg* 2006 Mar; 243(3): 321–28.

105. Lu MD, Kuang M, Liang LJ, et al. [Surgical resection versus percutaneous thermal ablation for early-stage hepatocellular carcinoma: a randomized clinical trial]. *Zhonghua Yi Xue Za Zhi* 2006 Mar 28; 86(12): 801–5.

106. Huang J, Yan L, Cheng Z, et al. A randomized trial comparing radiofrequency ablation and surgical resection for HCC conforming to the Milan criteria. *Ann Surg* 2010 Dec; 252(6): 903–12.

107. Livraghi T, Meloni F, Di Stasi M, et al. Sustained complete response and complications rates after radiofrequency ablation of very early hepatocellular carcinoma in cirrhosis: is resection still the treatment of choice? *Hepatology* 2008 Jan; 47(1): 82–89.

108. Montorsi M, Santambrogio R, Bianchi P, et al. Survival and recurrences after hepatic resection or radiofrequency for hepatocellular carcinoma in cirrhotic patients: a multivariate analysis. *J Gastrointest Surg* 2005 Jan; 9(1): 62–67; discussion 7–8.

109. Lupo L, Panzera P, Giannelli G, Single hepatocellular carcinoma ranging from 3 to 5 cm: radiofrequency ablation or resection? *HPB* (Oxford) 2007; 9(6): 429–34.

110. Hong SN, Lee SY, Choi MS, et al. Comparing the outcomes of radiofrequency ablation and surgery in patients with a single small hepatocellular carcinoma and well-preserved hepatic function. *J Clin Gastroenterol* 2005 Mar; 39(3): 247–52.

111. Guglielmi A, Ruzzenente A, Valdegamberi A, et al. Radiofrequency ablation versus surgical resection for the treatment of hepatocellular carcinoma in cirrhosis. *J Gastrointest Surg* 2008 Jan; 12(1): 192–98.

112. Abu-Hilal M, Primrose JN, Casaril A, McPhail MJ, Pearce NW, Nicoli N. Surgical resection versus radiofrequency ablation in the treatment of small unifocal hepatocellular carcinoma. *J Gastrointest Surg* 2008 Sep; 12(9): 1521–26.

113. Vivarelli M, Guglielmi A, Ruzzenente A, et al. Surgical resection versus percutaneous radiofrequency ablation in the treatment of hepatocellular carcinoma on cirrhotic liver. *Ann Surg* 2004 Jul; 240(1): 102–7.

114. Graham JA, Newman DA, Smirniotopolous J, Shetty K, Slidell MB, Johnson LB. Transplantation for hepatocellular carcinoma in younger patients has an equivocal survival advantage as compared with resection. *Transplant Proc* 2013 Jan–Feb; 45(1): 265–71.

115. Mazzaferro V, Romito R, Schiavo M, et al. Prevention of hepatocellular carcinoma recurrence with alpha-interferon after liver resection in HCV cirrhosis. *Hepatology* 2006 Dec; 44(6): 1543–54.

116. Yao FY. Liver transplantation for hepatocellular carcinoma: beyond the Milan criteria. *Am J Transplant* 2008 Oct; 8(10): 1982–89.

117. Yao FY, Ferrell L, Bass NM, et al. Liver transplantation for hepatocellular carcinoma: expansion of the tumor size limits does not adversely impact survival. *Hepatology* 2001 Jun; 33(6): 1394–403.

118. Ghobrial RM, Freise CE, Trotter JF, et al. Donor morbidity after living donation for liver transplantation. *Gastroenterology* 2008 Aug; 135(2): 468–76.

119. Lei J, Yan L, Wang W. Donor safety in living donor liver transplantation: a single-center analysis of 300 cases. *PloS One* 2013; 8(4): e61769.

120. Yi NJ, Suh KS, Suh SW, et al. Excellent outcome in 238 consecutive living donor liver transplantations using the right liver graft in a large volume single center. *World J Surg* 2013 Mar 7; 37(6): 1419–29.

121. Lo CM, Ngan H, Tso WK, et al. Randomized controlled trial of transarterial lipiodol chemoembolization for unresectable hepatocellular carcinoma. *Hepatology* 2002 May; 35(5): 1164–71.

122. Takayasu K, Arii S, Ikai I, et al. Overall survival after transarterial lipiodol infusion chemotherapy with or without embolization for unresectable hepatocellular carcinoma: propensity score analysis. *AJR Am J Roentgenol* 2010 Mar; 194(3): 830–37.

123. Raoul JL, Sangro B, Forner A, et al. Evolving strategies for the management of intermediate-stage hepatocellular carcinoma: available evidence and expert opinion on the use of transarterial chemoembolization. *Cancer Treat Rev* 2011 May; 37(3): 212–20.

124. Camma C, Schepis F, Orlando A, et al. Transarterial chemoembolization for unresectable hepatocellular carcinoma: meta-analysis of randomized controlled trials. *Radiology* 2002 Jul; 224(1): 47–54.

125. Chan AO, Yuen MF, Hui CK, Tso WK, Lai CL. A prospective study regarding the complications of transcatheter intraarterial lipiodol chemoembolization in patients with hepatocellular carcinoma. *Cancer* 2002 Mar 15; 94(6): 1747–52.

126. Llovet JM, Bruix J. Systematic review of randomized trials for unresectable hepatocellular carcinoma: chemoembolization improves survival. *Hepatology* 2003 Feb; 37(2): 429–42.

127. Varela M, Real MI, Burrel M, et al. Chemoembolization of hepatocellular carcinoma with drug eluting beads: efficacy and doxorubicin pharmacokinetics. *J Hepatol* 2007 Mar; 46(3): 474–81.

128. Hong K, Khwaja A, Liapi E, Torbenson MS, Georgiades CS, Geschwind JF. New intra-arterial drug delivery system for the treatment of liver cancer: preclinical assessment in a rabbit model of liver cancer. *Clin Cancer Res* 2006 Apr 15; 12(8): 2563–67.

129. Lammer J, Malagari K, Vogl T, et al. Prospective randomized study of doxorubicin-eluting-bead embolization in the treatment of hepatocellular carcinoma: results of the PRECISION V study. *Cardiovasc Intervent Radiol* 2010 Feb; 33(1): 41–52.

130. Song MJ, Chun HJ, Song do S, et al. Comparative study between doxorubicin-eluting beads and conventional transarterial chemoembolization for treatment of hepatocellular carcinoma. *J Hepatol* 2012 Dec; 57(6): 1244–50.

131. Burrel M, Reig M, Forner A, et al. Survival of patients with hepatocellular carcinoma treated by transarterial chemoembolisation (TACE) using Drug Eluting Beads. Implications for clinical practice and trial design. *J Hepatol* 2012 Jun; 56(6): 1330–35.

132. Kulik LM, Carr BI, Mulcahy MF, et al. Safety and efficacy of 90Y radiotherapy for hepatocellular carcinoma with and without portal vein thrombosis. *Hepatology* 2008 Jan; 47(1): 71–81.

133. Tsai AL, Burke CT, Kennedy AS, et al. Use of yttrium-90 microspheres in patients with advanced hepatocellular carcinoma and portal vein thrombosis. *J Vasc Interv Radiol* 2010 Sep; 21(9): 1377–84.

134. Sangro B, Bilbao JI, Boan J, et al. Radioembolization using 90Y-resin microspheres for patients with advanced hepatocellular carcinoma. *Int J Radiat Oncol Biol Phys* 2006 Nov 1; 66(3): 792–800.

135. Geschwind JF, Salem R, Carr BI, et al. Yttrium-90 microspheres for the treatment of hepatocellular carcinoma. *Gastroenterology* 2004 Nov; 127(5 Suppl 1): S194–S205.

136. Salem R, Lewandowski RJ, Atassi B, et al. Treatment of unresectable hepatocellular carcinoma with use of 90Y microspheres (TheraSphere): safety, tumor response, and survival. *J Vasc Interv Radiol* 2005 Dec; 16(12): 1627–39.

137. Riaz A, Lewandowski RJ, Kulik LM, et al. Complications following radioembolization with yttrium-90 microspheres: a comprehensive literature review. *J Vasc Interv Radiol* 2009 Sep; 20(9): 1121–30; quiz 31.

138. Mazzaferro V, Sposito C, Bhoori S, et al. Yttrium(90) radioembolization for intermediate-advanced hepatocarcinoma: a phase II study. *Hepatology* 2012 Aug 22; 57(5): 1826–37.

139. Salem R, Lewandowski RJ, Kulik L, et al. Radioembolization results in longer time-to-progression and reduced toxicity compared with chemoembolization in patients with hepatocellular carcinoma. *Gastroenterology* 2011 Feb; 140(2): 497–507 e2.

140. Kooby DA, Egnatashvili V, Srinivasan S, et al. Comparison of yttrium-90 radioembolization and transcatheter arterial chemoembolization for the treatment of unresectable hepatocellular carcinoma. *J Vasc Interv Radiol* 2010 Feb; 21(2): 224–30.

141. Moreno-Luna LE, Yang JD, Sanchez W, et al. Efficacy and safety of transarterial radioembolization versus chemoembolization in patients with hepatocellular carcinoma. *Cardiovasc Intervent Radiol* 2013 Jun; 36(3): 714–23.

142. Lai CL, Wu PC, Chan GC, Lok AS, Lin HJ. Doxorubicin versus no antitumor therapy in inoperable hepatocellular carcinoma. A prospective randomized trial. *Cancer* 1988 Aug 1; 62(3): 479–83.

143. Chlebowski RT, Brzechwa-Adjukiewicz A, Cowden A, Block JB, Tong M, Chan KK. Doxorubicin (75 mg/m$^2$) for hepatocellular carcinoma: clinical and pharmacokinetic results. *Cancer Treat Rep* 1984 Mar; 68(3): 487–91.

144. Yeo W, Mok TS, Zee B, et al. A randomized phase III study of doxorubicin versus cisplatin/interferon alpha-2b/doxorubicin/fluorouracil (PIAF) combination chemotherapy for unresectable hepatocellular carcinoma. *J Natl Cancer Inst* 2005 Oct 19; 97(20): 1532–38.

145. Nerenstone SR, Ihde DC, Friedman MA. Clinical trials in primary hepatocellular carcinoma: current status and future directions. *Cancer Treat Rev* 1988 Mar; 15(1): 1–31.

146. Wrzesinski SH, Taddei TH, Strazzabosco M. Systemic therapy in hepatocellular carcinoma. *Clin Liver Dis* 2011 May; 15(2): 423–41, vii-x.

147. Llovet JM, Ricci S, Mazzaferro V, et al. Sorafenib in advanced hepatocellular carcinoma. *N Engl J Med* 2008 Jul 24; 359(4): 378–90.

148. Cheng AL, Kang YK, Chen Z, et al. Efficacy and safety of sorafenib in patients in the Asia-Pacific region with advanced hepatocellular carcinoma: a phase III randomised, double-blind, placebo-controlled trial. *Lancet Oncol* 2009 Jan; 10(1): 25–34.

149. Muszbek N, Shah S, Carroll S, et al. Economic evaluation of sorafenib in the treatment of hepatocellular carcinoma in Canada. *Curr Med Res Opin* 2008 Dec; 24(12): 3559–69.

150. Abou-Alfa GK, Johnson P, Knox JJ, et al. Doxorubicin plus sorafenib vs doxorubicin alone in patients with advanced hepatocellular carcinoma: a randomized trial. *JAMA* 2010 Nov 17; 304(19): 2154–60.

151. Santoro A, Rimassa L, Borbath I, et al. Tivantinib for second-line treatment of advanced hepatocellular carcinoma: a randomised, placebo-controlled phase 2 study. *Lancet Oncol* 2013 Jan; 14(1): 55–63.

152. Lencioni R. Llovet JM, Han G., et al. Sorafenib or placebo in combination with transarterial chemoembolization (TACE) with doxorubicin-eluting beads (DEBDOX) for intermediate-stage hepatocellular carcinoma. *J Clin Oncol* 2012; 30(Suppl 4). Abstract LBA154.

153. Lin MH, Wu PY, Tsai ST, Lin CL, Chen TW, Hwang SJ. Hospice palliative care for patients with hepatocellular carcinoma in Taiwan. *Palliat Med* 2004 Mar; 18(2): 93–99.

154. Habermehl D, Haase K, Rieken S, Debus J, Combs SE. Defining the role of palliative radiotherapy in bone metastasis from primary liver cancer: an analysis of survival and treatment efficacy. *Tumori* 2011 Sep–Oct; 97(5): 609–13.

155. Ren Z. Zhu K, Kang H, et al. A randomized controlled study of the prophylactic effect of urea-based cream on the hand foot skin reaction associated with sorafenib in advanced hepatocellular carcinoma. *J Clin Oncol* 2012; 30(15) (May 20 Supplement). Abstract 4008.
156. Ferenci P, Fried M, Labrecque D, et al. World Gastroenterology Organisation Guideline. Hepatocellular carcinoma (HCC): a global perspective. *J Gastrointest Liver Dis* 2010 Sep; 19(3): 311–17.
157. Kung CM, Mo LR, Yan YH. Consumption of national health insurance medical resources by hepatocellular carcinoma patients treated using radiofrequency ablation therapy. *Asia Pac J Clin Oncol* 2012 Sep; 8(3): 275–81.

# 9

# Gynecologic Cancers

*Linus Chuang, Tania Sierra, Xiaohua Wu, and Fredric V. Price*

Gynecologic cancers have an important impact on women worldwide. In this chapter, we focus on cervical, endometrial, and ovarian cancers, as well as briefly cover vulvar and vaginal cancers and choriocarcinoma. Globally, cervical cancer is the most prevalent gynecologic malignancy with a disproportionate incidence and mortality in the developing world. This discrepancy is a result of the infrastructure that exists in developed countries, which allows for screening and detection of preinvasive disease. Endometrial cancer is the second most prevalent gynecologic malignancy, with a higher incidence in industrialized countries. It is associated with obesity and postmenopausal bleeding. Ovarian cancer is the third most prevalent gynecologic malignancy and the most lethal, with an almost equal distribution across underdeveloped and developed areas. Vulvar and vaginal cancers are rare, accounting for about 3% and 2% of all gynecologic malignancies, respectively. Choriocarcinoma accounts for only 0.6% of all gynecologic cancers, almost exclusively diagnosed in developed countries in conjunction with molar pregnancy. Treatment plans for gynecologic cancers differ between low- and high-resource settings due to the availability of advanced surgical care, radiation facilities, and chemotherapy drugs. In this chapter, we focus on both ideal and alternative treatment plans, when standard of care is not available.

## CERVICAL CANCER

### Global Epidemiology

Cervical cancer is the seventh most common cancer in the world and the third most common cancer in women. Globally, it is the most common gynecologic malignancy with a disproportionate burden, in terms of incidence and mortality, in low-resource settings. In 2008, there were an estimated

530,000 new cases worldwide with 275,000 deaths. Approximately 85% of these cases occurred in resource-poor regions.[1] The highest incidence rates are found in eastern, western, and southern Africa; South-Central Asia; and South America (Table 9.1). Mortality due to cervical cancer is also highest in these areas, accounting for 88% of all deaths. It was estimated in 2008 that 53,000, 31,000, and 159,000 women died in Africa, Latin America and the Caribbean, and Asia, respectively.[1] However, both the incidence and mortality are low in industrialized countries. This is attributable to infrastructures that support cervical cancer screening with Papanicolaou (Pap) smears and standard follow-up and treatment of abnormalities, leading to the detection of treatable, preinvasive disease. Early diagnosis leads to improved survival.

## Etiology

Cervical cancer is essentially a sexually transmitted disease caused by persistent human papillomavirus (HPV) infection. HPV is a non-enveloped, double-stranded, circular DNA virus. There are more than 100 genotypes, with at least 30 oncogenic strains that are responsible for preinvasive disease and cervical cancer. Approximately 610,000 of the world's 12.7 million cancers are attributed to HPV infection, which is equivalent to a Population

TABLE 9.1  Age-Standardized Rates of Cervical Cancer per 100,000 Population (Reference 17)

| Regions | Incidence | Mortality |
|---|---|---|
| Eastern Africa | 42.7 | 27.6 |
| Southern Africa | 31.5 | 17.9 |
| Western Africa | 29.3 | 18.5 |
| Middle Africa | 30.6 | 22.2 |
| Northern Africa | 6.6 | 3.2 |
| Central America | 23.5 | 8.9 |
| Caribbean | 21 | 8.6 |
| South America | 20.3 | 8.6 |
| Northern America | 6.6 | 2.6 |
| South-Central Asia | 19.3 | 10.9 |
| Southeastern Asia | 16.3 | 7.9 |
| Eastern Asia | 7.9 | 3.3 |
| Western Asia | 4.4 | 1.9 |
| Central and Eastern Europe | 16.3 | 6.2 |
| Northern Europe | 8.7 | 2.2 |
| Southern Europe | 8.5 | 2.4 |
| Western Europe | 7.3 | 1.8 |
| Australia/New Zealand | 5.5 | 1.5 |

Incidence and mortality are based on age-standardized rates per 100,000.

Attributable Fraction (PAF) of 4.8%.[2] HPV is a known precursor for six cancers: cervix, penis, vulva, vagina, anus, and oropharynx. The PAF is also higher in low-resource settings than in industrialized countries.

Risk factors for cervical cancer include early age of onset of sexual activity, multiple partners, cigarette smoking, oral contraceptive use, and immunosuppressed states such as HIV infection or transplantation. The male partner also plays an important role in the transmission of HPV infection. For example, the incidence of cervical cancer has been reported to be higher in women whose sexual partners have squamous cell penile cancer.[3] In summary, cervical cancer risk factors are those characteristics that increase exposure to HPV and/or magnify its oncogenicity.

## Prevention

It is estimated that more than half of women become infected with HPV within 2 to 3 years after onset of sexual activity. Most of these infections regress spontaneously; only 5% to 15% eventually develop into preinvasive cervical disease. The average time of initial infection to cervical cancer is 20 years. Early detection via Pap smears and treatment of persistent lesions result in decreased mortality. Given that 70% of cervical cancer is caused by two high-risk genotypes HPV 16 and 18, the quadrivalent vaccine Gardasil (HPV-16, 18, 6, 11) and bivalent vaccine Cervarix (HPV-16, 18), recently developed, are great preventive tools that have yet to be fully utilized globally. Several issues, such as cost, access, distribution, and regional policy making are factors that need to be addressed in order to implement vaccination programs. The World Health Organization estimates that a 5-year vaccination initiative could prevent 1 million cervical cancer deaths.[4]

Another tool in cancer prevention is earlier detection and treatment of premalignant lesions. Screening via Pap smears requires health-care infrastructure for cytological processing and pathological interpretation, as well as patient commitment to a regimen of follow-up. A more cost-efficient method for low-resource areas is "see-and-treat" algorithms that rely on visual inspection with acetic acid or Lugol's iodine and treatment with cryotherapy. DNA testing for HPV in cervical samples is another potential tool in high-risk women.[5] These methods have been studied in several settings, such as India and Africa, with single-visit or two-visit models of women in their thirties showing the best promise for lifetime reduction risk of 25% to 66%.[6,7]

## Treatment

Cervical cancer treatment is dependent on the extent of the disease. Staging is based on clinical examination of the patient and imaging, such as chest x-ray, intravenous pyelogram, barium enema, and skeletal x-ray. Various other imaging studies such as computerized axial tomography, magnetic resonance imaging, and positron emission tomography have been utilized to aid the staging of cervical cancer. The results of these additional studies are not included in the International Federation of Gynecology and Obstetrics (FIGO) staging of cervical cancer (Table 9.2), updated in 2009, as these tests may not be readily available in low-resource settings.

The treatment modalities used in cervical cancer management include surgery, radiation, and chemoradiation. Early cervical cancer (stages IA2, IB1, IIA1) can be managed by either surgery or chemoradiation with an excellent 5-year survival rate of 85%. In patients who are good surgical candidates, radical hysterectomy and bilateral pelvic with or without para-aortic lymphadenectomy can be a definitive treatment. In settings where the availability of radiation therapy is limited, surgical options are often recommended to patients with larger tumor size or more advanced diseases (stages IB2, IIA2, and IIB), as retrospective studies support this practice.[8] Postoperative adjuvant therapies are recommended to patients who are found to be at risk for developing recurrent disease. Adjuvant radiation for patients who have at least two of the following three risk factors has been shown to reduce tumor recurrence: greater than one-third stromal invasion, capillary lymphatic space involvement, and large tumor size.[9] Recently more conservative surgical management such as radical trachelectomy and large cone biopsy has been able to preserve fertility in patients with small early cervical cancers.[10,11]

Radiation therapy is the most commonly recommended treatment modality for patients with stage IIB and higher.[12] Radiation is delivered with

**TABLE 9.2  Staging for Carcinoma of the Cervix**

| | |
|---|---|
| IA1 | Confined to the cervix, diagnosed only by microscopy with invasion of <3 mm in depth and lateral spread <7 mm |
| IA2 | Confined to the cervix, diagnosed with microscopy with invasion of between 3 and 5 mm with lateral spread <7 mm |
| IB1 | Clinically visible lesion or greater than A2, ≤4 cm in greatest dimension |
| IB2 | Clinically visible lesion, >4 cm in greatest dimension |
| IIA1 | Involvement of the upper two-thirds of the vagina, without parametrial invasion, ≤4 cm in greatest dimension |
| IIA2 | Involvement of the upper two-thirds of the vagina, without parametrial invasion, >4 cm in greatest dimension |
| IIB | Involvement of the upper two-thirds of the vagina, with parametrial involvement |
| IIIA | Tumor involves lower one-third of the vagina, with no extension to the pelvic wall |
| IIIB | Extension to the pelvic wall or hydronephrosis or nonfunctioning kidney |
| IVA | Spread to adjacent organs |
| IVB | Spread to distant organs |

both external beam radiation therapy (EBRT) and brachytherapy. Concurrent chemotherapy (CCT) with radiation therapy is recommended. A study randomizing 500 patients to receive either CCT with radiation or radiation alone showed that of the 228 survivors at 6-year follow-up, there was a significant increase in survival (61% vs. 41% at 8 years) and a 51% decrease in tumor recurrence in favor of CCT. There was no significant increase in complications or treatment-related side effects.[13] EBRT is delivered by two types of megavoltage machines: linear accelerators, often referred to as *linacs*, and Cobalt-60 devices. Linacs are the more sophisticated of the two, as the components of the machine allow fine adjustments in depth, angle, and distance, resulting in a more precise contour of energy delivery. Cobalt devices are less expensive and require less maintenance, but cannot create treatment volume contours as well as those of the linacs. While linacs are readily available in most cancer centers in the United States and other developed countries, Cobalt is still used widely in low-resource settings. Brachytherapy can be administered by two dosing schedules: low-dose radiotherapy, which consists of treatment over consecutive days and requires hospitalization; and high-dose radiotherapy (HDR), which spans only minutes and can be administered weekly as an outpatient. HDR has become more popular because of its convenience for patients, but research shows equivalent results for tumor control.[14] Access to radiation therapy in low-resource settings is limited by various factors, such as the lack of equipment and trained staff, the availability of reliable power supply, and the ability to afford radiotherapy. Various strategies can be developed to overcome the shortages of radiotherapy equipment. One strategy would be to perform radical hysterectomy with pelvic and para-aortic lymphadenectomy for patients with larger locally advanced cervical cancers. Approximately 30% of these patients may benefit from additional chemoradiation therapies. Another strategy is to use a radiation "boost" after chemoradiation because of the lack of brachytherapy devices. Radical or simple hysterectomy have also been performed to complete the treatment in place of brachytherapy.[15]

## Survival

Cervical cancer survival is dependent on the clinical stage of the disease. The 5-year survival rate for early-stage disease is favorable, with 95% for stage IA and 85% for stage IB diseases. The survival worsens for stage II at 75%, stage III at 50%, and stage IVB at <10%.[16] The overall mortality to incidence ratio is about 50%. The survival rates are far lower in Asian and African countries. The overall survival in Western countries ranges from 66% to 72%, whereas it is between 29% and 68% in Asia and much lower in Africa, with 18% reported in Uganda.[17] Palliative care is an important component of patient management for women with advanced cervical cancers, especially in these low-resource settings.

## ENDOMETRIAL CANCER

### Global Epidemiology

Endometrial cancer is the second most common female pelvic cancer, following cervical cancer worldwide. By contrast, the highest incidence is in industrialized countries. There are an estimated 287,000 new cases annually.[18] The median age at diagnosis in the United States is 61 years, with a lifetime risk of 2.6%.[19] Most uterine cancers are adenocarcinomas of the endometrium. It is primarily a postmenopausal diagnosis (Table 9.3).

### Etiology

Endometrial cancers have been divided into types I and II based on clinical and histological presentations. Type I cancer is regarded as an estrogen-dependent malignancy of endometrioid histology (grade 1 or 2). It comprises approximately 80% of endometrial cancers. These patients are usually younger and obese; the survival is excellent. Type II cancer is typically

TABLE 9.3  Incidence of Endometrial Cancer in the World (Reference 17)

| Regions | Incidence | Mortality |
|---|---|---|
| Eastern Africa | 3.4 | 1.3 |
| Southern Africa | 6.5 | 1.8 |
| Western Africa | 3.3 | 1.4 |
| Middle Africa | 3.4 | 1.5 |
| Northern Africa | 3.1 | 0.9 |
| Central America | 6.6 | 1.7 |
| Caribbean | 10.4 | 3.3 |
| South America | 5.5 | 1.5 |
| Northern America | 19.1 | 2.2 |
| South-Central Asia | 2.7 | 1 |
| Southeastern Asia | 5.1 | 1.5 |
| Eastern Asia | 8.6 | 1.9 |
| Western Asia | 7.6 | 1.9 |
| Central and Eastern Europe | 15.6 | 3.4 |
| Northern Europe | 14.1 | 2.3 |
| Southern Europe | 12.9 | 2.1 |
| Western Europe | 11.6 | 1.9 |
| Australia/New Zealand | 12.4 | 1.5 |

Incidence and mortality are based on age-standardized rates per 100,000.

diagnosed in older women and carries a poorer prognosis. Histologically, they consist of grade 3 endometrioid tumors and non-endometrioid tumors, such as serous or clear cell type. Genetically, P53 mutations are more common in type II cancers, whereas PTEN mutations are usually seen in type I cancers. As obesity has become an increasingly common global problem, especially in industrialized countries, the incidence of endometrial cancer is rising.

The risk factors for endometrial cancer are rooted in increased estrogen, whether exogenous or endogenous, without progestin opposition. These include obesity, polycystic ovarian syndrome, estrogen intake (i.e., tamoxifen), estrogen-producing tumors, early menarche, late menopause, nulliparity (type I cancers), black race (type II cancers), diabetes, and hypertension.

There are also inherited genetic risk factors. About 2% to 5% of cancer cases are related to hereditary non-polyposis colorectal cancer (HNPCC) syndrome.[20] Otherwise known as Lynch syndrome, it is an autosomal dominant disorder, with germline mutations in DNA mismatch repair genes. Endometrial cancer is the most common extracolonic cancer in this syndrome. The age of onset is often less than 50 years and affected women are at 10-fold higher risk than the general population.[21] Another hereditary condition associated with endometrial cancer, albeit much rarer, is Cowden syndrome. It is an autosomal dominant PTEN mutation with characteristic mucocutaneous lesions, high prevalence of fibroids, and increased risk of other cancers such as breast, colorectal, thyroid, and renal. The lifetime risk of endometrial cancer for carriers is 13% to 19%.[22] However, the majority of endometrial cancer is sporadic in nature.

## Prevention

Hormonal contraceptives, through their utilization of progestin, offer protection against endometrial cancer. For example, combined oral contraceptives decrease the risk by 50%, with an effect that persists 10 to 20 years after cessation.[23] Other protective factors include smoking and coffee consumption. Obesity is the major modifiable risk factor. Weight control via dietary monitoring, exercise, and bariatric surgery (if necessary) may contribute to the prevention and reduction of endometrial cancers.

In patients with unopposed estrogen production secondary to polycystic ovarian syndrome, sequential progestin treatment for 10 to 14 days per month can protect against the development of endometrial cancer.[24]

Screening is important for high-risk populations. Women with HNPCC syndrome have a 40% to 60% lifetime risk of endometrial and 9% to 12% lifetime risk of ovarian cancer.[20] Awareness of this risk factor has been shown to be the most important predictor of compliance with screening for HNPCC.[25]

**TABLE 9.4  Staging for Endometrial Carcinoma**

| | |
|---|---|
| IA | Tumor confined to the uterus with <½ myometrial invasion |
| IB | Tumor confined to the uterus with >½ myometrial invasion |
| II | Cervical stromal invasion, but not beyond uterus |
| IIIA | Tumor invades serosa or adnexa |
| IIIB | Vaginal and/or parametrial involvement |
| IIIC1 | Pelvic node involvement |
| IIIC2 | Para-aortic involvement |
| IVA | Tumor invasion into bladder and/or bowel mucosa |
| IVB | Distant metastases including abdominal metastases and/or inguinal lymph nodes |

## Treatment

Surgery is the mainstay of treatment for patients with endometrial cancer. The standard procedure is hysterectomy and bilateral salpingo-oophorectomy with or without pelvic and para-aortic lymphadenectomy. Given that the incidence of lymphatic spread is minimal in patients with low-risk endometrial cancer (grades 1 to 2 with <50% myometrial invasion), the role of lymphadenectomy in these patients is questionable. Comprehensive pelvic and para-aortic lymphadenectomy should be performed in patients with intermediate- and high-risk (grade 3, invasion >50%; or serous or clear cell histologies) endometrial cancers. Ongoing clinical trials are under way to investigate whether an appropriate chemotherapy regimen with or without radiation therapy can improve survival in patients with high-risk diseases.[26]

## Survival

Endometrial cancer survival is dependent on multiple factors. FIGO surgical stage (as shown in Table 9.4), histologic types, and patient ethnicity are important prognostic factors for disease survival. Overall, 5-year survival ranges from 80% to 90% in stage I, 70% in stage II, between 32% and 60% in patients with stage III, and <20% in patients with stage IV endometrial cancers.[16] Rare endometrial cancers such as serous and clear cell carcinoma have a known propensity for distant metastasis and thus carry a poorer prognosis than endometrioid types. Studies from the United States showed a higher mortality rate and lower 5-year survival among African American women despite a lower overall incidence compared to white women.[27]

## OVARIAN CANCER

### Epidemiology across the Globe

Ovarian cancer is the seventh most common cancer among women worldwide and the fifth most common cancer among women in industrialized countries.[18] It is the third most common gynecologic malignancy.[18] In 2008, there were 225,000 new ovarian cancers reported; slightly more than half of the cases (125,000) occurred in low-resource settings.[18] It is the most lethal gynecologic malignancy in the United States, accounting for more deaths than all the other gynecologic cancers combined (Table 9.5).[28]

## Etiology

The etiology for the development of ovarian cancer is unclear. This is partly because the tissue of origin is uncertain—ovarian, fallopian, and primary peritoneal cancers are histologically similar. Recently, there has been increasing evidence that the precursor lesion for serous carcinoma may originate in the distal fallopian tube. This has important implications for screening and prophylactic surgery.

Some prominent theories include cellular damage caused by incessant ovulation, increased division secondary to gonadotropin stimulation, inflammation-induced injury, and androgen-induced carcinogenesis.[29] The known risk factors are highlighted by these theories. They include age, family history, nulliparity, early menarche, late menopause, white race, personal history of breast cancer, and ethnic background (i.e., Ashkenazi Jewish). The most important of these is family history of a first-degree relative. Additional postulated risk factors that have not consistently shown an increase

TABLE 9.5  Incidence of Ovarian Cancer in the World (Reference 17)

| Regions | Incidence | Mortality |
|---|---|---|
| Eastern Africa | 5.5 | 4.4 |
| Southern Africa | 5.2 | 3.8 |
| Western Africa | 3.6 | 3 |
| Middle Africa | 4.1 | 3.3 |
| Northern Africa | 5.6 | 4.1 |
| Central America | 5 | 3.4 |
| Caribbean | 5 | 3 |
| South America | 5.8 | 3.6 |
| Northern America | 8.1 | 5 |
| South-Central Asia | 4.9 | 3.7 |
| Southeastern Asia | 6.5 | 4.4 |
| Eastern Asia | 4.7 | 1.9 |
| Western Asia | 5.3 | 3.7 |
| Central and Eastern Europe | 11.4 | 6 |
| Northern Europe | 11 | 5.9 |
| Southern Europe | 9.1 | 4.4 |
| Western Europe | 7.5 | 4.7 |
| Australia/New Zealand | 7.6 | 4.5 |

Incidence and mortality are based on age-standardized rates per 100,000.

in cancer risk are talc use, fertility drug treatment, and hormone replacement therapy. Interestingly, residence in North America or industrialized European countries confers a higher probability of developing ovarian cancer. By comparison, Japan has lower rates despite being a developed country. The consumption of low-fat food may play a role in this discrepancy.

Genetic influences also contribute to the risk of developing ovarian cancer. Although only 10% of cases are related to genetic predispositions, awareness of this risk factor remains an important screening tool. More than 90% of inherited ovarian cancers result from germline mutations in the BRCA1 or BRCA2 genes. These are tumor suppressor genes that repair double-strand DNA breaks. Carriers infer a risk of ovarian cancer of approximately 39% for BRCA1 and 22% for BRCA2.[30] Patients with a family history of ovarian and/or breast cancer should be appropriately counseled. Patients with inheritance of HNPCC gene mutations have 9% to 12% lifetime risk of developing ovarian cancer.[20]

Protective factors against ovarian cancer include multiparity, use of oral contraceptives greater than 5 years, breastfeeding, tubal ligation, and hysterectomy.

## Prevention

Currently, no screening method is recommended for general populations. A recent U.S. Preventive Services Task Force recommended against screening for ovarian cancer based on the result of the Prostate, Lung, Colorectal, and Ovarian Cancer Screening Trial. Screening using transvaginal ultrasonography and serum CA 125 testing was not recommended because of the high ratio of surgeries to screen-detected cancers (19.5:1), and most detected cancers (72%) were stage III/V; most importantly, a follow-up study did not show a reduction in mortality.[31,32]

Screening strategies with a focus on high-risk women have been identified and may be used until more definitive testing is developed.[33] Oral contraceptive and prophylactic surgery have been shown to effectively reduce the risk of developing ovarian cancer. A 50% reduction of risk has been reported after taking oral contraceptives for 5 years, with a protective effect lasting 25 years after cessation.[34] In patients who carry BRCA1 or 2 gene mutations, prophylactic salpingo-oophorectomy is recommended after completion of childbearing or after 35 years. The risk reduction has been reported to be more than 90%.[35,36] In women who desire delayed oophorectomy, secondary to premature menopausal side effects, bilateral salpingectomy may be a cost-effective strategy for reduction of BRCA-related ovarian cancers.[37]

## Treatment

Surgical removal of the ovary and comprehensive staging, including pelvic washings for cytology, total omentectomy, and peritoneal and lymph node biopsies should be performed in patients who are diagnosed with ovarian cancers. Table 9.6 outlines the FIGO staging system for carcinoma of the ovary. Hysterectomy and bilateral salpingo-oophorectomy are recommended for women who have extensive ovarian cancers and/or who have completed childbearing. The surgery is traditionally carried out through a vertical incision. Laparoscopic management for patients with early or limited ovarian cancer has been reported.[38] The goal of surgery is to resect all metastatic deposits. Survival is improved by leaving <1 cm residual tumor, with the best long-term control of the disease when there is zero residual.[39] Vergote et al. conducted a phase III trial that randomized patients with stage IIIC or IV ovarian cancer to either primary cytoreduction followed by chemotherapy or neoadjuvant chemotherapy followed by surgery. Neoadjuvant chemotherapy followed by surgery was not inferior as a treatment option compared to the patients who underwent primary cytoreductive surgeries.[40] This approach may benefit patients who presented with advanced, unresectable disease or who have significant comorbid problems precluding from aggressive surgeries.

Adjuvant chemotherapy is recommended for all patients who have ovarian cancers except those diagnosed with early-stage disease (stage IA or IB grade 1 and 2). Despite ovarian cancer's relative sensitivity to chemotherapy, fewer than 20% of patients with advanced ovarian cancer are cured. Intravenous chemotherapy consisting of a combination of cisplatinum or carboplatinum and paclitaxel has been accepted as the standard of care for treatment of ovarian cancer across the world.[41,42] In Europe, two phase III trials compared single agent carboplatin to combination chemotherapy and were not able to show a survival difference between the two treatment regimens. Therefore, single agent carboplatin for six cycles can be considered in low-resource

**TABLE 9.6 Staging for Ovarian Cancer**

| | |
|---|---|
| IA | One ovary, without ascites or external tumor, capsule intact |
| IB | Both ovaries, without ascites or external tumor, capsule intact |
| IC | IA or IB with surface involvement, or capsule rupture, or ascites with malignant cells |
| IIA | Involvement of uterus and/or tubes |
| IIB | Involvement of other pelvic tissues |
| IIC | IIA or IIB with surface involvement, or capsule rupture, or ascites with malignant cells |
| IIIA | Tumor grossly limited to true pelvis with negative nodes, and microscopic seeding of abdominal peritoneal surfaces or extension to small bowel or mesentery |
| IIIB | Tumor of one or both ovaries with implants, metastasis of abdominal peritoneal surfaces not exceeding 2 cm in diameter, with negative nodes |
| IIIC | Peritoneal metastasis beyond pelvis >2 cm in diameter and/or positive retroperitoneal or inguinal nodes |
| IV | Distant metastasis, such as pleural effusion (positive cytology) or parenchymal liver metastasis |

settings as an alternative option.[43] In 2006, the finding from a phase III trial comparing systemic chemotherapy to intraperitoneal chemotherapy showed an improvement of median overall survival by 16 months in the group of patients who received intraperitoneal chemotherapy; however, toxic side effects were greater and fewer than half of the patients completed treatment.[44] More recently, a phase III study compared administration of paclitaxel and carboplatin in a weekly schedule versus the traditional schedule of every 3 weeks with a resultant survival benefit.[45] Further studies are being conducted comparing intraperitoneal and dose dense regimens to traditional chemotherapy. Results from recent large randomized trials have shown a nearly 4-month improvement in progression-free survival for women who received chemotherapy with bevacizumab as initial therapy for ovarian cancer,[46] as well as for treatment for advanced and recurrent ovarian cancer.[47,48] However, there is not yet enough evidence to support using bevacizumab to treat ovarian cancer. Further study is needed to demonstrate that the addition of this costly agent will have a significant impact on women.

Unfortunately, more than 80% of women with advanced ovarian cancer recur and require either additional surgery or chemotherapy treatments. The role of secondary cytoreductive surgery remains controversial. It is best reserved for patients who have platinum-sensitive disease (>6 to 12 months remission) and limited recurrence without ascites. Retrospective analysis has shown a survival benefit for those with residuals ≤0.5 cm.[39] Salvage chemotherapy is required to treat patients with recurrent ovarian cancers. The prognosis is unfortunately poor. For patients who present with end-stage ovarian cancer, palliative care including aggressive symptom control is important.

## Survival

In the United States, the overall 5-year survival rate for ovarian cancer is 44%. This is significantly lower than cervical (68%) and uterine (82%) cancers, according to the SEER database from 2002 to 2008. In addition, the 5-year survival rate for early-stage disease is between 80% to 90%, 65% to 70% for stage II, 30% to 45% for stage III, and 18% for stage IV cancers.[49] The survival is poorer where aggressive surgery or chemotherapy is not readily available. For example, in Uganda the 5-year survival has been reported to be as low as 16%.[17] The availability of quality surgical care and chemotherapy is needed to improve the outcomes of patients with ovarian cancer in low-resource settings.

## Other Ovarian Cancers

In Western industrialized countries, epithelial ovarian cancer represents more than 90% of the new ovarian cancer cases. This is followed by sex cord stromal tumors (5% to 6%) and germ cell tumors (2% to 3%). Germ cell tumors are reported more often in Asian and African countries at a rate 10% to 15%.[17] Both of these tumors develop at a younger age and lower stage and thus carry a better prognosis following surgery and adjuvant chemotherapy (when indicated). Preservation of fertility is important as these patients develop these tumors in their reproductive age.

## OTHER GYNECOLOGIC CANCERS

Vulvar cancer represents about 3% of all gynecologic malignancies.[17] Worldwide, there are an estimated 26,800 cases, with 11,100 occurring in low-resource settings. Treatment of vulvar cancer usually includes radical vulvectomy and inguinal node dissection. Sentinel node biopsy of the inguinal lymphatic chain has been developed in the United States and Europe to minimize the potential complication of lymphedema after inguinal dissections. Cancer of the vagina is also rare, accounting for 2% of gynecologic malignancies. Globally, it accounts for 13,200 new cases each year.[17] It closely resembles cervical or vulvar cancer and often requires chemoradiation therapy. Choriocarcinoma accounts for only 0.6% of all gynecologic cancers. There are about 5,800 cases worldwide every year, with the overwhelming majority of these cases occurring in developing countries.[17] Curettage of molar pregnancies followed by close monitoring of the serum hCG levels is important. Adjuvant chemotherapy for gestational trophoblastic neoplasia is highly effective and cure rates are usually excellent.

## STORY

Isabella was from the town of La Ceiba in Honduras, famous for its beautiful beaches. However, the town has little primary-care resources, and women are not offered Pap smear screening. Isabella experienced abnormal vaginal bleeding between menses for more than a year. She was referred to Hospital San Felipe in Tegucigalpa. On exam, Isabella was noted to have a cervical mass, the size of an orange. Cervical biopsy and examination confirmed that she had cervical cancer at stage IIB. Because of the lack of brachytherapy units in Honduras, she was not able to receive concurrent chemoradiation, which is considered the standard of care in the industrialized countries. Isabella was recommended to undergo chemoradiation with external radiation followed by possible hysterectomy. She received her external radiation therapy at Hospital San Felipe over the duration of 5 weeks. Although weekly chemotherapy was recommended, she received only two doses because she was not able to afford the six indicated doses. After Isabella completed 70 Gy of external radiation, she underwent a simple hysterectomy. Follow-up examination after 2 years showed no evidence of recurrent disease, and she has kept regular follow-up for a total of 5 years. The alternative treatment plan allowed her to receive equivalent treatment that was necessary to cure her cervical cancer.

## REFERENCES

1. Globocan 2008. Cancer Fact Sheet. International Agency for Research on Cancer. Available at http://globocan.iarc.fr/factsheet.asp.
2. Forman D, de Martel C, Lacey CJ, et al. Global burden of human papillomavirus and related diseases. *Vaccine* 2012 Nov 20; 30(Suppl 5): F12–F23.
3. Iversen T, Tretli S, Johansen A, Holte T. Squamous cell carcinoma of the penis and of the cervix, vulva and vagina in spouses: is there any relationship? An epidemiological study from Norway, 1960–1992. *Br J Cancer* 1997; 76: 658–60.
4. WHO/ICO Information Centre on HPV and Cervical Cancer (HPV Information Centre). Human Papillomavirus and Related Cancers in World. Summary Report 2010.
5. Sherris J, Wittet S, Kleine A, et al. Evidence-based, alternative cervical cancer screening approaches in low-resource settings. *Int Perspect Sex Reprod Health* 2009 Sep; 35(3): 147–54.
6. Goldie SJ, Gaffikin L, Goldhaber-Fiebert JD, et al. Cost-effectiveness of cervical-cancer screening in five developing countries. *N Engl J Med* 2005, 353(20): 2158–68.
7. Sankaranarayanan R, Esmy PO, Rajkumar R, et al. Effect of visual screening on cervical cancer incidence and mortality in Tamil Nadu, India: a cluster randomised trial. *Lancet* 2007; 370(9585): 398–406.
8. Park JY, Kim DY, Kim JH, et al. Comparison of outcomes between radical hysterectomy followed by tailored adjuvant therapy versus primary chemoradiation therapy in IB2 and IIA2 cervical cancer. *J Gynecol Oncol* 2012 Oct; 23(4): 226–34.
9. Sedlis A, Bundy BN, Rotman MZ, Lentz SS, Muderspach LI, Zaino RJ. A randomized trial of pelvic radiation therapy versus no further therapy in selected patients with stage IB carcinoma of the cervix after radical hysterectomy and pelvic lymphadenectomy: a Gynecologic Oncology Group Study. *Gynecol Oncol* 1999 May; 73(2): 177–83.
10. Dursun P, LeBlanc E, Nogueira MC. Radical vaginal trachelectomy (Dargent's operation): a critical review of the literature. *Eur J Surg Oncol* 2007 Oct; 33(8): 933–41.
11. Schmeler KM, Frumovitz M, Ramirez PT. Conservative management of early stage cervical cancer: is there a role for less radical surgery? *Gynecol Oncol* 2011 Mar; 120(3): 321–25.
12. NCCN Guidelines 2011, Version 2, 2013. Available at http://www.tri-kobe.org /nccn/guideline/gynecological/english/cervical.pdf.
13. Eifel PJ, Winter K, Morris M, et al. Pelvic irradiation with concurrent chemotherapy versus pelvic and para-aortic irradiation for high-risk cervical cancer: an

update of radiation therapy oncology group trial (RTOG) 90–01. *J Clin Oncol* 2004 Mar 1; 22(5): 872–80.

14. Schorge J, Schaeffer J, Hoalvorson L, Hoffmen B, Bradshaw K, Cunningham F (Eds). *Williams Gynecology*. 1st ed. New York: McGraw-Hill, 2008.

15. Cetina L, Garcia-Arias A, Candelaria M, et al. Brachytherapy versus radical hysterectomy after external beam chemoradiation: a non-randomized matched comparison in IB2-IIB cervical cancer patients. *World J Surg Oncol* 2009; 7: 1–8.

16. Creasman WT, Odicino F, Maisonneuve P, et al. FIGO 26th Annual Report on the Results of Treatment in Gynecologic Cancer. *Int J Gynaecol Obstet* 2006 Nov; 95(Suppl 1): S105–43.

17. Sankaranarayanan R, Ferlay J. Worldwide burden of gynaecological cancer: the size of the problem. *Best Pract Res Clin Obstet Gynaecol* 2006 Apr; 20(2): 207–25.

18. Jemal A, Bray F, Center MM, Ferlay J, Ward E, Forman D. Global cancer statistics. *CA Cancer J Clin* 2011 Mar–Apr; 61(2): 69–90.

19. SEER Stat Fact Sheets: Corpus and Uterus, NOS. National Cancer Institute: Surveillance Epidemiology and End Results. Available at http://www.seer.cancer.gov/csr/1975_2009_pops09/results_single/sect_01_table.11_2pgs.pdf. 2013.

20. Lancaster JM, Powell CB, Kauff ND, et al. Society of Gynecologic Oncologists Education Committee statement on risk assessment for inherited gynecologic cancer predispositions. *Gynecol Oncol* 2007 Nov; 107(2): 159–62.

21. Watson P, Vasen HF, Mecklin JP, Järvinen H, Lynch HT. The risk of endometrial cancer in hereditary nonpolyposis colorectal cancer. *Am J Med* 1994 Jun; 96(6): 516–20.

22. Riegert-Johnson DL, Gleeson FC, Roberts M, et al. Cancer and Lhermitte-Duclos disease are common in Cowden syndrome patients. *Hered Cancer Clin Pract* 2010; 8(1): 6.

23. Mueck AO, Seeger H, Rabe T. Hormonal contraception and risk of endometrial cancer: a systematic review. *Endocr Relat Cancer* 2010 Dec; 17(4): R263–71.

24. Maxwell GL, Schildkraut JM, Calingaert B, et al. Progestin and estrogen potency of combination oral contraceptives and endometrial cancer risk. *Gynecol Oncol* 2006 Nov; 103(2): 535–40.

25. Ketabi Z, Mosgaard BJ, Gerdes AM, Ladelund S, Bernstein IT. Awareness of endometrial cancer risk and compliance with screening in hereditary nonpolyposis colorectal cancer. *Obstet Gynecol* 2012 Nov; 120(5): 1005–12.

26. Nezhat FR, Chuang L. Clinical commentary regarding endometrial cancer and lymphadenectomy. *J Minim Invasive Gynecol* 2009 Jul–Aug; 16(4): 381–83.

27. Yap OW, Matthews RP. Racial and ethnic disparities in cancers of the uterine corpus. *J Natl Med Assoc* 2006 Dec; 98(12): 1930–33.

28. Jemal A, Siegel R, Xu J, Ward E. Cancer statistics 2010. *CA Cancer J Clin* 2010; 60(5): 277–300.

29. Kindelberger D, Lee Y, Miron A, et al. Intraepithelial carcinoma of the fimbria and pelvic serous carcinoma: evidence for a causal relationship. *Am J Surg Pathol* 2007; 31: 161–169.

30. Chen S, Iversen ES, Friebel T, et al. Characterization of BRCA1 and BRCA2 mutations in a large United States sample. *J Clin Oncol* 2006 Feb 20; 24(6): 863–71.

31. Buys SS, Partridge E, Black A, et al. Effect of screening on ovarian cancer mortality: the Prostate, Lung, Colorectal and Ovarian (PLCO) Cancer Screening Randomized Controlled Trial. *JAMA* 2011 Jun 8; 305(22): 2295–303.

32. Partridge EE, Greenlee RT, Riley TL, et al. Assessing the risk of ovarian malignancy in asymptomatic women with abnormal CA 125 and transvaginal ultrasound scans in the prostate, lung, colorectal, and ovarian screening trial. *Obstet Gynecol* 2013 Jan; 121(1): 25–31.

33. Partridge EE, Kreimer AR, Greenlee RT, et al. Results from four rounds of ovarian cancer screening in a randomized trial. *Obstet Gynecol* 2009 Apr; 113(4): 775–82.

34. Riman T, Dickman PW, Nilsson S, et al. Risk factors for invasive epithelial ovarian cancer: results from a Swedish case-control study. *Am J Epidemiol* 2002 Aug 15; 156(4): 363–73.

35. Kauff ND, Satagopan JM, Robson ME et al. Risk-reducing salpingo-oophorectomy in women with a BRCA1 or BRCA2 mutation. *N Engl J Med* 2002 May 23; 346(21): 1609–15.

36. Rebbeck TR, Lynch HT, Neuhausen SL, et al. Prophylactic oophorectomy in carriers of BRCA1 or BRCA2 mutations. *N Engl J Med* 2002 May 23; 346(21): 1616–22.

37. Kwon JS, Tinker A, Pansegrau G, et al. Prophylactic salpingectomy and delayed oophorectomy as an alternative for BRCA mutation carriers. *Obstet Gynecol* 2013 Jan; 121(1): 14–24.

38. Nezhat FR, DeNoble SM, Liu CS, et al. The safety and efficacy of laparoscopic surgical staging and debulking of apparent advanced stage ovarian, fallopian tube, and primary peritoneal cancers. *JSLS* 2010 Apr–Jun; 14(2): 155–68.

39. Chi DS, McCaughty K, Diaz JP, et al. Guidelines and selection criteria for secondary cytoreductive surgery in patients with recurrent, platinum-sensitive epithelial ovarian carcinoma. *Cancer* 2006 May 1; 106(9): 1933–39.

40. Vergote I, Tropé CG, Amant F, et al. Neoadjuvant chemotherapy or primary surgery in stage IIIC or IV ovarian cancer. *N Engl J Med* 2010 Sep 2; 363(10): 943–53.

41. Du Bois A, Lück HJ, Meier W, et al. A randomized clinical trial of cisplatin/paclitaxel versus carboplatin/paclitaxel as first-line treatment of ovarian cancer. *J Natl Cancer Inst* 2003 Sep 3; 95(17): 1320–29.

42. Ozols RF, Bundy BN, Greer BE, et al. Phase III trial of carboplatin and paclitaxel compared with cisplatin and paclitaxel in patients with optimally resected stage III ovarian cancer: a Gynecologic Oncology Group study. *J Clin Oncol* 2003 Sep 1; 21(17): 3194–200.

43. International Collaborative Ovarian Neoplasm Group. Paclitaxel plus carboplatin versus standard chemotherapy with either single-agent carboplatin or cyclophosphamide, doxorubicin, and cisplatin in women with ovarian cancer: the ICON3 randomised trial. *Lancet* 2002 Aug 17; 360(9332): 505–15.

44. Armstrong DK, Bundy B, Wenzel L, et al. Intraperitoneal cisplatin and paclitaxel in ovarian cancer. *N Engl J Med* 2006 Jan 5; 354(1): 34–43.

45. Katsumata N, Yasuda M, Takahashi F, et al. Dose-dense paclitaxel once a week in combination with carboplatin every 3 weeks for advanced ovarian cancer: a phase 3, open-label, randomised controlled trial. *Lancet* 2009 Oct 17; 374(9698): 1331–38.

46. Burger RA, Brady MF, Bookman MA, et al. Incorporation of bevacizumab in the primary treatment of ovarian cancer. *N Engl J Med* 2011 Dec 29; 365(26): 2473–83.

47. Perren TJ, Swart AM, Pfisterer J, et al. A phase 3 trial of bevacizumab in ovarian cancer. *N Engl J Med* 2011 Dec 29; 365(26): 2484–96.

48. Aghajanian C, Blank SV, Goff BA, et al. OCEANS: a randomized, double-blind, placebo-controlled phase III trial of chemotherapy with or without bevacizumab in patients with platinum-sensitive recurrent epithelial ovarian, primary peritoneal, or fallopian tube cancer. *J Clin Oncol* 2012 Jun 10; 30(17): 2039–45.

49. SEER Stat Fact Sheets: Ovary. National Cancer Institute: Surveillance Epidemiology and End Results. Available at http://seer.cancer.gov/statfacts/html/ovary .html.

# 10

# Lymphoma

## Potjana Jitawatanarat and Francisco J. Hernandez-Ilizaliturri

### INTRODUCTION

Lymphoma is a heterogeneous group of lymphoid tissue malignancies with varied clinical, pathological, and biological features arising from B-, T-, or natural killer (NK)-cells. For its study, lymphomas are divided into Hodgkin lymphoma (HL) and non-Hodgkin lymphoma (NHL), which are subclassified based on the 2008 WHO classification to >60 subtypes (see Table 10.1).[1] There is a difference in etiology and epidemiology of specific subtypes of lymphoma in different areas around the world. The overall incidence of lymphoid malignancies in Asian countries is relatively low as compared to North America or Europe. The incidence and prevalence of histopathologic subtypes of lymphoma are different between the Eastern and Western hemispheres. Infectious-related lymphomas such as Epstein-Barr virus (EBV), human T-cell leukemia virus 1 (HTLV1), and hepatitis C-associated lymphomas are more common in Asia and Africa as compared to North America. Not only are there differences in the etiology and epidemiology between lymphomas occurring in different parts of the world, but the disparity in access to medical care and cutting-edge treatment modalities (i.e., monoclonal antibodies, radiation therapy, bone marrow transplantation) affects the clinical outcome of lymphoma patients across the world.

According to global statistics, there were an estimated 356,000 new cases of NHL and 191,000 deaths from NHL in 2008. In the same year, there were 68,000 new cases of HL and 30,000 deaths from HL worldwide. Areas of highest incidence of NHL and HL include North America, Northern and Western Europe, Australia, and New Zealand. The NHL incidence is higher in men than in women, but no differences in HL incidence between sexes had been observed.[2] Strong demographic associations are observed in lymphoma subtypes.

## TABLE 10.1 World Health Organization Classification of Lymphoid Malignancies 2008

| Mature B-Cell Neoplasm | Mature T-Cell/NK-Cell Neoplasm |
| --- | --- |
| Chronic lymphocytic leukemia/small lymphocytic lymphoma | T-cell prolymphocytic leukemia |
| B-cell prolymphocytic leukemia | T-cell large granular lymphocytic leukemia |
| Splenic marginal zone lymphoma | Chronic lymphoproliferative disorder of NK-cells* |
| Hairy cell leukemia | Aggressive NK-cell leukemia |
| Splenic lymphoma/leukemia, unclassifiable | Systemic EBV+ T-cell lymphoproliferative disease of childhood (associated with chronic active EBV infection) |
| Splenic diffuse red pulp small B-cell lymphoma* | Hydroa vacciniforme-like lymphoma |
| Hairy cell leukemia variant* | Adult T-cell leukemia/lymphoma |
| Lymphoplasmacytic lymphoma | Extranodal NK-/T-cell lymphoma, nasal type |
| Waldenström macroglobulinemia | Enteropathy-associated T-cell lymphoma |
| Heavy chain diseases | Hepatosplenic T-cell lymphoma |
| Alpha heavy chain disease | Subcutaneous panniculitis-like T-cell lymphoma |
| Gamma heavy chain disease | Mycosis fungoides |
| Mu heavy chain disease | Sézary syndrome |
| Plasma cell myeloma | Primary cutaneous CD30+ T-cell lymphoproliferative disorder |
| Solitary plasmacytoma of bone | Lymphomatoid papulosis |
| Extraosseous plasmacytoma | Primary cutaneous anaplastic large-cell lymphoma |
| Extranodal marginal zone B-cell lymphoma of mucosa-associated lymphoid tissue (MALT lymphoma) | Primary cutaneous aggressive epidermotropic CD8+ cytotoxic T-cell lymphoma* |
| Nodal marginal zone B-cell lymphoma (MZL) | Primary cutaneous gamma-delta T-cell lymphoma |
| Pediatric type nodal MZL | Primary cutaneous small/medium CD4+ T-cell lymphoma* |
| Follicular lymphoma | Peripheral T-cell lymphoma, not otherwise specified |
| Pediatric-type follicular lymphoma | Angioimmunoblastic T-cell lymphoma |
| Primary cutaneous follicle center lymphoma | Anaplastic large cell lymphoma (ALCL), ALK+ |
| Mantle cell lymphoma | Anaplastic large cell lymphoma (ALCL), ALK–* |
| Diffuse large B-cell lymphoma (DLBCL), not otherwise specified | |
| T-cell/histiocyte-rich large B-cell lymphoma | |
| DLBCL associated with chronic inflammation | |
| Epstein–Barr virus (EBV)+ DLBCL of the elderly | |

| Mature B-Cell Neoplasm | Mature T-Cell/NK-Cell Neoplasm |
| --- | --- |
| Lymphomatoid granulomatosis<br>Primary mediastinal (thymic) large B-cell<br>  lymphoma<br>Intravascular large B-cell lymphoma<br>Primary cutaneous DLBCL, leg type<br>ALK+ large B-cell lymphoma<br>Plasmablastic lymphoma<br>Primary effusion lymphoma<br>Large B-cell lymphoma arising in<br>  HHV8-associated multicentric<br>  Castleman disease<br>Burkitt's lymphoma<br>B-cell lymphoma, unclassifiable, with<br>  features intermediate between diffuse<br>  large B-cell lymphoma and Burkitt's<br>  lymphoma<br>B-cell lymphoma, unclassifiable, with<br>  features intermediate between diffuse<br>  large B-cell lymphoma and classical<br>  Hodgkin lymphoma<br>Hodgkin lymphoma<br>Nodular lymphocyte-predominant<br>  Hodgkin lymphoma<br>Classical Hodgkin lymphoma<br>  Nodular sclerosis classical Hodgkin<br>  lymphoma<br>  Lymphocyte-rich classical Hodgkin<br>  lymphoma<br>  Mixed cellularity classical Hodgkin<br>  lymphoma<br>  Lymphocyte-depleted classical Hodgkin<br>  lymphoma | |

*Represents provisional entities or provisional subtypes of other neoplasms.

Follicular lymphoma (FL) and diffuse large B-cell lymphoma (DLBCL) are more common in North America and Europe, but on the other hand, adult T-cell leukemia/lymphoma (ATLL), a disease of mature T-cell with a strong link to the human T-cell lymphotropic virus (HTLV-1), is endemic in parts of Japan, the Caribbean basin, and Central and West Africa.[3,4] It can account for >50% of NHL in these areas.[5] HL is relatively rare in Asian countries, and its subtypes are various in comparison with other areas.[6] T- and NK-cell lymphomas are more common among the Asian continent, with approximately 15% to 20% of all lymphoma classified as PTCL or NK-/T-cell lymphoma (NKTCL).[7-9] Endemic Burkitt's lymphoma (BL) that is associated with the EBV infection is common in the equatorial belt of Africa and accounts for 70% of childhood lymphoma in this region.[10] On the other hand, only 20% to 30% of BLs in North America are associated with EBV infection.

## INFECTION-RELATED LYMPHOMA

### Human Immunodeficiency Virus (HIV) Infection and Lymphoma

Among HIV-infected patients, the relative risk of developing NHL has been reported to be >100-fold higher than the general population, with greatest risk of B-cell origin lymphoma and high-grade histology.[11] Immune deficiency and chronic antigenic stimulation may be responsible for the increased risk observed in HIV-infected patients. Plasmablastic lymphoma and primary effusion lymphoma (PEL) are commonly associated with HIV infection. Plasmablastic lymphoma is a unique DLBCL subtype associated with EBV infection that mainly involves the jaw and oral cavity of HIV-infected patients.[12,13] Human herpes virus 8 is associated with PEL, a subtype of NHL that almost exclusively affects HIV-infected patients; many of them are also coinfected with EBV.[14]

Acquired immunodeficiency syndrome (AIDS)-related lymphoma is an AIDS-defining diagnosis in patients infected by HIV. The most common forms of systemic HIV-associated lymphoma, which accounts for 70% to 90% of cases, are DLBCL and BL. Primary central nervous system (CNS) lymphoma accounts for 10% to 30% of those cases.[15–17] EBV has been implicated as cofactor in the development of PEL, BL, HL, and posttransplant lymphoproliferative disorder. Mostly EBV-related B-cell and T-cell lymphomas occur in the context of immunosuppression, HIV infection, congenital immunodeficiency syndromes, use of immunosuppressive drugs, and/or any medical condition that could lead to the reactivation of a preexistent latent EBV infection.[18]

Highly active antiretroviral therapy (HAART), introduced in 1996, has altered the epidemiology and clinical outcome of HIV-related lymphoma.[19,20] The incidence of systemic AIDS-related lymphoma has decreased from 86 per 10,000 between 1993 and 1994 to 42.9 per 10,000 person-years between 1997 and 1998. The incidence of primary CNS lymphoma also declined from 27.8 per 10,000 to 9.7 per 10,000 person-years in the same period of time.[16] In the era of HAART, two-thirds of patients diagnosed with HIV-related systemic NHL survive for longer than 1 year after diagnosis.[15] On the other hand, the prognosis of primary CNS lymphoma in the context of HIV infection remains poor with a median overall survival (OS) <3 months both pre-HAART (1993 to 1994) and post-HAART era (1997 to 1998).[16] Despite improvements in oncologic care (i.e., incorporation of monoclonal antibodies, high-dose chemotherapy and autologous stem cell support [HDC-ASCS], radiation therapy, and/or functional imaging), HIV-associated lymphoma outcomes remain inferior when compared to non-HIV-associated lymphoma. The 2-year OS rates for patients with HIV-associated lymphomas treated in the HAART era (1996 to 2005) were reported to be 41% compared with 70% in lymphoma patients without HIV infections treated during the same decade. Of interest, the clinical outcomes for those patients who had a CD4 cell count of $\geq 200/mm^3$ and no prior AIDS-defining illness appeared to have comparable lymphoma-specific mortality with that of HIV-uninfected patients (relative risk = 1.1 [0.7–1.9], p = 0.66).[21] BL histology appears to be associated with poorer survival outcomes among patients with HIV-associated lymphoma even in the HAART era.[21,22] While the incorporation of rituximab, an anti-CD20 monoclonal antibody, to systemic chemotherapy improved the clinical outcome of FL and DLBCL, chemo-immunotherapy has been less successful in HIV-infected patients. Rituximab-based chemo-immunotherapy resulted in similar clinical outcomes than chemotherapy alone in FL/DLBCL HIV-infected patients, but an increased risk of infection(s) was observed in patients with a CD4+ count <50 to $100/mm^3$.[23] A randomized phase III clinical trial (AMC 010 study) compared the effects of adding rituximab (R) to standard doses of cyclophosphamide, doxorubicin, vincristine, and prednisone (CHOP) in patients with HIV-associated lymphoma. Although the addition of rituximab to CHOP chemotherapy improved the complete response (CR) rate (47% vs. 58%), median time to progression (TTP) (20 vs. 29 months), and OS (25 vs. 32 months), these outcomes were not statistically significantly different between treatment arms (CHOP vs. R-CHOP).[23] Multiple subsequent phase II studies have shown that the addition of rituximab is feasible, effective, and safe in patients with HIV-associated lymphomas.[24-26] Therefore, the National Comprehensive Cancer Network (NCCN) recommends that rituximab be omitted only for HIV-infected NHL patients who have a low CD4+ count of $<100/mm^3$ due to a higher risk of serious infectious complications.[27] An alternative regimen consisting of rituximab in combination with dose-adjusted etoposide, prednisone, vincristine, cyclophosphamide, and doxorubicin (R-DA-EPOCH) was found to be highly effective and tolerable in patients with HIV-associated DLBCL.[28-30] Dunleavy et al. demonstrated that R-DA-EPOCH resulted in CR rate of 100% in BL patients.[30] Similarly, in patients with HIV-associated DLBCL treated with the R-DA-EPOCH regimen, the CR rate was 91% after six cycles of therapy and the progression-free survival (PFS) and OS rates were 84% and 68%, respectively.[28] Therefore, in the United States, the NCCN suggests that R-DA-EPOCH is the preferred immunochemotherapy regimen in HIV-associated DLBCL.[27]

## Viral Hepatitis and Lymphoma

The prevalence of chronic hepatitis B virus (HBV) is 0.3% to 0.5% among U.S. residents and 47% to 70% if these people were born in other countries.[31] In areas of Africa and Asia, the overall HBV carrier rate is higher (10% to 15%).[32] HBV reactivation had been demonstrated in up to 25% of B-cell lymphoma patients treated with rituximab.[33] The reactivation of HBV may result in severe hepatitis, delay chemotherapy, or even cause death from fulminant liver failure. Screening all patients, including high-risk and low-risk patients, has shown to be the most effective strategies for patients with DLBCL or other subtypes of lymphomas before initiation of rituximab-based chemotherapy in terms of clinical outcomes and cost-effectiveness as compared to screening only high-risk patients or no screening at all.[34] The NCCN recommends screening testing for hepatitis B using the following studies: hepatitis B surface antigen (HBs Ag) and hepatitis B core antibody (HBc Ab). Quantitative hepatitis B viral load by polymerase chain reaction (PCR) should be done only if one of the screening tests is positive. Prophylactic antiviral therapy is recommended in addition to close monitoring on HBV viral load by PCR monthly through treatment and every 3 months thereafter. Prophylaxis antiviral therapy (tenofovir is preferred) should be maintained between 6 and 12 months after oncologic treatment completion.[27]

Hepatitis C virus (HCV) was recently recognized as being an etiological factor for the development of NHL. It has been estimated that 180 million people worldwide are currently infected with the HCV, accounting for 3% of the global population.[35] Epidemiological studies have clearly demonstrated a correlation between chronic HCV infection and the occurrence of B-cell NHL.[36-39] HCV is associated with certain B-NHL subtypes; in geographic areas with endemic HCV infection, like Italy, Japan, and Egypt, the prevalence rates of HCV in lymphoma patients range from 20% to 40%,[37,39-42] whereas in non-endemic areas, as Northern Europe, North America, and the United Kingdom, the prevalence rate is less than 5%.[43,44] The decrease in the incidence of HCV-associated lymphoproliferative disorders following antiviral therapy (i.e., interferon and/or ribavirin) especially of indolent B-cell NHL strongly supports a relationship between chronic HCV infection and B-cell lymphoma.[38,45] In a recent meta-analysis of 15 studies, the pooled relative risk of all B-NHL among HCV-positive persons was found to be 2.5 (95% CI 2.1–3.1) in case–control studies and 2.0 (95% CI, 1.8–2.2) in cohort studies. Relative risks were consistently increased for all major B-NHL subtypes.[46] The mechanism(s) by which HCV induces B-cell lymphoma have yet to be defined. Postulated mechanisms involve (1) chronic antigen stimulation, (2) high-affinity interaction between HCV-E2 protein and its cellular receptors, (3) direct HCV infection of B-cells, and (4) HCV-induced mutations in proto-oncogenes and tumor suppressor genes. Together all of them lead to an oncogenetic transformation of the infected B-cells in a so-called hit-and-run mechanism of cell transformation.[47] Recently approved antiviral agents against chronic HCV with genotype 1 demonstrated a high-rate of sustained virological response. According to the American Association of the Study of Liver Diseases, combined therapy with direct-acting antiviral agents should be considered in asymptomatic HCV genotype 1 patients diagnosed with low-grade B-cell NHL since antiviral therapy can result in a complete oncologic remission. For aggressive B-cell NHL patients who are HCV carriers, antiviral therapy should be considered after completion of lymphoma therapy.[27]

## CLINICAL AND HISTOLOGICAL SUBTYPES OF LYMPHOMA

### Peripheral T-Cell Lymphoma

Peripheral T-cell lymphomas (PTCLs) are a heterogeneous group of lymphoproliferative disorders arising from mature T-cells of post-thymic origin, accounting for about 10% of NHL cases.[48] PTCLs are clinically aggressive lymphoid malignancies associated with a poor clinical outcome. Complex and rare histological subtypes, delayed diagnosis, lack of robust evidence-based medicine treatment guidelines, and associated deregulation of the immune system commonly observed in T-cell lymphoma patients (i.e., opportunistic infections, autoimmune phenomena, and/or hemophagocytosis) are contributing factors that affect the treatment selection and clinical outcomes in PTCL. Aggressive T-cell lymphomas include the nodal, extra-nodal, and leukemic disease groups.[49] The nodal lymphoma group includes PTCL, not otherwise specified (PTCL-NOS), the most common PTCLs accounting for 25.9% of cases. PTCL-NOS is more common in North America and less common in the European and Asian countries. Angioimmunoblastic T-cell lymphoma (AITL) is the second most common form of PTCLs accounting for 18.5% of cases. AITL is more common in Europe than in Asia or North America, often associated with autoimmune phenomena. Anaplastic large cell lymphoma (ALCL), further separated into the anaplastic large cell kinase (ALK)+ and ALK− entities, represents the third most common type of nodal PTCL.[1,9] ALK− ALCL is slightly more common in Europe and is associated with extra-nodal involvement, but ALK+ ALCL is more common in North America.[50] The extra-nodal PTCL group is a less common group of T-cell malignancies. Hepatosplenic T-cell lymphoma accounts for 1.4% of PTCL cases.[9] The disease is common in children and young males who often present with B-symptoms and cytopenias.[51,52] Enteropathy-associated T-cell lymphoma accounts for 4.7% of cases of T-cell lymphoma but is more common in geographic areas where the incidence of celiac disease is higher such as in North America and Europe but less common in Asia.[9] Panniculitis-like T-cell lymphomas constitute only 0.9% of PTCL, are more common in men, and often are associated with hemophagocytosis.[9,49] The T-cell leukemia group consists of T-cell chronic large granular lymphocytic leukemia, ATLL associated with the HTLV-1, aggressive NK-cell leukemia/lymphoma, and T-cell pro-lymphocytic leukemia (T-cell PLL). Those with aggressive NK-cell leukemia and ATLL are more common in Asia and often have a poor outcome.[1,49] NK-cell nasal-type lymphomas are occurring more frequently in Asia and Latin America. The increased incidence of T/NK-cell lymphomas in East Asia is related to the frequency of endemic HTLV-1 and EBV infections in these parts of the world.[53,54]

The International Prognostic Index (IPI), derived historically from DLBCL patients, has been applied and validated as a prognostic indicator score in PTCL patients. In general, patients with PTCLs have a poorer prognosis when compared to B-cell lymphoma patients with similar IPI scores and receiving similar aggressive combination chemotherapy treatments with or without high-dose chemotherapy and autologous stem cell rescue.[55] In a retrospective GELA study, PTCLs compared to B-cell lymphoma are shown to have a poorer prognosis in all outcomes, including CR rates (54% vs. 63%), 5-year OS rate (41% vs. 52%), and 5-year event-free survival rates (32% vs. 45%). ALCL has a better CR rate (69% vs. 45%) and median OS (65 vs. 20 months) as compared to other PTCLs subtype in another retrospective study.[56] A new prognostic index specifically designed for PTCL, the prognostic index for PTCL, is similar to the IPI, including age, lactate dehydrogenase, performance status, and bone marrow involvement. When applied to patients with PTCL-NOS, the index separated patients into more specific prognostic groups than the IPI.[57]

T-cell lymphomas have traditionally been treated much like the B-cell lymphomas, with systemic combination chemotherapy regimens. CHOP is the most widely used, although there were no randomized studies that proved that it was the best therapy, and with the exception of ALK+ ALCL, outcomes are disappointing compared to the favorable results achieved with DLBCL (especially after the incorporation of rituximab in B-cell lymphoma treatment). A retrospective meta-analysis of 2,912 patients treated with CHOP or CHOP-like regimens reported a 5-year OS of 37% and median 5-year OS rates <40%.[58] Chemotherapy regimens more intensive than CHOP, including hyper-fractionated cyclophosphamide, vincristine, doxorubicin, and dexamethasone alternating with high-dose methotrexate and cytarabine regimen (hyper-CVAD/HD-MC)[59] and CHOP + etoposide (CHOEP),[60] have not shown any significant improvement in OS in patients with PTCL, with the exception of ALCL. Due to unfavorable results with conventional chemotherapy, several studies explore the role of HDC-ASCS as a first-line consolidation therapy option. Several retrospective studies have reported positive outcomes with HDC-ASCS in patients with PTCL during first or subsequent remission.[61-69] The 3-year OS rate and PFS rate ranged from 53% to 58% and 44% to 50%, respectively. Several prospective studies have also demonstrated improved treatment outcome in patients with PTCLs, except for ALK+ ALCL, utilizing HDC-ASCS as a consolidation treatment (especially in patients with ALK– ALCL).[70-77] The NLG-T-01 study evaluated dose-dense induction therapy with CHOEP in patients with previously untreated PTCL followed by HDC-ASCS responding to initial induction chemotherapy. Following induction therapy, 71% of patients underwent HDC-ASCS. The 5-year OS and PFS rates were 51% and 44%, respectively.[70,76,77] CHOP chemotherapy followed by HDC-ASCS results in an estimated 3-year OS, and PFS rates were 48% and 36%, respectively.[74] The NCCN recommends CHOP or CHOEP and involved field radiation therapy (IF-XRT) for patients with early-stage ALK+ ALCL or six cycles of CHOP/CHOEP for patients with advance-stage ALK+ ALCL. For other T-cell subtypes, multi-agent systemic chemotherapy with adjuvant locoregional radiation therapy to involved region is recommended for patients with low/low intermediate risk stage I–II disease, and additional consolidation with HDC-ASCS should be considered for high-risk stage I–II and all stage III–IV patients.[27] Several novel therapeutic agents have been studied in clinical trials and include novel and more potent histone deacetylase inhibitors, immunomodulatory agents, nucleoside analogs, proteasome inhibitors, and cell-signaling inhibitors.[49]

## Mature NK-/T-Cell Lymphoma

Mature NK-/T-cell lymphoma is a rare subtype of NHL. In the 2008 WHO classification, two subtypes were recognized: extra-nodal NK-/T-cell lymphoma (nasal type) and aggressive NK-cell leukemia.[1] Nevertheless, NK-/T-cell lymphoma nasal type can have extra-nasal presentation(s). From the International T-Cell Lymphoma Project, the largest population study of T-cell lymphoma patients, NK-/T-cell lymphomas were identified in 12% of patients; among these 68% were nasal type, 26% were extra-nasal, and 6% were aggressive or unclassifiable.[9,78] The frequency of mature NK-/T-cell lymphoma is higher in Asia than in Western countries (22% vs. 5%). EBV has been implicated in the pathogenesis of and has been found in the tumor cells of nasal/NK-cell lymphomas and aggressive NK-cell leukemia.[79] NK-/T-cell lymphoma is considered to have poor prognosis and generally is refractory to standard chemotherapy regimens (i.e., CHOP or CHOEP). Over-expression of P-glycoprotein in NK-/T-cell lymphomas has shown to contribute to the chemoresistant phenotype observed, and poor clinical outcomes were observed in those patients treated with CHOP-based therapies.[80,81] According to outcomes from the International T-Cell Lymphoma Project, the 5-year OS rates for all patients with NK-/T-cell lymphoma was 32%, and the median OS was about 8 months.[9,78] The IPI score is limited in patients with NK-/T-cell lymphoma partly because most patients have a dismal clinical outcome regardless of the stage of the disease. The new prognostic model specifically designed for patients with NK-/T-cell lymphoma identified four risk groups with different survival outcomes based on presence or absence of B-symptoms, stage of the disease, lactic dehydrogenase levels, and regional lymph node involvement.[82] The optimal treatment approach for patients with NK-/T-cell lymphoma have not yet been established. Several studies suggest that concurrent chemotherapy and IF-XRT is effective in patients with stage IE or contiguous stage IIE with cervical node involvement.[83-85] A phase II Korean clinical trial treated 30 patients with stage I/II NK-/T-cell lymphoma nasal type with concurrent chemotherapy (cisplatin) and radiotherapy (40% to 52.8 Gy) followed by three cycles of etoposide, ifosfamide, cisplatin, and dexamethasone (VIPD). The CR rate was 80% after chemotherapy. The estimated 3-year PFS and OS rates were 85% and 86%, respectively.[84] The phase I/II study conducted by the Japanese Clinical Oncology group showed similar results. A total of 33 patients were treated with concurrent IF-XRT (50 Gy) and three courses of chemotherapy with dexamethasone, etoposide, ifosfamide, and carboplatin (DeVIC). The CR rate was 77% and the 2-year OS was 78%.[83] Several studies showed that a L-asparaginase-based regimen was effective for patients with advanced, relapsed, or refractory NK-/T-cell lymphoma.[86-89] A recent phase II study from the NK-cell Tumor Study Group conducted in Japan evaluated the efficacy and safety of a novel regimen consisting of dexamethasone, methotrexate, ifosfamide, L-asparaginase, and etoposide (SMILE regimen) in 38 patients with newly diagnosed stage IV or relapsed or refractory NK-/T-cell lymphoma nasal type. The overall response rate (ORR) and CR rate were 79% and 45%, respectively. The 1-year OS rate was 55% (95% CI, 38% to 69%).[88] The EBV-DNA copy number was shown to be predictive factor of response after SMILE chemotherapy. The ORR was 88% in patients with less than $10^5$ EBV-DNA copies/mL as opposed to 44% in patients with >$10^5$ EBV-DNA copies/mL.[90] The efficacy and safety of the SMILE regimen were confirmed in an unselected patient population with previously untreated stage III/IV or relapsed/refractory NK-/T-cell lymphoma by the Asia Lymphoma Study Group. The ORR was reported to be 81%, and with a median follow-up of 31 months, the estimated 5-year OS was 50% and 4-year disease free survival was 64%.[91]

## Burkitt's Lymphoma (BL)

BL is a rare aggressive mature B-cell lymphoma typically involving extra-nodal sites. It was the first human tumor found to be associated with the EBV virus. In addition, it was the first lymphoma associated with a very specific chromosomal translocation (i.e., t(8;14) resulting in c-myc deregulation) and the first lymphoma reported to be associated with HIV infection.[92-94] Three clinical variants of BL are recognized: endemic BL, sporadic BL, and immunodeficiency-associated BL.[1] All three clinical variants are similar in morphology, immunophenotype, and genetic features. The endemic variant is associated with malaria and EBV infection (100% of the cases). It is the most common childhood cancer in areas where malaria is endemic (e.g., equatorial Africa, Brazil, and Papua New Guinea).[95] Sporadic BL accounts for 1% to 2% of all adult lymphomas in the United States and Western Europe. In contrast to endemic BL, sporadic BL is associated with EBV infection only in about 30% of cases.[96] Immunodeficiency-associated BL occurs mainly in patients infected with HIV, but can occur in post-solid organ or hematological transplant patients and/or in congenital immunodeficiency patients.[97,98] The risk of BL, in contrast to all other lymphomas, actually declines at the lowest CD4 counts. Immunodeficiency-related BL is associated with EBV infection in 40% of the cases.[99] The risk of BL increases 4 to 5 years after organ transplantation, but this risk is much less as compared to that associated with HIV infection.[100] The link between malaria infection, EBV, and endemic BL has been reported.[101] Two epidemiological studies showed that the risk of BL was greatest in people with the highest titers of antibodies against both EBV and *Plasmodium falciparum*.[102,103] Several studies have shown that malaria can cause profound deregulation of EBV infection and induces the immunoglobulin-MYC translocation characteristic of BL.[104-114] In EBV-infected B-cell, the cysteine-rich inter-domain 1 of the *P. falciparum* erythrocyte membrane protein induces reactivation of EBV infection.[111] In addition, *P. falciparum* has a ligand for toll-like receptor 9 that can induce the enzyme cytidine deaminase in human B-cells.[112-114] The over-expression of this enzyme induces immunoglobulin-MYC translocations.[110] In BL, extra-nodal sites are often involved. In all three clinical variants, patients are at risk of CNS involvement. Patients with endemic BL most frequently present with jaw and other facial bone lesions. Infiltration of bone marrow is rare.[115,116] In sporadic BL, approximately 60% to 80% of presentation involves the abdomen (retroperitoneal tissue, gut, ovary, or kidney). Presenting symptoms include abdominal pain, distension, nausea, vomiting, and gastrointestinal bleeding.[117] The next most common site is the head and neck and is manifested by rapidly growing lymphadenopathy and involvement of the nasal, oropharynx, tonsils, or sinus regions. Bone marrow is infiltrated in 20% of patients. Some cases are classified as Burkitt's leukemia and are characterized by more than 25% lymphoblasts in bone marrow specimen. The typical immunophenotype of BL is sIg+, CD10+, CD19+, CD20+, CD22+, TdT-, Ki67+ (>95%), BCL2+, BCL6+, and simple karyotype with MYC rearrangement. Translocations involving the MYC gene are detected in nearly all cases of BL.

In high-income countries, the diagnosis of BL can be done with a core or an excisional biopsy of lymph node. On the other hand, in some cases a laparotomy or laparoscopy is necessary to obtain adequate tissue. Several essential investigations including complete blood count, renal function, liver function test, and EBV status should be obtained. Computed tomography (CT-scan) of chest/abdomen/pelvis and bone marrow examination are necessary for staging purposes. Functional imaging with positron emission tomography scan is recommended but not essential and should not delay treatment if urgently indicated. After the confirmation of diagnosis, bone marrow (BM) aspiration and central system fluid (CSF) should be examined for the presence of malignant cells. In contrast, BL patients in underdeveloped countries face several diagnostic and therapeutic challenges. Diagnostic facilities in low-income countries are likely to be limited. The most common diagnostic test in some countries could be the cytological examination of tumor cells from a fine-needle aspirate. Results are usually not available at the time of treatment clinical decision-making. Common coinfection such as malaria or parasite infestation should be identified and treated before chemotherapy agents are administered. Concomitant HIV infection should be tested so that antiretroviral therapy can be given after planned chemotherapy. Tuberculosis (TB) and Kaposi's sarcoma should be ruled out.[118]

BL is curable in a significant subset of patients when treated with dose-intensive, multi-agent chemotherapy in combination with rituximab regimens that include CNS prophylaxis. Approximately 60% to 90% of pediatric and young adult patients with BL achieve durable remission.[119] However, the survival of older adult BL patients appears to be less favorable.[120] In low-income countries, treatment failure can be caused by incomplete treatment, treatment-related mortality, late presentation, or relapsed/refractory disease. The intensity of treatment is determined by the amount of available supportive care, tolerance of chemotherapy, and the extent of comorbidities. In Malawi, the treatment for BL of all stages is intravenous cyclophosphamide (40 mg/kg on day 1 and oral cyclophosphamide 60 mg/kg on days 8, 18, and 28) for four cycles. Intrathecal hydrocortisone 12.5 mg and methotrexate 12.5 mg are given with each treatment cycle for four cycles. The cost of this 28-day treatment is less than US$50. This regimen has 1-year EFS about 50% and treatment-related mortality was roughly 5%.[121] In a French-African Pediatric Oncology Group study, two moderately intensive modified LMB-89 protocols including high-dose methotrexate and cytarabine were used in several French-speaking African countries. Of 306 patients, 23.2% died during the induction therapy; 13.1% deaths were attributed to infection.[122] Adequate supportive care, nutritional support as endemic malnutrition is associated with chemotherapy-related neutropenia, management of tumor lysis syndrome, antiemetics, transfusion support, and antibiotic therapy are essential.[118,123] In developed countries, the regimens used in adult patients have been adapted from pediatric protocols and include intensive multi-agent chemotherapy along with CNS prophylaxis. A highly effective regimen involves cyclophosphamide, vincristine, doxorubicin, high-dose methotrexate (CODOX), alternating with ifosfamide, etoposide, and high-dose cytarabine (IVAC) either original or modified. In low-risk patients, the 2-year EFS and OS rates were 83% and 81%, respectively, compared with 60% and 70%, respectively, for high-risk patients.[124–126] The addition of the anti-CD20 monoclonal antibody (mAb), rituximab, has shown improvement in EFS and OS outcome.[127,128] Another effective regimen in BL patients combines rituximab with hyper-CVAD/HD-MC.[129,130] The 3-year DFS and OS were 88% and 88%, respectively, among BL patients treated with rituximab + hyper-CVAD/HD-MC. The Cancer and Leukemia Group B (CALGB) studied the CALGB10002 regimen in BL patients. The regimen included the administration of cyclophosphamide, cytarabine, dexamethasone, doxorubicin, etoposide, ifosfamide, methotrexate, vincristine, and prednisone.[131] The 2-year EFS and OS rates were 77% and 79%, respectively. Dose-adjusted R-DA-EPOCH has been studied in BL patients. This particular regimen is active and results in EFS and OS rates of 97% and 100%, respectively, at a median follow-up of 57 months.[132] The treatment approach for relapsed/refractory BL is yet to be defined, especially in countries where bone marrow transplantation is not available. Chemotherapy regimens are based on limited, retrospective studies with a few patients. The best options for patients who require therapy for relapsed or refractory disease are investigational treatments in the context of clinical trials. In low-income countries, better diagnostic testing and a higher standard of supportive care are necessary to deliver more effective therapies and improve clinical outcomes. In addition, novel, effective, less toxic, and inexpensive therapies are needed. The improvement in molecular profiling and a better understanding of the biology of BL as with other forms of NHL are paving the road for the development of novel targeted agents.[118]

## GLOBAL CHALLENGES IN THE MANAGEMENT OF LYMPHOMA

### The Impact of Rituximab in the Management of B-Cell Lymphoma

Rituximab is a chimeric IgG1 targeting antibody CD20 and was one of the first mAbs to be approved by the Food and Drug Association (FDA) for the treatment of hematological malignancies. Four weekly doses of rituximab are well tolerated and results in clinically meaningful responses in up to 50% of previously treated indolent NHL patients.[133,134] As a result of the initial clinical studies, rituximab became the first mAb to be approved by the FDA to treat patients with B-cell lymphoma.[135] However, in ~50% of indolent NHL patients treated with rituximab, little to no clinical benefit can be demonstrated. Scientific efforts to improve its antitumor activity are based on improving the understanding of the biology of CD20 and the mechanisms of action of rituximab. Historically, Czuczman et al. reported the first multicenter study evaluating rituximab in combination with standard doses of CHOP.[136,137] The study was a multi-institutional phase II clinical trial that evaluated the safety and efficacy of rituximab in combination with CHOP and enrolled 40 patients with either newly diagnosed or previously treated low-grade or follicular B-cell NHL expressing CD20. Patients with bulky disease (defined as any single mass >10 cm in its greater diameter) or with prior anthracycline therapy were excluded. The results of this study were impressive as initially reported and then updated after a 9-year follow-up period.[137] The ORR was 95% and 22 patients (55%) achieved a CR and 16 patients (40%) a partial response (PR). In the subsequent and final analysis of the study, responses were updated using the International Workshop Response Criteria (IWRC) developed for lymphomas as described.[138] According to IWRC, the ORR was 100%, with 87% of the patients achieving a CR or unconfirmed complete response and 13% a PR. The median TTP in all patients was 82.3 months (range 4.5 to 105.6+ months) and the median duration of response was 83.5 months (range 3.1 to 105.1+ months). At the time of the final analysis, 42% of the patients continue to be on long-term remission. The toxicity profile of the combination was comparable to that observed for CHOP alone. Moreover, the addition of rituximab and CHOP did not compromise the CHOP dose intensity or density.[136,137] Mature data from randomized clinical studies has demonstrated the superiority of rituximab in combination with chemotherapy against chemotherapy alone in terms of response rates, TTP, and OS in patients with indolent lymphomas.[139–141] Rituximab in combination with systemic chemotherapy has improved ORR, PFS, and OS in aggressive B-cell NHL when compared to chemotherapy alone.[142–145] Long-term results from the GELA study in treating diffuse large B-cell lymphoma are as follows: the 10-year PFS and OS were 36.5% and 43.5% in R-CHOP compared with 20% and 27.6% in CHOP alone.[142] Based on all the information generated from prospective clinical trials, rituximab in combination with systemic chemotherapy has become the standard of care for the treatment of aggressive B-cell lymphoma and in the majority of indolent B-cell lymphoma requiring systemic therapy in North America and European countries.

## Global Access to Effective Immunotherapy (mAbs)

The clinical benefit of rituximab is beyond dispute. However, the significant cost of rituximab creates a major barrier that limits access to this agent in the underdeveloped world. Bio-similars are protein products that are sufficiently similar to a biopharmaceutical agent already approved by a regulatory agency.[146] Since 2007, bio-similar products of rituximab had been developed. One of them, Reditux was developed by Dr. Reddy's Laboratories Ltd and has been used for the treatment of NHL in India and other countries.[146] This bio-similar product has a biochemical profile similar to rituximab, including molecular weight, N-amino acid terminal structure, and sequencing of the heavy chain and light chain similar. On the other hand, it has never been tested in clinical trial before marketing in large scale. Indian regulatory agencies accepted comparability studies from Dr. Reddy's Laboratories based on circular dichromism (CD) studies. There are some concerns regarding the accuracy of CD studies in terms of sensitivity/specificity in detecting sequence variants problems due to mutations of bio-similar rituximab product during the production process.[147] Currently, two other manufacturers of generic drugs are conducting clinical trials comparing the pharmacokinetics, pharmacodynamics, safety, and efficacy between rituximab and anti-CD20 mAb bio-similars for the treatment of rheumatoid arthritis.[146] It is uncertain if the approval and clinical use of bio-similars will decrease the cost of anti-CD20 mAbs and improve the access of this agent in poor countries.

## Challenges in the Management of Lymphoma in the African Continent

In sub-Saharan Africa, most NHLs are BL or HIV-associated NHL and the treatment outcomes are very poor.[148] In Uganda, NHL treated with CHOP chemotherapy results in a median OS of only 61 days.[149] Lack of trained health workers and equipment leads the development of pragmatic approaches to the treatment of B-cell lymphoma in Africa, such as the development of oral regimens. One prospective study in Kenya and Uganda evaluated an oral regimen consisting of lomustine, etoposide, cyclophosphamide, and procarbazine given as first-line therapy in HIV-associated NHL resulting in a median OS of 12.3 months.[150] Radiotherapy access is also limited. Only 18% of radiotherapy needed for the management of lymphoma is provided. Moreover, 21 countries in sub-Saharan Africa have no operational radiotherapy units available.[151] Besides the limited access to immunotherapy, chemotherapy, and radiation therapy, resources to diagnoses, supportive care, and palliation are also scarce.[148] In sub-Saharan Africa where the patients frequently have HIV and other immunosuppressive conditions such as malnutrition, infectious complications from cancer therapy present a significant obstacle. Cancer treatment increases the risk of TB reactivation in endemic areas.[152,153] Bacterial infection is also another major obstacle following chemotherapy; gram-negative enteric pathogens are likely to predominate as the source of febrile neutropenia episodes.[123] Available intravenous antibiotics include penicillin, ampicillin, ceftriaxone, chloramphenicol, ciprofloxacin, gentamicin, metronidazole, and sulfamethoxazole-trimethoprim.[154] However, the antibiotics used for empiric treatment for febrile neutropenia (i.e., vancomycin, ceftazidime, and imipenem) in developed countries, are not usually available.[148] In addition, antifungal agents against invasive molds are lacking. Furthermore, access to growth factor support is extremely limited. Lack of transfusion support is another major obstacle; as an example, only 41.5% of transfusions requested for patients in Africa were met in 2006. Most countries rely on hospital-based systems that require a family member to donate blood products as a replacement for an individual patient.[155,156] There is even less capacity for platelet transfusion due to technical barriers to preparation of pooled products from multiple donors or apheresis products from single donors. In addition, there remains a persistent risk of acquiring infectious agents (i.e., HIV, HBV, or HCV) via transfusion.[155,156]

## Disparities in the Management of Relapsed/Refractory Aggressive B-Cell Lymphoma

Patients with intermediate- or high-grade NHL who relapse after initial response or are refractory to initial therapy have a poor overall clinical outcome.[157,158] Salvage chemotherapy followed by HDC-ASCS is the most effective therapy in relapsed/refractory DLBCL patients as long as they are eligible, and this aggressive approach is available. Comorbid conditions, duration of initial response, IPI score at relapse, response to salvage chemotherapy, and experience of the treating center play a role in the clinical outcome of relapsed/refractory DLBCL patients. Given the risks involved in HDC-ASCS, patients with suspected relapsed/refractory DLBCL should undergo a repeat biopsy to document recurrent/persistent active disease. Repeat biopsy is also important to further characterize and identify key regulatory pathways for which novel targeted agents may be available.[159] HDC-ASCS and to a lesser degree allogeneic stem cell transplantation (allo-SCT) play an important role both in first-line (i.e., mantle cell lymphoma and T-cell lymphoma), high-risk aggressive lymphoma and in relapsed refractory disease (i.e., DLBCL).[70–74,160–171] HDC-ASCS was initially evaluated in patients with relapsed/refractory DLBCL. In 1995, the PARMA trial randomized 215 patients with chemotherapy-sensitive relapsed DLBCL to salvage chemotherapy consisting of dexamethasone, cisplatin, and high-dose cytarabine (DHAP) followed by observation or HDC-ASCS. Both EFS and OS were significantly superior in patients receiving HDC-ASCS following salvage chemotherapy when compared to the chemotherapy-alone group (46% vs. 12%, p = 0.001 and 53% vs. 12%, p = 0.038).[161] As rituximab changed the treatment paradigm of patients with DLBCL, it has been postulated that the current subset of patients with refractory or relapsed DLBCL represents a different patient population to the one studied in pre-rituximab clinical trials. Several investigators are questioning if response to second-line chemotherapy or if the value of HDC-ASCS in patients relapsing or primary refractory DLBCL previously treated with R-CHOP has decreased when compared to historical controls. The need to develop novel salvage chemotherapy regimens after rituximab-CHOP failures was further demonstrated by the results of the prospective multicenter phase III Collaborative trial in relapsed aggressive lymphoma (CORAL) study. This study was aimed to define the most appropriate salvage chemotherapy regimen and the role, if any, of rituximab maintenance after HDC-ASCS. In this study, patients with relapsed/refractory after/to CHOP or R-CHOP DLBCL were randomized to receive three cycles of R-ICE or R-DHAP followed by high-dose chemotherapy with carmustine, etoposide, cytarabine and melphalan (BEAM) and ASCS. Subsequently, patients were randomized to rituximab maintenance or observation. The study enrolled 396 patients stratified on basis of prior exposure to rituximab, relapsed (within 12 months or after 12 months following frontline therapy) versus refractory. The investigators demonstrated that factors affecting EFS include second-line age-adjusted international prognostic index (aaIPI) of 0 to 1 (39% vs. 56%, p = 0.0084), relapsed <12 months after completion of first-line therapy (36% vs. 68%, p < 0.001), and prior rituximab exposure in the frontline setting (34% vs. 66%, p < 0.001).[172] While no significant differences in terms of response rates were observed between patients treated with R-ICE and R-DHAP, the response to salvage chemotherapy was lower among patients previously treated with R-CHOP (51%) when compared to those patients treated with CHOP in the frontline setting (83%). Moreover, the CR rate in R-CHOP pretreated patients to either R-ICE or R-DHAP was only 38%.[172,173] The results of the CORAL study validated the predictive value of the aaIPI in the relapsed/refractory setting, and rituximab chemotherapy used as a frontline therapy appears to select for a DLBCL phenotype that is refractory to standard salvage regimens. Because drug costs of R-DHAP are significantly less than that of R-ICE, R-DHAP is the preferred salvage therapy before HDC-ASCS.[159] There were no differences in 4-year EFS rates between rituximab maintenance after HDC-ASCT as compared to observation (52% vs. 53%, p = 0.7).[174] Although, there are encouraging results in relapsed and refractory DLBCL, HDC-ASCT has not shown a benefit as first-line consolidation in first remission.[175] The Cochrane Hematological Malignancies Group performed a meta-analysis in 2008, which included data from 15 randomized controlled trials with a total of 3,079 aggressive NHL patients treated with HDC-ASCS in first remission versus observation following first-line therapy. There was no evidence that HDC-ASCS improves OS (HR 1.05; CI 0.92 to 1.19) or EFS (HR 0.92; CI 0.80 to 1.05) in this clinical setting.[176] However, there is evidence that high-risk DLBCL patients may benefit from HDC-ASCS in first remission. Now, up-front HDC-ASCS following R-CHOP therapy is recommended only in selected high-risk patients or in the context of a clinical trial.[27] Allo-HCT has been used as a salvage strategy, with encouraging results for patients who failed previous HDC-ASCS.[159] The European Group for Blood and Marrow Transplantation analyzed retrospectively the outcome of DLBCL patients receiving allo-BMT after failing HDC-ASCS. This study included 101 patients; conditioning regimens were non-myeloablative in 64 patients. The 3-year PFS was 41% and OS was 53%. Patients with a long remission after HDC-ASCT and with chemosensitive disease at the time of allo-BMT seem to benefit the most from this elaborate and complicated procedure.[177] While HDC-ASCS has shown to improve the OS of relapsed/refractory DLBCL, this treatment modality is not fully accessible in many parts of the world, for instance, sub-Saharan Africa or certain regions in Asia. The Center for International Blood and Marrow Transplant Research (CIBMTR) has more than 300 centers worldwide, but the majority of centers are located in North America. In 2012, CIBMTR reported that approximately 12,000 patients underwent HDC-ASCS and 7,000 had an allo-BMT.[178] The CIBMTR has availability to international data in order to assess outcomes in rare indications outside the United States, to understand international differences in access and outcomes, and/or to determine the outcome of HDC-ASCS performed with U.S. products in international centers. The CIBMTR has active voluntary participation from 17 centers in Canada, 24 in Latin America, 46 in Europe, 7 in the Middle East, 14 in Asia, 2 in Africa, and 18 in Australia/New Zealand. Providing cutting-edge treatment is not the only problem encountered in underdeveloped countries; proper data collection and documentation needs significant improvement. A recently published study demonstrated deficiencies in the care of DLBCL patients in India. Vidyasagar et al. analyzed 303 cases of DLBCL treated between 2000 and 2006. Only 100 patients had a complete pretreatment evaluation and received some form of treatment. Several factors contributed to suboptimal management of the remaining 203 patients: (1) financial constraint, (2) distance from treatment center, (3) miscommunication between the treating physician and the patient/caregivers, (4) poor prognosis/fear of relapse, or (5) preferences for alternate medicine. Despite all of these factors, the OS of the cohort studied at 5 years was 50%.[179]

In summary, the improvement in our understanding in the biology of lymphoma, the incorporation of mAbs to systemic chemotherapy, development of more effective and less toxic chemotherapy regimens, the discovery of novel targeted agents, risk-stratified chemotherapy selection, identification and validation of biomarkers predictive of prognosis, the use of HDC-ASCS, and monitoring treatment response by functional imaging are factors that have contributed to the improvement in clinical outcomes in patients with various subtypes of NHL. On the other hand, a significant population in the world is not receiving the benefit from such advances. There is a dire need to globalize the medical knowledge and training so that better care and infrastructure can be developed in underdeveloped countries. Moreover, a global effort needs to be organized in order to assure that curative therapeutic approaches and/or effective therapeutic interventions reach lymphoma patients not only in developed countries but also in poorer countries where abundant areas with limited medical care access exist and lack of education is prevalent. As practicing oncologists and academicians, we have an obligation to assist in improving the concept of global health care.

## REFERENCES

1. Steven H. Swerdlow EC, Harris NL, et al. *WHO Classification of Tumours of Haematopoietic and Lymphoid Tissues*. 4th ed. Lyon, France: International Agency for Research on Cancer, 2008.
2. Ferlay J, Shin H, Bray F, Forman D, Mathers C, Parkin DM. *GLOBOCAN 2008 v2.0, Cancer Incidence and Mortality Worldwide: IARC CancerBase No. 10*. Lyon, France: International Agency for Research on Cancer, 2010. Available at http://globocan.iarc.fr. Accessed 18 April, 2013.
3. Arisawa K, Soda M, Endo S, et al. Evaluation of adult T-cell leukemia/lymphoma incidence and its impact on non-Hodgkin lymphoma incidence in southwestern Japan. *Int J Cancer* 2000; 85: 319–24.
4. Boffetta P. I. Epidemiology of adult non-Hodgkin lymphoma. *Ann Oncol* 2011; 22(Suppl 4): iv27–iv31.
5. Newton R. *Epidemiology of Exogenous Human Retroviruses Associated with Hematologic Malignancies*. 3rd ed. London: Hodder Arnold, 2010, pp. 99–115.
6. Zahra M. *Epidemiology of Lymphoid Malignancy in Asia, Epidemiology Insights*, Dr. Maria De Lourdes Ribeiro De Souza Da Cunha (Ed.), 2012. ISBN: 978–953–51–0565–7, InTech, doi:10.5772/31746. Available at http://www.in techopen.com/books/epidemiology-insights/epidemiology-of-lymphoid-ma lignancy-in-asia. Accessed April 2, 2013.
7. Anderson JR, Armitage JO, Weisenburger DD. Epidemiology of the non-Hodgkin's lymphomas: distributions of the major subtypes differ by geographic locations. Non-Hodgkin's Lymphoma Classification Project. *Ann Oncol* 1998; 9: 717–20.
8. Nakamura S, Koshikawa T, Koike K, et al. Phenotypic analysis of peripheral T cell lymphoma among the Japanese. *Acta Pathol Jpn* 1993; 43: 396–412.
9. Vose J, Armitage J, Weisenburger D. International peripheral T-cell and natural killer/T-cell lymphoma study: pathology findings and clinical outcomes. *J Clin Oncol* 2008; 26: 4124–30.
10. Mannucci S, Luzzi A, Carugi A, et al. EBV reactivation and chromosomal polysomies: Euphorbia tirucalli as a possible cofactor in endemic Burkitt lymphoma. *Adv Hematol* 2012; 149780.

11. Cote TR, Biggar RJ, Rosenberg PS, et al. Non-Hodgkin's lymphoma among people with AIDS: incidence, presentation and public health burden. AIDS/Cancer Study Group. *Int J Cancer* 1997; 73: 645–50.

12. Dong HY, Scadden DT, de Leval L, Tang Z, Isaacson PG, Harris NL. Plasmablastic lymphoma in HIV-positive patients: an aggressive Epstein-Barr virus-associated extramedullary plasmacytic neoplasm. *Am J Surg Pathol* 2005; 29: 1633–41.

13. Delecluse HJ, Anagnostopoulos I, Dallenbach F, et al. Plasmablastic lymphomas of the oral cavity: a new entity associated with the human immunodeficiency virus infection. *Blood* 1997; 89: 1413–20.

14. Ascoli V, Lo Coco F, Torelli G, et al. Human herpesvirus 8-associated primary effusion lymphoma in HIV—patients: a clinicopidemiologic variant resembling classic Kaposi's sarcoma. *Haematologica* 2002; 87: 339–43.

15. Bohlius J, Schmidlin K, Costagliola D, et al. Prognosis of HIV-associated non-Hodgkin lymphoma in patients starting combination antiretroviral therapy. *AIDS* 2009; 23: 2029–37.

16. Besson C, Goubar A, Gabarre J, et al. Changes in AIDS-related lymphoma since the era of highly active antiretroviral therapy. *Blood* 2001; 98: 2339–44.

17. Levine AM, Seneviratne L, Espina BM, et al. Evolving characteristics of AIDS-related lymphoma. *Blood* 2000; 96: 4084–90.

18. Ambinder R. Herpesvirus and lymphoma. In: Magrath IT (Ed). *The Lymphoid Neoplasms*. 3rd ed. London: Hodder Arnold, 2010, pp. 116–25.

19. Clarke CA, Glaser SL. Epidemiologic trends in HIV-associated lymphomas. *Curr Opin Oncol* 2001; 13: 354–59.

20. Cancer ICoHa. Highly active antiretroviral therapy and incidence of cancer in human immunodeficiency virus-infected adults. *J Natl Cancer Inst* 2000; 92: 1823–30.

21. Chao C, Xu L, Abrams D, et al. Survival of non-Hodgkin lymphoma patients with and without HIV infection in the era of combined antiretroviral therapy. *AIDS* 2010; 24: 1765–70.

22. Lim ST, Karim R, Nathwani BN, Tulpule A, Espina B, Levine AM. AIDS-related Burkitt's lymphoma versus diffuse large-cell lymphoma in the pre-highly active antiretroviral therapy (HAART) and HAART eras: significant differences in survival with standard chemotherapy. *J Clin Oncol* 2005; 23: 4430–38.

23. Kaplan LD, Lee JY, Ambinder RF, et al. Rituximab does not improve clinical outcome in a randomized phase 3 trial of CHOP with or without rituximab in patients with HIV-associated non-Hodgkin lymphoma: AIDS-Malignancies Consortium Trial 010. *Blood* 2005; 106: 1538–43.

24. Boue F, Gabarre J, Gisselbrecht C, et al. Phase II trial of CHOP plus rituximab in patients with HIV-associated non-Hodgkin's lymphoma. *J Clin Oncol* 2006; 24: 4123–28.

25. Ribera JM, Oriol A, Morgades M, et al. Safety and efficacy of cyclophosphamide, adriamycin, vincristine, prednisone and rituximab in patients with human immunodeficiency virus-associated diffuse large B-cell lymphoma: results of a phase II trial. *Br J Haematol* 2008; 140: 411–19.

26. Spina M, Jaeger U, Sparano JA, et al. Rituximab plus infusional cyclophosphamide, doxorubicin, and etoposide in HIV-associated non-Hodgkin lymphoma: pooled results from 3 phase 2 trials. *Blood* 2005; 105: 1891–97.

27. National Comprehensive Cancer Network guidelines: Non-Hodgkin's Lymphoma version 1.2013. Available at http://www.nccn.org/professionals/physician_gls/pdf/nhl.pdf. Accessed March 9, 2013.

28. Dunleavy K, Little RF, Pittaluga S, et al. The role of tumor histogenesis, FDG-PET, and short-course EPOCH with dose-dense rituximab (SC-EPOCH-RR) in HIV-associated diffuse large B-cell lymphoma. *Blood* 2010; 115: 3017–24.

29. Sparano JA, Lee JY, Kaplan LD, et al. Rituximab plus concurrent infusional EPOCH chemotherapy is highly effective in HIV-associated B-cell non-Hodgkin lymphoma. *Blood* 2010; 115: 3008–16.

30. Dunleavy K, Little RF, Pittaluga S. A prospective study of dose-adjusted (DA) EPOCH with rituximab in adult with newly diagnosed Burkitt lymphoma: a regimen with high efficacy and low toxicity. *Ann Oncol* 2008; 19(Suppl 4): iv83–iv84.

31. Weinbaum CM, Williams I, Mast EE, et al. Recommendations for identification and public health management of persons with chronic hepatitis B virus infection. *MMWR Recomm Rep* 2008; 57: 1–20.

32. World Health Organization. Available at http://www.who.int/csr/disease/hepatitis/whocdscsrlyo20022/en/index3.html. Accessed January 2, 2013.

33. Yeo W, Chan TC, Leung NW, et al. Hepatitis B virus reactivation in lymphoma patients with prior resolved hepatitis B undergoing anticancer therapy with or without rituximab. *J Clin Oncol* 2009; 27: 605–11.

34. Zurawska U, Hicks LK, Woo G, et al. Hepatitis B virus screening before chemotherapy for lymphoma: a cost-effectiveness analysis. *J Clin Oncol* 2012; 30: 3167–73.

35. Rosen HR. Clinical practice. Chronic hepatitis C infection. *N Engl J Med* 2011; 364: 2429–38.

36. Ferri C, Caracciolo F, Zignego AL, et al. Hepatitis C virus infection in patients with non-Hodgkin's lymphoma. *Br J Haematol* 1994; 88: 392–94.

37. Luppi M, Longo G, Ferrari MG, et al. Clinico-pathological characterization of hepatitis C virus-related B-cell non-Hodgkin's lymphomas without symptomatic cryoglobulinemia. *Ann Oncol* 1998; 9: 495–98.

38. Marcucci F, Mele A. Hepatitis viruses and non-Hodgkin lymphoma: epidemiology, mechanisms of tumorigenesis, and therapeutic opportunities. *Blood* 2011; 117: 1792–98.

39. Mele A, Pulsoni A, Bianco E, et al. Hepatitis C virus and B-cell non-Hodgkin lymphomas: an Italian multicenter case-control study. *Blood* 2003; 102: 996–99.

40. Goldman L, Ezzat S, Mokhtar N, et al. Viral and non-viral risk factors for non-Hodgkin's lymphoma in Egypt: heterogeneity by histological and immunological subtypes. *Cancer Causes Control* 2009; 20: 981–87.

41. Pellicelli AM, Marignani M, Zoli V, et al. Hepatitis C virus-related B cell subtypes in non Hodgkin's lymphoma. *World J Hepatol* 2011; 3: 278–84.

42. Mizorogi F, Hiramoto J, Nozato A, et al. Hepatitis C virus infection in patients with B-cell non-Hodgkin's lymphoma. *Intern Med* 2000; 39: 112–17.

43. Hausfater P, Cacoub P, Sterkers Y, et al. Hepatitis C virus infection and lymphoproliferative diseases: prospective study on 1,576 patients in France. *Am J Hematol* 2001; 67: 168–71.

44. Sy T, Jamal MM. Epidemiology of hepatitis C virus (HCV) infection. *Int J Med Sci* 2006; 3: 41–46.

45. Luppi M, Barozzi P, Potenza L, Riva G, Morselli M, Torelli G. Is it now the time to update treatment protocols for lymphomas with new anti-virus systems? *Leukemia* 2004; 18: 1572–75.

46. Dal Maso L, Franceschi S. Hepatitis C virus and risk of lymphoma and other lymphoid neoplasms: a meta-analysis of epidemiologic studies. *Cancer Epidemiol Biomarkers Prev* 2006; 15: 2078–85.

47. Forghieri F, Luppi M, Barozzi P, et al. Pathogenetic mechanisms of hepatitis C virus-induced B-cell lymphomagenesis. *Clin Dev Immunol* 2012:807351.

48. Savage KJ. Peripheral T-cell lymphomas. *Blood Rev* 2007; 21: 201–16.

49. Foss FM, Zinzani PL, Vose JM, et al. Peripheral T-cell lymphoma. *Blood* 2011; 117: 6756–67.

50. Savage KJ, Harris NL, Vose JM, et al. ALK-anaplastic large-cell lymphoma is clinically and immunophenotypically different from both ALK+ ALCL and peripheral T-cell lymphoma, not otherwise specified: report from the International Peripheral T-Cell Lymphoma Project. *Blood* 2008; 111: 5496–504.

51. Charton-Bain MC, Brousset P, Bouabdallah R, et al. Variation in the histological pattern of nodal involvement by gamma/delta T-cell lymphoma. *Histopathology* 2000; 36: 233–39.

52. Gaulard P, Belhadj K, Reyes F. Gammadelta T-cell lymphomas. *Semin Hematol* 2003; 40: 233–43.

53. Yoshida M, Miyoshi I, Hinuma Y. Isolation and characterization of retrovirus from cell lines of human adult T-cell leukemia and its implication in the disease. *Proc Natl Acad Sci USA* 1982; 79: 2031–35.

54. Posner LE, Robert-Guroff M, Kalyanaraman VS, et al. Natural antibodies to the human T cell lymphoma virus in patients with cutaneous T cell lymphomas. *J Exp Med* 1981; 154: 333–46.

55. Gisselbrecht C, Gaulard P, Lepage E, et al. Prognostic significance of T-cell phenotype in aggressive non-Hodgkin's lymphomas. Groupe d'Etudes des Lymphomes de l'Adulte (GELA). *Blood* 1998; 92: 76–82.

56. Lopez-Guillermo A, Cid J, Salar A, et al. Peripheral T-cell lymphomas: initial features, natural history, and prognostic factors in a series of 174 patients diagnosed according to the R.E.A.L. Classification. *Ann Oncol* 1998; 9: 849–55.

57. Gallamini A, Stelitano C, Calvi R, et al. Peripheral T-cell lymphoma unspecified (PTCL-U): a new prognostic model from a retrospective multicentric clinical study. *Blood* 2004; 103: 2474–79.

58. Abouyabis AN SP, Flowers C, Lechowicz MJ. Response and survival rates in patients with peripheral T-cell lymphoma treated with anthracycline-based regimens: a comprehensive meta-analysis. Blood 2007; 110(11). Abstract 3452.

59. Escalon MP, Liu NS, Yang Y, et al. Prognostic factors and treatment of patients with T-cell non-Hodgkin lymphoma: the M. D. Anderson Cancer Center experience. *Cancer* 2005; 103: 2091–98.

60. Schmitz N, Trumper L, Ziepert M, et al. Treatment and prognosis of mature T-cell and NK-cell lymphoma: an analysis of patients with T-cell lymphoma treated in studies of the German High-Grade Non-Hodgkin Lymphoma Study Group. *Blood* 2010; 116: 3418–25.

61. Feyler S, Prince HM, Pearce R, et al. The role of high-dose therapy and stem cell rescue in the management of T-cell malignant lymphomas: a BSBMT and ABMTRR study. *Bone Marrow Transplant* 2007; 40: 443–50.

62. Kyriakou C, Canals C, Goldstone A, et al. High-dose therapy and autologous stem-cell transplantation in angioimmunoblastic lymphoma: complete remission at transplantation is the major determinant of Outcome-Lymphoma Working Party of the European Group for Blood and Marrow Transplantation. *J Clin Oncol* 2008; 26: 218–24.

63. Yang DH, Kim WS, Kim SJ, et al. Prognostic factors and clinical outcomes of high-dose chemotherapy followed by autologous stem cell transplantation in patients with peripheral T cell lymphoma, unspecified: complete remission at transplantation and the prognostic index of peripheral T cell lymphoma are the major factors predictive of outcome. *Biol Blood Marrow Transplant* 2009; 15: 118–25.

64. Kim MK, Kim S, Lee SS, et al. High-dose chemotherapy and autologous stem cell transplantation for peripheral T-cell lymphoma: complete response at transplant predicts survival. *Ann Hematol* 2007; 86: 435–42.

65. Rodriguez J, Conde E, Gutierrez A, et al. The adjusted International Prognostic Index and beta-2-microglobulin predict the outcome after autologous stem cell transplantation in relapsing/refractory peripheral T-cell lymphoma. *Haematologica* 2007; 92: 1067–74.

66. Rodriguez J, Conde E, Gutierrez A, et al. The results of consolidation with autologous stem-cell transplantation in patients with peripheral T-cell lymphoma (PTCL) in first complete remission: the Spanish Lymphoma and Autologous Transplantation Group experience. *Ann Oncol* 2007; 18: 652–57.

67. Yamazaki T, Sawada U, Kura Y, et al. Treatment of high-risk peripheral T-cell lymphomas other than anaplastic large-cell lymphoma with a dose-intensified CHOP regimen followed by high-dose chemotherapy. A single institution study. *Acta Haematol* 2006; 116: 90–95.

68. Jantunen E, Wiklund T, Juvonen E, et al. Autologous stem cell transplantation in adult patients with peripheral T-cell lymphoma: a nation-wide survey. *Bone Marrow Transplant* 2004; 33: 405–10.

69. Schetelig J, Fetscher S, Reichle A, et al. Long-term disease-free survival in patients with angioimmunoblastic T-cell lymphoma after high-dose chemotherapy and autologous stem cell transplantation. *Haematologica* 2003; 88: 1272–78.

70. d'Amore F, Relander T, Lauritzsen G, et al. Dose-dense induction followed by autologous stem cell transplantation (ASCT) as 1st line treatment in peripheral t-cell lymphoma (PTCL)—a phase II study of the Nordic Lymphoma Group (NLG). *Blood* 2006; 108. Abstract 401.

71. Corradini P, Tarella C, Zallio F, et al. Long-term follow-up of patients with peripheral T-cell lymphomas treated up-front with high-dose chemotherapy followed by autologous stem cell transplantation. *Leukemia* 2006; 20: 1533–38.

72. Rodriguez J, Conde E, Gutierrez A, et al. Frontline autologous stem cell transplantation in high-risk peripheral T-cell lymphoma: a prospective study from The Gel-Tamo Study Group. *Eur J Haematol* 2007; 79: 32–38.

73. Mercadal S, Briones J, Xicoy B, et al. Intensive chemotherapy (high-dose CHOP/ ESHAP regimen) followed by autologous stem-cell transplantation in previously untreated patients with peripheral T-cell lymphoma. *Ann Oncol* 2008; 19: 958–63.

74. Reimer P, Rudiger T, Geissinger E, et al. Autologous stem-cell transplantation as first-line therapy in peripheral T-cell lymphomas: results of a prospective multicenter study. *J Clin Oncol* 2009; 27: 106–13.

75. Sieniawski M, Lennard J, Millar C, et al. Aggressive primary chemotherapy plus autologous stem cell transplantation improves outcome for peripheral T cell lymphomas compared with CHOP-like regimens. *Blood* 2009; 114. Abstract 1660.

76. Relander T, Lauritzsen G, Jantunen E, et al. Favorable outcome in ALK-negative anaplastic large-cell lymphoma following intensive induction chemotherapy and autologous stem cell transplantation (ASCT): a prospective study by the Nordic Lymphoma Group (NLG-T-01). *Blood* 2010; 116. Abstract 3566.

77. d'Amore F, Relander T, Lauritzsen GF, et al. High-dose chemotherapy and autologous stem cell transplantation in previously untreated peripheral T-cell lymphoma—final analysis of a large prospective multicenter study (NLG-T-01). *Blood* 2011; 118. Abstract 331.

78. Au WY, Weisenburger DD, Intragumtornchai T, et al. Clinical differences between nasal and extranasal natural killer/T-cell lymphoma: a study of 136 cases from the International Peripheral T-Cell Lymphoma Project. *Blood* 2009; 113: 3931–37.

79. Yachie A, Kanegane H, Kasahara Y. Epstein-Barr virus-associated T-/natural killer cell lymphoproliferative diseases. *Semin Hematol* 2003; 40: 124–32.

80. Pescarmona E, Pignoloni P, Puopolo M, et al. p53 over-expression identifies a subset of nodal peripheral T-cell lymphomas with a distinctive biological profile and poor clinical outcome. *J Pathol* 2001; 195: 361–66.

81. Yong W, Zheng W, Zhang Y, et al. L-asparaginase-based regimen in the treatment of refractory midline nasal/nasal-type T/NK-cell lymphoma. *Int J Hematol* 2003; 78: 163–67.

82. Lee J, Suh C, Park YH, et al. Extranodal natural killer T-cell lymphoma, nasal-type: a prognostic model from a retrospective multicenter study. *J Clin Oncol* 2006; 24: 612–18.

83. Yamaguchi M, Tobinai K, Oguchi M, et al. Phase I/II study of concurrent chemoradiotherapy for localized nasal natural killer/T-cell lymphoma: Japan Clinical Oncology Group Study JCOG0211. *J Clin Oncol* 2009; 27: 5594–600.

84. Kim SJ, Kim K, Kim BS, et al. Phase II trial of concurrent radiation and weekly cisplatin followed by VIPD chemotherapy in newly diagnosed, stage IE to IIE, nasal, extranodal NK/T-cell lymphoma: Consortium for Improving Survival of Lymphoma study. *J Clin Oncol* 2009; 27: 6027–32.

85. Yamaguchi M. Current and future management of NK/T-cell lymphoma based on clinical trials. *Int J Hematol* 2012; 96: 562–71.

86. Jaccard A, Gachard N, Marin B, et al. Efficacy of L-asparaginase with methotrexate and dexamethasone (AspaMetDex regimen) in patients with refractory or relapsing extranodal NK/T-cell lymphoma, a phase 2 study. *Blood* 2011; 117: 1834–39.

87. Jaccard A, Petit B, Girault S, et al. L-asparaginase-based treatment of 15 western patients with extranodal NK/T-cell lymphoma and leukemia and a review of the literature. *Ann Oncol* 2009; 20: 110–16.

88. Yamaguchi M, Kwong YL, Kim WS, et al. Phase II study of SMILE chemotherapy for newly diagnosed stage IV, relapsed, or refractory extranodal natural killer (NK)/T-cell lymphoma, nasal type: the NK-Cell Tumor Study Group study. *J Clin Oncol* 2011; 29: 4410–16.

89. Yong W, Zheng W, Zhu J, et al. L-asparaginase in the treatment of refractory and relapsed extranodal NK/T-cell lymphoma, nasal type. *Ann Hematol* 2009; 88: 647–52.

90. Suzuki R, Kimura H, Kwong Y-L, et al. Pretreatment EBV-DNA copy number is predictive for response to SMILE chemotherapy for newly-diagnosed stage IV, relapsed or refractory extranodal NK/T-cell lymphoma, nasal type: results of NKTSG Phase II study. *Blood* 2010; 116. Abstract 2873.

91. Kwong YL, Kim WS, Lim ST, et al. SMILE for natural killer/T-cell lymphoma: analysis of safety and efficacy from the Asia Lymphoma Study Group. *Blood* 2012; 120: 2973–80.

92. Epstein MA, Achong BG, Barr YM. Virus particles in cultured lymphoblasts from Burkitt's lymphoma. *Lancet* 1964; 1: 702–3.

93. Zech L, Haglund U, Nilsson K, Klein G. Characteristic chromosomal abnormalities in biopsies and lymphoid-cell lines from patients with Burkitt and non-Burkitt lymphomas. *Int J Cancer* 1976; 17: 47–56.

94. Schulz TF, Boshoff CH, Weiss RA. HIV infection and neoplasia. *Lancet* 1996; 348: 587–91.

95. Parkin DM, Hamdi-Cherif M, Sita F, et al. Cancer in Africa: epidemiology and prevalence. Burkitt lymphoma. International Agency for Cancer Research (IARC) Scientific Publications 2003; 153: 324–28. Available at http://www.iarc.fr/en/publications/pdfs-online/epi/sp153/index.php.

96. Mbulaiteye SM, Biggar RJ, Bhatia K, Linet MS, Devesa SS. Sporadic childhood Burkitt lymphoma incidence in the United States during 1992–2005. *Pediatr Blood Cancer* 2009; 53: 366–70.

97. Knowles DM. Etiology and pathogenesis of AIDS-related non-Hodgkin's lymphoma. *Hematol Oncol Clin North Am* 2003; 17: 785–820.

98. Martinez-Maza O, Breen EC. B-cell activation and lymphoma in patients with HIV. *Curr Opin Oncol* 2002; 14: 528–32.

99. Newton R, Ziegler J, Beral V, et al. A case-control study of human immunodeficiency virus infection and cancer in adults and children residing in Kampala, Uganda. *Int J Cancer* 2001; 92: 622–27.

100. Ferry JA. Burkitt's lymphoma: clinicopathologic features and differential diagnosis. *Oncologist* 2006; 11: 375–83.

101. Carpenter LM, Newton R, Casabonne D, et al. Antibodies against malaria and Epstein-Barr virus in childhood Burkitt lymphoma: a case-control study in Uganda. *Int J Cancer* 2008; 122: 1319–23.

102. Rochford R, Cannon MJ, Moormann AM. Endemic Burkitt's lymphoma: a polymicrobial disease? *Nat Rev Microbiol* 2005; 3: 182–87.

103. Chene A, Donati D, Orem J, et al. Endemic Burkitt's lymphoma as a polymicrobial disease: new insights on the interaction between Plasmodium falciparum and Epstein-Barr virus. *Semin Cancer Biol* 2009; 19: 411–20.

104. Lam KM, Syed N, Whittle H, Crawford DH. Circulating Epstein-Barr virus-carrying B cells in acute malaria. *Lancet* 1991; 337: 876–78.

105. Njie R, Bell AI, Jia H, et al. The effects of acute malaria on Epstein-Barr virus (EBV) load and EBV-specific T cell immunity in Gambian children. *J Infect Dis* 2009; 199: 31–38.

106. Yone CL, Kube D, Kremsner PG, Luty AJ. Persistent Epstein-Barr viral reactivation in young African children with a history of severe Plasmodium falciparum malaria. *Trans R Soc Trop Med Hyg* 2006; 100: 669–76.

107. Rasti N, Falk KI, Donati D, et al. Circulating Epstein-Barr virus in children living in malaria-endemic areas. *Scand J Immunol* 2005; 61: 461–65.

108. Moormann AM, Chelimo K, Sumba OP, et al. Exposure to holoendemic malaria results in elevated Epstein-Barr virus loads in children. 2005; *J Infect Dis* 191: 1233–38.

109. Donati D, Espmark E, Kironde F, et al. Clearance of circulating Epstein-Barr virus DNA in children with acute malaria after antimalaria treatment. *J Infect Dis* 2006; 193: 971–77.

110. Ramiro AR, Jankovic M, Callen E, et al. Role of genomic instability and p53 in AID-induced c-myc-Igh translocations. *Nature* 2006; 440: 105–9.

111. Donati D, Zhang LP, Chene A, et al. Identification of a polyclonal B-cell activator in Plasmodium falciparum. *Infect Immun* 2004; 72: 5412–18.

112. Parroche P, Lauw FN, Goutagny N, et al. Malaria hemozoin is immunologically inert but radically enhances innate responses by presenting malaria DNA to Toll-like receptor 9. *Proc Natl Acad Sci USA* 2007; 104: 1919–24.

113. Capolunghi F, Cascioli S, Giorda E, et al. CpG drives human transitional B cells to terminal differentiation and production of natural antibodies. *J Immunol* 2008; 180: 800–808.

114. Potup P, Kumsiri R, Kano S, et al. Blood stage Plasmodium falciparum antigens induce immunoglobulin class switching in human enriched B cell culture. *Southeast Asian J Trop Med Public Health* 2009; 40: 651–64.

115. Magrath IT. African Burkitt's lymphoma. History, biology, clinical features, and treatment. *Am J Pediatr Hematol Oncol* 1991; 13: 222–46.

116. Hesseling P, Molyneux E, Kamiza S, Israels T, Broadhead R. Endemic Burkitt lymphoma: a 28-day treatment schedule with cyclophosphamide and intrathecal methotrexate. *Ann Trop Paediatr* 2009; 29: 29–34.

117. Patte C, Auperin A, Michon J, et al. The Societe Francaise d'Oncologie Pediatrique LMB89 protocol: highly effective multiagent chemotherapy tailored to the tumor burden and initial response in 561 unselected children with B-cell lymphomas and L3 leukemia. *Blood* 2001; 97: 3370–79.

118. Molyneux EM, Rochford R, Griffin B, et al. Burkitt's lymphoma. *Lancet* 2012; 379: 1234–44.

119. Gerrard M, Cairo MS, Weston C, et al. Excellent survival following two courses of COPAD chemotherapy in children and adolescents with resected localized B-cell non-Hodgkin's lymphoma: results of the FAB/LMB 96 international study. *Br J Haematol* 2008; 141: 840–47.

120. Kelly JL, Toothaker SR, Ciminello L, et al. Outcomes of patients with Burkitt lymphoma older than age 40 treated with intensive chemotherapeutic regimens. *Clin Lymphoma Myeloma* 2009; 9: 307–10.

121. Hesseling P, Broadhead R, Mansvelt E, et al. The 2000 Burkitt lymphoma trial in Malawi. *Pediatr Blood Cancer* 2005; 44: 245–50.

122. Harif M, Barsaoui S, Benchekroun S, et al. Treatment of B-cell lymphoma with LMB modified protocols in Africa—report of the French-African Pediatric Oncology Group (GFAOP). *Pediatr Blood Cancer* 2008; 50: 1138–42.

123. Israels T, van de Wetering MD, Hesseling P, van Geloven N, Caron HN, Molyneux EM. Malnutrition and neutropenia in children treated for Burkitt lymphoma in Malawi. *Pediatr Blood Cancer* 2009; 53: 47–52.

124. Adde M, Shad A, Venzon D, et al. Additional chemotherapy agents improve treatment outcome for children and adults with advanced B-cell lymphomas. *Semin Oncol* 1998; 25: 33–39; discussion 45–8.

125. Mead GM, Sydes MR, Walewski J, et al. An international evaluation of CODOX-M and CODOX-M alternating with IVAC in adult Burkitt's lymphoma: results of United Kingdom Lymphoma Group LY06 study. *Ann Oncol* 2002; 13: 1264–74.

126. Mead GM, Barrans SL, Qian W, et al. A prospective clinicopathologic study of dose-modified CODOX-M/IVAC in patients with sporadic Burkitt lymphoma defined using cytogenetic and immunophenotypic criteria (MRC/NCRI LY10 trial). *Blood* 2008; 112: 2248–60.

127. Barnes JA, Lacasce AS, Feng Y, et al. Evaluation of the addition of rituximab to CODOX-M/IVAC for Burkitt's lymphoma: a retrospective analysis. *Ann Oncol* 2011; 22: 1859–64.

128. Maruyama D, Watanabe T, Maeshima AM, et al. Modified cyclophosphamide, vincristine, doxorubicin, and methotrexate (CODOX-M)/ifosfamide, etoposide, and cytarabine (IVAC) therapy with or without rituximab in Japanese adult patients with Burkitt lymphoma (BL) and B cell lymphoma, unclassifiable, with features intermediate between diffuse large B cell lymphoma and BL. *Int J Hematol* 2010; 92: 732–43.

129. Thomas DA, Cortes J, O'Brien S, et al. Hyper-CVAD program in Burkitt's-type adult acute lymphoblastic leukemia. *J Clin Oncol* 1999; 17: 2461–70.

130. Thomas DA, Faderl S, O'Brien S, et al. Chemoimmunotherapy with hyper-CVAD plus rituximab for the treatment of adult Burkitt and Burkitt-type lymphoma or acute lymphoblastic leukemia. *Cancer* 2006; 106: 1569–80.

131. Rizzieri DA JJ, Byrd JC, et al. Efficacy and toxicity of rituximab and brief duration, high intensity chemotherapy with filgrastim support for Burkitt or Burkitt-like leukemia/lymphoma: Cancer and Leukemia Group B (CALGB) Study 10002. *Blood* 2010; 116. Abstract 858.

132. Dunleavy K, Pittaluga S, Wayne AS, et al. MYC+ aggressive B-cell lymphomas: a novel therapy of untreated Burkitt lymphoma (BL) and MYC+ diffuse large B-cell lymphoma (DLBCL) with DA-EPOCH-R. *Ann Oncol* 2011; 22 (Suppl 4). Abstract 71.

133. Piro LD, White CA, Grillo-Lopez AJ, et al. Extended Rituximab (anti-CD20 monoclonal antibody) therapy for relapsed or refractory low-grade or follicular non-Hodgkin's lymphoma. *Ann Oncol* 1999; 10: 655–61.

134. McLaughlin P, Grillo-Lopez AJ, Link BK, et al. Rituximab chimeric anti-CD20 monoclonal antibody therapy for relapsed indolent lymphoma: half of patients respond to a four-dose treatment program. *J Clin Oncol* 1998; 16: 2825–33.

135. Leget GA, Czuczman MS. Use of rituximab, the new FDA-approved antibody. *Curr Opin Oncol* 1998; 10: 548–51.

136. Czuczman MS, Grillo-Lopez AJ, White CA, et al. Treatment of patients with low-grade B-cell lymphoma with the combination of chimeric anti-CD20 monoclonal antibody and CHOP chemotherapy. *J Clin Oncol* 1999; 17: 268–76.

137. Czuczman MS, Weaver R, Alkuzweny B, Berlfein J, Grillo-López AJ. Prolonged clinical and molecular remission in patients with low-grade or follicular non-Hodgkin's lymphoma treated with rituximab plus CHOP chemotherapy: 9-year follow-up. *J Clin Oncol* 2004; 22: 4711–16.

138. Cheson BD, Horning SJ, Coiffier B, et al. Report of an international workshop to standardize response criteria for non-Hodgkin's lymphomas. NCI Sponsored International Working Group. *J Clin Oncol* 1999; 17: 1244.

139. Forstpointner R, Dreyling M, Repp R, et al. The addition of rituximab to a combination of fludarabine, cyclophosphamide, mitoxantrone (FCM) significantly increases the response rate and prolongs survival as compared with FCM alone in patients with relapsed and refractory follicular and mantle cell lymphomas: results of a prospective randomized study of the German Low-Grade Lymphoma Study Group. *Blood* 2004; 104: 3064–71.

140. Marcus R, Imrie K, Belch A, et al. CVP chemotherapy plus rituximab compared with CVP as first-line treatment for advanced follicular lymphoma. *Blood* 2005; 105: 1417–23.

141. Hiddemann W, Kneba M, Dreyling M, et al. Frontline therapy with rituximab added to the combination of cyclophosphamide, doxorubicin, vincristine, and prednisone (CHOP) significantly improves the outcome for patients with advanced-stage follicular lymphoma compared with therapy with CHOP alone: results of a prospective randomized study of the German Low-Grade Lymphoma Study Group. *Blood* 2005; 106: 3725–32.

142. Coiffier B, Thieblemont C, Van Den Neste E, et al. Long-term outcome of patients in the LNH-98.5 trial, the first randomized study comparing rituximab-CHOP to standard CHOP chemotherapy in DLBCL patients: a study by the Groupe d'Etudes des Lymphomes de l'Adulte. *Blood* 2010; 116: 2040–45.

143. Pfreundschuh M, Schubert J, Ziepert M, et al. Six versus eight cycles of bi-weekly CHOP-14 with or without rituximab in elderly patients with aggressive CD20+ B-cell lymphomas: a randomised controlled trial (RICOVER-60). *Lancet Oncol* 2008; 9: 105–16.

144. Pfreundschuh M, Trumper L, Osterborg A, et al. CHOP-like chemotherapy plus rituximab versus CHOP-like chemotherapy alone in young patients with good-prognosis diffuse large-B-cell lymphoma: a randomised controlled trial by the MabThera International Trial (MInT) Group. *Lancet Oncol* 2006; 7: 379–91.

145. Feugier P, Van Hoof A, Sebban C, et al. Long-term results of the R-CHOP study in the treatment of elderly patients with diffuse large B-cell lymphoma:

a study by the Groupe d'Etude des Lymphomes de l'Adulte. *J Clin Oncol* 2005; 23: 4117–26.

146. Kay J. Biosimilars: a regulatory perspective from America. *Arthritis Res Ther* 2011; 13: 112.

147. Harris R. Comparability Assessment Strategies and Techinques for Post-Approval CMC Changes. Available at http://www.bioanalyse.org/slides/08S02.pdf. Accessed April 2, 2013.

148. Gopal S, Wood WA, Lee SJ, et al. Meeting the challenge of hematologic malignancies in sub-Saharan Africa. *Blood* 2012; 119: 5078–87.

149. Bateganya MH, Stanaway J, Brentlinger PE, et al. Predictors of survival after a diagnosis of non-Hodgkin lymphoma in a resource-limited setting: a retrospective study on the impact of HIV infection and its treatment. *J Acquir Immune Defic Syndr* 2011; 56: 312–19.

150. Mwanda WO, Orem J, Fu P, et al. Dose-modified oral chemotherapy in the treatment of AIDS-related non-Hodgkin's lymphoma in East Africa. *J Clin Oncol* 2009; 27: 3480–88.

151. Salminen EK, Kiel K, Ibbott GS, et al. International Conference on Advances in Radiation Oncology (ICARO): outcomes of an IAEA meeting. *Radiat Oncol* 2011; 6: 11.

152. Wu CY, Hu HY, Pu CY, et al. Aerodigestive tract, lung and haematological cancers are risk factors for tuberculosis: an 8-year population-based study. *Int J Tuberc Lung Dis* 2011; 15: 125–30.

153. Stefan DC, Kruis AL, Schaaf HS, Wessels G. Tuberculosis in oncology patients. *Ann Trop Paediatr* 2008; 28: 111–16.

154. World Health Organization. WHO Model Lists of Essential Medicines. Available at http://www.who.int/medicines/publications/essentialmedicines/en/index.html. Accessed March 28, 2013.

155. Bloch EM, Vermeulen M, Murphy E. Blood transfusion safety in Africa: a literature review of infectious disease and organizational challenges. *Transfus Med Rev* 2012; 26: 164–80.

156. Tapko J, Mainuka P, Diarra-Nama AJ. Status of Blood Safety in the WHO African Region: Report of the 2006 Survey. Available at http://www.afro.who.int/en/clusters-a-programmes/hss/blood-safetylaboratories-a-health-technology.html. Accessed March 27, 2013.

157. Rosenberg SA. Autologous bone marrow transplantation in non-Hodgkin's lymphoma. *N Engl J Med* 1987; 316: 1541–42.

158. Philip T, Armitage JO, Spitzer G, et al. High-dose therapy and autologous bone marrow transplantation after failure of conventional chemotherapy in adults with intermediate-grade or high-grade non-Hodgkin's lymphoma. *N Engl J Med* 1987; 316: 1493–98.

159. Friedberg JW. Relapsed/refractory diffuse large B-cell lymphoma. *Hematology Am Soc Hematol Educ Program* 2011: 498–505.

160. Schetelig J, van Biezen A, Brand R, et al. Allogeneic hematopoietic stem-cell transplantation for chronic lymphocytic leukemia with 17p deletion: a retrospective European Group for Blood and Marrow Transplantation analysis. *J Clin Oncol* 2008; 26: 5094–100.

161. Philip T, Guglielmi C, Hagenbeek A, et al. Autologous bone marrow transplantation as compared with salvage chemotherapy in relapses of chemotherapy-sensitive non-Hodgkin's lymphoma. *N Engl J Med* 1995; 333: 1540–45.

162. Khouri IF, Romaguera J, Kantarjian H, et al. Hyper-CVAD and high-dose methotrexate/cytarabine followed by stem-cell transplantation: an active regimen for aggressive mantle-cell lymphoma. *J Clin Oncol* 1998; 16: 3803–9.

163. Khouri IF, Saliba RM, Okoroji GJ, Acholonu SA, Champlin RE. Long-term follow-up of autologous stem cell transplantation in patients with diffuse mantle cell lymphoma in first disease remission: the prognostic value of beta2-microglobulin and the tumor score. *Cancer* 2003; 98: 2630–35.

164. Lefrere F, Delmer A, Suzan F, et al. Sequential chemotherapy by CHOP and DHAP regimens followed by high-dose therapy with stem cell transplantation induces a high rate of complete response and improves event-free survival in mantle cell lymphoma: a prospective study. *Leukemia* 2002; 16: 587–93.

165. Dreyling M, Lenz G, Hoster E, et al. Early consolidation by myeloablative radiochemotherapy followed by autologous stem cell transplantation in first remission significantly prolongs progression-free survival in mantle-cell lymphoma: results of a prospective randomized trial of the European MCL Network. *Blood* 2005; 105: 2677–84.

166. Ritchie DS, Seymour JF, Grigg AP, et al. The hyper-CVAD-rituximab chemotherapy programme followed by high-dose busulfan, melphalan and autologous stem cell transplantation produces excellent event-free survival in patients with previously untreated mantle cell lymphoma. *Ann Hematol* 2007; 86: 101–5.

167. van 't Veer MB, de Jong D, MacKenzie M, et al. High-dose Ara-C and beam with autograft rescue in R-CHOP responsive mantle cell lymphoma patients. *Br J Haematol* 2009; 144: 524–30.

168. Till BG, Gooley TA, Crawford N, et al. Effect of remission status and induction chemotherapy regimen on outcome of autologous stem cell transplantation for mantle cell lymphoma. *Leuk Lymphoma* 2008; 49: 1062–73.

169. Choi I, Tanosaki R, Uike N, et al. Long-term outcomes after hematopoietic SCT for adult T-cell leukemia/lymphoma: results of prospective trials. *Bone Marrow Transplant* 2011; 46: 116–18.

170. Okamura J, Uike N, Utsunomiya A, et al. Allogeneic stem cell transplantation for adult T-cell leukemia/lymphoma. *Int J Hematol* 2007; 86: 118–25.

171. Fukushima T, Miyazaki Y, Honda S, et al. Allogeneic hematopoietic stem cell transplantation provides sustained long-term survival for patients with adult T-cell leukemia/lymphoma. *Leukemia* 2005; 19: 829–34.

172. Thieblemont C, Briere J, Mounier N, et al. The germinal center/activated B-cell subclassification has a prognostic impact for response to salvage therapy in relapsed/refractory diffuse large B-cell lymphoma: a Bio-CORAL study. *J Clin Oncol* 2011; 29:4079–87.

173. Gisselbrecht C, Glass B, Mounier N, et al. Salvage regimens with autologous transplantation for relapsed large B-cell lymphoma in the rituximab era. *J Clin Oncol* 2010; 28: 4184–90.

174. Gisselbrecht C, Schmitz N, Mounier N, et al. Rituximab maintenance therapy after autologous stem-cell transplantation in patients with relapsed CD20(+)

diffuse large B-cell lymphoma: final analysis of the collaborative trial in relapsed aggressive lymphoma. *J Clin Oncol* 2012; 30: 4462–69.

175. Visani G, Picardi P, Tosi P, et al. Autologous stem cell transplantation for aggressive lymphomas. *Mediterr J Hematol Infect Dis* 2012; 4: e2012075.

176. Greb A, Bohlius J, Schiefer D, Schwarzer G, Schulz H, Engert A. High-dose chemotherapy with autologous stem cell transplantation in the first line treatment of aggressive non-Hodgkin lymphoma (NHL) in adults. *Cochrane Database Syst Rev* 2008: CD004024.

177. van Kampen RJ, Canals C, Schouten HC, et al. Allogeneic stem-cell transplantation as salvage therapy for patients with diffuse large B-cell non-Hodgkin's lymphoma relapsing after an autologous stem-cell transplantation: an analysis of the European Group for Blood and Marrow Transplantation Registry. *J Clin Oncol* 2011; 29: 1342–48.

178. Center for International Blood and Marrow Transplant Research. Available at http://www.cibmtr.org/About/ProceduresProgress/Pages/index.aspx. Accessed April 1, 2013.

179. Vallabhajosyula S, Baijal G, Vadhiraja BM, Fernandes DJ, Vidyasagar MS. Non-Hodgkin's lymphoma: is India ready to incorporate recent advances in day to day practice? *J Cancer Res Ther* 2010; 6: 36–40.

# 11

# Genitourinary Cancers

## Matthew M. Cooney, Gregory MacLennan, and Fred Okuku

## PROSTATE CANCER

Prostate cancer is a tumor in older men, with the average age at diagnosis above 70 years.[1] Although the majority of prostate cancers grow slowly, some men may experience rapid growth and disease dissemination. If the prostate cancer is localized, it usually can be cured. However, after metastatic disease occurs, prostate cancer can be palliated from a variety of therapies but is incurable. All men with prostate cancer should be informed of the benefit of treatment with the risks and treatment side effects to make informed decisions about their care.

### Prostate Anatomy and Physiology

The prostate is a walnut-sized gland located between the bladder, penis, and anterior to the rectum. The prostate completely encircles the urethra, allowing urine to empty through the bladder into the penis. Neurovascular bundles that are responsible for erectile function and the urinary sphincter that controls passive urinary flow are contiguous with the prostate.

The prostate gland is formed by branching tubule-alveolar glands, which are arranged in a lobular fashion and are surrounded by stroma. The acinal unit of the prostate is made up of epithelial, neuroendocrine and basal cells, and a stromal component. The stromal compartment is composed of fibroblasts and smooth-muscle cells. Prostate-specific antigen (PSA) and acid phosphatase are both produced by the epithelial cells. Androgen receptors promote both prostate epithelial and stromal cell growth. 5α-reductase converts testosterone to dihydrotestosterone in the prostate gland. Functionally, the prostate gland produces a fluid that nourishes the sperm as semen during ejaculation.

The central area of the prostate, the peri-urethral zone, enlarges with age and may cause urinary voiding symptoms over time. The peripheral zone is where most prostate cancers occur and can be palpated on a digital rectal exam (DRE).

## Epidemiology

Globally prostate cancer is the second most frequently diagnosed cancer in men (899,000 new cases, 13.6% of the total) and the fifth most common cancer overall.[2] High-income countries account for approximately 75% of the registered cases (644,000 cases). There are enormous variations in prostate cancer incidence worldwide. In areas with widespread prostate cancer screening (Europe, North America, Australia, and New Zealand), high rates of prostate cancer incidence are observed (up to 104 per 100,000). Asia and North Africa have the lowest incidence rates (4.1 per 100,000).

Prostate cancer in sub-Saharan Africa presents a unique and growing problem. Despite essentially no cancer screening programs and the relative young average age in sub-Saharan African countries, prostate cancer has become the most frequently diagnosed cancer in men.[3] Prostate cancer incidence in Uganda between 1991 and 2006 increased by 4.5% annually. The vast majority of these African men present with locally advanced or distant metastatic disease, and the treatments are only palliative.[4] Although the exact etiology for the increased incidence of prostate cancer in sub-Saharan Africa is unclear, factors such as urbanization, genetic predisposition, diet, and increased obesity may all be contributing to increased incidence.

In 2008 there were an estimated 258,000 deaths, making prostate cancer the sixth leading cause of death from cancer in men (6.1% of the total). Mortality rates are strikingly different depending on which region of the world is examined. For example, in the United States where prostate cancer screening is offered and surgery and radiation are readily available, the 5-year survival rate with men localized or regional disease was 100%.[5] In contrast, in Uganda, where there is no national prostate cancer screening program and limited urology access, the 5-year absolute survival rate was 29.5%.[6]

## Clinical Presentation: Diagnosis and Staging

In countries with screening programs, most men are diagnosed with prostate cancer before being symptomatic.[7] However, tumor growth can create symptoms such as decreased urinary stream, urgency, hesitancy, nocturia, incomplete bladder emptying, and erectile dysfunction. In many instances it is difficult to determine if these symptoms are related to cancer or to benign hypertrophy of the gland. If the patient presents later in the prostate cancer course with metastatic disease, he may have symptoms of bone pain, urinary obstruction, cord compression, hypercalcemia, or renal failure (Table 11.1).

The DRE can detect palpable prostate cancer, especially in the peripheral portion of the gland. The DRE is a mandatory evaluation for a patient suspected to have prostate cancer and should not be omitted. Exam findings can vary from a focal nodule for localized tumors to abnormal irregular anatomy which can denote locally advanced disease.

Diagnosis of prostate cancer via an ultrasound-guided prostate biopsy is the standard of care. This procedure is performed by a transrectal ultrasound-guided approach using a tru-cut needle. Currently, it is recommended that at least 12 cores be taken. Occasionally, when prostate cancer is not found after 12 biopsies are performed and the clinical index of suspicion is high for prostate cancer, a "saturation biopsy" may be undertaken, which may include up to 24 to 30 cores for further evaluation. In many resource-limited areas globally, a patient presenting with prostate symptoms and an elevated PSA is considered diagnostic of prostate cancer. However, the lack of a prostate biopsy is suboptimal and should be avoided whenever possible.

The majority of prostate cancers are adenocarcinoma (95%) and are frequently multifocal and heterogeneous in patterns of differentiation. The remaining 5% of prostate cancer cases histologically include small-cell tumors, introlobular acinar carcinomas, ductal carcinomas, clear cell carcinomas, and mucinous carcinomas. Prostate cancers are staged both clinically by DRE and prostate biopsy (Table 11.2) and pathologically at the time of prostatectomy.[8]

**TABLE 11.1  Presenting Symptoms for Prostate Cancer**

| Local Symptoms | Metastatic Symptoms |
|---|---|
| Nocturia | Bone pain |
| Frequency | Anemia |
| Urgency | Hypercalcemia |
| Hematuria | Lower extremity edema |
| Hematospermia | Fracture |
| Erectile dysfunction | Cord compression |

**TABLE 11.2  Clinical Staging of Prostate Cancer by Digital Rectal Exam and Prostate Biopsy**

| | |
|---|---|
| T1a | Tumor incidental histologic finding in ≤5% of tissue resected |
| T1b | Tumor incidental histologic finding in >5% of tissue resected |
| T1c | Tumor identified by needle biopsy (e.g., because of elevated PSA) |
| T2 | Palpable tumor confined within prostate |
| T3 | Tumor extends through the prostate capsule |
| T4 | Tumor is fixed or invades adjacent structures other than seminal vesicles such as external sphincter, rectum, bladder, levator muscles, and/or pelvic wall |

The Gleason system provides a grade score based on the dominant histological grades ranging from 1 (well differentiated) to 5 (poorly differentiated) (Figure 11.1). The Gleason score is obtained by adding the most prevalent grade first to the second most prevalent grade second (e.g., Gleason score 4 + 4 = 8).[9] Over time pathologists have tended to award a higher Gleason score in current versus historical series.[10,11] This increase in higher Gleason score over time has been called "grade inflation."

Prostate-specific antigen can be produced by either prostatic epithelium or prostate cancer cells. Many factors can elevate the PSA besides cancer, including benign prostatic hypertrophy, infections, trauma, and urethral instrumentation. The PSA increases with aging and levels of <4.0 up to 10.0 ng/mL can be considered normal based on the individual's age.

Prostate cancer can be divided into low, intermediate, and high risk. These risk groups not only predict which patients at time of diagnosis may develop metastatic disease but also help group patients into risk categories for research purposes. Although there is no one grouping strategy, low risk may be considered T1a-T2a, Gleason score ≤ 6, PSA ≤ 10 ng/mL, intermediate risk

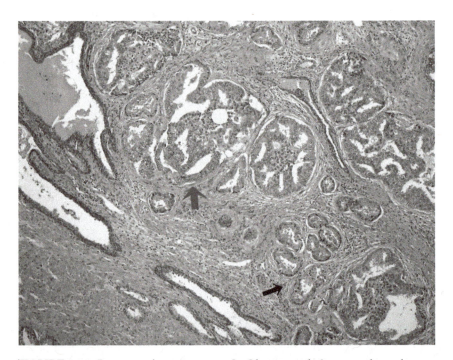

**FIGURE 11.1** Prostatic adenocarcinoma. In Gleason grade 3 cancer, the malignant glands are separated from one another by fibromuscular stroma (bottom arrow). In Gleason grade 4 cancer, the malignant glands are "fused"; that is, they do not have stroma between them and they form cribriform ("sieve-like") structures (top arrow).

TABLE 11.3  Risk Stratification of Prostate Cancer by Stage, PSA, and
            Gleason Score

| Risk | Clinical Stage | PSA | Gleason Score |
|------|----------------|-----|---------------|
| Low | T1a-T2a | ≤10 ng/mL | ≤6 |
| Intermediate | T2b-T2c | ≥10.0 and ≤20 ng/mL | 7 |
| High | T3a | PSA ≥ 20 ng/mL | ≥8 |

being T2b-T2c, Gleason score 7 and PSA ≥ 10.0 and ≤20 ng/mL, and high
risk T3, Gleason score ≥ 8, with a PSA ≥ 20 ng/mL (Table 11.3).

The role of prostate cancer screening is highly controversial. The evidence is insufficient to determine whether screening for prostate cancer with
PSA or DRE reduces mortality. After decades of screening the United States
Preventative Task Force has now recommended against PSA screening in
healthy asymptomatic men. This task force stated that there was insufficient
evidence to determine if screening decreased mortality from prostate cancer and the morbidity of prostate cancer therapies outweighs the benefit of
screening.[12] It is unknown, however, if this recommendation will be followed
in the United States and if the detection rates of prostate cancer will decrease
accordingly in the future.

Several imaging modalities are used frequently with the diagnosis of prostate cancer. CT scans lack sensitivity and specificity of detecting extracap-
sular prostatic capsule invasion and lymph node involvement. MRI scans
using an endorectal coil are superior to CT scans in determining local extent
of disease and presence of regional lymph node spread. Bone scans can be
used to evaluate for systemic spread but are rarely positive with PSA levels
<20 ng/mL.

## Clinically Localized Prostate Cancer

Once a patient is diagnosed with prostate cancer, the first step is to determine if the patient should be treated. Asymptomatic patients of advanced age
or significant concomitant illness may just be carefully observed without any
therapeutic intervention unless they become symptomatic from their prostate cancer.

For patients with low-risk disease, generally defined as PSA < 10 ng/mL
and Gleason score 6, *active surveillance* should be considered.[13,14] The basis for
active surveillance is watching the low-risk individual closely and initiating
curative intent therapy if there are any signs of tumor progression. The goal
of active surveillance is to avoid the morbidity of therapy in men who have
indolent tumors but preserve the ability to cure them if the tumor should
progress. Although there are no uniformly accepted guidelines for active

surveillance patient visits with PSA every 6 months, DRE examinations and ultrasound-guided trans-rectal needle biopsies every other year are reasonable.[15,16] Indications to consider curative intent therapy to a patient on active surveillance include a change in the DRE, increase in the PSA velocity or the doubling time, increase in Gleason grade, or increase in the tumor volume on the biopsy.

Although an imperfect tumor marker, the higher the PSA at baseline, the higher risk for subsequent metastatic disease progression.[17,18] The Gleason score and PSA, when evaluated together, may help predict outcomes before radical prostatectomy or chance of recurrence after surgery.[19-24] Although imperfect, these nonograms may help the physician and patient make a more informed decision about the risks and benefits of pursuing surgery based on the patient's prostate cancer risk.

A variety of technologies are trying to improve on the Gleason score and PSA risk assessment for prostate cancer. The majority of these technologies use genetic analysis of the individual tumor and try and predict the future risk of harm from prostate cancer. Examples include a technology called Prolaris, which analyzes cell cycle progression and housekeeping genes and attempts to predict those tumors that are indolent versus those that may become aggressive. Another example is Oncotype DX, which analyzes specific genes from the prostate biopsy tissue. By analyzing these genes, the patient is then given a risk score, which attempts to predict the chance the individual's prostate cancer will metastasize. It is unclear how these technologies will be adapted in the future and what role they will have in influencing patient and physician treatment decisions.

## Surgery

The goal of radical prostatectomy is the complete removal of the tumor with preservation of urinary, erectile, and bowel functions. For considering a patient for radical prostatectomy, the patient should be in good health with a life expectancy of at least 10 years and with the disease localized to the prostate gland. The procedure can be undertaken via a perineal, retropubic, or laparoscopic approach. For tumors with a high Gleason score and/or elevation of PSA, lymph node dissection may be considered at the time of surgery.[25] The use of hormonal agents to lower testosterone before surgery has not resulted in an increase in survival from prostate cancer.

Robotic-assisted laparoscopic prostatectomy is rapidly becoming the treatment of choice for prostate surgery over an open retropubic approach in high-income countries. Over 1,000 robotic units are now deployed throughout the United States. Although with the robotic surgery there are smaller incisions and less blood loss, this minimally invasive procedure still has complications. In a survey comparing men who had either a robotic-assisted prostatectomy or an open surgery, no statistical difference was observed between the rates of incontinence or erectile dysfunction.[26]

In centers of excellence that perform a high volume of prostate surgeries, there may be a decrease in complications compared to lower volume hospitals. However, even with the most capable surgeons, complications from prostatectomy do occur. Erectile dysfunction can occur in over 50% of patients even with nerve-sparing procedures.[27] Factors associated with a decrease in the risk of erectile dysfunction after surgery include younger age, level of potency before surgery, and nerve-sparing approach. Medications such as PDE5 inhibitors, e.g., sildenafil, vacuum assist devices, and intra-cavernosal injections of vasodilators may improve potency after surgery. Other complications from prostate surgery include urinary incontinence, penile shortening (up to 2 cm), perioperative infections, bleeding, stricture, and rectal injury.

## Radiotherapy

A variety of radiation therapy techniques can deliver precise dosing with minimal toxicity for the treatment of prostate cancer. Unfortunately, in many areas globally, the access to radiotherapy technology is limited or nonexistent. Also in many regions the radiotherapy devices, such as cobalt units, cause exceptionally high toxicity rates, limiting their use. Currently over 23 countries with a population of 1 million or more do not have access to radiotherapy.[28]

Where available the modern external beam radiotherapy unit uses image-guided systems to better visualize the prostate and surrounding tissues. Image-guided radiotherapy (IGRT) is a technique that allows the prostate gland to be visualized daily via a CT scan to set the correct position of each treatment. Intensity modulated radiotherapy (IMRT) delivers the radiation dose that is sculpted around the prostate and spares normal tissues, thus limiting side effects. Taken together, IGRT and IMRT can deliver very high doses of radiotherapy to the cancer with minimal side effects. Toxicity, however, can still occur, including lower urinary tract symptoms, rectal bleeding, and erectile dysfunction.

In addition to external beam radiotherapy, there are several other curative intent treatment methods for prostate cancer. None of these technologies have been studied in a randomized prospective manner demonstrating superiority over each other. These techniques include brachytherapy, which is the placement of radioactive seeds into the prostate that emit gamma rays to kill the prostate cancer. Cyberknife is an image-guided stereotactic system that uses a linear accelerator attached to a robotic arm allowing for increased degrees of freedom that delivers high-intensity radiation. Cryotherapy uses probes that are temporarily inserted into the prostate causing an ice ball that kills the cancer cells. High-intensity frequency ultrasound uses focused ultrasound waves to cause prostate cancer tissue necrosis and cell death. Proton therapy units deliver charged particles that can deliver extremely focused radiation deposits with no exit dose beyond the target.

## Rising PSA after Definitive Local Therapy

Since the 1940s lowering the testosterone to treat prostate cancer has been a mainstay of treatment for men with advanced disease. The surgical removal of the testicles (orchiectomy) provides rapid lowering of 95% of the testosterone in the body. Low levels of androgens are maintained primarily in the adrenal glands even after orchiectomy. Although surgical orchiectomy is permanent and inexpensive, many men do not wish to undertake this procedure. Medical castration, primarily with luteinizing hormone-releasing hormone (LHRH) agonists, was introduced in the 1980s. These LHRH medications disrupt the ability of the pituitary gland to release luteinizing hormone, which decreases the ability of the Leydig cells of the testes to produce testosterone. Both orchiectomy and LHRH agonists are equally effective in lowering the testosterone level and palliating men with advanced prostate cancer. There is no survival difference between orchiectomy and LHRH agonists in the treatment of advanced prostate cancer.

Although the lowering of testosterone helps the vast majority of men with the treatment of their prostate cancer, however, this hypogonadal state can cause many significant side effects. Hot flashes, sweats, weight gain, osteoporosis, and decreased energy can all occur. Also, a significant decrease in libido and erectile dysfunction is almost universal in men on LHRH agonists. Finally, with the decreased energy, weight gain, and decrease in muscle mass, there is a concern of increased risk of cardiovascular complications for these men. Patients on LHRH therapy should be strongly encouraged to exercise several times a week and eat a balanced diet to help avoid some of the side effects of a low testosterone state.

Since men after orchiectomy or on LHRH agonists can experience a variety of side effects, there has been interest in exploring intermittent LHRH treatment schedules to help limit the toxicity. However, in a large randomized trial it was reported that intermittent LHRH agonist treatment may not be inferior to continuous androgen suppression. Thus, the investigators could not rule out up to a 20% increased risk in the relative risk of death in men receiving androgen suppression intermittently versus those receiving the treatment continuously. The current recommendation for treatment of patients with advanced prostate cancer is continuous androgen suppression with orchiectomy or LHRH therapy.[29] However, this continuous androgen suppression must be weighed against the toxicity related to treatment.

The time that prostate cancer is controlled by lowering the testosterone can vary widely between patients. When patients are given LHRH agonists when they still have localized tumors, they may have no tumor growth for years.[30] However, when LHRH agonists are initiated at the time of metastatic disease, the average time until the tumor becomes "castrate resistant" is approximately 2 years. Castrate-resistant prostate cancer occurs when the testosterone is lowered via orchiectomy or via LHRH agonists and the tumor exhibits growth. This progression occurs if there are at least two different PSA increases at least 2 weeks apart, progressive lesions on imaging scans, clinical exam findings of tumor progression, or worsening local symptoms due to tumor.

Fortunately, there are numerous medications in different drug classes to help treat men with castrate-resistant metastatic prostate cancer (Table 11.4). Many of these agents can help palliate the symptoms related to this advanced cancer; however, none are curative. The majority of these medications can be classified as antiandrogens, androgen receptor inhibitors, immune therapy, chemotherapy, or radioactive isotopes.

Antiandrogens are medications that either inhibit the production of androgens or block the tumor use of androgens in circulation. The first antiandrogen in clinical use was the antifungal medication ketoconazole. However, due to ketoconazole's side effects and interactions with a variety of other medications, its use has been limited. Abiraterone acetate is an oral medication that blocks cytochrome P450 which also decreases adrenal androgen production. This medication has demonstrated efficacy for men with castrate-resistant prostate cancer both before and after taxane-based chemotherapy.[31,32] Overall abiraterone is well tolerated, and side effects such as edema, hypertension, and hyperkalemia can be averted with low-dose prednisone.

The androgen receptor plays a key role in the division and dissemination of prostate cancer cells. When circulating androgens bind to the androgen receptor, the receptor is translocated to the DNA. The androgen receptor then activates the DNA promoting tumor growth. Bicalutamide and flutamide are first-generation androgen receptor inhibitors for the treatment of prostate

**TABLE 11.4 Medications for Castrate-Resistant Metastatic Prostate Cancer**

| Medication | Mechanism of Action | Comments |
| --- | --- | --- |
| Abiraterone Acetate | Inhibits androgen production | Oral agent, well tolerated |
| Enzalutamide | Androgen receptor inhibitor | Oral agent, well tolerated |
| Sipuleucel-T | Immunotherapy | Requires leukapheresis |
| Docetaxel | Taxane chemotherapy | Available in generic forms |
| Cabazitaxel | Taxane chemotherapy | Active in docetaxel-treated patients |
| Radium-223 | Radioisotope | Relieves bone pain |

cancer. Although they both are well tolerated, they provide only minimal clinical benefit. Enzalutamide, however, is a second-generation drug that binds with great affinity the androgen receptor. In randomized clinical trials, enzalutamide has also demonstrated an improvement in overall survival for men with castrate-resistant prostate cancer after docetaxel chemotherapy.[33]

Immunotherapy has become an option for men with advanced castrate-resistant disease. Sipuleucel-T is a novel immunotherapy approved for the treatment of advanced prostate cancer. To obtain this therapy, a patient must undergo leukapheresis and a collection of their immune cells and are transported within 24 hours to the processing factory. There these autologous peripheral blood mononuclear cells are activated *ex vivo* via a recombinant fusion protein composed of prostatic acid phosphatase fused to granulocyte-macrophage colony-stimulating factor. This activated cellular immunity is then returned after 48 hours and infused into the patient. The process is repeated 3 times. Side effects are generally mild and mimic a transfusion reaction. Although the PSA and imaging studies do not change in response to a sipuleucel-T infusion, this treatment has demonstrated an increase in overall survival.[34] Other prostate cancer vaccine–based immunotherapies that do not require *ex vivo* approaches, such as Prostavac, are currently in late-stage clinical evaluation.

Chemotherapy has demonstrated the ability to palliate symptoms and increase the overall survival for men with metastatic castrate-resistant prostate cancer. Docetaxel and cabazitaxel are tubulin inhibitors in the taxane family. These cytotoxic agents can decrease the PSA, relieve bone pain, and provide tumor responses on imaging studies. Side effects include myelosuppression, nausea, vomiting, alopecia, fatigue, and neuropathy. However, both of these agents are well tolerated and can provide a significant benefit to the patients in regard to both their symptoms and improvement in overall survival.[35,36]

Bone pain can be a significant problem for men with advanced prostate cancer. A variety of therapies can be helpful, including low-dose prednisone, focal palliative external beam radiotherapy, and appropriate analgesics including narcotics. Medications to help decrease bone fractures and to limit the osteoporotic effects of low testosterone are also important. Agents such as the bisphosphonate zoledronic acid and denosumab, a monoclonal antibody that inhibits osteoclast function, have demonstrated the ability to decrease skeletal events.[37]

Radioisotopes are agents that release energy within the bone marrow to help palliate bone pain from metastatic lesions. Older compounds including strontium chloride Sr 89 have demonstrated palliation of pain but not an increase in prostate cancer survival. However, a new agent, radium-223, has demonstrated an improvement in overall survival in metastatic prostate cancer. The skeletal system cannot differentiate between calcium and radium-223 and therefore rapidly absorbs radium into the bone. Radium-223 then releases energy, killing prostate cancer cells in the marrow and helping to alleviate pain.[38] Overall radium-223 is well tolerated, with tolerable side effects including nausea and myelosuppresion.

## KIDNEY CANCER

Kidney cancer is the 14th most common cancer worldwide with an estimated 274,000 cases in 2008.[39] In higher-income countries, the age-standardized rate for kidney cancer is 8.6 per 100,000 and only occurs 1.9 per 100,000 in lower-income nations. Although the exact etiology for kidney cancer is unknown, in most cases risk factors include Von Hippel–Lindau disease, chronic dialysis, obesity, tobacco use, hypertension, and polycystic kidney disease. Cancers of the kidney can include a variety of tumors with differing clinical presentation, histology, and response to therapy. In general when the tumor is localized to the kidney, nephrectomy can cure the vast majority of patients (Figure 11.2). Unfortunately, when the cancer arising from the kidney metastasizes, the cancer is rarely curable and 5-year survival rates are poor.

### Signs and Symptoms

In high-income countries with the proliferation of CT, ultrasound, and MRI scans, there has been an increase in finding incidental renal masses. This

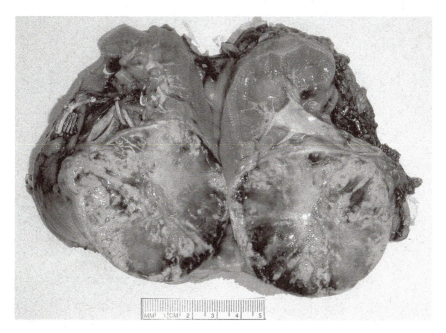

**FIGURE 11.2** Renal cell carcinoma. Tumors are typically well circumscribed, with a variegated cut surface, exhibiting golden yellow viable tumor interspersed with areas of hemorrhage and necrosis.

discovery of early-stage tumors has allowed for more partial-nephrectomy surgeries sparing renal function.

The classic triad of flank pain, hematuria, and flank mass occurs only in 10% to 20% of patients. Other presenting signs include weight loss, anemia, fever, hypertension, and an elevation of the erythrocyte sedimentation rate. Paraneoplastic syndromes can occur, including hypercalcemia, abnormal renal or liver function tests (Stauffer's syndrome), erythrocytosis, and acquired fibrinogen abnormalities.

Evaluation should include CT scan of the chest, abdomen, and pelvis, urinalysis, and urine cytology. If patient is having headaches or other findings concerning neurological involvement, an MRI of the head should be ordered. Also an MRI of the kidney can be helpful to assess tumor involvement of the inferior vena cava. If the patient is having bone pain, a nuclear bone scan can be helpful in documenting the extent of osseous metastatic disease. Findings that present on imaging similar to renal cell carcinomas include oncocytoma, benign adenoma, abscesses, pyelonephritis, or other metastatic cancers. Common metastatic lesions to the kidney include primary lung tumors, sarcoma, and lymphoma.

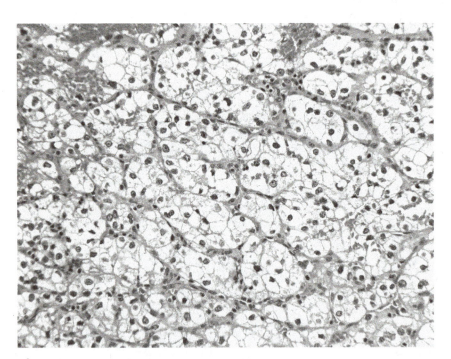

**FIGURE 11.3** Renal cell carcinoma, clear cell type. The tumor cells form small nests, surrounded by delicate blood vessels. The cytoplasm appears optically clear because glycogen and lipids are removed from the cytoplasm by chemicals used in histologic processing.

## Pathology

Clear cell (>85%) is the most common cancer of the kidney followed by papillary tumors (Figures 11.3 and 11.4). For practical purposes, clear cell kidney cancer and renal cell cancer are synonymous. Less common renal cell neoplasms include sarcomatoid variants, squamous cell, clear-cell sarcoma, Wilm's tumor, and medullary. It is crucial for the pathological diagnosis to be accurate for kidney cancer because of the varied prognosis and treatment options available depending on the tumor histology. Also it is important to rule out transitional cell carcinoma arising from the renal pelvis as a differential diagnosis of a kidney mass because of the need for cytotoxic chemotherapy for uroepithelial tumors.

## Staging and Prognosis

The American Joint Committee on Cancer staging system lists stage I tumors as being ≤7 cm and confined to the kidney and stage II tumors as being

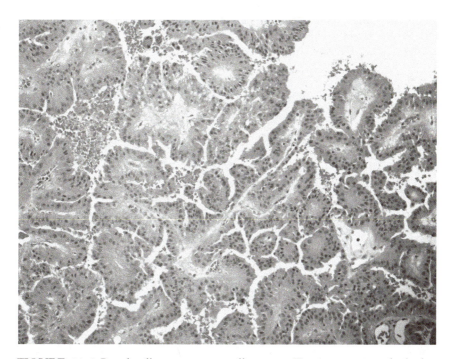

**FIGURE 11.4** Renal cell carcinoma, papillary type. Tumor is composed of arborizing fibrovascular cores lined by a single layer of malignant cells. By definition, papillary renal cell carcinoma must be greater than 5 mm in diameter; renal lesions with similar architecture, less than or equal to 5 mm in diameter, are designated as papillary adenomas.

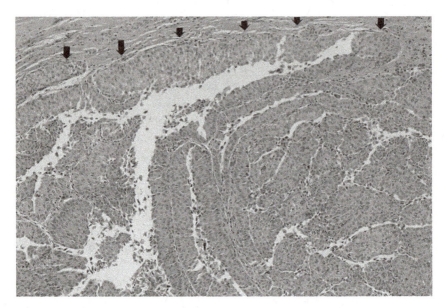

**FIGURE 11.5** Urothelial carcinoma, noninvasive. Tumor is composed of branching fibrovascular cores lined by multiple layers of urothelial cells with varying degrees of cytologic atypia. Tumor rests upon a collagenous basement membrane and does not infiltrate into the underlying lamina propria. The junction between tumor and lamina propria is indicated by the black arrows.

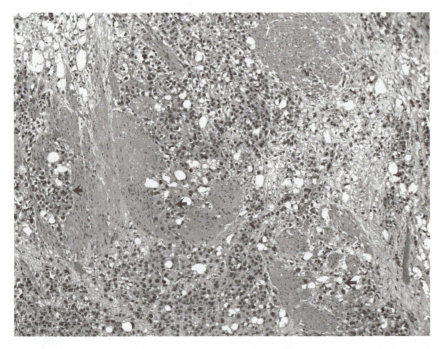

**FIGURE 11.6** Urothelial carcinoma, invasive. Ragged bands of tumor cells (arrows) intersect and invade thick bundles of muscularis propria.

≥7 cm also confined to the kidney. Stage III are tumors regardless of size that is confined to the kidney and involves a regional lymph node, tumors that involve the renal vein within Gerota's fascia, or tumors that involve the inferior vena cava with or without regional lymph node involvement. Stage IV is a tumor that extends beyond Gerota's fascia, with or without lymph node involvement, or any primary tumor size with a metastatic lesion.[40]

Factors associated with a poor prognosis include hypercalcemia, elevation of the LDH, poor performance status, and anemia. The 5-year survival rates differ based on the presenting stage. Stage I patients have a 5-year survival of >90%, stage II has >85% survival, stage III has approximately 60% survival, and stage IV has 10% survival.

## Surgery

Surgery is the primary treatment of stage I or stage II tumors. A radical nephrectomy includes the resection of the kidney, adrenal gland, perirenal fat, and Gerota's fascia with or without regional lymph node dissection. To spare kidney function partial nephrectomy can be considered for carefully selected patients. Stage III patients with large vein involvement can still be considered for surgery. These cases require a multidisciplinary approach with urology, vascular surgery, and anesthesia for optimal results. For patients who are not surgical candidates due to other comorbidities, external-beam radiotherapy or arterial embolization can be considered but are suboptimal procedures compared to surgery. Adjuvant therapy for high-risk patients using immunotherapy or tyrosine kinase inhibitors has not yet demonstrated any survival advantage.

In patients with a good performance status in the setting of stage IV disease, a nephrectomy of the primary tumor should be considered. Older data, before the use of tyrosine kinase inhibitors, demonstrated a survival advantage for patients with stage IV disease having a nephrectomy.[41] However, primary nephrectomy in the setting of advanced disease has not been studied in a randomized way with tyrosine kinase inhibitors. Even with this limitation, the removal of the primary tumor should still be considered in patients with an excellent performance status.

## Metastatic Disease

In general patients with metastatic kidney cancer require systemic therapy (Table 11.5). However, a subset of patients may significantly benefit from metastectomy of isolated renal tumor lesions. In patients with two or fewer metastatic lesions, consideration of removal of these tumors can provide some patients with prolonged disease-free intervals. Areas for isolated lesions amenable for metastectomy include the brain, thyroid, lung, and ovaries. The

TABLE 11.5  Summary of Available Agents for Advanced Kidney Carcinoma

| Treatment | Mechanism of Action | Indication | Comments |
|---|---|---|---|
| Interleukin-2 | Immunotherapy | First line | 5% cure rate |
| Sunitinib | VEGF inhibition | First line | Clear cell patients |
| Pazopanib | VEGF inhibition | First line | Clear cell patients |
| Axitinib | VEGF inhibition | Second line | Active after prior VEGF inhibitors |
| Temsirolimus | mTOR inhibitors | First line | Poor performance status patients |
| Everolimus | mTOR inhibitors | Second line | Option after prior use of VEGF inhibitor |

likelihood of achieving a benefit from surgical removal of isolated tumor deposits increases with long disease-free interval between the initial nephrectomy and the development of metastases.[42–46]

Although the overall response rate was very low immunotherapy from either interferon-α or interluekin-2, these treatments were the mainstay for advanced kidney cancer for over 20 years. Currently, the use of interferon-α is quite limited due to lack of efficacy. High-dose interluekin-2, however, is still used in very selective cases. Appropriate patients for interluekin-2 include those with an excellent performance status, clear cell histology, and non-bulky pulmonary or soft tissue lesions. For optimal results, all of these patients should also have a nephrectomy of their primary tumor. Patients with a poor performance status, non-clear cell histology, large tumor burden, or brain lesions are not good candidates for interluekin-2. Although the overall response rate for high-dose interluekin-2 is low (approximately 15%), approximately 5% of patients have a complete durable remission. Due to the significant toxicities related to high-dose interleukin-2, it should be given only by institutions experienced with handling the side effects. Thus, for the minority of patients with metastatic clear cell kidney carcinoma, interluekin-2 can be considered.[47]

## Targeting Vascular Endothelial Growth Factor

Clear cell kidney cancer has a preponderance to have overstimulation for angiogenesis, and multiple agents are now available to target the vascular endothelial growth factor (VEGF)–mediated pathways. The two main classes of drugs currently in use include the oral, small molecule, tyrosine kinase inhibitors (pazopanib, sorafenib, axitinib, and sunitinib) as well as the anti-VEGF monoclonal antibody (bevacizumab).

The tyrosine kinase inhibitors provide a dramatic increase in response rate when compared to immunotherapy. Patients with advanced kidney cancer can respond to these agents with improvements in quality of life and a delay in disease progression. However, these tyrosine kinase inhibitors are not curative. The treatment strategy must include the use of these agents sequentially over a period of time. After the first agent selected is no longer controlling the cancer, or the patient has intolerable side effects, moving to another VEGF targeted therapy or to an mTOR inhibitor should be considered.

Patients with clear cell and good performance status are appropriate candidates for either sunitinib or pazopanib. Both agents have demonstrated an improved survival advantage for patients with advanced kidney cancer.[48,49] Although their side effects are similar they are not the same. A randomized, double-blinded trial demonstrated that the efficacy and overall progression-free survival of Sutent and pazopanib were similar. However, pazopanib appeared to be better tolerated in regard to less fatigue, hand-foot syndrome, and thrombocytopenia. Also on the quality of life, patient questionnaire favored pazopanib over sunitinib.[50]

Once the patient has progression on pazopanib or sunitinib, axitinib as a second-line therapy of changing to a different class of drugs (mTOR inhibitor) should be considered. Axitinib, a highly potent VEGF inhibitor, has demonstrated efficacy by prolonging disease progression after first-line therapy even after use of prior tyrosine kinase inhibitors.[51]

Although the tyrosine kinase inhibitors are not cytotoxic agents, they can still have toxicity. Common side effects include hypertension, rash, thyroid abnormalities, taste alterations, fatigue, and myelosuppresion. If patients experience side effects, the medication can be withheld and restarted at a lower dose with acceptable results.

Bevacizumab, a monoclonal antibody that binds to and neutralizes circulating VEGF protein, has demonstrated the ability to delay progression of clear-cell renal cell carcinoma.[52] In addition bevacizumab and interferon-$\alpha$ resulted in longer progression-free survival compared to interferon-$\alpha$ alone.[53] In clinical practice, however, bevacizumab, if prescribed for the advanced kidney cancer patient, is usually given alone and without the interferon-$\alpha$.

## Mammalian Target of Rapamycin (mTOR) Inhibitors

The mTOR inhibitors are serine/threonine protein kinases that target regulators of cell growth, division, and survival. The two approved mTOR inhibiting agents include temsirolimus, an intravenously administered medication, and everolimus, an oral agent. Temsirolimus, evaluated as a first-line therapy, demonstrated an improvement in overall survival in patients with advanced kidney cancer who had intermediate- to poor-risk features.[54] Everolimus, studied as a second-line agent, has demonstrated efficacy in improving progression-free survival in patients after a VEGF tyrosine kinase inhibitor.[55]

Both agents are generally well tolerated and are excellent options for patients with advanced kidney cancer.

## Treatment of Non-clear Cell Kidney Cancer

The treatment of non-clear cell kidney cancer, such as papillary tumors, can be quite difficult. VEGF inhibition, either with oral tyrosine kinase inhibitors or with bevacizumab, has demonstrated very poor results for papillary renal tumors. Temsirolimus, studied as a first-line therapy for patients with suboptimal performance status, may have some efficacy against papillary tumors, but the results are modest. There is no one standard regimen for papillary tumors that has significant clinical activity.

Sarcomatoid kidney cancer is rapidly growing and usually a fatal tumor. The majorities of these patients are diagnosed with advanced disease and experience significant morbidity related to the tumor. Common presentations include fatigue, weight loss, and bone pain. Chemotherapy regimens using doxorubicin, gemcitabine, and taxanes for sarcomatoid kidney cancer can be used but unfortunately have only modest efficacy.

## BLADDER CANCER

Bladder cancer is the ninth most common cancer worldwide (over 350,000 cases per year) and the 13th most cause of cancer death (145,000 per year). Bladder cancer occurs in males at rates 3 to 4 times higher than females. Globally bladder cancer is highest in southern and Eastern Europe and in select locations in Africa, the Middle East, and North America. The highest mortality rates are in Egypt, being 8 times higher than those in North America. Tobacco and schistosomiasis are the leading risk factors. Although tobacco causes 50% of bladder cancer in men and 35% in women, the incidence rates of bladder cancer are stable or decreasing.[56,57] Bladder cancer most frequently presenting with superficial disease can be a tumor that recurs many times over a number of years. Over 90% of bladder carcinomas are transitional cell carcinomas derived from the uroepithelium (Figures 11.5 and 11.6). Other subtypes include squamous cell carcinomas (8%) and adenocarcinomas (2%).[58]

Bladder cancer in Africa presents a unique challenge for prevention and control. Since there are a limited number of tumor registries, the incidence and mortality of bladder cancer for much of Africa are not well known. The two distinct tumors arising from the bladder that occur in Africa, transitional cell and squamous cell, have different risk factors, age of presentation and prognosis.

Historically in areas of rural Africa, where there was less risk for carcinogens and tobacco use, the incidence of transitional cell bladder cancer was relatively low. However, with increase in industrialization and cigarette smoking, there is an increase in incidence of transitional cell carcinoma. Patients who develop transitional cell cancer from the bladder are typically older males who present with locally advanced or metastatic disease.

In contrast, squamous cell carcinoma of the bladder is related to fluke infection from areas with endemic schistosomiasis (bilharzia). Squamous cell carcinoma on average presents 10 to 20 years earlier than those with transitional cell carcinoma. In North African countries, including Egypt, squamous cell carcinoma is more prevalent in men performing agricultural work. However, in sub-Saharan countries, men and women present with equal incidence of squamous cell carcinoma. When the tumor is still localized to the bladder, many patients may be candidates for curative cystectomy. Unfortunately, due to limited resources and lack of access to health care, many patients in Africa present with inoperable or metastatic disease and ultimately succumb to their tumor.[59]

Bladder cancer can be divided into superficial non-muscle-invading tumors, tumors that invade into the muscle, and metastatic lesions. The prognostic factors important for bladder cancer include depth of invasion into the bladder wall and the degree of differentiation of the tumor. Superficial tumors that are poorly differentiated, large, multiple, or associated with carcinoma in situ (Tis) are at greatest risk for recurrence and the development of invasive cancer. Such patients may be considered to have the entire urothelial surface at risk for the development of recurrent tumors.

## Clinical Presentation and Staging

The most common presentation of a patient with bladder cancer is microscopic or gross hematuria. Urinary frequency, infection, pelvic pain, or urinary obstruction may also be present. Deterioration of kidney function may signal locally advanced disease. Patients should be evaluated with cystoscopy and urine cytology. Transurethral resection (TUR) of the tumor, with adequate muscle in the sample, should be obtained of any abnormal areas, and accurate histological diagnosis is critical for staging and prognosis. In patients with high-grade or invasive lesions, abdominal and pelvis imaging with a CT scan or MRI should be considered. Imaging of the upper tracts can be accomplished by renal ultrasound, intravenous pyelogram, CT urography, or ureteroscopy.

Transitional cell cancer arises from the bladder approximately 90% of the time. Less often the tumor can arise from the renal pelvis (8%) or the ureters

(2%). Outside of the areas prone to schistosomiasis infection, the majority of bladder cancers are urothelial (transitional) cell cancers, with less than 10% of the time being squamous cell, micropapillary, sarcomatoid, or adenocarcinoma. Adenocarcinoma usually arises from the dome of the bladder from a remnant related to the urachus. The staging of bladder cancer (Table 11.6) focuses on tumor depth, presence of lymph nodes, and absence or presence of metastatic lesions.[60]

## Superficial Bladder Cancer

Stage 0 (Ta, Tis, N0, M0) and stage I (T1, N0, M0) bladder cancer are both highly curable (image 5). Transurethral resection and fulguration can remove the vast majority of tumors, but the relapse rates are high. The risk of bladder cancer recurrence after resection is 30% to 80%.[61,62] Increased risk of recurrence includes large poorly differentiated tumors, multiple lesions, over-expression of nuclear p53, or carcinoma in situ.[63] Although carcinoma in situ is not common, it has a very high relapse rate and can recur in any location of the uroepithelium. After discovering a superficial bladder cancer, the recommendation is to repeat the cystoscopy every 3 months for the first 2 years and less frequently thereafter.[64] If the repeat biopsy demonstrates that the tumor is high grade or there is inadequate muscle in the specimen, another repeat TUR should be performed within 6 weeks.

Patients with high-risk superficial disease are candidates for intravesical therapy. Bacillus Calmette-Guérin (BCG) is most often used in patients with

**TABLE 11.6  Staging of Bladder Cancer**

| | |
|---|---|
| **Primary Tumor** | |
| Ta | Noninvasive papillary |
| Tis | Carcinoma in situ |
| T1 | Invades subepithelial tissue |
| T2 | Invades muscularis propria |
| T3 | Invades peri-vesical tissue |
| T4 | Involves (any) prostate, seminal vesicles, vagina, uterus, pelvic wall, abdominal wall |
| **Lymph Nodes** | |
| N0 | None |
| N1 | Single lymph node in pelvis |
| N2 | Multiple lymph nodes in pelvis |
| **Distant Metastasis** | |
| M0 | None |
| M1 | Distant metastases |

multiple tumors, recurrent tumors, high-grade lesions, and carcinoma in situ as a prophylactic measure after TUR of the tumor. BCG has been demonstrated to decrease both tumor recurrence and progression to muscle-invasive disease, improve bladder preservation, and decrease risk of death from bladder cancer.[65-67] Two non-consecutive 6-week BCG therapies may be necessary for optimal response.[68] Maintenance therapies up to 1 year are also common. Individuals who have persistent T1 or Tis after BCG therapy or those with persistent multifocal or high-grade lesions should be considered for radical cystectomy.[69]

Additional intravesical agents for superficial bladder cancer are available. These include thiotepa, mitomycin, doxorubicin, and interferon. Some of these agents may be better tolerated by the patient but generally are not considered superior to BCG for superficial bladder cancer.[70-72]

Carcinoma in situ is a unique and difficult problem. Patients who experience a complete response to BCG still have a 20% risk of recurrence at 5 years. Those who have an incomplete response to BCG with carcinoma in situ have a 95% risk of disease progression.[73] If the patient has recurrent carcinoma in situ after BCG or other intravesical therapies, consideration of radical cystectomy is a reasonable option.

## Muscle-Invasive Bladder Cancer

Muscle-invasive bladder cancer consists of stage II (T2a, T2b, N0, M0) and stage III (T3a, T3b, T4a, N0, M0) tumors. Invasive tumors that are confined to the bladder have a 5-year 75% progression-free survival compared to a more deeply invasive tumor where the 5-year survival rates decrease to 30% to 50%.[74,75] Initial evaluation should include CT scans of the abdomen and pelvis and either a chest x-ray or a CT scan of the chest.

Although muscle-invasive bladder cancer may be controlled in some patients by TUR, the standard of care is radical cystectomy for tumor control. Some select patients, with isolated tumor such as in the dome of the bladder, may be candidates for partial cystectomy. Radical cystectomy includes removal of the bladder, peri-vesical tissues, prostate, and seminal vesicles in men and the uterus, tubes, ovaries, anterior vaginal wall, and urethra in women with associated pelvic lymph node dissection. The decision for a urostomy, or the creation of an internalized neo-bladder, is dependent on the patient's tumor presentation, comorbidities, and surgeon's experience. Elderly patients in good health (≥70 years) can have excellent results after cystectomy, and age alone should not preclude a decision to offer surgery for these patients.[76] Preoperative radiotherapy has not been shown to increase overall survival in muscle-invasive bladder cancer and should not be considered standard of care.

Unfortunately, between 25% and over 50% of patients will have recurrence of their muscle-invasive bladder cancer after radical cystectomy. The role of neoadjuvant chemotherapy, which is chemotherapy given before surgical resection, has been studied extensively in muscle-invasive bladder cancer. A meta-analysis of over 2,600 patients demonstrated a 13% relative reduction in the risk of death and an improvement in the 5-year survival for combination cisplatin-based chemotherapy regimens.[77] Neoadjuvant chemotherapy given before surgery is preferred over adjuvant therapy because chemotherapy given neoadjuvantly may downstage the tumor, increase ability to remove the entire tumor, treat distant occult metastases, and may be better tolerated than given after surgery.

The most common neoadjuvant regimens studied included cisplatin, methotrexate, vinblastine, and doxorubicin (MVAC) and cisplatin, vinblastine, and methotrexate. Of note common chemotherapy regimens, such as cisplatin and gemcitabine or carboplatin and gemcitabine, have never been studied in a randomized fashion to improve survival given in the neoadjuvant setting. Also, single agent cisplatin has not been shown to improve overall survival when given before surgery.

Adjuvant chemotherapy after cystectomy is not well defined. The trials completed have been underpowered to determine if giving cisplatin combination chemotherapy in the adjuvant setting improves overall survival. However in high-risk patients with positive surgical margins or with malignant adenopathy, the consideration of cisplatin combination chemotherapy is reasonable.[78]

Patients with muscle-invasive disease who are poor surgical candidates or desire to avoid a cystectomy may be considered for bladder preservation. Ideal patients for bladder preservation include completely resected tumor at the time of the TUR, no evidence of carcinoma in situ, and no hydronephrosis seen on imaging studies. Appropriate patients should receive either concurrent radiotherapy with cisplatin or a regimen consisting of 5-FU and mitomycin C. After approximately 40 Gy of radiation, the patient should have a repeat cystoscopy. If there is no tumor present, the patient should finish the 65-Gy dose. If however the tumor is still present after 40 Gy, then the patient should be considered for cystectomy if the patient is a surgical candidate. Appropriate selected patients given bladder preservation therapy with chemotherapy and radiation have 5-year survival rates approaching 50%. Of these long-term survivors, approximately 75% are able to avoid future cystectomy.[79,80]

Patients who are treated with chemotherapy and radiation for muscle-invasive bladder cancer must undergo regular cystoscopic evaluations to look for disease recurrence. If the tumor recurs after bladder preservation therapy almost always, the correct next course of action is radical cystectomy. Since bladder preservation using chemotherapy and radiation has never been directly compared to cystectomy for muscle-invasive bladder cancer, the choice of treatment should be guided by the patient's overall health, disease status, and physician's clinical judgment.

## Metastatic Bladder Cancer

Stage IV bladder cancer (T4b, N0, M0; any T, N1–3, M0; any T, any N, M1) is not generally considered curable, although a small percentage of patients may be rendered disease free after aggressive local control and systemic chemotherapy. If a patient presents with advanced disease and has local bladder symptoms such as pain, bleeding, infections, and urgency, aggressive local therapy should be considered. Depending on the patient's symptoms and overall health, local control can be managed with TUR of the tumor, urinary diversion, cystectomy, palliative urinary diversion, or radiotherapy.

Palliative chemotherapy is the mainstay for advanced bladder cancer. Although the vast majority of patients will succumb to their illness in approximately 12 months' illness, dramatic responses can also be observed. Gemcitabine and cisplatin are considered the standard for patients who have appropriate renal function. Although MVAC has a similar response and overall survival as compared to gemcitabine and cisplatin, the latter is preferred based on a better side effect profile.[81] No triplet chemotherapy regimen has ever demonstrated improved overall survival over gemcitabine and cisplatin and should not be considered standard of care.

Unfortunately, for patients with a poor renal function, there is a lack of data guiding what regimens should be considered. Two small randomized studies were underpowered to answer if carboplatin is equivalent to cisplatin when given with gemcitabine. However, substituting carboplatin, in combination with gemcitabine, is a reasonable option for elderly patients or those who do not have adequate renal function. Carboplatin and paclitaxel combination also has demonstrated some efficacy in a phase II trial. Single agents studied in phase II trials include docetaxel, doxorubicin, premetrexed, and paclitaxel, but their impact on overall survival is unknown. These agents should be considered as second-line treatments in the setting of advanced disease, and it is unknown which, if any, of these chemotherapies may benefit.

## Non-urothelial Cell Carcinomas of the Bladder

Although rare, non-urothelial cell cancers can occur including small cell sarcomatoid and adenocarcinoma. Small cell tumors of the bladder are localized to the bladder and are generally treated with combination platinum-based chemotherapy followed by radiotherapy. If the tumor persists after radiation, then radical cystectomy should be considered. Sarcomatoid cancers of the bladder are highly aggressive and rarely present with localized disease. Standard sarcoma chemotherapy regimens are preferred for this lethal tumor.

## Upper Urinary Tract Tumors

Tumors arising from the ureters or renal pelvis are not common. These cancers are sometimes found after a positive urine cytology and a negative bladder cystoscopy are further explored. Many of these lesions can be seen on upper tract imaging using a CT scan, MRI, or retrograde pyelogram. The primary goal of tumor removal is usually performed by a nephroureterectomy. Neoadjuvant or adjuvant chemotherapy has not been studied enough to routinely recommend its use in this setting. In the metastatic setting of upper urinary tract tumors, the chemotherapy regimens similar to those used to tumors arising from the bladder are recommended.[82]

## REFERENCES

1. Howlader N, Noone AM, Krapcho M, et al. (Eds). *SEER Cancer Statistics Review, 1975–2008*. Bethesda, MD: National Cancer Institute, 2011.
2. International Agency for the Research and Treatment on Cancer. Globalcan 2008 Cancer Fact Sheet. Available at http://globocan.iarc.fr/factsheet.asp. Accessed August 19, 2013.
3. Jemal A, Bray F, Forman D, et al. Cancer burden in Africa and opportunities for prevention. *Cancer* 2012 Sep 15; 118(18): 4372–84. doi:10.1002/cncr.27410. Epub Jan 17, 2012.
4. Parkin DM, Nambooze S, Wabwire-Mangen F, Wabinga HR. Changing cancer incidence in Kampala, Uganda, 1991–2006. *Int J Cancer* 2010 Mar 1; 126(5): 1187–95. doi:10.1002/ijc.24838.
5. American Cancer Society. *Cancer Facts and Figures 2012*. Atlanta, GA: American Cancer Society, 2012. Accessed January 4, 2013.
6. Gondos A, Brenner H, Wabinga H, Parkin DM. Cancer survival in Kampala, Uganda. *Br J Cancer* 2005 May 9; 92(9): 1808–12.
7. Zelefsky MJ, Eastham JA, Sartor AO. Cancer of the prostate. In: DeVita VT Jr, Lawrence TS, Rosenberg SA (Eds). *Cancer: Principles and Practice of Oncology*. 9th ed. Philadelphia, PA: Lippincott Williams & Wilkins, 2011, pp. 1220–71.
8. Compton CC, Byrd DR, Garcia-Aguilar J, Kurtzman SH, Olawaiye A, Washington MK (Eds). *A Companion to the Seventh Editions of the AJCC Cancer Staging Manual and Handbook*. New York: Springer, 2013.
9. Chan TY, Partin AW, Walsh PC, et al. Prognostic significance of Gleason score 3+4 versus Gleason score 4+3 tumor at radical prostatectomy. *Urology* 2000; 56(5): 823–27.
10. Albertsen PC, Hanley JA, Barrows GH, et al. Prostate cancer and the Will Rogers phenomenon. *J Natl Cancer Inst* 2005; 97(17): 1248–53.
11. Thompson IM, Canby-Hagino E, Lucia MS. Stage migration and grade inflation in prostate cancer: will Rogers meets Garrison Keillor. *J Natl Cancer Inst* 2005; 97(17): 1236–37.
12. U.S. Preventative Services Task Force. Screening for Prostate Cancer Recommendation Statement. Available at http://www.uspreventiveservicestaskforce .org/prostatecancerscreening/prostatefinalrs.htm. Accessed August 19, 2013.

13. Chodak GW, Thisted RA, Gerber GS, et al. Results of conservative management of clinically localized prostate cancer. *N Engl J Med* 1994; 330(4): 242–48.

14. Whitmore WF Jr. Expectant management of clinically localized prostatic cancer. *Semin Oncol* 1994; 21(5): 560–68.

15. Johansson JE, Holmberg L, Johansson S, Bergström R, Adami HO. Fifteen-year survival in prostate cancer. A prospective, population-based study in Sweden. *JAMA* 1997; 277(6): 467–71.

16. Johansson JE, Andrén O, Andersson SO, et al. Natural history of early, localized prostate cancer. *JAMA* 2004; 291(22): 2713–19.

17. Matzkin H, Eber P, Todd B, van der Zwaag R, Soloway MS. Prognostic significance of changes in prostate-specific markers after endocrine treatment of stage D2 prostatic cancer. *Cancer* 1992; 70(9): 2302–9.

18. Pisansky TM, Cha SS, Earle JD, et al. Prostate-specific antigen as a pretherapy prognostic factor in patients treated with radiation therapy for clinically localized prostate cancer. *J Clin Oncol* 1993; 11(11): 2158–66.

19. Partin AW, Kattan MW, Subong EN, et al. Combination of prostate-specific antigen, clinical stage, and Gleason score to predict pathological stage of localized prostate cancer. A multi-institutional update. *JAMA* 1997; 277(18): 1445–51.

20. Partin AW, Mangold LA, Lamm DM, Walsh PC, Epstein JI, Pearson JD. Contemporary update of prostate cancer staging nomograms (Partin Tables) for the new millennium. *Urology* 2001; 58(6): 843–48.

21. Kattan MW, Eastham JA, Stapleton AM, Wheeler TM, Scardino PT. A preoperative nomogram for disease recurrence following radical prostatectomy for prostate cancer. *J Natl Cancer Inst* 1998; 90(10): 766–71.

22. Stephenson AJ, Scardino PT, Eastham JA, et al. Preoperative nomogram predicting the 10-year probability of prostate cancer recurrence after radical prostatectomy. *J Natl Cancer Inst* 2006; 98(10): 715–17.

23. Kattan MW, Wheeler TM, Scardino PT. Postoperative nomogram for disease recurrence after radical prostatectomy for prostate cancer. *J Clin Oncol* 1999; 17(5): 1499–507.

24. Stephenson AJ, Scardino PT, Eastham JA, et al. Postoperative nomogram predicting the 10-year probability of prostate cancer recurrence after radical prostatectomy. *J Clin Oncol* 2005; 23(28): 7005–12.

25. Fournier GR Jr, Narayan P. Re-evaluation of the need for pelvic lymphadenectomy in low grade prostate cancer. *Br J Urol* 1993; 72(4): 484–88.

26. Barry MJ, Gallagher PM, Skinner JS, Fowler FJ Jr. Adverse effects of robotic-assisted laparoscopic versus open retropubic radical prostatectomy among a nationwide random sample of medicare-age men. *J Clin Oncol* 2012 Feb 10; 30(5): 513–18. doi:10.1200/JCO.2011.36.8621. Epub Jan 3, 2012.

27. Potosky AL, Davis WW, Hoffman RM, et al. Five-year outcomes after prostatectomy or radiotherapy for prostate cancer: the prostate cancer outcomes study. *J Natl Cancer Inst* 2004; 96(18): 1358–67.

28. International Atomic Energy Agency. Directory of Radiotherapy Centers (DIRAC). Available at http://www-naweb.iaea.org/nahu/dirac/default.shtm. Accessed August 7, 2011.

29. Hussain M, Tangen CM, Berry DL, et al. Intermittent versus continuous androgen deprivation in prostate cancer. *N Engl J Med* 2013; 368(14): 1314–25.

30. Schröder FH, Kurth KH, Fosså SD, et al. Early versus delayed endocrine treatment of pN1–3 M0 prostate cancer without local treatment of the primary tumor: results of European Organisation for the Research and Treatment of Cancer 30846—a phase III study. *J Urol* 2004 Sep; 172(3): 923–27.

31. Ryan CJ, Smith MR, de Bono JS, et al. Abiraterone in metastatic prostate cancer without previous chemotherapy. *N Engl J Med* 2013; 368(2): 138–48..

32. de Bono JS, Logothetis CJ, Molina A, et al. Abiraterone and increased survival in metastatic prostate cancer. *N Engl J Med* 2011; 364(21): 1995–2005.

33. Scher HI, Fizazi K, Saad F, et al. Increased survival with enzalutamide in prostate cancer after chemotherapy. *N Engl J Med* 2012; 367(13): 1187–97.

34. Kantoff PW, Higano CS, Shore ND, et al. Sipuleucel-T immunotherapy for castration-resistant prostate cancer. *N Engl J Med* 2010; 363(5): 411–22.

35. Tannock IF, de Wit R, Berry WR, et al. Docetaxel plus prednisone or mitoxantrone plus prednisone for advanced prostate cancer. *N Engl J Med* 2004; 351(15): 1502–12.

36. de Bono JS, Oudard S, Ozguroglu M, et al. Prednisone plus cabazitaxel or mitoxantrone for metastatic castration-resistant prostate cancer progressing after docetaxel treatment: a randomised open-label trial. *Lancet* 2010; 376(9747): 1147–54.

37. Fizazi K, Carducci M, Smith M, et al. Denosumab versus zoledronic acid for treatment of bone metastases in men with castration-resistant prostate cancer: a randomised, double-blind study. *Lancet* 2011; 377(9768): 813–22.

38. Parker C, Nilsson S, Heinrich D, et al. Alpha emitter radium-223 and survival in metastatic prostate cancer. *N Engl J Med* 2013 Jul 18; 369(3): 213–23. doi:10.1056/NEJMoa1213755.

39. World Cancer Research Fund International. Cancer Statistics. Available at http://www.wcrf.org/cancer_statistics/data_specific_cancers/kidney_cancer_statistics.php. Accessed August 26, 2013.

40. Kidney. In: Edge SB, Byrd DR, Compton CC, et al. (Eds). *AJCC Cancer Staging Manual.* 7th ed. New York, NY: Springer, 2010, pp. 479–89.

41. Flanigan RC, Salmon SE, Blumenstein BA, et al. Nephrectomy followed by interferon alfa-2b compared with interferon alfa-2b alone for metastatic renal-cell cancer. *N Engl J Med* 2001; 345(23): 1655–59.

42. Murthy SC, Kim K, Rice TW, et al. Can we predict long-term survival after pulmonary metastasectomy for renal cell carcinoma? *Ann Thorac Surg* 2005; 79(3): 996–1003.

43. Eggener SE, Yossepowitch O, Kundu S, Motzer RJ, Russo P. Risk score and metastasectomy independently impact prognosis of patients with recurrent renal cell carcinoma. *J Urol* 2008; 180(3): 873–78; discussion 878.

44. Kwak C, Park YH, Jeong CW, Lee SE, Ku JH. Metastasectomy without systemic therapy in metastatic renal cell carcinoma: comparison with conservative treatment. *Urol Int* 2007; 79(2): 145–51.

45. Russo P, O'Brien MF. Surgical intervention in patients with metastatic renal cancer: metastasectomy and cytoreductive nephrectomy. *Urol Clin North Am* 2008; 35(4): 679–86; viii.

46. Hofmann HS, Neef H, Krohe K, Andreev P, Silber RE. Prognostic factors and survival after pulmonary resection of metastatic renal cell carcinoma. *Eur Urol* 2005; 48(1): 77–81; discussion 81–82.

47. McDermott DF, Regan MM, Clark JI, et al. Randomized phase III trial of high-dose interleukin-2 versus subcutaneous interleukin-2 and interferon in patients with metastatic renal cell carcinoma. *J Clin Oncol* 2005; 23(1): 133–41.

48. Motzer RJ, Hutson TE, Tomczak P, et al. Sunitinib versus interferon alfa in metastatic renal-cell carcinoma. *N Engl J Med* 2007; 356(2): 115–24.

49. Sternberg CN, Davis ID, Mardiak J, et al. Pazopanib in locally advanced or metastatic renal cell carcinoma: results of a randomized phase III trial. *J Clin Oncol* 2010; 28(6): 1061–68.

50. Motzer RJ, Hutson TE, Cella D, et al. Pazopanib versus Sunitinib in metastatic renal-cell carcinoma. *N Engl J Med* 2013 Aug 22; 369: 722–31. doi:10.1056/NEJMoa1303989.

51. Motzer RJ, Escudier B, Tomczak P, et al. Axitinib versus sorafenib as second-line treatment for advanced renal cell carcinoma: overall survival analysis and updated results from a randomised phase 3 trial. *Lancet Oncol* 2013; 14(6): 552–62.

52. Yang JC, Haworth L, Sherry RM, et al. A randomized trial of bevacizumab, an anti-vascular endothelial growth factor antibody, for metastatic renal cancer. *N Engl J Med* 2003; 349(5): 427–34.

53. Escudier B, Pluzanska A, Koralewski P, et al. Bevacizumab plus interferon alfa-2a for treatment of metastatic renal cell carcinoma: a randomised, double-blind phase III trial. *Lancet* 2007; 370(9605): 2103–11.

54. Hudes G, Carducci M, Tomczak P, et al. Temsirolimus, interferon alfa, or both for advanced renal-cell carcinoma. *N Engl J Med* 2007; 356(22): 2271–81.

55. Motzer RJ, Escudier B, Oudard S, et al. Efficacy of everolimus in advanced renal cell carcinoma: a double-blind, randomised, placebo-controlled phase III trial. *Lancet* 2008; 372(9637): 449–56.

56. Zeegers MP, Tan FE, Dorant E, van Den Brandt PA. The impact of characteristics of cigarette smoking on urinary tract cancer risk: a meta-analysis of epidemiologic studies. *Cancer* 2000; 89(3): 630–39. doi:10.1002/1097–0142(20000801)89.

57. Parkin DM. The global burden of urinary bladder cancer. *Can J Urol* 2008 Feb; 15(1): 3899–908.

58. Mostofi FK, Davis CJ, Sesterhenn IA. Pathology of tumors of the urinary tract. In: Skinner DG, Lieskovsky G (Eds). *Diagnosis and Management of Genitourinary Cancer*. Philadelphia, PA: WB Saunders, 1988, pp. 83–117.

59. Heyns CF, van der Merwe A. Bladder cancer in Africa. *Scand J Urol Nephrol Suppl* 2008 Sep; 218: 12–20.

60. American Joint Committee on Cancer (AJCC). *Bladder Cancer Staging (AJCC Staging Manual)*. 7th ed. New York: Springer, 2010.

61. Holmäng S, Hedelin H, Anderström C, Johansson SL. The relationship among multiple recurrences, progression and prognosis of patients with stages Ta and T1 transitional cell cancer of the bladder followed for at least 20 years. *J Urol* 1995; 153(6): 1823–26; discussion 1826–7.

62. Sylvester RJ, van der Meijden AP, Oosterlinck W, et al. Predicting recurrence and progression in individual patients with stage Ta T1 bladder cancer using EORTC risk tables: a combined analysis of 2596 patients from seven EORTC trials. *Eur Urol* 2006 Mar; 49(3): 466–475; discussion 475–77. Epub Jan 17, 2006.

63. Lacombe L, Dalbagni G, Zhang ZF, et al. Overexpression of p53 protein in a high-risk population of patients with superficial bladder cancer before and after

bacillus Calmette-Guérin therapy: correlation to clinical outcome. *J Clin Oncol* 1996; 14(10): 2646–52.

64. Herr HW. The value of a second transurethral resection in evaluating patients with bladder tumors. *J Urol* 1999; 162(1): 74–76.

65. Herr HW, Schwalb DM, Zhang ZF, et al. Intravesical bacillus Calmette-Guérin therapy prevents tumor progression and death from superficial bladder cancer: ten-year follow-up of a prospective randomized trial. *J Clin Oncol* 1995; 13(6): 1404–8.

66. Lamm DL, Griffith JG. Intravesical therapy: does it affect the natural history of superficial bladder cancer? *Semin Urol* 1992; 10(1): 39–44.

67. Shelley MD, Wilt TJ, Court J, Coles B, Kynaston H, Mason MD. Intravesical bacillus Calmette-Guérin is superior to mitomycin C in reducing tumour recurrence in high-risk superficial bladder cancer: a meta-analysis of randomized trials. *BJU Int* 2004 Mar; 93(4): 485–90.

68. Coplen DE, Marcus MD, Myers JA, Ratliff TL, Catalona WJ. Long-term followup of patients treated with 1 or 2, 6-week courses of intravesical bacillus Calmette-Guerin: analysis of possible predictors of response free of tumor. *J Urol* 1990; 144(3): 652–57.

69. Amling CL, Thrasher JB, Frazier HA, et al. Radical cystectomy for stages Ta, Tis and T1 transitional cell carcinoma of the bladder. *J Urol* 1994; 151(1): 31–35; discussion 35–36.

70. Lamm DL, Blumenstein BA, Crawford ED, et al. A randomized trial of intravesical doxorubicin and immunotherapy with bacille Calmette-Guérin for transitional-cell carcinoma of the bladder. *N Engl J Med* 1991; 325(17): 1205–9.

71. Malmström PU, Wijkström H, Lundholm C, Wester K, Busch C, Norlén BJ. 5-year followup of a randomized prospective study comparing mitomycin C and bacillus Calmette-Guerin in patients with superficial bladder carcinoma. Swedish-Norwegian Bladder Cancer Study Group. *J Urol* 1999; 161(4): 1124–27.

72. Boccardo F, Cannata D, Rubagotti A, et al. Prophylaxis of superficial bladder cancer with mitomycin or interferon alfa-2b: results of a multicentric Italian study. *J Clin Oncol* 1994; 12(1): 7–13.

73. Hudson MA, Herr HW. Carcinoma in situ of the bladder. *J Urol* 1995; 153(3 Pt 1): 564–72.

74. Quek ML, Stein JP, Nichols PW, et al. Prognostic significance of lymphovascular invasion of bladder cancer treated with radical cystectomy. *J Urol* 2005; 174(1): 103–6.

75. Thrasher JB, Crawford ED. Current management of invasive and metastatic transitional cell carcinoma of the bladder. *J Urol* 1993; 149(5): 957–72.

76. Figueroa AJ, Stein JP, Dickinson M, et al. Radical cystectomy for elderly patients with bladder carcinoma: an updated experience with 404 patients. *Cancer* 1998; 83(1): 141–47.

77. Advanced Bladder Cancer Meta-analysis Collaboration. Neoadjuvant chemotherapy in invasive bladder cancer: a systematic review and meta-analysis. *Lancet* 2003; 361(9373): 1927–34.

78. Advanced Bladder Cancer (ABC) Meta-analysis Collaboration. Adjuvant chemotherapy in invasive bladder cancer: a systematic review and meta-analysis

of individual patient data. *Eur Urol* 2005 Aug; 48(2): 189–99; discussion 199–201. Epub Apr 25, 2005.

79. Rödel C, Grabenbauer GG, Kühn R, et al. Combined-modality treatment and selective organ preservation in invasive bladder cancer: long-term results. *J Clin Oncol* 2002; 20(14): 3061–71.

80. James ND, Hussain SA, Hall E, et al. Radiotherapy with or without chemotherapy in muscle-invasive bladder cancer. *N Engl J Med* 2012 Apr 19; 366(16): 1477–88. doi:10.1056/NEJMoa1106106.

81. von der Maase H, Hansen SW, Roberts JT, et al. Gemcitabine and cisplatin versus methotrexate, vinblastine, doxorubicin, and cisplatin in advanced or metastatic bladder cancer: results of a large, randomized, multinational, multicenter, phase III study. *J Clin Oncol* 2000; 18(17): 3068–77.

82. Audenet F, Yates DR, Cussenot O, Rouprêt M. The role of chemotherapy in the treatment of urothelial cell carcinoma of the upper urinary tract (UUT-UCC). *Urol Oncol* 2013 May; 31(4): 407–13. doi:10.1016/j.urolonc.2010.07.016. Epub Sep 29, 2010.

# 12

# Pediatric Cancer

## *Aziza Shad, Luca Szalontay, and Miya Shitama*

## INTRODUCTION

"Cancer Control in Low and Middle-Income Countries," a 2007 consensus study conducted by the Institute of Medicine, identified pediatric cancer care in the developing world as a field that demanded the attention of the global health community, both because of the great burden that exists—approximately 80% of the world's children with cancer live in the developing world—and because of the great opportunity that exists to cure children with cancer.[1] In the United States, 5-year survival rates for the most common childhood cancers now range from 80% to 99%.[2] These high survival rates provide hope that the diseases themselves are not what stand in the way of curing children with cancer. Rather, it is a question of equipping medical professionals in the developing world with the tools and training that have been so successful elsewhere across the globe. The little data we currently possess on low- and middle-income countries (LMICs) (scarcity of data is a huge problem) points to the fact that medical infrastructure is grossly underdeveloped. In Africa, for example, where reliable cancer registries cover only about 1% of the population, only 20% of patients are reportedly cured.[3]

The potential to achieve substantial survival rates is demonstrated by the upward climb of survival rates in the United States throughout the latter half of the 20th century and into the 21st century. Acute lymphoblastic leukemia (ALL), the most common childhood cancer, is now considered cured in close to 90% of children, up from just 4% in 1962. Significant improvement in survival has occurred for each curable childhood cancer. Five diseases (including ALL), have seen survival rates grow by 60% or more; five have seen those rates grow by at least 30%.[2,4] Elsewhere in the developed world, improvement in care has yielded similar exciting results. In the United Kingdom, 5-year survival rates for ALL as well as non-Hodgkin's and Hodgkin's lymphoma, have increased on average 42% since 1971, with survival rates for these cancers all currently above 80%.[5]

This success is now being mirrored by a slow but steady increase in cure rates in selected pediatric oncology programs in LMICs in Asia, Africa, Middle East, and Latin America through collaborative projects with high-income countries (HICs), focused on capacity building through training and education.[6,7]

In this chapter, we address the challenges to pediatric cancer care in LMICs and discuss possible solutions and opportunities.

## UNDERSTANDING THE CHALLENGES AND BARRIERS

The United Nations General Assembly in May 2002 in its Special Session on Children dreamed of a "world fit for children" and set its millennium development goals.[13] Global initiatives in pediatric cancer care are urgently needed. However, before embarking on any program to improve survival in pediatric cancer in LMICs, it is important to understand some of the barriers that currently exist to providing adequate care to children.

1. *Accurately assessing the tumor burden:*

    The sheer numbers of children with cancer in LMICs, most of whom go undiagnosed or are diagnosed late, are overwhelming. The proportion of the childhood cancer burden borne by LMICs continues to rise with a current approximate of 80%,[11] stemming primarily from the fact that most of the world's population less than 18 years lives in low-income countries.[12] The absolute number of incident cases is also growing faster in the developing countries than in industrialized societies. Epidemiologic studies and local cancer registries play a crucial part in enabling health-care professionals to address the cancer burden more effectively. There are only a few, truly population-based registries in LMICs; underdiagnosis and under-reporting are common. For example, clinical records from the TASGH Radiotherapy Center estimate that there are 120,500 new cancer cases per year in Ethiopia, although Globocan estimates are much lower (51,000 per year).[22] Similarly, based on extrapolating estimates from another East African nation, Tanzania, with an incidence of pediatric cancer of 134 cancer cases per million,[43] Ethiopia probably has close to 6,000 new cases of pediatric cancer each year.[22] Establishing population-based cancer registries should be a priority in planning programs for LMICs.

2. *Understanding differences in incidence and characteristics of cancer:*

    The incidence and unique characteristics of various cancers differ from country to country. For instance, there is a significant difference between the incidences of different types of cancers in LMICs and HICs, as shown in Figure 12.1.[14,15] Incidence rates vary among different ethnic groups in the same country and between the same ethnic groups in different countries. This reflects differences in cancer biology, both in the host and in the environment, which helps in understanding the disease process.[16] This phenomenon is well exemplified by the incidence rates of Burkitt's lymphoma and retinoblastoma in different parts of the world and should be taken into consideration when resources are being allocated.

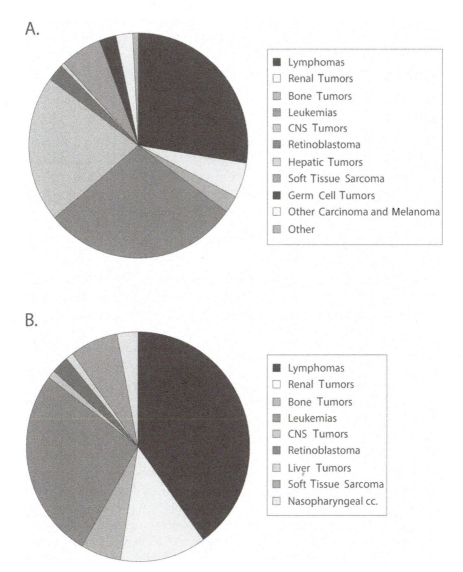

**FIGURE 12.1** Incidence rates of different types of childhood cancer in the United Kingdom between 2001 and 2005 based on National Registry of Childhood Tumours (A) and in Sudan between 1999 and 2004 based on the patient population of Institute of Nuclear Medicine, Molecular Biology and Oncology in Central Sudan (B).

3. *Relationship between infection and cancer:*

Mortality related to infection, malnutrition, and diarrheal dehydration continues to remain high in LMICs, although recently there has been a noticeable increase in the relative importance of cancer in childhood. There are important interactions between infections, nutritional status, and cancer in early life. The association between Epstein–Barr virus infection, Burkitt's lymphoma and nasopharyngeal carcinoma, hepatitis B infection and hepatocellular carcinoma, and human papillomavirus (HPV) and carcinoma of the cervix is well recognized, as are HIV-associated malignancies. Immunizations, timely anti-infective therapy, and management of malnutrition might decrease the incidence of some cancers and definitively contribute to improved outcome.

4. *Cultural differences:*

Cultural differences and adjusting strategies to them is one of the key elements of success. Preference for traditional forms of health-care intervention is rooted deep in developing countries and must be respected, as it has many advantages, including trust and compliance. This also explains the widespread use of complementary and alternative medicines among families of children with cancer in HICs.[18] In many communities, local/traditional "medicine-men" have been enlisted to help children with cancer get appropriate care.

5. *Socioeconomic status and education:*

Both these factors impact heavily on morbidity and mortality in pediatric oncology. Disadvantaged members of the society are less likely to seek conventional health care for themselves or their children, hence the late presentation at diagnosis. For those, who live in a rural area, travel is expensive and access to centralized medical systems is more difficult. Cost of treatment, inability to support the family while one child is in treatment away from home, lack of understanding of the disease, all contribute to early abandonment of treatment. Educational status is another significant factor that plays a role in motivation to undergo treatment and compliance.

6. *Lack of infrastructure and resources:*

One of the biggest barriers to cancer care in LMICs is the lack of trained medical personnel, poor diagnostic facilities, inadequate units for treatment, insufficient supply of essential chemotherapy drugs and simple pain medications necessary to treat cancer patients, and a weak and overburdened health-care system. Human resources are scant—few pediatricians, no trained oncologists, nurses, or pharmacists—all of whom make meager salaries without incentives.

As a result of all these barriers, there is little public awareness that cancer can be cured, little public demand that health systems address cancer, and, consequently, few government medical resources devoted to cancer treatment.

## PALLIATIVE CARE

Improving pediatric cancer care in LMICs is not just about increasing survival rates, but also quality of life. Palliative care is an essential component of cancer care and must be treated as a priority in the developing world. Many children in resource-poor settings arrive at treatment centers with very advanced cancers that leave doctors with little hope of doing anything but treating pain. Meanwhile, health-care providers at these centers are not trained to recognize or treat pain adequately; basic pain medication such as morphine is either not available or not used secondary to misconceptions about addiction; ultimately the child dies after great suffering. The pediatric palliative care program that began in Pakistan in 2008 with the support of the International Network for Cancer Treatment and Research (INCTR) and other global health organizations presents an example of a partnership-based program aiming to address this crucial issue in an LMIC.[44] The Middle East Cancer Consortium initiative in pediatric palliative care has successfully focused on education and awareness in health-care providers.[10]

## CHALLENGES AND PROGRESS IN GLOBAL PEDIATRIC ONCOLOGY NURSING

In many HICs, such as the United Kingdom, overall childhood survival rates are approaching 80%[23] due in part to clinical trials and significant resources for biomedical and supportive care. In fact, in some HICs, nurses are participating in the development and conduct of clinical trials in the Children's Oncology Group (COG).[24] Therapies can include biological therapies (such as monoclonal antibodies or therapeutic vaccines), targeted therapies, and bone marrow transplant. Together with a multidisciplinary team including nutritionists, psychologists, and pharmacists, HIC nurses support the family and child throughout the high-tech intensive cancer treatment.

Nurses in HICs must also understand cancer genetics and the particular challenges of families with children with a family history of cancer or who are at high risk for cancer. Examples include children who are at risk for retinoblastoma, and children with Down's syndrome or neurofibromatosis. Evidenced-based nursing practice is expected in most HICs. Nursing researchers, both quantitative and qualitative, have contributed to a substantial body of work that supports standards of care and nursing protocols based on documented investigation of issues such as central venous catheter care, pain assessment and management, and patient/family education strategies (i.e., Oncology Nursing Society in the United States and the European Oncology Nursing Society).

Recently, the specific needs of teens and young adults with cancer have been recognized and addressed. The United Kingdom has led this area of specialty care with the Teenage Cancer Trust.[25] COG in the United States and in other countries has initiated action to ensure that this population no longer falls through the crack between pediatrics and adult care, but rather is identified for special nursing attention.[26]

Long-term follow-up for survivors of childhood cancer is another area of importance for nurses in HICs. Many cancer survivors develop serious morbidity, die at a young age from non-cancer causes, and experience diminished health status.[27] Nurses working with children, teens, and young adults must be aware of the potential disabilities of late effects from cancer treatment and inform the family and former patient of the need to seek ongoing surveillance after therapy is completed.[28]

Nurses caring for children with cancer in LMICs, however, face another reality. Children are generally diagnosed with a late stage of disease due to the lack of health-care and financial resources and community awareness.[29] Therefore, cure is rarely possible, and palliative care forms the larger part of the nurses' practice.[30] Although pediatric oncology nurses have been found to be instrumental in successful palliative care,[31] unfortunately, most nurses caring for children in LMICs do not receive specialty training or multidisciplinary support. Units treating children with cancer may also have children with infectious diseases and other medical conditions. Staffing is usually poor due to migration, shortfalls in preservice training,[32] low salaries, heavy workloads, and the absence of other incentives as well as dual practice.[33]

Due to the lack of oncology pharmacists in LMICs, the burden of preparing and administering chemotherapy as well as symptom management for the child with cancer and educating the family overwhelms the limited nursing staff. However, programs such as AMPATH-Oncology Pharmacy Service training in western Kenya is working to address patient safety, practitioner safety, inventory, procurement centralization, and environmental containment of hazardous drugs,[34] thus increasing nursing care time by introducing oncology pharmacists even in a low-income setting.

Many families of children with cancer in LMICs live in extreme poverty and sell their assets or borrow from family members to just arrive at the hospital for cancer treatment, which is usually in the capital of their country. Most LMICs do not offer free cancer treatment; thus, there is a significant rate of abandonment of care since the families cannot afford the cost of complex and lengthy cancer treatment.[35] Nurses can have a significant role in educating families and providing ongoing support to decrease abandonment of treatment and the effects of stigma and misconceptions about cancer.[36] LMICs often have multiple local languages, so it is possible that the pediatric oncology nurses have communication troubles with families of children under their care. Families have often visited traditional healers in LMICs before arriving at the hospital and receiving a cancer diagnosis for their child. Even during treatment, families may continue to rely on traditional and complementary medical approaches.[37] Therefore, nurses must be aware of these practices and sensitive to the families' choices, while collaborating with the family to ensure that the child does not have treatments that might negatively affect his or her biomedical cancer treatment.

Across the world regardless of income status, all nurses caring for children with cancer must participate in raising awareness of cancer signs and symptoms and cancer's potential curability. Nurses must advocate for specialized training and continuing education to ensure that their nursing care remains optimal. In addition, nurses must work to improve communication with the medical team as well as ancillary personnel since only a well-coordinated multidisciplinary team with strong interdisciplinary communication can ensure the safest and most effective cancer care.[38]

Nurses caring for children, teens, and young adults with cancer must strive to be expert clinicians capable of professional collaboration with the medical team and support families to exploit their own strengths and those of their community when facing the challenge of childhood cancer. One powerful ally in this struggle is a parent group as evidenced by the significant role of the International Cooperative of Childhood Cancer Parent Organizations in LMICs.[39]

Twinning and international partnerships in pediatric oncology have shown that collaboration can improve the nursing care of children with cancer.[40-42] Visiting nurses from HICs learn much from their partners in LMICs, who are resourceful at addressing complex care with few resources and patient populations who are extremely diverse, are undereducated, and live in extreme poverty. HIC nurses share technical skills and critical thinking skills that help their local nursing partners to creatively solve the many challenges in nursing care of children with cancer in LMICs. Together nurses work to ensure that children being treated for cancer everywhere receive the best nursing care in the context of their local setting with the resources available.

## PREVENTION AND SCREENING

There are very few opportunities to prevent cancers that occur during childhood and adolescence. Educational programs aiming at reducing direct sun exposure, avoiding unprotected sex, and changing some regional habits could affect the prevalence of some types of cancer later in life. Adequate immunization, especially directed against hepatitis B and HPV, is an example.

Cancer screening, the best tool for early detection in adults, faces numerous challenges in developing countries. Symptoms and signs of cancer in children are often vague and difficult to recognize, and the knowledge among community health workers is poor.[20] One of the cancers prevalent in many LMICs is retinoblastoma. Successful efforts to raise awareness of retinoblastoma, a cancer that is curable if detected early, are resulting in an improvement in survival in Mexico and Brazil.

## OPPORTUNITIES AND SOLUTIONS

Cancer is set to become the newest epidemic in the developing world.[19] The United Nations and the World Health Organization have put forth their millennium goals, and governments, international cancer agencies, and cancer centers in HICs face a moral responsibility to help stave this looming crisis.

One such solution is the establishment of partnerships between cancer control programs in HICs and LMICs focused on training, education, and infrastructure support. The goal of these partnerships would be to help improve diagnosis, increase knowledge in health-care professionals, raise awareness for early recognition, encourage a national cancer control plan that is evidence based and adapted to local needs, facilitate availability of chemotherapy agents and anti-infective drugs, and establish palliative care. This has been demonstrated very successfully in pediatric oncology through twinning programs.

### Twinning

Sharing knowledge and resources is the basis of a successful "twinning" program wherein a medical institution from a HIC partners with a local institution in a LMIC to create or expand their capacity to treat pediatric cancer (Table 12.1). The vast majority of successful pediatric cancer programs in LMICs have embraced twinning. One of the earliest, celebrated twinning programs began in 1986 as a partnership between the Monza group of Italy led by Dr. Giuseppe Masera and the La Mascota Children's Hospital in Nicaragua.[6] Measured in terms of increased patient load as well as survival rates, the early successes in these programs have been encouraging. At Ocean Road Cancer Institute, a pediatric cancer center in Tanzania, supported in part by the INCTR, patient intake nearly tripled from 2005 to 2010, a period that saw the 1-year survival rate for Burkitt's lymphoma increase from 5–10% to 60%.[7]

Another pioneer of twinning is St. Jude Children's Hospital. Through its International Outreach Program, it has provided an early standard for how to succeed in low-income settings using twinning, which it published in "A Guide for Establishing a Pediatric Oncology Twinning Program" (2008). With partner sites in over 20 countries, St. Jude has supported programs that have been very successful at working closely with local institutions to substantially increase pediatric cancer survival rates.[8] For example, a St. Jude-supported twinning program in Guatemala led to a 50% increase,

**TABLE 12.1  Pediatric Oncology Twinnings as of August 2013**

| | |
|---|---|
| St. Jude Children's Research Hospital (United States) | Costa Rica—Hospital Nacional de Niños in San Jose |
| | Honduras—Hospital Escuela Materno Infantilin Tegucigalpa, Honduras |
| | Guatemala—Unidad Nacional de Oncología Pediátrica, Guatemala City |
| | El Salvador—Benjamin Bloom Children's Hospital, San Salvador |
| | Panama—Panama Children's Hospital, Panama City |
| | Morocco—Hôpital 20 Août 1953, Casablanca |
| | Hôpital d'Enfants, Rabat |
| | Chile—Calvo Mackenna Hospital in Santiago, Chile |
| | Ecuador—Hospital de la Sociedad de Lucha Contra el Cáncer Núcleo de Quito (SOLCA), Quito |
| | Jordan—King Hussein Cancer Center, Amman |
| | Brasil—Centro de Hematologica e Oncologia Pediatrica de Pernambuco (CEHOPE), Recife |
| | Lebanon—American University of Beirut/Children's Cancer Center of Lebanon, Beirut |
| | China—Beijing Children's Hospital, Beijing |
| | Shanghai Children's Medical Center, Shanghai |
| | Venezuela—Hospital de Niños J.M. de los Ríos, Caracas |
| | Hospital de Especialidades Pediátricas, Maracaibo |
| | Philippines—South Philippines Medical Centre, Davao City, Mindanao |
| | Mexico—Hospital General de Tijuana, Tijuana |
| | Hospital Pediátrico de Sinaloa, Culiacán |
| | Hospital Civil de Guadalajara, Guadalajara |
| Georgetown University Medical Center/ International Network of Cancer Treatment and Research | Ethiopia—Tikur Anbessa Specialized General Hospital, Addis Ababa |
| Boston Children's Hospital/ Dana Farber Cancer Institute, Boston, MA, United States | Children's Cancer Center of Egypt, Cairo, Egypt Instituto Nacional de Cancerología, Bogotá |
| Texas Children's Cancer and Hematology Center, Baylor, TX, United States | Botswana—Princess Marina Hospital, Gabarone |
| University of Texas Health Science Center, San Antonio, TX, United States | Children's Hospital No. 2 in Ho Chi Minh City, Vietnam |
| Fred Hutchinson Cancer Research Center, Seattle, WA,United States | Uganda Cancer Institute in Kampala, Uganda |

*(Continued)*

**TABLE 12.1** (*Continued*)

| | |
|---|---|
| Hospital for Sick Kids, Toronto, Canada | Trinidad & Tobago |
| World Child Cancer (United Kingdom) | Bangladesh—Bangabandhu Sheik Mujab Medical University, Dhaka |
| | Philippines—South Philippines Medical Centre, Davao City, Mindanao |
| | Cameroon—Banso Baptist Hospital, Northwest Province |
| | Mbingo Baptist Hospital, Northwest Province |
| | Mutengene Baptist Hospital, Southwest Province |
| | Colombia—Instituto Nacional de Cancerología, Bogotá |
| | Ghana—Korle Bu Teaching Hospital, Accra |
| | Malawi—Queen Elizabeth Central Hospital, Blantyre |
| Royal Sick Children's Hospital, Edinburgh, United Kingdom | Ghana—Korle Bu Teaching Hospital, Accra |
| Victoria Royal Infirmary, Newcastle, United Kingdom | Malawi—Queen Elizabeth Central Hospital, Blantyre |
| Lund University Hospital, Lund, Sweden | National Hospital of Pediatrics in Hanoi, Vietnam |
| Hospital Universitario Niño Jesús, Madrid, Spain | Servicio de Oncología Pediátrica, Instituto Nacional de Cáncer in Asunción, Paraguay |
| | Departamento de Hemato-Oncología Pediátrica, Hospital de Clínicas San Lorenzo, Facultad de Medicina, Universidad Nacional de Asunción in Asunción, Paraguay |
| Vrije University Medical Center, Amsterdam, the Netherlands | Malawi—Queen Elizabeth Central Hospital, Blantyre |
| | Gadjah Mada University, Yogyakarta, Indonesia |
| French African Pediatric Oncology Group/Institut de Cancérologie Gustave Roussy in Villejuif, France | Algeria—Algiers, Oran |
| | Cameroon—Yaoundé |
| | Madagascar—Antananarivo |
| | Morocco—Rabat, Casablanca |
| | Senegal—Dakar |
| | Tunisia—Tunis |
| | Mali, Burkina Faso, Ivory Coast, Togo, Congo, Mauritania |
| San Gerardo Hospital, Monza, Italy | Nicaragua—Hospital Infantil Manual de Jesús Rivera "La Mascot," Managua |
| New Zealand Paediatric Oncology Group | Children's Haematology Oncology Centre, Christchurch Hospital, Christchurch |
| | Starship Children's Health, Aukland |
| | Pacific Island Workstream—Fiji, Samoa, Tonga, Vanuatu, Rarotonga |
| Tygerberg Children's Hospital, Stellenbosch University, Cape Town, South Africa | Windhoek Central Hospital in Windhoek, Namibia |

| | Cameroon—Banso Baptist Hospital, Northwest Province |
|---|---|
| | Mbingo Baptist Hospital, Northwest Province |
| | Mutengene Baptist Hospital, Southwest Province |
| Hospital de Pediatría Samic "JP Garrahan," Buenos Aires, Argentina | Hospital de Niños de La Paz, in La Paz, Bolivia |

from 10% to 60%, in the survival rates of children with ALL between 1994 and 1996.[9]

Improving diagnostic capacity is another key element of twinning. The INCTR "iPath" program is an Internet-based pathology and diagnostic support system currently used in many parts of Africa, including Kenya and Ethiopia, to improve diagnosis by training pathologists and technicians and providing Internet and hands-on consultation.[22]

In January 2012, the INCTR, USA, in collaboration with the Division of Pediatric Hematology Oncology, Blood and Marrow Transplantation Program, Lombardi Comprehensive Cancer Center, Georgetown University Hospital, Washington DC, signed an agreement with the Federal Ministry of Health, Ethiopia, Addis Ababa University Medical Faculty, and the Tikur Anbessa Specialized General Hospital (TASGH), Addis Ababa, to establish the first pediatric cancer program in Ethiopia.[22] As a result, there is now a dedicated pediatric cancer unit (PCU) for children, a fellowship program to train doctors in pediatric oncology is under way, training for nurses and pharmacists has been established, and morphine is available as part of palliative care.

Early successes in twinning indicate that it is an approach that will continue to be replicated throughout the resource-poor global community. Prospects for this expansion of twinning programs will no doubt be aided by the investment that St. Jude has made in its Cure4Kids platform. This vital educational tool allows its worldwide population of users to access a wealth of scholarship on pediatric cancer, as well as provides a space for interactive learning through its virtual classrooms. Similarly crucial is the creation of databases that allow for the collection and sharing of data from cancer centers in the developing world. St. Jude's Pediatric Oncology Networked Data system is one such system but not the only one. Making use of these types of tools will no doubt prove vital to the success of future initiatives that seek to establish substantial and sustainable improvements to care.

## Pediatric Cancer Units (PCU)

The twinning approach also encourages the development of dedicated PCUs to improve accessibility and cure rates.[21] A PCU represents the

**TABLE 12.2 Function of a Pediatric Cancer Unit (PCU)**

Function of a Pediatric Cancer Unit (PCU)
1. Increase capacity and expertise in pediatric cancer through training doctors, nurses, pharmacists, and other staff.
2. Standardize care through the introduction of low-cost, effective treatment protocols designed for LMICs.
3. Educate pharmacists and nurses in preparation and safe handling and delivery of chemotherapy.
4. Focus on infection control and management of treatment-related toxicity
5. Ensure all staff have a working knowledge of palliative care, especially pain management
6. Improve diagnostic capacity through support for pathology
7. Encourage multidisciplinary teamwork
8. As expertise improves, encourage academic activities, including research

assembly of dedicated resources and staff to coordinate inpatient and outpatient childhood cancer care. Not only are PCUs a physical space where children can get treatment, they also create opportunities for education and conduct of research, bringing together all specialists and ancillary personnel crucial for the successful management of these young patients (Table 12.2).

## Pediatric Oncology Research in LMICs

Many believe, incorrectly, that research cannot be conducted in LMICs. In fact, it is only through research that we can better understand the biology of different cancers in those countries, which clearly present differently and cannot necessarily be treated similar to HICs. Most progress in pediatric cancer treatment has been stimulated by research involving children in HICs. Since the susceptibility to and pathogenesis of cancer are heavily influenced by genetic background, environmental exposure, and lifestyle, we must extend this research to LMICs. The INCTR treatment protocol for Burkitt's lymphoma in Africa is an example—in addition to treatment, it includes specimen collection, iPath diagnosis, and data collection.[7] All training of medical personnel should include an introduction to research. Pediatric oncologists in training could benefit from short research electives in HICs.

## CONCLUSION

Unprecedented gains have been made in the cure rates for childhood cancer in HICs in the last 40 years. This progress reflects steady improvement in treatment protocols, a multidisciplinary approach to patient care, adequate hospital infrastructure, and psychosocial and economic support for affected families. As a result, almost 80% of these children are survivors today, who go on to live productive lives. The situation in LMICs is very different, with more than 60 percent of the world's children with cancer having little or no access to effective therapy or pain management and survival rates well below those in HICs. Efforts in the last decade through partnerships and twinning programs between academic institutions, cancer centers, nongovernmental organizations, private sector, and civil society in HICs and LMICs are slowly beginning to bear fruit. Much still needs to be done, but the first steps to improve survival have already been taken and the future looks brighter today.

## REFERENCES

1. Institute of Medicine (U.S.), Sloan FA, Gelband H. *Cancer control opportunities in low- and middle-income countries*. Washington, DC: National Academies Press, 2007.
2. St. Jude's, Five-Year Cancer Survival Rates—1962 vs. present, 2012. Available at http://www.stjude.org/stjude/v/index.jsp?vgnextoid=5b25e64c5b470110Vgn VCM1000001e0215acRCRD&vgnextchannel=4bbafe08dc835110VgnVCM 1000001e0215acRCRD.
3. Sullivan R, Kowalczyk JR, Agarwal B, et al. New policies to address the global burden of childhood cancers. *Lancet Oncol* 2013; 14: 125–35.
4. Kaatsch P. Epidemiology of childhood cancer. *Cancer Treat Rev* 2010; 36: 277–85.
5. Childhood Cancer Research Group, Survival from Childhood Cancer, Great Britain, 1971–2005. 2010. Available at http://www.ccrg.ox.ac.uk/datasets/sur vivalrates.shtml. Accessed August 26, 2013.
6. Masera G, Baez F, Biondi A, et al. North–South twinning in paediatric haemato-oncology: the La Mascota programme, Nicaragua. *Lancet* 1998; 352: 1923–26.
7. Scanlan T, Kaijage J. From Denis Burkitt to Dar es Salaam. What happened next in East Africa?—Tanzania's story. *Br J Haematol* 2012; 156: 704–8.
8. St. Judes' Children's Hospital, About International Outreach, 2013. Available at http://www.stjude.org/stjude/v/index.jsp?vgnextoid=2f166f9523e70110Vgn VCM1000001e0215acRCRD&vgnextchannel=e41e6fa0a9118010VgnVCM 1000000e2015acRCRD.
9. Wilimas JA, Ribeiro RC. Pediatric hematology-oncology outreach for developing countries. *Hematol Oncol Clin North Am* 2001; 15: 775–87.
10. Silbermann M, Arnaout M, Sayed HAR, et al. Pediatric palliative care in the Middle East. In: Knapp C, Madden V, Fowler-Kerry S (Eds). *Pediatric Palliative Care: Global Perspectives*. Netherlands: Springer, 2012, pp. 127–59.
11. Howard SC, Metzger ML, Wilimas JA, et al. Childhood cancer epidemiology in low-income countries. *Cancer* 2008; 112: 461–72.
12. Population Reference Bureau—2012 World Population Data Sheet.
13. A world fit for children. Millennium development goals. Special session on children. Documents and Convention on the Rights of the Child. New York, NY: UNICEF, 2002; 14: 16.

14. Haroun HM, Mahfouz MS, Elhaj AM. Patterns of childhood cancer in children admitted to the institute of nuclear medicine, molecular biology and oncology (inmo), wad medani, gezira state. *J Family Community Med* 2006; 13: 71–74.

15. http://www.childrenwithcancer.org.uk/incidence-of-childhood-cancerhttp://www.ccrg.ox.ac.uk/datasets/registrations.htm.

16. Pizzo P, Poplack D. *Principles and Practices of Pediatric Oncology*. 6th ed. Philadelphia: Lippincott Williams & Wilkins, 2010.

17. Barr RD, Kasili EG. Caring for children with cancer in the developing world. In: Pochedly C (Ed). *Neoplastic Diseases of Childhood*. Chur: Harwood Academic Publishers, 1994, pp. 1535–58.

18. Weitzman S. Complementary and alternative (CAM) dietary therapies for cancer. In: Barr RD (Ed). Nutrition and Cancer in Children. The Second International Workshop. *Pediatr Blood Cancer* 2008; 50: 494–97.

19. Lingwood RJ, Boyle P, Milburn A, et al. The challenge of cancer control in Africa. *Nat Rev Cancer* 2008; 8: 398–403.

20. Workman GM, Ribeiro RC, Rai SN, Pedrosa A, Workman DE, Pedrosa F. Pediatric cancer knowledge: assessment of knowledge of warning signs and symptoms for pediatric cancer among Brazilian community health workers. *J Cancer Educ* 2007; 22: 181–85.

21. St. Jude Children's Research Hospital. International Outreach Program: guide to establishing a Pediatric Oncology Twinning Program.

22. Shad A, Challinor J, Cohen ML. Paediatric oncology in Ethiopia: an INCTR-USA and Georgetown University Hospital twinning initiative with Tikur Anbessa Specialized Hospital. *Cancer Control* 2013; 1: 108–12.

23. Cancer Research UK. "Childhood Cancer Statistics." Available at http://cancerresearchuk.org/cancer-info/cancerstats/childhoodcancer. Accessed September 17, 2013.

24. Landier W, Leonard M, Ruccione KS. Children's Oncology Group's 2013 blueprint for research: nursing discipline. *Pediatr Blood Cancer* 2013; 60: 1031–36.

25. www.teenagecancertrust.org.

26. Freyer DR, Felgenhauer J, Perentesis J, COG Adolescent and Young Adult Oncology Discipline Committee. Children's Oncology Group's 2013 blueprint for research: adolescent and young adult oncology. *Pediatr Blood Cancer* 2013; 60: 1055–58.

27. Oeffinger KC, Nathan PC, Kremer LC. Challenges after curative treatment for childhood cancer and long-term follow up of survivors. *Pediatr Clin North Am* 2008; 55: 251–73.

28. COG Long-Term Follow-Up Guidelines for Survivors of Childhood, Adolescent, and Young Adult Cancers. Available at http://www.survivorshipguidelines.org.

29. Israëls T. *Aspects of the Management of Children with Cancer in Malawi*. Amsterdam: University of Amsterdam, 2010.

30. Knaul FM, Frenk J, Shulman L, for the Global task force on expanded access to cancer care and control in developing countries. Closing the cancer divide: a blueprint to expand access in low and middle income countries. Harvard Global Equity Initiative, Boston, MA, October 2011.

31. Foster TL, Lafond, DA, Reggio C, Hinds PS. Pediatric palliative care in childhood cancer nursing: from diagnosis to cure or end of life. *Semin Oncol Nurs* 2010; 26: 205–11.

32. Kinfu Y, Dal Poz MR, Mercer H, Evans D. The health worker shortage in Africa: Are enough physicians and nurses being trained? *Bull World Health Organ* 2009; 87: 225–30.

33. Ranson MK, Chopra M, Atkins S, Dal Poz MR, Bennett S. Priorities for research into human resources for health in low- and middle-income countries. *Bull World Health Organ* 2010; 88: 435–43.

34. Strother RM, Rao KV, Gregory KM, et al. The oncology pharmacy in cancer care delivery in a resource-constrained setting in western Kenya. *J Oncol Pharm Pract* 2012; 18: 406–16.

35. Arora RS, Pizer B, Eden T. Understanding refusal and abandonment in the treatment of childhood cancer. *Indian Pediatr* 2010; 47: 1005–10.

36. Knaul F, Anderson B, Bradley C, Kerr D. Access to cancer treatment in low-and middle-income countries—an essential part of global cancer control: CanTreat International.

37. Ben-Arye E, Visser A. The role of health care communication in the development of complementary and integrative medicine. *Patient Educ Couns* 2012; 89: 363–67.

38. Tulsky JA. Interventions to enhance communication among patients, providers, and families. *J Palliat Med* 2005; 8(Suppl 1): S95–S102.

39. www.icccpo.org.

40. Lemerle J. Traiter les cancers des enfants en Afrique. *Archives De Pédiatrie* 2003; 10: s247–49.

41. Day SW, Segovia L, Viveros P, Banfi A, Rivera GK, Ribeiro RC. Development of the Latin American Center for pediatric oncology nursing education. *Pediatr Blood Cancer* 2011; 56: 5–6.

42. Hesseling P, Israels T, Harif M, Chantada G, Molyneux E. Pediatric oncology in developing countries. Practical recommendations for the management of children with endemic Burkitt lymphoma (BL) in a resource limited setting. *Pediatr Blood Cancer* 2013; 60: 357–62.

43. Ribeiro RC, Steliarova-Foucher E, Magrath I, et al. Baseline status of paediatric oncology care in ten low-income or mid-income countries receiving My Child Matters support: a descriptive study. *Lancet Oncol* 2008; 9: 721–29. doi:10.1016/S1470-2045(08)70194-3.

44. Shad A, Ashraf MS, Hafeez H. Development of palliative-care services in a developing country: Pakistan. *J Pediatr Hematol Oncol* 2011 Apr; 33(Suppl 1): S62–S63.

# 13

# Adult Soft Tissue Sarcoma

## Aman Opneja, Rohit Gosain, Fred Okuku, and Kenneth D. Miller

## INTRODUCTION

Soft tissue sarcomas (STS) is a diverse group of tumors that account for approximately 1% of adult and 15% of pediatric malignancies.[1] The WHO has described more than 50 histological subtypes,[2] and variable interpretations of histology results make accurate estimate of incidence difficult. Various groups have studied the incidence of sarcoma in specific countries or regions, but consolidated data on global epidemiology is not available. In the United States, sarcomas are diagnosed in 10,600 patients per year, and approximately 4,000 patients die each year from STS.[3]

## GLOBAL SOFT TISSUE SARCOMA EPIDEMIOLOGY

Soft tissue sarcomas (STS) are rare tumors, and their incidence per 100,000 population in several countries is summarized in Table 13.1 (though the methodology in interpreting histology and in collecting these data precludes a complete comparison of the rates). Most histologic types of sarcoma are more common among men.[4]

In the United States the incidence of STS is at 1.4 per 100,000; however, after age 80, it rises to 8 per 100,000. As demonstrated in the SEER analysis, Kaposi's sarcoma (KS) has the highest incidence followed by undifferentiated sarcomas and leiomyosarcomas. RARECARE, in Europe, similarly reported that KS was the most common STS observed in the adult population.[10]

## STS ANATOMIC DISTRIBUTION

STS are most commonly found in limb or limb girdle, while the second most common site in the abdomen.[11] Anatomic distribution and common

TABLE 13.1  Global Incidence of
STS

| | |
|---|---|
| Europe (EU 27) | 5.6 |
| France | 6.4 |
| Austria | 2.4 |
| Japan | 2.5 |
| Switzerland | 6 |
| United States | 1.4 |
| Global | 0.6 |

TABLE 13.2  **Anatomic Distribution of STS**

| Site | Total Percentage | Most Common Histology |
|---|---|---|
| Lower extremity | 34 | Liposarcoma (28%) |
| Retroperitoneal | 15 | Liposarcoma (42%) |
| Visceral | 14 | Leiomyosarcoma (59%) |
| Upper extremity | 14 | Malignant fibrous histiocytoma (32%) |

*Source:* Anatomic distribution and site-specific histiotypes of 4,207 adult patients with soft-tissue sarcomas seen at the University of Texas MD Anderson Cancer Center, 1996 to 2003.

histologic subtypes are summarized in Table 13.2. Histopathology is correlated with the site of presentation and also the stage. More specifically, the percentage of patients presenting with local presentation of STS is more common than systemic or regional presentation.

## ETIOLOGY

Most of the STS have no clear etiology, but several predisposing factors have been described here and summarized in Table 13.3.

*Genetic syndromes:* In a prospective study performed on STS, 2.8% cases were associated with genetic syndromes,[12] including Li–Fraumeni syndrome, neurofibromatosis type 1, and hereditary retinoblastoma.

*Therapeutic radiation:* A small percentage of sarcomas are secondary to therapeutic radiation. Exposure of 1 Gy doubled the risk of soft tissue sarcoma.[13] In a study of women with breast cancer treated with radiation, a small subset developed angiosarcoma within the radiation field. Chronic lymphedema, after radical mastectomy for breast cancer (Stewart–Treves syndrome), or idiopathic or hereditary lymphedema has also been associated with cutaneous angiosarcoma. For other subtypes of sarcoma, the dose of radiotherapy was a predictor of the risk.[14] Survivors of retinoblastoma who underwent radiotherapy were also found to have an increased rate of sarcomas.[15]

*Viral infections:* Some viral infections in immunocompromised patients have been associated with the development of sarcomas. HHV-8 infection

**TABLE 13.3  Etiology of STS**

| Genetic | • Li-Fraumeni neurofibromatosis 1 |
|---|---|
| | • Retinoblastoma |
| Exposure | • Radiation |
| | • Chemicals |
| | ○ Phenoxyherbicides |
| | ○ Chlorophenols |
| | ○ Dioxin |
| Virus | • HHV-8 |
| | • EBV |

has been found to be associated with the development of KS[16] and EBV with a subset of leiomyosarcoma.[17]

*Chemical agents:* Exposure to chemical agents like phenoxyherbicides, chlorophenols, and dioxin has been thought to be associated with development of different types of sarcoma.

## KAPOSI'S SARCOMA: GLOBALLY, THE MOST COMMON STS

### Pathogenesis

Kaposi's sarcoma is the most common HIV-associated malignancy worldwide. KS has received great amount of attention when it was first recognized for its association with HIV/AIDS in 1981. Description of eight young men in New York City with previously rare cancer heralded the beginning of HIV epidemic. KS cells are endothelial in origin. In addition to proliferation of spindle cells that are latently infected with Kaposi's sarcoma herpesvirus (KSHV), tumors also are often characterized by an inflammatory infiltrate and leaky vasculature.[18] Infection with KSHV affects the host's vascular endothelial cells and upregulates lymphatic vessel endothelial factor and vascular growth factor receptor 3.[19] Like other herpesviruses, HHV-8 remains latent within cells and develops a variety of mechanisms to evade the host immune system. However, KSHV infection is necessary but insufficient cause of KS. The disease progresses or regresses based on the host immune system.

### Epidemiology

Before the AIDS epidemic, KS was regarded as extremely rare other than exceptionally high rates observed in the Mediterranean, mid-East, or eastern European descent, predominantly in males over age 50, and those residing in sub-Saharan Africa.[20] Table 13.4 depicts distribution of KS in Africa.

**TABLE 13.4  Estimated Number of Cases of KS in Africa**

|                     | Men | | Women | |
| --- | --- | --- | --- | --- |
|                     | Number | Rate per 100,000 | Number | Rate per 100,000 |
| Eastern Africa      | 16,000 | 14.9 | 9,000  | 6.8 |
| Western Africa      | 2,000  | 1.9  | 1,500  | 1.2 |
| Southern Africa     | 2,700  | 11.5 | 1,600  | 5.1 |
| Middle Africa       | 1,500  | 4.1  | 300    | 0.6 |
| Sub-Saharan Africa  | 22,000 | 8.1  | 12,000 | 3.6 |

*Source:* Global Cancer Statistics, reference 20.

Since the 1980s Kaposi's sarcoma has been a common cancer in Africa even before the era of HIV/AIDS. Central Africa is the most affected region. In sub-Saharan Africa, KS is most common cancer in males constituting 15.9% of all cancers. In females, it is third most common cancer constituting 6.2%.[21] In Africa, the highest rates of more than 6 per 1,000 are found in a broad strip across equatorial Africa, with particularly high rates in northeastern Zaire and in western Uganda and Tanzania.[22] In Uganda, the crude annual incidence rate per million for the country as a whole was 7.9 for both sexes combined.[23] Antiretroviral therapies (HAART) have caused a decline in the incidence of KS in Western countries. In the United States, the incidence of KS has declined over time due to advent of better treatment of HIV/AIDS as demonstrated in SEER data and depicted in Figure 13.1.[24] Incidence rates of classic KS in Europe were found to be markedly variable, with Sardinia[25] and Sicily[26] having the highest rate.

The four variants of KS that differ epidemiologically and clinically include classical, African which is endemically based, AIDS-associated epidemically based, and iatrogenic (or transplant-associated) KS. Different types of KS have different epidemiology and behavior, as detailed in Table 13.5.

The occurrence of KS reflects the seroprevalence of KSHV in the population, with KS more prevalent in areas with high KSHV seropositivity. Seroprevalence of HHV-8 virus among healthy adults in southern Europe, Africa, and the Middle East is between 30% and 100%, but is uncommon in U.S. population (5% blood donors). Classical KS occurs in elderly men of Mediterranean or eastern European descent, predominantly involving the skin of the lower extremities and occasionally involving mucosal and visceral prevalent areas of the body. Endemic KS also known as African type occurs in certain sub-Saharan African countries. This form is one of the aggressive forms involving skin, lower extremities, and sometimes lymph nodes. Epidemic KS, which refers to KS in HIV-infected individuals, tends to be aggressive, commonly involving the mucocutaneous and visceral areas such

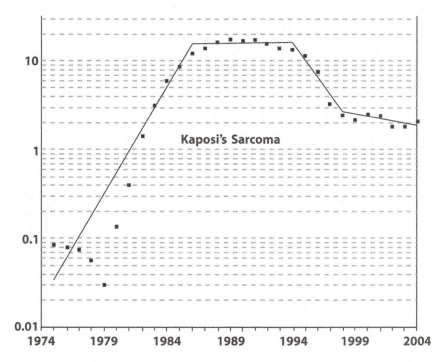

**FIGURE 13.1** Kaposi rate per 100,000 (SEER cancer statistics review).

**TABLE 13.5 Types of KS and Their Behavior**

| KS Type | Epidemiology | Behavior |
|---|---|---|
| Classical | Men 40 to 70 years | Indolent |
| | Mediterranean, Jewish | |
| African | Middle-aged adults | Progressive, aggressive |
| HIV | IVDA, HIV+ | Aggressive, Rxn to HAART |
| Iatrogenic | Therapeutic immunosuppressed | Variable, may regress |

as skin, gastrointestinal tract, and respiratory tract. In contrast to classical KS, lesions commonly involve the mucosal and visceral areas like, face (often the nose), genitalia, and oral cavity (palatal and gingival), in addition to the lower extremities.[27] Iatrogenic KS tends to be aggressive and occurs in individuals who are immunocompromised such as from organ transplantation or multiple comorbidities.

## Clinical Presentation

KS usually involves the skin and presents as lesions that enlarge from patches to plaques to nodules.[28,29] The highly vascular nature of KS can create a violaceous color, and then with hemosiderin deposition, lesions may change color from violaceous to brown.

In the African subtype of KS, significant leg edema can develop as well with skin ulceration, which is presumed to be secondary to obstruction of lymphatics. As described earlier, KSHV works on the host's vascular endothelial cells.

Kidney allograft recipients appear to be at higher risk for developing KS compared to other transplant recipients.[26] Of note, KS regressed in renal transplant patients with KS who were switched from cyclosporine to rapamycin (sirolimus) immunosuppression, and therefore, considering rapamycin (or one of its analogues) as an immunosuppressive choice is encouraged for transplant recipients with KS.[30,31] Interestingly, reduction of immunosuppression can lead to KS remission, highlighting the critical role played by the immune system in this infection. Similarly, epidemic KS often responds well to boosting of the immune response with HAART therapy.[29,32] The incidence of KS in HIV infection has decreased in developed countries since the introduction of HAART regimen, but the standardized incidence rate remains highest for KS compared to other cancers in HIV infection.[33,34]

Although KS can often be recognized by a trained observer, the diagnosis is confirmed by biopsy.[27,29] Early stages of KS can be more difficult to recognize. The skin manifestations of KS often resemble that from bacillary angiomatosis, which is caused by *Bartonella* species. Skin lesions of bacillary angiomatosis are more commonly vascular in nature and may mimic those caused by KS.[29]

### Treatment

At present there is no cure for KS. Surgical excision is restricted for cosmetically disturbing KS lesions, to alleviate discomfort or to control local tumor growth, but typically is not curative. Treatment goals of KS include symptom palliation, prevention of KS progression, improvement of cosmesis, and abatement of associated edema, organ compromise, and psychologic stress.[35]

A graduated approach to systemic therapy has been used in the treatment of KS. A common approach in the first line for treatment in HIV-positive patients who are symptomatic or have visceral disease is HAART (if not already initiated) to improve immune function and local therapy, which potentially includes surgery or radiation if the disease is localized or Interferon and pegylated-doxorubicin (Doxil) if the disease is systemic. For patients with disease progression, other cytotoxic drugs have been used either as single agents or in combination, including vinca-alkaloids, doxorubicin, bleomycin, and paclitaxel. Treatment is palliative, and newer approaches are being investigated including, angiogenesis inhibitors.

Optimal control of HIV infection, using antiretroviral therapy, is a key component in the treatment of AIDS-KS. HAART has greatly decreased the incidence of AIDS-KS dramatically in countries such as the United States, where HAART is widely available.[36] Yet despite the availability of HAART, risk of KS remains elevated in people infected with HIV, and KS is the second most common tumor in people with HIV/AIDS in the United States.[36] This decrease in incidence has not been reflected in sub-Saharan Africa[38,39] perhaps because of limited access of HAART therapy in sub-Saharan Africa.[40] However, the results should improve as HAART therapy is more readily available, and patients are more aware about the options available. This is reflected in one study from KwaZulu Natal, South Africa—where HAART therapy has become increasingly available, and as a result there has been decline in incidence of KS.[41-43] In sub-Saharan Africa, the burden of HIV and KSHV coinfection is high, and widespread access to HAART in some areas is still limited, surveillance programs for KS are lacking, and KS remains a growing public health problem.[36,37]

## SARCOMAS OF BONE

### Introduction

In the United States, among adults primary bone tumors are rare and account for 0.2% of all cancers, have an incidence of 0.8 per 100,000, and are more common in African Americans.[48,51] Approximately 2,500 new malignant sarcomas of bone are diagnosed each year in the United States, and in adults, chondrosarcoma, osteosarcoma, and Ewing's sarcoma are the most common.[44,48] Sarcoma can develop in any bone, but the femur is the most common site. Osteosarcoma is the most common though a rare primary sarcoma of bone. Despite the rarity, it accounts for 750 to 900 new cases in the United States annually and has a bimodal age distribution, with one peak of incidence seen in early adolescence and another peak observed in adults older than 65 years.[45-47] In adults it is sometimes associated with Paget's disease or other underlying disease process, whereas in childhood, it rather occurs sporadically.

The incidence of bone sarcomas in Europe is similar to that in the United States. A higher incidence of osteosarcoma has been observed in two African countries, Sudan and Uganda, compared with the United States and Europe. This is consistent with the finding of higher rate of osteosarcoma in individuals of African American descent.[52] Higher rates were also observed in males in Argentina and Brazil.[49]

Reports from other countries are as follows:

In the United Kingdom, between 1996 and 2000, an average of 427 new cases were diagnosed each year in England and Wales (National Institute

for Health and Clinical Excellence) 2006. In England, incidence of osteosarcoma under age 40 was highest in the age group 15 to 29.

In Finland, during 1991 to 2005 there were 144 cases of histologically
diagnosed osteosarcoma, constituting incidence of 1.8 new cases
per million.[50]

In Australia over a period of 25 years (1972 to 1996), 94 cases of sarcoma
were recorded.[53] In the age group 0 to 14 years, it was 2.5 per million per
year, for the age group 15 to 29 years, it was 4.5, and for the age group
30 to 39, it was 1.0.[54]

In the Philippines and Ecuador, higher rate of incidence was observed in
all age groups.[55]

Due to paucity of data, complete and accurate global data is not available on
bone sarcomas in general though data for osteosarcoma is better studied.

## Anatomic Distribution

Osteosarcoma generally occurs in areas around the knee. Of total osteosarcoma, 60% is found in this region, with maximum occurring in distal femur.
OS is found in areas of rapid bone growth and classically in long bones. This
finding is supported by the observation that there is an earlier peak of incidence of OS in adolescent girls and more common occurrence of tumor in
long bones.

## Etiology

For most OS, etiology is unknown though certain factors have been associated with an increased incidence of OS (Table 13.6). Various studies have reported increased incidence of OS after radiation exposure. OS usually occurs
on the edge of radiation field and is usually difficult to manage. Post radiation
therapy for breast cancer, bone sarcomas have been reported and OS is the
most common type.[56] Various studies reported different rate of occurrence of
OS, but in most of them an increased rate of OS was observed. Paget's disease

TABLE 13.6 Etiology of Osteosarcoma

| Exposure | Radiation |
|---|---|
| Preexisting disease | Paget's disease |
| Genetic factors | 1. Li–Fraumeni syndrome and p5 |
| | 2. Retinoblastoma |
| | 3. Werner syndrome |
| | 4. Bloom's syndrome |
| | 5. Rothmund–Thomson syndrome |

has been linked to the development of OS, but the occurrence is rare. Tumor arising in such circumstances has a poor prognosis.

## Pathogenesis

Osteosarcoma is a high-grade sarcoma, which consists of malignant osteoblast cells. It is a vascular tumor in which osteoblasts produce osteoid (immature bone) or woven bone; in addition, these tumors may demonstrate areas of fibrous tissue, cartilage, and bone differentiation. The tumor follows vascular Haversian and Volkmann canals in the cortex. This irregular growth and woven bone production replaces the cortex with the tumor bone. With this irregular growth, the periosteum is lifted and in response to that, it forms Codman's triangle.

Osteosarcoma is divided into two main categories—conventional and surface.[57] Conventional type accounts for majority of the cases. Surface osteosarcoma is divided into parosteal, periosteal, and high-grade surface.[58,59] On the other hand, conventional osteosarcoma is divided into osteoblastic, chondroblastic, fibroblastic, and other mixed types.

## Clinical Presentation

There is no specific clinical presentation of osteosarcoma. Most patients complain of localized pain in the affected bone, which may wax and wane over several months. The symptoms are often misinterpreted on initial presentations; this is to isolate other more common causes of bone pains. Usual site of osteosarcoma is the metaphysis of long bones, with the knee being the most common site. Other common sites are proximal humerus, and mild and proximal femur.[60]

Plain radiograph is the best diagnostic tool for diagnosing osteosarcoma. Some of the analogies used to describe the radiological findings of osteosarcoma are "fir-tree," "moth-eaten," or "sun-burst" appearance. The tumor spicules form a right angle, which is also known as Codman's triangle. There are no blood lab studies that help in diagnosing osteosarcoma, but it has been observed in large groups of patients that an elevated alkaline phosphatase and/or lactic dehydrogenase is associated with worse prognosis.[61–63] Osteosarcomas may either completely destroy the bone or replace it with blastic lesions. Osteosarcoma is usually large enough to destroy the cortex and further associate deep with soft tissue.

## Treatment

For low-grade bone sarcoma, treatment with surgery alone may be adequate if the risk of developing metastases is low, and overall 80% to 90% long-term survival can be expected.[66] Chemotherapy is often a major component of the management of patients with osteosarcoma because of the high risk of developing metastatic disease. Before effective chemotherapy, majority of the patients (80% to 90%) develop distant metastases and die of their disease despite achieving local disease control.[64] A common approach is neoadjuvant chemotherapy followed by surgery and then treatment with postoperative adjuvant chemotherapy that is informed by the response to the neoadjuvant therapy. Given this approach, 60% to 70% of patients without overt metastases at diagnosis are expected to be long-term survivors.[65]

## REFERENCES

1. Borden EC, Baker LH, Bell RS, et al. Soft tissue sarcomas of adults: state of the translational science. *Clin Cancer Res* 2003 Jun; 9(6):1941–56.
2. Fletcher CDM, Unni KK, Mertens F. *World Health Organization Classification of Tumors. Pathology and Genetics of Tumors of Soft Tissue and Bone.* Lyon: IARC Press, 2002.
3. Samuel Singer. Sarcoma. In: Townsend CM (Ed). *Sabiston Textbook of Surgery: The Biological Basis of Modern Surgical Practice.* 19th ed, Chapter 33. Philadelphia: Elsevier. Available at http://www.amazon.com/Sabiston-Textbook-Surgery-Biological-Surgical/dp/1437715605#reader_1437715605.
4. Morrison, BA. Soft tissue sarcomas of the extremities. *Proceedings* (Baylor University. Medical Center) 2003; 16(3): 285–90. Available at http://www.ncbi.nlm.nih.gov/pubmed/?term=Morrison%20BA%5Bauth%5D.
5. Stiller CA, Trama A, Serraino D, et al. Descriptive epidemiology of sarcoma in Europe: report from the RARECARE project. *Eur J Cancer* 2013 Feb; 49(3): 684–95.
6. Ducimetière F, Lurkin A, Ranchère-Vince D, et al. Incidence of sarcoma histotypes and molecular subtypes in a prospective epidemiological study with central pathology review and molecular testing. *PLoS One* 2011; 6(8): e20294.
7. Wibmer C, Leithner A, Zielonke N, Sperl M, Windhanger R. Increasing incidence rates of soft tissue sarcomas? A population-based epidemiologic study and literature review. *Ann Oncol* 2010; 21: 1106–11.
8. Nomura E, Ioka A, Tsukuma H. Incidence of soft tissue sarcoma focusing on gastrointestinal stromal sarcoma in Osaka, Japan, during 1978–2007. *Jpn J Clin Oncol* 2013; 43(8), 841–45.
9. Levi F, La Vecchia C, Randimbison L, Te VC. Descriptive epidemiology of soft tissue sarcomas in Vaud, Switzerland. *Eur J Cancer* 1999; 35: 1711–16.
10. RARECARE—Surveillance of Rare Cancers in Europe. Available at http://www.rarecare.eu/resources/RARECARE_WP_5_Report.pdfhttp://www.rarecare.eu/resources/RARECARE_WP_5_Report.pdf.
11. Clark MA, Fisher C, Judson I, Thomas JM. Soft tissue sarcoma in adults. *N Engl J Med* 2005 Aug 18; 353: 701.
12. Penel N, Grosjean J, Robin YM, Vanseymortier L, Clisant S, Adenis A. Frequency of certain established risk factors in soft tissue sarcomas in adults: a

prospective descriptive study of 658 cases. *Sarcoma* 2008; 2008:459386. doi:10.1155/2008/459386.

13. Samartzis D. Ionizing radiation exposure and the development of soft-tissue sarcomas in atomic-bomb survivors. *J Bone Joint Surg* 2013 Feb 6; 95(3): 222.

14. Karlsson P, Holmberg E, Samuelsson A, Johansson KA, Wallgren A. Soft tissue sarcoma after treatment for breast cancer—a Swedish population-based study. *Eur J Cancer* 1998 Dec; 34(13): 2068–75.

15. Cumber H. Risk of sarcoma increased in survivors of retinoblastoma. *Lancet Oncol* Feb 2007; 8(2): 104.

16. Raab-Traub N, Webster-Cyriaque J. Epstein-Barr virus infection and expression in oral lesions. *Oral Dis* 1997 May; 3(Suppl 1): S164–70.

17. Lee ES, Locker J, Nalesnik M, et al. The association of Epstein-Barr virus with smooth-muscle tumors occurring after organ transplantation. *N Engl J Med* 1995; 332: 19–25.

18. Uldrick TS, Whitby D. Update on KSHV epidemiology, Kaposi sarcoma pathogenesis, and treatment of Kaposi Sarcoma. *Cancer Lett* 2011; 305(2): 150–62. Available at http://ehis.ebscohost.com.ezproxy.welch.jhmi.edu/ehost /pdfviewer/pdfviewer?sid=76cdd671-c9f1-4eac-8a3b-986e66fa13e7%40 sessionmgr13&vid=1&hid=6http://ehis.ebscohost.com.ezproxy.welch.jhmi .edu/ehost/pdfviewer/pdfviewer?sid=76cdd671-c9f1-4eac-8a3b-986e66fa13e7% 40sessionmgr13&vid=1&hid=6.

19. Hong YK, Foreman K, Shin JW, et al. Lymphatic reprogramming of blood vascular endothelium by Kaposi sarcoma-associated herpesvirus. *Nat Genet* 2004; 36(7): 683–85.

20. Jemal A, Bray F, Center MM, Ferlay J, Ward E, Forman D. Global cancer statistics. *CA Cancer J Clin* 2011 Mar–Apr; 61(2): 69–90.

21. Jamison DT, Feachem RG, Makgoba MW, et al. *Disease and Mortality in Sub-Saharan Africa*. 2nd ed. Washington, DC: World Bank, 2006.

22. Cook-Mozaffari P, Newton R, Beral V, Burkitt DP. The geographical distribution of Kaposi's sarcoma and of lymphomas in Africa before the AIDS epidemic. *Br J Cancer* 1998 Dec; 78, 1521–28. doi:10.1038/bjc.1998.717.

23. Taylor JF, Smith PG, Bull D, Pike MC. Kaposi's sarcoma in Uganda: geographic and ethnic distribution. *Br J Cancer* 1972 Dec; 26: 483–97. doi:10.1038/bjc .1972.66.

24. Ries LAG, Eisner MP, Kosary CL, et al. (Eds). *SEER Cancer Statistics Review, 1975–2001*. Bethesda, MD: National Cancer Institute, 2004.

25. Cottoni F, De Marco R, Montesu MA. Classical Kaposi's sarcoma in north-east Sardinia: an overview from 1977 to 1991. *Br J Cancer* 1996; 73: 1132–33.

26. Iscovich J, Boffetta P, Franceschi S, Azizi E, Sarid R. Classic Kaposi sarcoma: epidemiology and risk factors. *Cancer* 2000; 88: 500–517.

27. Dezube BJ, Groopman JE. AIDS-related Kaposi's sarcoma: clinical features and treatment, 2003. Available at www.uptodate.com. Accessed November 12, 2003.

28. Habif TP. *Clinical Dermatology*. St. Louis: Mosby-Year Book, 1996.

29. Hengge UR, Ruzicka T, Tyring SK, et al. Update on Kaposi's sarcoma and other HHV8 associated diseases. Part 1: epidemiology, environmental predispositions, clinical manifestations, and therapy. *Lancet Infect Dis* 2002; 2: 281–92.

30. Sullivan RJ, Pantanowitz L, Casper C, Stebbing J, Dezube BJ. HIV/AIDS: epidemiology, pathophysiology, and treatment of Kaposi sarcoma-associated herpesvirus disease: Kaposi sarcoma, primary effusion lymphoma, and multicentric Castleman disease. *Clin Infect Dis* 2008; 47: 1209–15.

31. Stallone G, Schena A, Infante B, et al. Sirolimus for Kaposi's sarcoma in renal-transplant recipients. *N Engl J Med* 2005; 352: 1317–23.

32. Scadden DT. AIDS-related malignancies. *Annu Rev Med* 2003; 54: 285–303.

33. Patel P, Hanson DL, Sullivan PS, et al. Incidence of types of cancer among HIV-infected persons compared with the general population in the United States, 1992–2003. *Ann Intern Med* 2008; 148: 728–36.

34. Engels EA, Biggar RJ, Hall HI, et al. Cancer risk in people infected with human immunodeficiency virus in the United States. *Int J Cancer* 2008; 123: 187–94.

35. Di Lorenzo G, Konstantinopoulos PA, Pantanowitz L, Di Trolio R, De Placido S, Dezube BJ. Management of AIDS-related Kaposi's sarcoma. *Lancet Oncol* 2007; 8(2): 167–76.

36. Mbulaiteye SM, Katabira ET, Wabinga H, et al. Engels spectrum of cancers among HIV-infected persons in Africa: the Uganda AIDS–cancer registry match study. *Int J Cancer* 2006; 118: 985–90.

37. Mosam A, Carrara H, Shaik F, et al. Increasing incidence of Kaposi's sarcoma in black South Africans in KwaZulu-Natal, South Africa (1983–2006). *Int J STD AIDS* 2009; 20: 553–56.

38. Casper C. The increasing burden of HIV-associated malignancies in resource limited regions. *Ann Rev Med* 2011; 62: 157–70.

39. Goldman JD, Mutyaba I, Okuku F, et al. Measurement of the impact of antiretroviral therapy coverage on incidence of AIDS-defining malignancies in sub-Saharan Africa. Abstract. *Lancet* 2011 [published online March 14]. doi:10.1016/S0140–6736(11)60169–4.

40. Krown SE. Treatment strategies for Kaposi sarcoma in sub-Saharan Africa: challenges and opportunities. *Curr Opin Oncol* 2011 Sep; 23(5): 463–68.

41. Mosam A, Uldrick T, Shaik F, et al. Availability of highly active antiretroviral therapy improves the ability to treat Kaposi's sarcoma in South Africa. *Int J STD AIDS* (in press).

42. Mosam A, Shaik F, Uldrick TS, et al. The KAART Trial: a randomized controlled trial of HAART compared to the combination of HAART and chemotherapy in treatment-naïve patients with HIV-associated Kaposi sarcoma (HIV-KS) in KwaZulu-Natal (KSN) South Africa. 12th International Conference on Malignancies in AIDS and Other Acquired Immunodeficiencies (ICMAOI). Bethesda, MD, April 26–27, 2010. Abstract 09, page 39.

43. Mosam A, Shaik F, Uldrick T, et al. The KAART Trial: a randomised controlled trial of HAART compared to the combination of HAART and chemotherapy in treatment naive patients with HIV-associated Kaposi's sarcoma (HIV-KS) in KwaZulu-Natal (KZN), South Africa NCT 00380770. 17th Conference on Retroviruses and Opportunistic Infections, San Francisco, CA, 2010. Paper #32.

44. Landis S, Murray T, Bolden S, Wingo P. Cancer statistics, 1999. *CA Cancer J Clin* 1999; 49: 31.

45. Stiller CA, Bielack SS, Jundt G, Steliarova-Foucher E. Bone tumours in European children and adolescents, 1978–1997. Report from the Automated Childhood Cancer Information System project. *Eur J Cancer* 2006; 42(13): 2124.

46. Gurney JG, Swensen AR, Bulterys M. SEER Pediatric Monograph. Available at http://seer.cancer.gov/publications/childhood/bone.pdf. Accessed August 1, 2011.

47. Dahlin DC, Unni KK. Osteosarcoma of bone and its important recognizable varieties. *Am J Surg Pathol* 1977; 1(1): 61–72.

48. American Cancer Society website. What Are the Key Statistics about Bone Cancer? Available at www.cancer.org/Cancer/BoneCancer/DetailedGuide/bone-cancer-key-statistics. Accessed October 10, 2012.

49. Parkin DM, Whelan SL, Ferlay J, Raymond L, Young J. *Cancer Incidence in Five Continents.* Lyon: IARC Press, 1997.

50. Sampo M, Koivikko M, Taskinen M, et al. Incidence, epidemiology and treatment results of osteosarcoma in Finland—a nationwide population-based study. *Acta Oncol* Nov 2011;50(8): 1206–14. doi:10.3109/0284186X.2011.615339.

51. Mirabello L, Troisi RJ, Savage SA. Osteosarcoma incidence and survival rates from 1973 to 2004. *Cancer* 2009; 115: 1531–43. doi:10.1002/cncr.24121.

52. Mirabello L, Troisi RJ, Savage SA. International osteosarcoma incidence patterns in children and adolescents, middle ages and elderly persons. *Int J Cancer* 2009; 125(1): 229–34.

53. Blackwell JB, Threlfall TJ, McCaul KA. Primary malignant bone tumours in Western Australia, 1972–1996. *Pathology* 2005; 37(4): 278–83.

54. Rachel E, Feltbower RG, James PW, et al. Research article. The epidemiology of bone cancer in 0–39 year olds in northern England, 1981–2002. *BMC Cancer* 2010; 10: 357.

55. Beckingsale TB, Gerrand CG. Osteosarcoma. *Orthopaed Trauma* 2010; 24(5): 321–31.

56. Pendlebury SC, Bilous M, Langlands AO. Sarcomas following radiation therapy for breast cancer. A report of three cases and a review of the literature. *Int J Radiat Oncol Biol Phys* 1995; 31: 405–10.

57. Inwards CY, Unni KK. Classification and grading of bone sarcomas. *Hematol Oncol Clin North Am* 1995; 9(3): 545.

58. Schajowicz F, McGuire MH, Santini Araujo E, Muscolo DL, Gitelis S. Osteosarcomas arising on the surfaces of long bones. *J Bone Joint Surg Am* 1988; 70(4): 555.

59. Raymond AK. Surface osteosarcoma. *Clin Orthop Relat Res* 1991; 270: 140–48.

60. Meyers PA, Gorlick R. Osteosarcoma. *Pediatr Clin North Am* 1997; 44(4): 973.

61. Bacci G, Longhi A, Ferrari S, et al. Prognostic significance of serum alkaline phosphatase in osteosarcoma of the extremity treated with neoadjuvant chemotherapy: recent experience at Rizzoli Institute. *Oncol Rep* 2002; 9: 171.

62. Gorlick R, Anderson P, Andrulis I, et al. Biology of childhood osteogenic sarcoma and potential targets for therapeutic development: meeting summary. *Clin Cancer Res* 2003; 9: 5442.

63. Bacci G, Longhi A, Versari M, Mercuri M, Briccoli A, Picci P. Prognostic factors for osteosarcoma of the extremity treated with neoadjuvant chemotherapy: 15-year experience in 789 patients treated at a single institution. *Cancer* 2006; 106: 1154.

64. Bruland OS, Høifødt H, Saeter G, Smeland S, Fodstad O. Hematogenous micrometastases in osteosarcoma patients. *Clin Cancer Res* 2005; 11(13): 4666.

65. Bacci G, Ferrari S, Donati D, et al. Neoadjuvant chemotherapy for osteosarcoma of the extremity in patients in the fourth and fifth decade of life. *Oncol Rep* 1998; 5(5): 1259.

66. Cesari M, Alberghini M, Vanel D, et al. Periosteal osteosarcoma: a single-insti tution experience. *Cancer* 2011; 117(8): 1731–35.

# Part II

## Cancers by Country or Region

# 14

# Abu Dhabi and United Arab Emirates: An Overview of Breast Cancer

## *Rola Shaheen*

### INTRODUCTION

Cancer is the third leading cause of death in Abu Dhabi Emirate, with cardiovascular diseases and road accidents ranked as the first and second causes, respectively; however, breast cancer is the second leading cause of death in women following cardiovascular disease.[1] There is no doubt that breast cancer has gained a compound recognition over the past decade in the Middle East region and particularly in the United Arab Emirates (UAE). This chapter sheds some light on the current status of breast cancer management in Abu Dhabi and the UAE, with focus on efforts and initiatives committed to improve breast cancer care outcomes (i.e., reduce mortality rates). Challenges and barriers for early detection and treatment of breast cancer are revealed. A brief regional overview on breast cancer care is provided in an effort to describe realistic insight into relevant regional challenges and opportunities. Lessons learned on how to improve breast health care are mainly drawn from local experience and research in light of international benchmarks. The bottom line is that to date breast cancer remains a major unforeseen burden on health-care systems in the region, and without collaborative interventions with multi-stakeholders, women in the Middle East will continue to die from a disease that has a high cure rate in other parts of the world.

### BREAST CANCER STATUS IN ABU DHABI AND UNITED ARAB EMIRATES

The Emirate of Abu Dhabi is the federal capital of the UAE and the largest among the seven emirates in the UAE, with an estimated population of 2.1 million in 2009 out of a total population of 7.5 million in the UAE.[25] Abu

Dhabi extends over an area of 67,340 square kilometers, equivalent to 86.7% of the country's total area, excluding the islands.[2]

Approximately 21.9% are nationals and the rest are expatriates. The UAE has one of the most diverse populations in the Middle East. About one-fifth of the population is non-Emirati Arabs or Persians, and the majority of the population (about 50%) is from South Asia. The population of the UAE has a skewed gender distribution, with female to male ratio being 1:3. The average life expectancy is 78.24 years, higher than any other Arab country. Health-care insurance is mandatory for Abu Dhabi residents. Abu Dhabi has established strong collaboration with internationally recognized health-care providers with an aim to transfer knowledge and know-how to the local market. SEHA is Abu Dhabi's health services company founded to manage the public hospitals and clinics of the Emirate of Abu Dhabi. As part of the government of Abu Dhabi's health-care sector reform initiatives, SEHA overlooks eight health system facilities, including multiple ambulatory health clinics throughout Abu Dhabi. Ten breast screening clinics are under the umbrella of SEHA, with the majority of screening mammograms performed at Tawam Hospital, a leading tertiary center for oncology affiliated with John Hopkins Medical Centers.[3]

The Health Authority of Abu Dhabi (HAAD), the regulatory body of the health-care sector at the Emirate of Abu Dhabi, defines the strategy for the health system and monitors and analyzes the status of the population and the performance of the system.[4] In 2012 HAAD has rated the cancer prevention and control plan at the fourth rank in its public health priorities following cardiovascular diseases prevention and control, road safety, and tobacco control. The HAAD Comprehensive Cancer Control Plan includes prevention, early detection, diagnosis and treatment, and palliative care. Cancers given top priority are breast, colorectal, and cervical cancers. HAAD started by developing the breast cancer management standards, which was a collaborative effort in partnership with local and external experts to match best practices.[5] Specific standards for breast cancer screening and diagnosis, such as screening for high-risk cases, were also addressed, including genetic counseling.

Breast cancer is the most common cancer affecting women in the UAE and constitutes almost 20% of all cancer cases annually and 38% of all cancers in women.[6] Approximately 130 to 150 women (almost half of all UAE cancer cases) are newly diagnosed with breast cancer annually. Recent estimates were 26 new cases of breast cancer per 100,000 among women.[7] The highest incidence rate occurs in the age group 45 to 54. Of these breast cancer cases, 47.9% present with regional lymph node involvement, 27.5% present with localized tumors, and 9% present with distant metastasis. More women die from breast cancer (44%) than in other countries such as the United States or the United Kingdom (15% to 20%). Regardless of nationality, more than 64% of breast cancer cases from Abu Dhabi Emirate presented late had either regional extension of the breast cancer or metastasis to other organs. Breast cancer was common among Arabs, followed by nationals and least among Asians. Fifty percent of women diagnosed with breast cancer are below the age of 46 years, compared to 61 years in the United States. No difference is seen in the mean and median age at diagnosis between Emirati and those of other nationalities.[2]

More recent data from HAAD 2012[1] confirmed that breast cancer is the leading cancer in females in the UAE, accounting for 25% of all cancers and 44.7% of female cancer, and proved to be the second killer in women after cardiovascular diseases in Abu Dhabi.[8] Rigorous efforts and focused HAAD cancer control strategy in the past 5 years had resulted in increased number of visitors by over 50% to the breast cancer awareness governmental link "simply check," which increased the number of screening mammograms from 4,323 in 2007 to 15,749 in 2012. More important is the noticeable reduction in women with late-stage breast cancer from 64% in 2007 to 25% in 2011. The current practice in Abu Dhabi recommends biannual screening mammograms starting at the age of 40, with a mandatory requirement of double reading by qualified radiologists per HAAD and National Breast Screening Program (NBSP) guidelines.

A remarkable milestone in the process of developing health-care services in the UAE is the establishment of the NBSP in 1995, which is operated by the, a division of the health policy affairs sector at the Ministry of Health in the UAE.[9] The program's mission is to reduce mortality from breast cancer by delivering high-quality breast screening service to UAE women as part of the overall spectrum of women's health. The program has been accredited by the WHO and the Nottingham Breast Institute in the United Kingdom in 2005. A WHO assignment report prepared by Dr. Wilson along with data from the UAE cancer register identified breast cancer as a significant alarming problem in the UAE, particularly in the age group 40 to 50.[10] This alarming result was a pivotal finding, leading experts and policy makers in the UAE to recommend the screening mammograms for asymptomatic women at the age of 40 in the UAE. The cancer detection rate for women aged 40 and above was 6.3 per 1,000, with the highest cancer detection rate present in women aged 45 to 49 and in women aged 60 years and above. Another finding to reflect upon is the fact that the percentage of invasive cancers <10 mm in NBSP (25.5%) fulfill the international standards (>20%), yet that of invasive cancers free of lymph node metastasis (42.5%) does not meet the expected international standard rate of 70% or above. This may be attributed to the fact that the program detects small but more aggressive tumors. In 2006 Marraaoui et al. concluded through a retrospective study on breast cancer patients at Mafraq Hospital in Abu Dhabi (largest tertiary hospital in the UAE at the time) that breast cancer tends to occur in the younger age group with more aggressive biology and histopathology in the

UAE. The majority of breast cancer patients included in the study (62%) were premenopausal.[11]

The NBSP screening center in Abu Dhabi (Maternal and Child Health Care Center) is the referral regional screening center for the Emirates for double readings of screening mammograms, consultation, biopsy, and training. The program has the support of political leadership and has joint committee with federal and nongovernmental sectors from variable sectors and partners in the UAE to promote breast cancer awareness and in turn increase the number of target women for screening. The goal of the NBSP is to screen 70% of women aged 40 and above. A participation rate of 70% and over in trials was linked to substantial mortality reduction.[12] NBCP uniquely offers screening mammograms free of charge to all UAE resident women (UAE nationals and nonnationals). Currently in Abu Dhabi, the national health insurance companies cover screening mammograms for nationals but not for nonnationals. However, diagnostic mammogram or any workup for breast complaints including breast interventions and treatment is covered for both nationals and nonnationals with national health insurance from Abu Dhabi.

## INITIATIVES TO IMPROVE BREAST CANCER CARE IN ABU DHABI AND THE UAE

In Abu Dhabi HAAD took the lead to increase awareness about breast cancer among health-care providers and the public. HAAD conducted multiple workshops and Continuing Medical Education–accredited training sessions for health-care professionals working on breast cancer management in Abu Dhabi in 2012 to ensure that the developed standards are well understood and properly implemented. HAAD has collaborated at national level with both governmental and private sectors to improve the delivery of quality management of breast cancer. In November 2008 the Global Initiative in the UAE was launched as a collaborative initiative between HAAD and Susan G. Komen for the Cure Foundation. Twenty-two partner organizations across Abu Dhabi participated in 2008. A community profile report was issued in 2008, which presented a snapshot of the status of breast health and breast cancer in three communities in Abu Dhabi.[2]

HAAD has facilitated screening mammogram bookings through its user-friendly website (www.simplycheck.ae), where booking at 18 screening centers is possible. The website also provides interactive questions and answers from public with instant reply, donation for breast cancer, health educational material, and list of cancer support groups. The website also offers mobile phone awareness application, linked to online booking. HAAD's future direction is to ensure the implementation of breast cancer management standards through quality audits and to continue with the training for health-care professionals on any newly updated standards. SEHA supported the development of the multidisciplinary breast care clinic at Tawam Hospital in 2007.[13] The free-standing center is equipped with state-of-the-art screening and diagnostic equipment. A mobile breast screening unit is utilized to extend the outreach of mammography screening to remote communities in Abu Dhabi. SEHA's vision is to establish consolidated breast imaging services that will be standardized across all SEHA business entities armed with quality assurance program to absorb the increasing numbers of breast cancer patients and to provide treatment in a multidisciplinary fashion approach comparable to international best practices. In addition, since 2005 the NBSP has offered structured training to radiologists and radiographers and conducted mammography courses through collaboration with international experts from the United Kingdom and the United States.

Recently, the role of nongovernmental organizations has been emphasized in the UAE in raising breast cancer awareness; an example of an active society in the past decade is the Friends of Cancer Patients Society, a UAE registered charity that has continuously delivered moral, financial, and clinical support to over 850 patients and families who have been affected by cancer regardless of their nationality, gender, age, religion, and ethnicity with a primary focus on promoting awareness about early detectable cancers.[14] The society has many contributions and achievements, including the launching of the Pink Caravan campaign across the UAE to promote breast cancer screening and the Kashf program that promotes screening methods and prevention for the seven early detectable cancers including breast cancer.[15]

National insurance companies play a pivotal role in improving breast health care in the UAE. Daman is UAE's first specialized National Health Insurance Company established in 2005.[16] Daman has developed breast cancer support program since March 2011 with a team of case coordinators who ensure timely quality management of breast cancer patients.

## CHALLENGES AND BARRIERS TO EARLY DETECTION OF BREAST CANCER

Breast cancer has an overall good prognosis; however, it remains the leading cause of women's cancer mortality globally. The high survival rate from the disease in the United States is mainly attributed to early detection through breast cancer screening and the timely effective treatment.[17] Although strong strides have been made in the UAE toward reducing mortality from breast cancer in the past two decades, many challenges exist, including barriers to early detection of the disease. Major barriers that affect the utilization of breast health services, ranked in order of importance, are fear, lack of awareness, cultural barriers, ignorance and delay because of busy schedules, cost, and finally accessibility.[2]

An interesting study conducted in Abu Dhabi by Sabih and colleagues on barriers to early detection and treatment showed that women were generally unaware of the common risk factors for breast cancer regardless of nationality, age, and educational level, and they have poor screening practices.[18] One of the greatest barriers to mammography screening identified by women in this study was the social stigma that would impact their lives and their families. The authors concluded that the new information revealed by this qualitative study targeting women of different backgrounds in Abu Dhabi can be used as a guidance to design the awareness messages to focus on overcoming certain common barriers, such as decreasing fear and shame, discouraging the practice of cauterization and herbal preparations that can delay treatment, and finally emphasizing the role of older female peers in favor of breast screening. These barriers to early detection of breast cancer are not unique to Abu Dhabi or the UAE; in fact the low popularity of screening utilization is a regional cultural challenge in the Middle East, which needs to be addressed by creating awareness programs focusing on benefits of screening (i.e., early detection), and many women in the UAE believe mammograms cause cancer, which is a myth. A study on Gaza women by Shaheen et al.[19] concluded that participating Gaza women regardless of their residing places were not keen on having screening mammograms despite acknowledging that screening mammogram is a tool for early detection, thus having higher chance of curability. Interestingly enough, the majority of Gaza women were willing to have diagnostic workup when and if a breast complaint arises. It is intriguing that the Middle East region shares similar cultural barriers to early detection of breast cancer; however, the economic and resources barriers vary considerably from one country to another in the Middle East. Some countries in the region like the UAE and other Gulf countries have the financial resources and economic growth rates to build the infrastructure needed to serve the rising number of breast cancer patients, but they are still short of human resources and the expertise to provide the needed multidisciplinary breast care. Other countries in the region, such as Egypt, Jordan, and Lebanon, might be equipped with the skilled labor force but lack the financial resources to build the infrastructure necessary to absorb the demand of cancer patients. These varying needs call for regional cooperation to ensure that solutions are crafted to make optimal use of the variable-scattered available resources, in terms of both human capital and financial assets.[20]

In November 2009 in Boston, at a Harvard conference on breast cancer awareness in developing countries, a regional breakout session for the Middle East and North Africa region was conducted.[21] Recommendations from expert participants were meant to serve as a blueprint to collaboratively improve breast cancer care in the region. Research recommendations had focused on conducting a multi-central baseline needs assessment, that is, community profile including statistics and barriers to early detection of breast cancer treatment and development of a cancer registry. Educational recommendations included the following: (1) develop multidisciplinary health-care teams that provide local training and increase opportunity for international exchange, (2) reverse the brain drain, (3) utilize available resources to build on and move forward, (4) emphasize the crucial role and need for treatment and palliative care services along with establishing a screening program, (5) utilize media, public power of survivors, civil and religious leadership to increase awareness about breast cancer, and target all policy makers, women, men, and their health-care providers. The recommendations had also encouraged efforts on affiliations and partnerships locally and internationally. A need for developing quality assurance programs tailored to the local needs and barriers, yet meeting international guidelines, was emphasized. Adaption of Breast Health Global Initiative guidelines, which provide flexible framework that can address differences in resources in different countries, was also suggested.[22,23]

## CONCLUSION

Breast cancer is the most common cancer in women and the second leading cause of death in women in the UAE. The burden of breast cancer with the relatively high mortality rate has been recognized and prioritized by policy makers in the health-care sectors in the UAE. Serious efforts and organized strategic plans to improve breast health care in Abu Dhabi have been discussed. Major barriers to early detection and treatment of breast cancer exist in Abu Dhabi, most of which are cultural rather than economic. Drawing conclusions from internal research to shape the awareness messages to promote for early detection and enhance early treatment of breast cancer is an innovative smart strategy, which is most suitable for such a unique country like the UAE where over 202 nationalities live in harmony.[24]

## ACKNOWLEDGMENT

Dr. Mohamad Al Jaloudi (Tawam Hospital, UAE), Dr. Jalaa Taher (HAAD, UAE), Dr. Nehad Kazem (NBSP-MOH, UAE), Dr. Sawsan Madhi (Friends of Cancer Patients Society, UAE), Ms. Thikra Abdulla (Daman, UAE), and Ms. Sophia Michelen (Research Assistant, Boston USA).

## REFERENCES

1. United Arab Emirates. Health Authority Abu Dhabi. *Health Statistics 2011.* HAAD, October 2012. Available at www.haad.ae/statistics.

2. The Global Initiative for Breast Cancer Team—Abu Dhabi, Al Neyadi, Ghuwaya, and Walaa Khaled Sabih. *2008 Community Profile Summary of Findings.* Comp. Jalaa Taher. Susan G. Komen for the Cure Global Initiative for Breast Cancer Awareness, Emirate of Abu Dhabi, UAE, n.d. March–July 2008. Available at http://www.haad.ae/SimplyCheck/LinkClick.aspx?fileticket=RTg9flTx MPQ%3D&tabid=86.

3. Abu Dhabi Health Services Company (SEHA). N.p., n.d. Aug 1, 2013. Available at http://www.seha.ae/seha/en/Pages/WelcomeMessage.aspx.

4. Health Authority—Abu Dhabi. N.p., n.d. Aug 1, 2013. Available at http://www.haad.ae.

5. United Arab Emirates. Health Authority Abu Dhabi. *HAAD Standard for the Management of Breast Cancer.* Public Health and Policy, Non Communicable Diseases Section, Health Authority—Abu Dhabi, December 2011. Available at http://www.haad.ae/HAAD/LinkClick.aspx?fileticket=DlZAqNMBOdk%3D&tabid=820.

6. United Arab Emirates. Ministry of Health. Preventive Medicine Sector. *National Breast Screening Program—Annual Report 2006.* N.p.: n.p., n.d.

7. United Arab Emirates. Health Authority Abu Dhabi. Surveillance Section, HAAD. *Abu Dhabi Cancer Report, 2010 Internal Report.* N.p., n.d.

8. United Arab Emirates. Health Authority Abu Dhabi. *2008–2010 Health Authority Abu Dhabi Mortality Record.* N.p., n.d.

9. United Arab Emirates. UAE Ministry of Health. Central Department of Maternal and Child Health. *Review 1999–2006 on The National Breast Screening Program.* N.p., n.d.

10. *Review of Breast Cancer Screening, Abu Dhabi UAE.* Rep. WHO—EMRO, April 2005.

11. American Society of Clinical Oncology. ASCO Annual Meeting Proceedings (Post-Meeting Edition). *J Clin Oncol* 2006; 24: 18S. June 20 Supplement.

12. Tabar L, Fagerberg G, Duffy SE, Day NE, Gad A, Gröntoft O. Update of the two county program of mammographic screening for breast cancer radiologic clinics of North America. *Radiol Clin North Am* 1992, 30: 187–210.

13. Tawam Hospital. *Breast Care Centre.* Abu Dhabi: Tawam Hospital, n.d. Available at http://www.tawamhospital.ae/raceagainstcancer/breastCare/Breast%20Care%20Center%20english.pdf.

14. Friends of Cancer Patients Society (FOCP). N.p., January 2012. 01 Aug. 2013. Available at http://www.focp.ae/.

15. "Breast Cancer." *Pink Caravan.* PinkCaravan.AE, January 2013. 01 Aug. 2013. Available at http://www.pinkcaravan.ae/ar/awareness/breast-cancer/?lang=en.

16. "About Us." *About Us.* Daman, n.d. 01 Aug. 2013. Available at http://www.damanhealth.ae/eDamanApp/en/AboutDaman/DamanOverview/about_daman.html?version=R110.11.12.

17. Weir HK, Thun MJ, Hankey BF, et al. Annual report to the nation on the status of cancer, 1975—2000, featuring the uses of surveillance data for cancer prevention and control. *J Natl Cancer Inst* 2003; 95(17): 1276–99.

18. Sabih WK, Taher JA, El Jabari C, Hajat C, Adib SM, Harrison O. Barriers to breast cancer screening and treatment among women in Emirate of Abu Dhabi. *Ethn Dis* 2012; 22(2): 148–54.

19. Shaheen R, Slanetz PJ, Raza S, Rosen MP. Barriers and opportunities for early detection of breast cancer in Gaza women. *Breast* 2011; 20(Suppl 2): S30–S34.

20. Bitar ZA, El-Malak L. A Middle East Viewpoint: We've Got to Talk about . . . the C-Word—Prioritizing Cancer at a Time When It Is Not a Priority. Tech. Deloitte, March–April 2012. Available at http://www.deloitte.com/assets /Dcom-MiddleEast/Local%20Assets/Documents/Insights/ME%20PoV/ ME%20PoV%20Spring%202012/me_pov8_Cancer.pdf.

21. Breast Cancer in the Developing World: Meeting the Unforeseen Challenge to Women, Health and Equity Conference, Harvard University, Boston, MA. Harvard Global Equity Initiative, November 3–5, 2009. Available at http://isites .harvard.edu/icb/icb.do?keyword=k62597&tabgroupid=icb.tabgroup96975.

22. Anderson BO, Braun S, Carlson RW, et al. Overview of breast health care guidelines for countries with limited resources. *Breast J* 2003; 9: S42–S50.

23. Anderson BO, Cazap E, El Saghir NS, et al. Optimisation of breast cancer management in low-resource and middle resource countries: executive summary of the Breast Health Global Initiative consensus, 2010. *Lancet Oncol* 2011; 12(4): 387–98.

24. "202 Nationalities in Labour Market." August 25, 2006. *Khalej Times* (Dubai) n.d. Available at http://www.khaleejtimes.ae/DisplayArticleNew.asp?xfile=data/the uae/2006/August/theuae_August735.xml.

25. World Health Organization (Ed). *Noncommunicable Diseases Country Profiles 2011 WHO Global Report*. Rep. N.p., September 2011. Available at http:// www.who.int/nmh/publications/ncd_profiles2011/en/.

# 15

# Cancer in Argentina

## Eduardo Cazap

## MAGNITUDE OF THE PROBLEM

In Argentina, cancer is the main cause of mortality in the age group between 45 and 64 years and comprises more than 100,000 new cases and close to 60,000 deaths per year, which is equivalent to 145 per 100,000 individuals per year. Poverty and educational level strongly influence mortality rates.[1]

## CANCER INCIDENCE

The International Agency for Research on Cancer (IARC) has estimated that in 2008 Argentina had 104,859 new cases of malignant tumors (excluding those located in skin histology other than melanoma). This estimate gives, for both genders, an incidence of 206 new cases per year per 100,000 population. These estimates determine that, in relation to the rest of the world, Argentina has a medium-to-high cancer incidence. In magnitude, the larger volume of cases corresponds to breast cancer with more than 18,000 new cases per year (18% of total), followed by prostate cancer (13,000 cases, 13%). The incidence of cancer, considering all sites except skin non-melanoma, is higher in men. However, the incidence of breast cancer in women is higher than that of prostate cancer in men[2] (Figure 15.1).

## CANCER MORTALITY

The number of deaths from cancer has increased approximately 9% in the last decade because of population growth and aging. However, the cause of mortality was exactly the opposite; standardized mortality rate (SMR) for cancer has decreased from 118.82 cases per 100,000 inhabitants in 2001 to 107.49 cases per 100,000 inhabitants in 2011 (−10%).

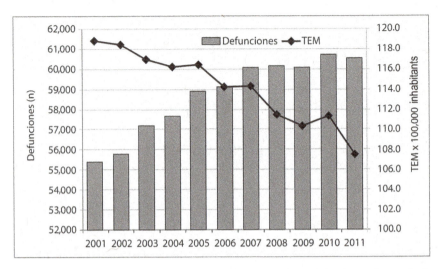

**FIGURE 15.1** Evolution of cancer mortality—number of deaths and standardized mortality rate (SMR) according to world population per 100,000 inhabitants, 2001–2011. (SIVER/INC according to DEIS database. Argentina, 2013.)

In 2011 about 58,000 men and women in Argentina died of cancer. The central region of the country, being the most populated, reported more than 70% of these deaths. Lung cancer occupies the first place in all regions. Next in order of frequency are colorectal cancer and breast cancer, except in the south and northwest where prostate cancer and stomach cancer occupy the third and fourth positions, respectively. Cervical cancer is ranked 10th in the country and is among the five leading causes of cancer death in the northeast region[3] (Figure 15.2).

## Mortality from Lung Cancer: Decreased in Men and Increased in Women

In Argentina mortality from lung cancer in men has declined since 1980 at a sustained rate of 1.3% annually. However, it increased in women—even at a steady pace—to nearly 2%. In this way, whereas in 1980 the gap between the genders was 37.7, in 2010 it decreased to 19.7 deaths per 100,000 individuals.[4]

## Mortality from Colorectal Cancer: Decreased in Women and Increased in Men

Colorectal cancer mortality decreased in women since 1980 at a sustained rate of 0.8% annually. However, in men this cancer mortality increased during the period 2002–2010 with an estimated annual change of 1%.[4]

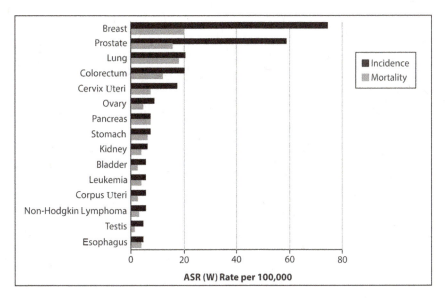

**FIGURE 15.2** Argentina: estimated age-standardized incidence and mortality rates: both sexes (Globocan 2008).

## Pediatric Cancer

According to the Argentine Oncology Pediatric Registry (ROHA), the annual incidence rate in Argentina is about 124 cases per million in children under 15 years. The cancers most frequently observed in the period 2000–2007 were leukemia (30% to 40%, about 470 cases annually), brain tumors (20%, about 240 cases annually), and lymphomas (13%). The chance of survival of these children in developed countries has been increasing to rates of 70%–80% because of early diagnosis, proper treatment, and comprehensive care. However, in Argentina the survival rate of children with cancer is around 65% because of various conditions, including loss of opportunity for proper diagnosis, lack of timely referral, treatment complications, and, in some cases, lack of comprehensive patient care.[5]

It is important to emphasize that all new cases of pediatric cancer are registered at the country level by ROHA. With respect to access to treatment, the best care is available in big cities (Buenos Aires, Cordoba, Santa Fe, and Mendoza). In several provinces or cities that lack pediatric oncology care, patients must be transferred to specialized centers in the main cities.

## NATIONAL CANCER INSTITUTE OF ARGENTINA (INC)

The National Cancer Institute of Argentina (INC) depends on the Ministry of Health (MoH). Created on September 9, 2010, by Presidential Decree 1286, it is responsible for the development and implementation of health policies and standards for the comprehensive care of cancer patients; the coordination of integrated prevention and cancer control actions; defining strategies for early detection, treatment, and rehabilitation; reducing risk factors; cancer research; and training professionals and establishing surveillance systems and epidemiological analysis. Thus, its main objective is to reduce cancer incidence and mortality in Argentina, as well as improve the quality of life of those affected by the disease.

The creation of the INC in Argentina was a decision of great significance in the health agenda of the government, and the primary reason was to promote cancer control at the policy level, with the coordination of all actions nationwide, according to the available resources, culturally adapted, and taking advantage of the existing resources of the health system of the country.

The main programs of INC are as follows: National Program for Cervical, Colon and Breast Cancers, together with a National Plan for Familiar and Hereditary Tumors, whose primary mission is "to improve the detection, management and prevention of high-risk groups in the Argentinean population," contributing to the development of a hereditary tumor registry and the national development of a comprehensive network of care. The pediatric area aims at improving the morbidity and mortality of children and adolescents with childhood cancer and their social rehabilitation after specific treatment, through equitable access to quality health care. The Palliative Care Program promotes continuous and integrated care for all cancer patients, with particular emphasis on reducing suffering and improving quality of life for patients and families. Getting pain relief and access to opioid medication is an effective reality for all patients in the country, removing barriers to access of drugs. The Tobacco Control Program's general objective is to promote scientific knowledge among policy makers for formulating public policies planned to protect people from the effects of tobacco and the exposure to smoke snuff.

In collaboration with the Departments of Cancer Research, Epidemiological Surveillance, Evaluation of Health Technologies, Communication, and Cancer Registries, the INC awards fellowships and conducts educational workshops.

INC maintains continuous collaboration with national, regional, and international organizations, such as the Pan American Health Organization, National Cancer Institute-US (NCI-US), IARC, International Atomic Energy Agency through the Program for Action for Cancer Therapy, and the Network of Latin-American Cancer Institutes.[6]

## HPV VACCINATION

In Argentina, human papillomavirus (HPV) vaccination was approved in 2006, but not included in the National Immunization Program (NIP). In 2008 a mass media campaign was carried out by a cancer nongovernmental organization, but it was stopped due to criticisms about the publicity. In October 2011 the MoH introduced HPV vaccination in the NIP. It is mandatory and free to all girls aged 11 years, and according to data from the NIP, the compliance to the vaccine is currently over 90%.[7]

## HEALTH SYSTEM

Argentina's health system is financed by three sectors: public health, social security, and private insurance. A fourth subsystem, known as the National Institute of Social Security and Retirement Fund (INSSJP-PAMI), specifically covers retirees, similar to Medicare in the United States. Although this matrix structure is intended to provide universal coverage, its multiple independent systems lack vertical and horizontal integration, resulting in inadequate coverage for many. In the social security and private systems, health care can be contracted from different sources, some of which own their health-care facilities. In the public sector, financing is provided by the provincial or municipal government. The national government has an oversight role, including specific programs to reduce provincial differences. Financing of the public system comes from national and provincial taxes, and coverage is open to all; however, it is mainly used by people who lack any other type of health coverage. Employers must provide health insurance for all workers. In addition, social insurance is mandatory for all government employees and is usually provided by workers' unions. This insurance is funded by employers' contributions and can include copayments. The system includes the National and Provincial Social Security and the INSSJP-PAMI. By contrast, the private system consists of direct contributions and prepayments to medical companies. Both the social security system and the private insurance are regulated by the superintendent of Health Services, reporting to the MoH, and by the Compulsory Medical Program. Any resident of Argentina has, according to the law, the right to medical care for catastrophic diseases, including cancer. Funding sources for cancer differ according to the health sector responsible for the patient. If a patient does not have private or social security insurance, the patient's province must cover costs. The national government also has resources to provide coverage for patients, including nonresidents. High-cost medications and treatments are covered by a special fund as part of the Special Programs Administration, supported by the superintendent of Health Services.[8]

## COSTS AND FINANCING OF THE HEALTH SECTOR

In 2007, the total health expenditures in Argentina were estimated at 10% of gross domestic product (GDP), which represented a per capita expenditure of approximately US$663. The largest external funding comes from loans for projects funded by the Inter-American Development Bank and the World Bank.[9] It is important to mention that cancer costs are included in the total budget of the different subsystems, making it very difficult to know the real costs of cancer treatment in the country.

## CONCLUSION

Cancer is a public health problem in Argentina, influenced by poverty and educational levels, and is the main cause of mortality in the age group between 45 and 64 years. Breast, prostate, colorectal, and lung cancers are the most relevant cancers in the country, whereas cervical cancer has high incidence in the poorest provinces, usually in the northeast part of Argentina. Pediatric cancers are fully covered by a National Pediatric Cancer registry (ROHA). The INC was created in 2010. HPV vaccination is mandatory since 2011 through the NIP. Argentina's health system is financed by public health, social security, and private insurance sectors, and a subsystem, known as the National Institute of Social Security and Retirement Fund (INSSJP-PAMI), specifically covers individuals aged 65 years and older, younger people with disabilities, and war veterans. The system is fragmented and many persons have double or even triple affiliations. The specific costs for cancer care are unknown.

## ACKNOWLEDGMENT

The author would like to thank Dr. Roberto Pradier, director general, INC, Dr. Maria Viniegra, technical coordinator, INC, and Dr. Maria Graciela Abriata, coordinator of Cancer Epidemiology and Surveillance, INC, for their helpful comments on earlier drafts of the manuscript.

## REFERENCES

1. http://www.msal.gov.ar/inc/index.php/acerca-del-cancer/estadisticas.
2. http://globocan.iarc.fr.
3. Abriata MG. Análisis de Situación en Salud—ASIS-Cáncer en Argentina, 2011 (in press).
4. http://www.baires-salud.com.ar/institucional-23/radiografia-actual-del-cancer-en-argentina-4538.html.
5. http://www.msal.gov.ar/inc/index.php/investigacion-y-epidemiologia/registro-/roha.
6. http://www.msal.gov.ar/inc/.

7. Arrossi S, Maceira V, Paolino M, Sankaranarayanan R. Acceptability and uptake of HPV vaccine in Argentina before its inclusion in the immunization program: a population-based survey. *Vaccine* 2012 Mar 23; 30(14): 2467–74.
8. Goss PE, Lee BL, Badovinac-Crnjevic T, et al. Planning cancer control in Latin America and the Caribbean. *Lancet Oncol* 2013 Apr; 14(5): 391–436.
9. Report of World Health Statistics, World Health Organization (WHO), 2010.

# 16

# Bhutan

## Tashi Dendup Wangdi

Bhutan is located on the southern slopes of the eastern Himalayas. With a land size of 38,394 km$^2$, it is roughly the size of Switzerland and people are predominantly Buddhists. Bhutan has a total population of 708,265 per the 2011 National Population and Census Report. Besides Buddhism, the other religions most common are Hinduism and Christianity. The birth rate is stated to be 19.7 per 1,000 people, and life expectancy for males is 66 years and for females 66.2 years. The infant mortality rate is only 102.56 per 1,000 live births. The sanitation coverage is 62% and the piped water coverage is almost 90%. Bhutan still has an acute shortage of medical personnel, with the ratio being 3 doctors per 10,000 people. The gross domestic product (GDP) at current market price is 85,580.6, but the government, under the visionary leadership of the fourth Druk Gyalpo, has developed a philosophy based on gross national happiness rather than GDP. The idea is that socioeconomic development based on happiness principles is more realistic than that based on monetary indicators. Bhutan is basically an agrarian-based economy, with more than 80% of the population dependent on agriculture for livelihood. At the moment, the engine fuelling economic growth is green energy or hydropower, as Bhutan is blessed with an abundance of rivers running down the glacier-fed streams and rivulets into the wide valleys. Bhutan transited into a democratic constitutional monarchy, holding its first ever general election in 2008.

Despite the availability of basic health services throughout the country, a delay in the diagnosis and treatment of patients with cancer still exists, which leads to detrimental effects. This delay is probably due to certain deep-seated beliefs, where some patients take the opinion of local healers and astrologers, and the initial period is spent taking recourse to these alternative therapies. Moreover, time is also lost sometimes performing rituals, which are also deeply grounded in the culture. Over the years, this scenario has changed to some extent, because of the initiatives taken by the government to integrate the local healers and educate them about the necessity of early referral, as they may still serve as the initial point of contact for patients in remote villages. Though health-care centers across the country are easily accessible, the majority of cancers are still diagnosed at advanced stages because of reasons such as late presentation, ignorance of patients, and lack of education of the health workers to detect the early signs and symptoms of cancers.

Reviewing the journey of modern health services in Bhutan, it should be mentioned that the first 20-bedded hospital was completed in 1956 in Thimphu. By 1961 there were still just two hospitals: the Thimphu hospital with 20 beds and the Samtse hospital with 10 beds, along with 11 dispensaries. By 2008, however, Bhutan had 29 hospitals and 176 basic health units, along with 485 outreach clinics. With 1,078 hospital beds in 2011, there are now 31 hospitals, 181 basic health units, and 38 dispensaries. As per the current statistics, there are 187 doctors and 556 nurses, 2.7 doctors per 10,000 persons, and 587 persons per hospital bed. Access to safe drinking water is 90%. Currently, two modern referral hospitals exist: the 150-bedded Eastern Referral Hospital in Mongar located at the east of the country and the 350-bedded Apex Referral Hospital in Thimphu, the capital city of Bhutan.

## CANCER STATISTICS

Until 2008, no reliable data was available for cancer incidence in Bhutan. Even Globocan did not have any realistic cancer information from Bhutan, and the cancer figures related to Bhutan in Globocan were derived from the averages of the neighboring countries. The interesting point was that breast cancer was reflected as the most common cancer among women, whereas in reality, cervical cancer was the most common one. For quite some time, it was indeed difficult to obtain authentic medical statistics, as the hospitals had no proper medical record system in place. Though it made access to health care easy, as there was no requirement for any identification while availing health care in the country, it was an impediment to generating authentic medical statistics. Thus, it was a common practice for patients to be admitted in the hospitals with different names at different times with different addresses and different diagnoses. It was only from 1995 that a computerized, unique numbering system for inpatients was established in the National Referral Hospital at Thimphu. Once a patient got admitted, it was easy to retrieve prior information for subsequent admissions, and the same number was reflected in subsequent admissions. This system helped prevent double reporting of cases and made the data collection more reliable than in the past. Moreover, from 2005, an International Classification of Diseases–based system for coding of diseases was introduced at the National Referral Hospital at Thimphu, which made it easier for data collection and interpretation. Hence, in 2008, a corrected version of the data was published in the Globocan after Dr. Hai Rim Shin of the International Agency for Research on Cancer (IARC) and I completed a detailed screening of the data. Data presented in Figures 16.1–16.4 was the data prior to the corrections in the Globocan directory.

Stomach cancer is the most common malignancy in Bhutan, and a study on the dietary risk factors leading to gastric cancer is currently in process. Recently a *Helicobacter pylori* incidence study at the National Referral Hospital in Thimphu was concluded, and it revealed an infection rate of almost 80%. Therefore, it seems probable that the high incidence of *H. pylori* in the Bhutanese population plays a role in the development of gastric cancer, in addition to other dietary factors, such as lack of consumption of fresh fruits and vegetables and intake of salty food. Stomach cancer has thus surfaced

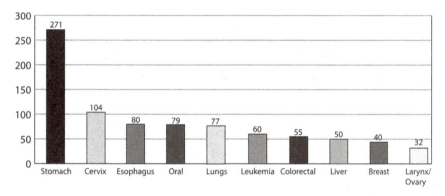

**FIGURE 16.1** Top 10 cancers in Bhutan (June 2006–April 2009) (Medical Records, JDW/NRH).

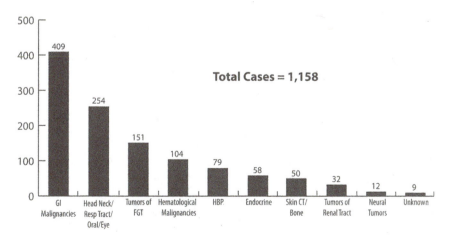

**FIGURE 16.2** Total number of cancer patients reported at JDW/NRH (June 2006–April 2009) (Medical Records, JDW/NRH).

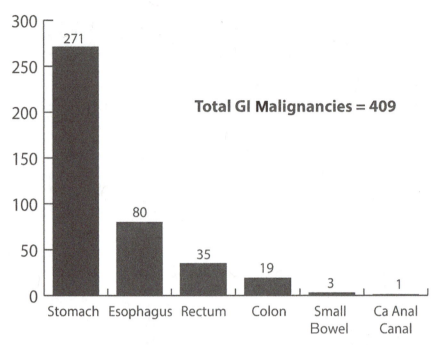

**FIGURE 16.3** Types of gastrointestinal cancers reported at JDW/NRH (June 2006–April 2009) (Medical Records, JDW/NRH).

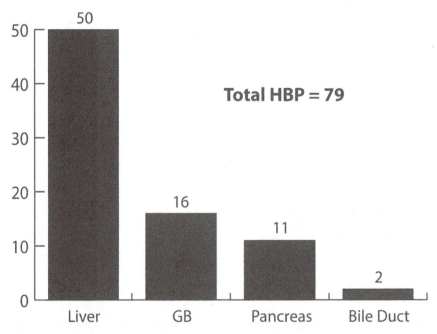

**FIGURE 16.4** Hepatobiliary malignancies (June 2006–April 2009) (Medical Records, JDW/NRH).

as one of the most lethal cancers in Bhutan, as the mortality is the highest, among all types of cancer. The second most common gastrointestinal malignancy is esophageal cancer with squamous cell histology. This cancer is also mostly related to behavior and lifestyle, caused by the consumption of betel nut and tobacco, alcohol usage, and the absence of protective factors in the diet. The third cancer commonly encountered is oral cancer, with betel nut, tobacco, and alcohol being the predisposing agents. In women, however, cervical cancer is the most common cancer, and poor socioeconomic conditions including poor hygiene, repeated child birth, common prevalence of sexually transmitted disease, and now recently human papillomavirus (HPV) infection are the contributing factors. Breast cancers among the women are also on the rise. Although the numbers are not alarming at present, almost 99% of the breast cancers detected are either locally advanced on presentation or diagnosed with distant metastasis. The most common hepatobiliary malignancies are hepatomas, diagnosed in hepatitis B–positive patients where the malignancies have actually developed in a background of chronic hepatitis. The prevalence of hepatitis B in Bhutan is higher than that estimated earlier. Interestingly, lung cancer, which is a global epidemic, is relatively low in Bhutan, and the common histology encountered is adenocarcinoma, which occurs in nonsmokers. With the legislation of ban on tobacco sales firmly in place, along with the religious teachings that discourage smoking, Bhutan is well positioned in preventing smoking-related deaths in decades to come. Colorectal malignancies are encountered sporadically and have not been a major problem in Bhutan; however, in the near future with the changing lifestyle and dietary habits, it could become a common cancer too, like in the West. Bhutan is actually at the crossroads where the health system is grappling with the burden of cancers because of infection and poor sanitation, as encountered in the developing countries; however, at the same time due to an era of modern development, Bhutan could see cancers in the near future, which are more common in the developed world, like colorectal and breast malignancies.

## MANAGEMENT

Bhutan has only one trained surgical and gynecologist oncologist and does not have a medical oncologist or a radiation oncologist. All cancer cases are worked up at the National Referral Hospital where adequate staging and treatment take place. Here, only surgery and chemotherapy can be offered as a treatment modality for cancer patients. Because Bhutan does not have a radiotherapy center, all patients requiring radiation are sent to Kolkata, a city in West Bengal, India, at the government's expenses. Some hesitancy is seen inpatients when they have to go to India for radiotherapy, probably because of the distance involved in travel and having to cope with a different culture. Referral of cancer cases for advanced treatment to India has a major cost implication to the government, but this referral practice would continue for several decades due to the acute shortage of trained and skilled manpower in health services. Earlier, the practice of administering chemotherapy was not uniform, because there were no guidelines, trained staff, or a designated area where patients received chemotherapy. Patients with cancer would be all over the hospital, receiving chemotherapy from nursing staff who are not trained to mix and deliver chemotherapy. Recognizing the special needs for cancer patients, in 2012 the National Referral Hospital opened an oncology unit run by trained oncological nurses for delivering chemotherapy to cancer patients. Since establishing the oncology unit, pharmacy technicians have also been trained to mix the drugs in a biological safety cabinet, therefore preventing exposure from the chemotherapy drugs and improving the safety of the staff who work in the oncology unit. This procedure has improved the overall quality of care to the patients undergoing chemotherapy, bringing satisfaction to both the patients and their caregivers. The majority of cancer surgeries are performed at the National Referral Hospital. Almost 90% cancer patients are diagnosed very late due to either ignorance on the part of the patient or lack of knowledge of the health workers, not recognizing the subtle signs and symptoms some cancer patients present at their health center. Occasionally, cancer patients may receive treatment early on from traditional healers or may resort to faith healing by religious practitioners. This late presentation results in a very high mortality from cancers in Bhutan, and the common belief is that once an individual gets cancer, he or she will certainly die. This opinion about cancer needs to change, but early diagnosis and prevention programs are the only ways to convince people that most cancers are curable if detected early and that a significant number of cancers can also be prevented. Due to the high number of advanced cancer patients, it would be beneficial to have a palliative care unit, where the needs of the terminally ill patients and their caregivers can be served. The majority of the doctors and nurses working in the National Referral Hospital have no exposure in palliative care, and due to the shortage of the health staff, adequate time cannot be given to the cancer patients and their caregivers to address their concerns. Most of the terminally ill patients are admitted to the hospital in the final stages of their illness, as their caregivers believe that their beloved ones would receive better care at the hospital. This practice has resulted in hospital beds being occupied for varying lengths of time by terminal ill patients, and in a setting where nurses are not yet trained on palliative care or end-of-life care issues. For this practice to change, establishing a palliative care unit would address these concerns.

Though morphine availability has been regulated in the past few years, acquiring long-acting morphine tablets has been difficult, and frequency of dosing, due to the short-acting morphine, still remains a problem. In Bhutan, there have been no reliable statistics on cancer incidences, and the National Referral Hospital in Thimphu was the only source of information. Even the National Referral Hospital data was not reliable, due to patients being admitted several times with different names and showing different admissions, as no single unique number was used for patient registration.

In 2008, a workshop on cancer registry was held in Thimphu, where the importance of having a cancer registry was emphasized. The data from the National Referral Hospital was scrutinized, and after proper screening of data with the help of the IARC staff, credible cancer data for the first time was published in Globocan 2008. From the data, it was found out that gastrointestinal malignancies were number one, followed by cervical and head and neck malignancies. This reflects a strong dietary and infectious etiology to the causes of malignancies in Bhutan. This situation is probably related to the socioeconomic status, such as poor hygiene, water, and sanitation, where bacteria such as *H. pylori* and viruses like HPV thrive.

Despite the challenges, the government has been making consistent efforts in cancer control, such as the cervical cancer screening program, with both PAP smear and visual inspection with acetic acid application technique. Bhutan became the first developing country to roll out a national vaccination program against HPV, along with introduction of the free nationwide HPV vaccine in May 2010, targeting girls between 12 and 18 years of age. Hepatitis B vaccination was also introduced in 1997 and administered to all newborns as part of the immunization schedule. To win a major battle against cancer, the legislation enacted the Tobacco Control Act of Bhutan 2010, banning the cultivation, harvesting, production, and sale of tobacco and tobacco-related products. Compared to other countries, it was easier to introduce this bill, as the national religion supported the antitobacco drive and was against the use of any form of tobacco products. Moreover, Bhutan did not manufacture any tobacco-related products in the past, so there were no industries to close. Although this has already resulted in less exposure to smoking among younger generations, the long-term benefit of this antitobacco law would be only seen several decades later.

## REFERENCES

1. Annual Health Bulletin 2012, Ministry of Health, Royal Government of Bhutan.
2. Bhutan at a Glance 2012, National Statistics Bureau, October 2012.
3. Wangdi TD. Gastric cancer prevalence, a preliminary study according to the cancer registry data at the Jigme Dorji Wangchuck National Referral Hospital, Thimphu, Bhutan, Cancer Registry Unit JDWNRH2011.
4. Lepcha P. Jigme Dorji Wangchuck National Referral Hospital Medical Record Data Base, 2010.

# 17

# Cancer Care in Canada

## Rahul Gosain, Amitoj S. Gill, and Kenneth D. Miller

## CANCER IN CANADA

### Cancer Statistics

A steady rise in cancer incidence can be attributed to better screening measures over the years. The Canadian Cancer Statistics published by the Public Health Agency of Canada estimated the incidence of cancer to be 187,600 and the mortality associated with cancer to be 75,500 in 2013. With increasing incidence, the statisticians report that about two in five Canadians will develop cancer in their lifetime and approximately one in four Canadians will die of cancer.[1]

It is estimated that there are 1 million Canadians diagnosed with cancer in the past 15 years. This translates into $22.5 billion burden to the economy in 2009 itself, with a direct cost of $6 billion for hospitalizations and treatments for cancer patients. Cancer charities alone accounted for $1.9 billion directed toward research on early detection, prevention, and treatment of cancer. Looking at the current trends in 2005, it was estimated that $1.17 trillion would go toward cancer in the next 30 years in Canada alone. The biggest cost of cancer, however, is that of human life. When calculated on the potential years of life lost scale, it is approximated that the average Canadian with diagnosis of cancer dies more than 15 potential years of life lost. Along with this, the families of patients provide caregiving time and medical expenses out of their own pockets.

### History of Cancer in Canada

Canada's first cancer committee "Canadian Cancer Society" was officially formed in 1938 to educate Canadians about the early warning signs of cancer.

In 2012, the committee included 140,000 volunteers around the nation and 1,200 full-time staff with the goal of eradicating cancer and enhancing the quality of life for people living with cancer.[2]

In recent years, efforts by Statistics Canada (SC) have provided large data to study cancer patterns and trends in Canada. The Canadian Cancer Registry (CCR) is an administrative survey maintained by SC that collects information about cancer incidence and survival in Canada. CCR was adopted in 1992 from National Cancer Incidence Reporting System, which was established in 1969. The data collected by CCR is used to identify risk factors for the cancer, monitor and evaluate broad range of cancer control programs, and conduct research in health services.[3]

## The Workforce of Oncologists in Canada

Cancer has been one of the leading causes of death in Canada for decades. Radiation and medical oncologists have largely carried out its nonsurgical management in recent years, taking the responsibility over from primary-care physicians.

In 2012, 450 medical oncologists were practicing in Canada. A total of 59% of practicing medical oncologists are men and 41% are women. Over half of medical oncologists (60%) work in an academic health sciences center, 35% work in a university, 20% work in community hospitals, and only 6% are in private settings. Medical oncologists work on an average of 58 hours per week (excluding overnight on-call).[4] Oncologists reported seeing an average of 66 patients a week.

With increase in cancer incidence, the need of medical oncologists remains high; however, with limited funding, securing a position remains a concern for newly trained medical oncologists. Provincial governments have paid millions of dollars to train more specialists to expand services and reduce patient delays, but hospitals and health regions often lack the money to hire specialists. Medical oncologists are not alone to face this bizarre conundrum in Canadian health job market. Given these circumstances, many specialists trained in Canada explore job opportunities around the world, with their main hub being the United States.[5]

## Cancer Trends in Canada

The most prevalent cancers continue to be of lung, breast, colorectal, and prostate origin (Tables 17.1 and 17.2). Prostate cancer accounts for the largest number of newly diagnosed cases.[1] However, compared to lung, colorectal, and breast cancers, prostate cancer causes the fewest deaths. Lung cancer is the most common cause of cancer death, causing more cancer deaths among

**TABLE 17.1  Percent Distribution of Top 10 Types of Cancer in Canadian Men**[1]

| Cancer Type | Estimated Percentage of New Cancer Cases |
| --- | --- |
| Prostate | 24.5 |
| Lung | 13.8 |
| Colorectal | 13.8 |
| Bladder | 6.1 |
| Non-Hodgkin's lymphoma | 4.4 |
| Kidney | 3.8 |
| Leukemia | 3.4 |
| Melanoma | 3.4 |
| Oral | 2.9 |
| Pancreas | 2.4 |

**TABLE 17.2  Percent Distribution of Top 10 Types of Cancer in Canadian Women**[1]

| Cancer Type | Estimated Percentage of New Cancer Cases |
| --- | --- |
| Breast | 26.1 |
| Lung | 13.3 |
| Colorectal | 11.6 |
| Body of uterus | 6.1 |
| Thyroid | 4.8 |
| Non-Hodgkin's lymphoma | 3.9 |
| Melanoma | 3.0 |
| Ovary | 2.9 |
| Leukemia | 2.7 |
| Pancreas | 2.6 |

Canadians than the other three (prostate, colorectal, and breast) cancer types combined.

There has been a constant increase in the incidence of cancer among men and women in the past decade in Canada. Among men, the peak in 2000 was due to the rising screening trend in prostate cancer. From 1998 to 2007, the overall incidence of cancer in women has increased approximately by 0.3% per year. In women, the cancer incidence rate primarily reflects the steady rise in lung, thyroid, and breast cancer incidence rates.[1]

In contrast, cancer mortality has been trending down after a peak in the late 1980s. Between 1988 and 2007, mortality rates from most forms of cancer dropped by 21% in men and 9% in women.[6] The decrease in men has largely been due to the decrease in mortality rate for lung cancer but also in prostate and colorectal cancers.[1]

For women, the decrease in age-specific mortality rate has largely been due to decreased mortality rate for breast and colorectal cancers. In Canada, the overall decline in the mortality rate has been noticed, but there has been a steady increase in lung cancer mortality in women.[1]

### Breast Cancer

Incidence of breast cancer increased in the period of the early 1990s, which may be due to the increased awareness about mammography screening. The incidence had a downward slope in the early 2000s, which may reflect the decrease in usage of hormonal replacement therapy in postmenopausal women.[1]

### Colorectal Cancer

There has been a drop in the incidence of colorectal cancer starting mid-1980s but then a rise again in the early 2000s.[1] The increase can be linked to increased awareness about screening colonoscopies.

### Lung Cancer

Lung cancer has been on a decline since the 1980s among males, but the incidence among females has been increasing due to the increasing prevalence of cigarette smoking among women. There has been a significant drop in lung cancer death rate, especially for men over the past 20 years, which has driven a decline in the overall cancer death rate.[1]

### Prostate Cancer

The incidence rate of prostate cancer has been following a decline. There have been two peaks, however, in 1993 and 2001, respectively. These peaks are related to the increased screening activity using the prostate-specific antigen testing. The mortality rate associated with prostate cancer initially increased but has been declining through 2001 to 2009.[1] This reflects the increased usage of hormonal therapy in both early and advanced prostate cancer.

## Cancer Research

Cancer research in Canada is funded by the government and by multiple charitable groups. The government-funded federal agency, the Canadian Institutes of Health Research (CIHR), is composed of 13 further subgroups, including the Institute of Cancer Research.[6] This is further divided on a provincial level, such as the Ontario Institute for Cancer Research and the

British Columbia Cancer Agency. Charitable groups are another major contributor, and before the CIHR came into existence, they were the largest funders for cancer research. The Canadian Cancer Society along with the Terry Fox Foundation and major hospital systems and pharmaceutical companies are leaders in funding cancer care and research.[6] The Canadian Cancer Research Alliance promotes a more coordinated and collaborative effort for cancer research.

Over the recent years, Canada has shown a progressive increase in funding for cancer-related research. A total of $545.5 million was dedicated to cancer research in Canada in 2009.[7] The allocation of funds was equally divided between general and specific cancer types. A total of $265.3 million was dedicated to specific cancers, of which breast cancer received 28%, leukemia 12%, prostate 9%, brain 8%, and lung and colorectal cancers 7%.[7] These statistics reflect the underfunding of stomach, pancreatic, colorectal, and lung cancers. However, this overall increase in research is evident by the 3-fold increase in publications from Canada between 2000 and 2008. Canada is also the world leader in biomedical articles published per $1 billion dollars spent.[7]

## REFERENCES

1. Canadian Cancer Society's Advisory Committee on Cancer Statistics. Canadian Cancer Statistics 2013.
2. Canadian Cancer Society, Public Health Agency of Canada. Available at www.cancer.ca. Retrieved August 8, 2013.
3. Canadian Cancer Registry. Statistics Canada. Available at Canada.gc.ca. Retrieved August 8, 2013.
4. General Information—Medical Oncology. Canadian Association of Medical Oncologists 2012.
5. Demand High but Medical Specialists Not Finding Work in Canada. *National Post*, November 2009.
6. Cancer research funding in Canada—Dr. Michael Wosnick in Cancer Research 101, published August 2012.
7. Canadian Cancer Research Alliance—in the report, Cancer Research in Canada, 2005–2009.

# 18

# Cancer Care in China

## Xinsheng Michael Liao

### COMMUNICABLE DISEASES AND NONCOMMUNICABLE DISEASES

Control of many communicable diseases has been touted as one of the most successful achievements of the current Chinese government since 1949. Many diseases, such as small pox, plague, cholera, and tuberculosis, have been eradicated or substantially brought under control. This control may be the most important reason for improvement of life expectancy among mainland Chinese. As for noncommunicable diseases, cardiovascular disease occupies the second-highest mortality rate next to cancer. In addition, hypertension and stroke are common, and diabetes is fast rising.[1]

### CANCER ETIOLOGIES

In addition to common etiologies that apply to the rest of the world, China does have a few cancers that stand out as "special." High incidence of hepatocellular carcinoma is linked to widespread hepatitis B infection.[2] In some areas, aflatoxin is a prominent culprit.[3] Esophageal cancer, which is believed to be associated with certain foods, has a very high incidence in China, especially in Henan Province.[4] Stomach cancer is still a prominent cause of cancer mortality in China, which is probably due to *Helicobacter pylori* infection and diet.[5] There used to be "poor" cancers, such as cancers of the stomach, liver, and esophagus. Now there are increasing "rich" cancers, such as lung, breast, and colorectal cancers. In general, higher incidence of cancer is suspected to be caused by industrialization, environmental pollution, diet, and so on. The incidence of lung cancer has risen 56% in the past 10 years in Beijing, for which air pollution is believed to be the cause.[7] The incidence of these rich cancers in China is not as high as that in Western countries, but the trend is certainly alarming.

## CANCER STATISTICS IN CHINA

Until 2002, no cancer registry system was available in China to accurately account for the number of cancer types; when the National Cancer Registry Center was set up, it allowed for more accurate comparison of cancer incidence between countries.[6] The government provided funding to set up more than 220 surveillance sites across the country, covering some 200 million people. Incidence of cancers in China has been steadily increasing in the past 30 years, with an estimate of 3.12 million cases a year, about 6 cases a minute, with a mortality of 2.5 million, reflecting an 80% mortality rate.[7] Although most types of cancers occur throughout different regions in China, some types of cancers occur in the form of clusters, reflecting a strong environmental influence. For example, lung cancer was 56% higher from 2001 to 2010 in Beijing, mostly because of smoking and air pollution. Hepatoma is very high in a part of Canton Province, whereas esophageal cancer is very high in a small region in Henan Province. There are many "cancer villages" in China as a consequence of pollution.

## HISTORY OF CANCER CARE

Organized anticancer medical care in China started with the establishment of the Cancer Institute and Hospital, Chinese Academy of Medical Sciences in 1963. To a large degree, the diagnosis of cancer carries a great deal of emotional stress because it is incurable. Therefore, an open labeling of "cancer" diagnosis has been avoided most of the time. Cancer hospitals in China are all called "tumor" hospitals. Most of the time, patients are not informed of their diagnosis. This situation is changing so that direct communication with patients is increasingly possible. Patients are becoming more resilient than before and therefore are more involved in treating their cancers.

## CANCER INFRASTRUCTURE

Nowadays each province in China has at least one hospital dedicated to cancer care. These hospitals have a complete setup for cancer care, including surgical oncology, medical oncology, radiation oncology, and imaging studies such as CT, MRI, and PET. In addition, almost all the general hospitals have a department for medical oncology, though surgeons are not dedicated to oncology. Not all hospitals have a radiation facility. Anticancer drugs are much more available than 20 years ago. Unlike in the past where there was a longer delay, new drugs made in the United States or Europe now take only 2 or 3 years to enter the Chinese market. However, there is a substantial disparity among hospitals in big cities and small cities.

A major challenge in infrastructure is the reimbursement system. Because medical care is regarded as social welfare, the fee standard has to be affordable to ordinary people. This results in a skewed fee structure for medical care in general and cancer care in particular. For example, although chemotherapy is more expensive in China than in the United States (new drugs are imported mostly from the United States and the price is higher than that in the United States), surgery may be the most economical way of treating cancer in China. As of 2014, the official price of lobectomy for lung cancer is $138, a hospital bed is $4.9 per day, breast biopsy is $3.27, and liver biopsy is $4.91.[8] The price of a hospital bed is much cheaper than that of any room in a hotel in Beijing, though this price level obviously does not reflect the cost of care in modern China. Patients and family members need to bribe physicians in order to get hospitalized. Therefore, all the hospitals are trying to prescribe expensive tests and expensive imported drugs to patients to make up the income deficit. All pharmaceutical companies, domestic or foreign, are routinely giving physicians kickbacks, though there is no official literature to document this. This is one of the reasons why surgeons are prescribing chemotherapy in China. In addition, the patient and family members need to give a so-called red bag (money) under the table to surgeons before the surgery. I believe the fee structure is one of the major reasons why the rapport between physicians and patients has been deteriorating in China in the past decade. Stories of doctors being killed, disfigured, or beaten by their patients or their families often emerge. In his book titled *Surviving Diary*, Ling Zhi Jun, a Chinese reporter, describes his personal experience of cancer treatment in the Chinese health-care system.[9]

## MEDICAL AND SURGICAL ONCOLOGY

The typical training for medical and surgical oncologists involves spending time in internal medicine and medical oncology. By the end of their 3 years of training, they are certified in both specialties. As residents, they are responsible for admitting patients, writing progress notes and orders, making hospital rounds, and performing operations with the attending physicians. Formal lectures are rare. There is no emphasis on following guidelines. Many well-known physicians teach their residents based on their personal experiences, rather than on evidence-based medicine. Because there is no habit of independent literature reading by the residents, or physicians in practice, personal opinions from authoritative figures can be quite influential. Different medical schools and hospitals have various authoritative figures. These so-called experts generate different approaches for cancer treatment. It is always hard to talk about "standard of care" among Chinese physicians. There is now a board for medical licensure in China, but there is still no board examination for any subspecialty.

Most surgeons in China consider themselves authoritative figures. They prescribe chemotherapy, and they don't prefer to listen to pathologists even regarding surgical margins. The margin determination on pathology reports can serve only as "reference" at best for surgeons, but not for any decision-making purpose. Obviously, there is no legal ramification against physicians even if they give a drastically different treatment to patients or if they don't follow any guidelines. There is no system in China for litigation, or expert witnesses. A positive development in the past 10 years is that many department heads or senior physicians have opportunities to travel to the United States for oncology meetings. This might help Chinese physicians adopt evidence-based approaches for cancer treatment. In addition, the National Comprehensive Cancer Network Guidelines have recently been translated into Chinese, giving Chinese physicians a new reference tool.

## RADIATION THERAPY

Compared to surgical oncology and medical oncology, radiation oncology is a relatively recent development in China. Because of the high cost of treatment and special training for personnel, radiation therapy is available only in big cities. This situation is expected to improve significantly because of continuous economic development and broader coverage by medical insurance plans.

## PALLIATIVE CARE

Pain control in the cancer setting has not been fully addressed with pain medication. Morphine and meperidine are the best available pain medications in the Chinese market. Fear of addiction to narcotics exists among patients, family members, and doctors. There is no home nursing system in China. For most patients, their family members and friends generally provide supportive care.

## ALTERNATIVE CANCER THERAPIES IN CHINA

As one would expect, a number of Chinese herb preparations and acupuncture strategies are available in China for cancer treatment. Many clinical trials in China incorporate Chinese herbs in the treatment plan. Astraga has been shown to increase the response rate to cisplatin-based chemo regimen for lung cancer.[10] In general, efficacy of alternative therapies remains to be demonstrated in strictly controlled clinical trials.

## PREVENTION

China employs many resources in preventing cancer. Much information is provided in the news media on prevention of cancers. The Chinese Center for Disease Control spends a great deal of effort in prevention. Its function is similar to that of the Centers for Disease Control and Prevention in the United States. In addition, the Chinese Academy of Preventive Medicine, which was formed in 1983, plays a role in cancer prevention.

## SCREENING

Pap smear has not been widely used in China for cervical cancer screening because of economic constraints and lack of resources.[11] Mammograms are offered only in big cities.[12] In the past few years, there has been a sharp rise in annual screening exams. These examinations cost between $100 and $30,000, indicating a wide variation in screening measures.

## FUTURE DIRECTIONS AND RESEARCH

China has employed significant resources for cancer research, though it is relatively quite small compared to the United States. One of the major contributions of China was the discovery of all-trans-retinoic acid and arsenic trioxide for treating acute promyelocytic leukemia[13,14] and the development of epidermal growth factor receptor inhibitor for lung cancer.[15] It is anticipated that more new drugs will be developed in China for cancer treatment in the coming years.

## REFERENCES

1. Ma RC, Chan JC. Type 2 diabetes in East Asians: similarities and differences with populations in Europe and the United States. *Ann N Y Acad Sci* Apr 2013; 1281: 64–91.
2. Gao J, Xie L, Yang WS, et al. Risk factors of hepatocellular carcinoma—current status and perspectives. *Asian Pac J Cancer Prev* 2012; 13(3): 743–52.
3. Liu Y, Chang CC, Marsh GM, Wu F. Population attributable risk of aflatoxin-related liver cancer: systematic review and meta-analysis. *Eur J Cancer* 2012; 48(14): 2125–36.
4. Yang CS. Research on esophageal cancer in China: a review. *Cancer Res* 1980; 40(8 Pt 1): 2633–44.
5. Roder DM. The epidemiology of gastric cancer. *Gastric Cancer* 2002; 5 (Suppl 1): 5–11.
6. Wang YC, Wei LJ, Liu JT, Li SX, Wang QS. Comparison of cancer incidence between China and the USA. *Cancer Biol Med* 2012; 9(2): 128–32.

7. Chinese Cancer Registry Annual Report 2012, edited by Hao Jie and Chen Wan Qing.

8. Fee Schedule of Medical Services in Beijing. Available at http://wenku.baidu .com/view/7bad2715a300a6c30c229fcb.html.

9. Jun, LZ. *Surviving Diary*, 2012.

10. McCulloch M, See C, Shu XJ, et al. Astragalus-based Chinese herbs and platinum-based chemotherapy for advanced non-small-cell lung cancer: meta-analysis of randomized trials. *J Clin Oncol* 2006 Jan 20; 24(3): 419–30.

11. Shi JF, Qiao YL, Smith JS, et al. Epidemiology and prevention of human papillomavirus and cervical cancer in China and Mongolia. *Vaccine* 2008 Aug 19; 26 (Suppl 12): M53–M59. Erratum in: *Vaccine* 2010 Mar 16; 28(13):2573–74.

12. Hu ZJ, Fan ZX. Status of breast cancer screening in China. Chinese *J Breast Dis* (electronic version) October 2007; 1: 5.

13. Huang ME, Ye YC, Chen SR, et al. Use of all-trans retinoic acid in the treatment of acute promyelocytic leukemia. *Blood* 1988; 72(2): 567–72.

14. Zhang P. The use of arsenic trioxide ($As_2O_3$) in the treatment of acute promyelocytic leukemia. *J Biol Regul Homeost Agents* 1999; 13(4): 195–200.

15. Shi Y, Zhang L, Liu X, et al. Icotinib versus gefitinib in previously treated advanced non-small-cell lung cancer (ICOGEN): a randomised, double-blind phase 3 non-inferiority trial. *Lancet Oncol* 2013; 14(10): 953–61.

# 19

# Central and Eastern Europe

*György Bodoky and Ágota Petrányi*

## PUBLIC HEALTH PERSPECTIVE

Enormous progress in health was achieved in Europe during the second half of the 20th century. The decrease in infant and early child mortality and the shift in the composition of mortality risk from communicable to noncommunicable diseases led to the increase of cancer and cardiovascular diseases (CVDs) resulting in the leading causes of death among adults. Adult health was so deteriorated in the East that by 1990 males overall lived 5 years less, and females 4 years less, than their counterparts in the West.[1]

Nowadays, in Central and Eastern European countries, infectious diseases represent a relatively minor cause of death, particularly in young adulthood and middle age. Similar rates were observed as in EU-15 countries (countries in the European Union before May 1, 2004). Despite this situation in Lithuania, Latvia, and Romania, the mortality from infectious diseases was 2 to 3 times higher than that in the EU-15 countries, which is likely to be due to the higher incidence of AIDS and tuberculosis and poorer therapy.[4]

Instead, chronic noncommunicable diseases and injuries have reemerged as the primary causes of premature death in the European population.[11] In developed countries, diseases of the heart and circulatory system (CVD) are the main cause of death, an important cause of disability and of large economic and social cost to the society. CVD has been the leading cause of death since the 1970s, but its mortality rate has declined in many high-income countries. CVD mortality among men is higher than among women in all European countries. In the Central and Eastern European countries, the ratio of men to women is high, except in Romania, where the CVD death rate is one of the highest, but with one of the lowest men to women ratio.[10]

In the 1970s and 1980s, Eastern Europe was the highest risk region for vascular diseases, as the CVD mortality rate was still increasing. The causes likely included increased consumption of tobacco, alcohol, and salt, as well as low consumption of fish and fruit.[4]

Since the 1990s, death rates from CVD have fallen, and cancer has emerged as the most common cause of death among young and middle-aged women (20 to 64 years) in these countries. In the coming decade, it seems likely that cancer will be the leading cause of death among young and middle-aged men as well, although now CVDs are still dominant in this group.[13]

On a global scale, cancer has become a major public health problem and an increasingly important factor in the burden of disease.

## CANCER ETIOLOGY

Increased cancer incidence in the Central and Eastern European countries cannot be completely explained by an aging population. Other nonmodifiable factors such as genetic susceptibility are likely to play an important role. Behavioral factors, such as cigarette smoking, alcohol consumption, exposure to occupational and environmental carcinogens, sexual behavior, obesity, diet, and physical activity, are crucial in the development of cancer. After World War II, in Central and Eastern Europe the consumption of tobacco and alcohol increased steadily. These products were easily accessible and their prices were kept at very low levels. For example, between the 1950s and 1980s, the consumption of tobacco increased linearly in Poland, from around 1,000 to 2,700 cigarettes/capita/year, reaching the highest contemporary level in the world,[37] and per capita alcohol consumption went from about 3 L to 8.4 L.[13,14] Traditionally, in Central and Eastern European countries, homemade alcohol is made not only from grapes but from other fruits (plums, peaches, apricots)[40] as well, yielding fruit brandy, such as rakija and pálinka, with high alcohol concentrations.[42,45] At the beginning of the 21st century, these countries had the highest levels of cirrhosis mortality in Europe. The drinking pattern in these countries can be characterized by the consumption of wine and hard fruit alcohol during meals. These are not binge-drinking countries, such as the Russian Federation and other "vodka" countries. A large portion of alcohol consumed in this region is homemade. A general lack of data exists about chemical constituents of homemade alcohol, which may be especially hepatotoxic. Recent studies from Hungary showed that the concentration of some short-chain aliphatic alcohols (methanol, isobutanol, 1-propanol, 1-butanol, 2-butanol, and isoamyl alcohol) was significantly higher in homemade alcohol than in commercial alcohol.[41] These alcohols have much more pronounced hepatotoxic effects.[43,44]

Diet was characterized by high (and increasing) consumption of animal fat (also butter) and very low consumption of vegetable oil, fish, and fruit.

Subsidies in Eastern Europe made meat and dairy prices low, creating higher consumption through the 1970s. This also likely resulted in Eastern Europe being the first of these two regions to develop an obesity problem.

Important and far-reaching environmental changes occurred in the past three decades in Central and Eastern European countries, although environmental protection remained low. Industrialization of agriculture, opening of several coal mines, and establishment of a series of chemical plants were major factors that negatively influenced the health status of the population, including cancer mortality.

## CANCER STATISTICS

In 2011, the South Eastern European Research Oncology Group collected and analyzed epidemiological data (on incidence and mortality) to evaluate the oncological care in selected Central and Eastern European countries (Figures 19.1-19.17). Population estimates of individual countries for 2002 to 2006 were generally based on official consensuses that were obtained from the World Health Organization (WHO) database. Analyzing the data, the highest cancer incidence among men has been found in Hungary, whereas in Poland it has been found to be lower by one-third, and in Romania by one-half. Among women, the highest incidence rates have been detected in the Czech Republic and Slovakia.[16]

Although the incidence of cancer is higher in Western European countries than in Central and Eastern Europe, the mortality rate is lower for men but equal for women. A decreasing mortality trend can be seen only in cases of children and youth (up to age 20) in both sexes, but their mortality level is still significantly higher than that in the Western European countries. In the Central and Eastern European countries, an increase in the mortality rates was witnessed until the 1990s, and then, it started to decline. Hungary and the Czech Republic are the leading countries in the list of cancer mortality, ranking first and second, respectively, followed by the Baltic countries, Poland and Slovenia.

Despite the relatively low incidence, the high, all-cancer mortality rates in most of the Central and Eastern European countries reflect the distribution of the most frequent cancers and the poor survival of these patients in the region. It is most likely lower-quality registered mortality rates, mandatory reporting practices, cause-of-death reporting, screening, health care, and management that create the differences.[52]

Lung cancer is the most frequent cancer in the Central and Eastern European countries, representing 25% of all cancers reported, and it causes more deaths than any other cancer in this region. Nearly 33% of all cancer deaths in males in Central and Eastern Europe are caused by lung cancer. The next most common overall causes of cancer deaths in the region are cancers of the colon and rectum, stomach, prostate, and bladder. Breast, colorectal, ovarian, and cervical cancer are the next most frequent causes of death in women.[16]

Death rates from breast cancer for all age groups are lower in the Central and Eastern European countries than in the EU-15. However, increases have stopped since 1990, and in some cases even declined for both the EU-15 and the Central and Eastern European region.

In Romania and the Baltic countries, colorectal cancers cause more deaths in men, women, and all age groups than the diseases do in EU-15 countries. For both genders, the lowest morality rate is in Romania, and the death rate in the Czech Republic, Hungary, and Slovakia is almost double that of other Central and Eastern European countries. Deaths from colorectal cancers are twice as frequent among men as among women in the Central and Eastern European countries.

In the second half of the 20th century in Europe, the decrease in mortality from cervical cancer was continuing and was significantly higher in each Central and Eastern European country. While mortality has declined in Slovenia, Czech Republic, Slovakia, Hungary, Estonia, and Poland, cervical cancer deaths are increasing in Latvia, Bulgaria, Lithuania, and, most strikingly, in Romania, which has mortality rates six times higher than that in the EU-15 region, the highest rates ever recorded in Europe.

## CANCER CARE

It is proven that there is a correlation between per capita total national expenditure for health and 5-year relative survival for all cancers combined.[59] Higher survival in a region compared to another one can be due to higher proportions of tumors diagnosed at early stage, availability of adequate treatment, and lower prevalence of comorbidity. All these factors reflect the investment of resources in health, thus explaining its relationship with cancer survival.[58] The analysis of cancer survival data can indicate the quality of treatment and the average stage at diagnosis.

The EUROCARE studies—the largest population-based investigation on cancer patient survival—showed that for most cancer sites there were marked differences in cancer survival between European countries. Population-based cancer survival gives us an average measurer of cancer care performance. Socioeconomic factors that have been shown to correlate with survival for two most treatable cancers—breast and colon—include per capita health expenditure and infant mortality. Conversely, geographic differences in survival are not remarkable for rare cancers that are treatable,[56] such as leukemia and testicular cancers, apparently because effective treatments are widely accessible because the rarity of these cancers means there are no major costs to implement treatment. In the case of fatal cancers that are not yet treatable, such as cancers of the liver and pancreas, survival rates do not vary greatly between geographical regions and do not reflect information on the national health system.[24]

The fluctuating levels of regional cancer care are the result of the following shortcomings:

- an absence of oncology teams, leading to mosaic-like uncoordinated treatment
- a lack of radiation therapy equipment
- limited access to reconstructive surgery
- a lack of rehabilitation opportunities
- not enough pain clinics
- insufficient hospice facilities
- a lack of a reliable register of continuous care

Compared to the rest of Europe, childhood cancer mortality is more than 20% higher in the Central and Eastern European region.[54] International clinical trials with almost all primary treatments incorporating long-standing medications in off-label uses included pediatric oncologists from the Central and Eastern European countries before they joined the EU. Regulatory agencies overall accepted the off-label situation. Later, the implementation of European directives produced new and stricter interpretations of regulations. Infrastructure changes needed for compliance were not funded, so not made.[53]

## CANCER CARE CONTINUUM

Although the WHO estimates that one-third of all cancers are preventable and another third can be cured if detected in time and treated adequately, to fight cancer with the best result, one must look beyond early detection and treatment and into the overall organization of health systems to comprehensively deliver cancer control.[27] In the Central and Eastern European countries, deficiency of primary prevention is a main reason of poor health consciousness (consequences of smoking, fatty diet, low physical activity) and late introduction of secondary prevention responses results in worse survival of the cancer patient.[1]

Primary prevention means eliminating the effects that are known, assumed causal or risk factors, and that play roles in the evolvement of cancer from artificial or natural environments or ways of life of individual people. Significant opportunities exist in primary prevention. Tobacco control offers the most potential for primary prevention. Pricing is widely known as the most effective form of smoking control (so cancer control), but in some places, cigarettes remain cheaper than staples such as a loaf of bread. Central and Eastern European countries in the past 10 years have seen some success with tobacco control preceding decreased cancer rates in young adults, even though the rates remain higher than those of Western Europe.[22]

In the Central and Eastern European countries, a general ban on advertising tobacco products is in place, which also prohibits indirect forms of advertising (e.g., brand stretching and brand sharing), but permits some specific forms of tobacco advertising (e.g., information displayed at points of sale). It also prohibits the sale of tobacco products through vending machines, the free distribution of tobacco products, and tobacco advertising on the television and radio.

Early detection increases the chance of successful treatment for most cancers.[12]

In health-care practice, we distinguish between organized mass and ad hoc screenings. In organized mass screenings, the methods used must already have been proven effective in large groups of average-risk people. The only acceptable evidence of effectiveness is a significant decline in mortality from the disease being screened for in the community being screened, a result that can be attributed to the screening. The most obvious illustration of this need is the dramatic increase in death from cervical cancer in some countries of Central and Eastern Europe over half a century—deaths that are now almost entirely preventable.[14] However, colorectal cancer screening is proven to be completely effective although there are some difficulties to overcome, mainly the very high cost of this type of screening (training of staff, purchase of equipment) and the preparation of the colon.[36]

The lack of emphasis on screening across years in the Central and Eastern European countries worked against effective cancer control, as did the lack of cancer literacy among the populace.

## CONCLUSION

Because of the lack of a uniform data source, quantitative data on health services is based on a number of different sources, including the WHO, the Regional Office for Europe's European Health for All database, data from national statistical offices, Eurostat, the Organization for Economic Co-operation and Development Health Data, data from the International Monetary Fund, the database of EUROCARE project, the GLOBOCAN 2008 website by the International Agency for Research on Cancer, the World Bank's World Development Indicators, and any other relevant sources considered useful for us (Tables 19.1-19.7).

**TABLE 19.1** Population and Human Development Indicators in Central and Eastern European Countries (data from: World Health Organization Statistical Information System. WHO database of mortality and population estimates [online]; http://apps.who.int/gho/data/node.country)

| | Population (in thousands) total | Total Area of the Country (sq. km) | Gross National Income per Capita (PPP int. $) | Total Expenditure on Health per Capita (int. $, 2011) | Total Expenditure on Health as a Percentage of Gross Domestic Product | General Government Expenditure on Health as a Percentage of Total Government Expenditure | General Government expenditure on Health as a Percentage of Total Expenditure on Health | Per Capita Total Expenditure on Health at Average Exchange Rate (US$) |
|---|---|---|---|---|---|---|---|---|
| Bulgaria | 7,278 | 110,994 | 1,416 | 1,064 | 7.30 | 11.30 | 55.30 | 521.50 |
| Czech Republic | 10,660 | 78,866 | 24,370 | 1,923 | 7.40 | 14.20 | 83.50 | 1922.80 |
| Estonia | 1,291 | 45,226 | 20,850 | 1,334 | 6.00 | 12.30 | 78.90 | 986.90 |
| Hungary | 9,932 | 93,036 | 20,310 | | 7.70 | 10.20 | 64.80 | 1669.00 |
| Latvia | 2,060 | 64,589 | 17,700 | 1,179 | 6.20 | 9.30 | 58.50 | 1178.70 |
| Lithuania | 3,028 | 65,200 | 19,640 | 1,337 | 6.60 | 12.60 | 71.30 | 1337.00 |
| Poland | 38,211 | 312,679 | 20,430 | 1,423 | 6.70 | 11.00 | 71.20 | 1422.70 |
| Romania | 21,755 | 238,391 | 15,120 | 902 | 5.80 | 12.14 | 82.88 | 457.23 |
| Slovakia | 5,446 | 49,035 | 22,130 | 978 | 8,70 | 14.5 | 63.8 | 2087.9 |
| Slovenia | 2,068 | 20,273 | 26,510 | 18,336 | 9.1 | 13.0 | 72.8 | 1615.0 |

TABLE 19.2 Life Expectancy Statistics and Demographics in Central and Eastern European Countries. (data from World Health Organization Statistical Information System. WHO database of mortality and population estimates [online]; http://apps.who.int/gho/data/node.country)

| | Average Life Expectancy at Birth | Healthy Life Expectancy | Population Living in Urban Areas (%) | Population Proportion under 15 (%) | Population Proportion over 60 (%) | Population Median Age (years) |
|---|---|---|---|---|---|---|
| Bulgaria | 71/78 | 66 | 73 | 13.53 | 26.11 | 42.84 |
| Czech Republic | 75/81 | 70 | 73 | 14.56 | 23.23 | 40.07 |
| Estonia | 71/81 | 66 | 69 | 15.69 | 23.92 | 40.78 |
| Hungary | 71/79 | 66 | 69 | 14.62 | 23.41 | 40.35 |
| Latvia | 69/78 | 64 | 68 | 14.57 | 24.14 | 41.44 |
| Lithuania | 68/79 | 63 | 67 | 15.13 | 20.57 | 39.09 |
| Poland | 72/81 | 67 | 61 | 14.91 | 20.48 | 38.55 |
| Romania | 70/78 | 65 | 53 | 15.5 | 14.7 | |
| Slovakia | 72/80 | 67 | 55 | 15.00 | 18.6 | 37.87 |
| Slovenia | 77/83 | 71 | 50 | 14.16 | 23.16 | 42.1 |

TABLE 19.3 Age-Standardized Death Rate per 100,000 (2008)

| | Age-Standardized Death Rate per 100,000 (2008) | | | | | | Proportional Mortality (percentage of total deaths, all ages) | | | |
| | All Noncommunicable Diseases | | Cardiovascular Diseases and Diabetes | | Cancer | | | | | |
| | Male | Female | Male | Female | Male | Female | CVD | Cancers | Respiratory Diseases | Injuries |
|---|---|---|---|---|---|---|---|---|---|---|
| Bulgaria | 849.2 | 513.9 | 566.6 | 367.7 | 179.1 | 100.6 | 66 | 17 | 2 | 4 |
| Czech Republic | 603.7 | 366.2 | 315.1 | 203.1 | 202.4 | 116.3 | 50 | 27 | 3 | 6 |
| Estonia | 823.9 | 391.0 | 469.4 | 233.4 | 219.9 | 103.1 | 56 | 22 | 2 | 8 |
| Hungary | 844.6 | 457.2 | 415.8 | 241.4 | 254.8 | 133.7 | 50 | 25 | 4 | 6 |
| Latvia | 921.2 | 458.9 | 566.8 | 295.0 | 233.6 | 107.9 | 59 | 20 | 1 | 9 |
| Lithuania | 875.5 | 438.0 | 503.2 | 263.7 | 219.9 | 110.1 | 55 | 19 | 2 | 11 |
| Poland | 713.6 | 377.8 | 366.4 | 204.5 | 229.2 | 120.9 | 48 | 26 | 3 | 7 |
| Romania | 788.7 | 483.0 | 476.9 | 322.5 | 188.9 | 100.1 | 59 | 19 | 3 | 5 |
| Slovakia | 767.9 | 425.2 | 430.8 | 259.4 | 218.9 | 110.3 | 53 | 23 | 2 | 6 |
| Slovenia | 517.3 | 287.2 | 209.9 | 127.8 | 207.3 | 112.7 | 40 | 31 | 3 | 8 |

Source: WHO database.

**TABLE 19.4** Smoking and Excessive Weight Prevalence, and Overall per Capita Recorded Alcohol Consumption in Liters of Pure Alcohol in Central and Eastern European Countries (data from: Global Health Observatory Data Repository; http://apps.who.int/gho/data/node.country)

| | Smoking Percentage | | Obesity Percentage | | |
|---|---|---|---|---|---|
| | Male | Female | Male | Female | Alcohol (L) |
| Bulgaria | 47.5 | 27.8 | 22.1 | 28.3 | 9.4 |
| Czech Republic | 36.6 | 25.4 | 26.8 | 30.9 | 13.9 |
| Estonia | 49.9 | 27.5 | 11.2 | 12.6 | 11.0 |
| Hungary | 45.7 | 33.9 | 22.5 | 23.4 | 17.4 |
| Latvia | 54.4 | 24.1 | 13.5 | 22.0 | 11.6 |
| Lithuania | 45.1 | 20.8 | 22.0 | 20.4 | 14.2 |
| Poland | 43.9 | 27.2 | 18.8 | 26.9 | 10.9 |
| Romania | 40.6 | 24.5 | 8.1 | 17.7 | 14.7 |
| Slovakia | 41.6 | 20.1 | 14.9 | 29.0 | 14.6 |
| Slovenia | 31.8 | 21.1 | 17.3 | 31.7 | 9.9 |

**TABLE 19.5** Mortality and Health Indicators in Hungary, 1970–2010

| | 1970 | 1980 | 1990 | 1995 | 2000 | 2005 | 2009 |
|---|---|---|---|---|---|---|---|
| Life expectancy at birth, total (years) | 69.3 | 69.1 | 69.5 | 70.1 | 71.9 | 73.0 | 74.5 |
| Life expectancy at birth, male (years) | 66.4 | 65.5 | 65.2 | 65.5 | 67.6 | 68.8 | 70.3 |
| Life expectancy at birth, female (years) | 72.2 | 72.8 | 73.9 | 74.8 | 76.3 | 77.2 | 78.5 |
| Crude death rate per 1,000 population, total | 11.6 | 13.6 | 14.0 | 14.1 | 13.3 | 13.5 | 13.0 |
| Crude death rate per 1,000 population, male | 12.5 | 14.8 | 15.4 | 15.7 | 14.5 | 14.6 | 13.9 |
| Crude death rate per 1,000 population, female | 10.8 | 12.4 | 12.8 | 12.6 | 12.2 | 12.5 | 12.1 |

**TABLE 19.6** The Main Data of Health Infrastructure in Central and Eastern European Countries (data from World Health Organization Statistical Information System. WHO database of mortality and population estimates [online]; http://apps.who.int/gho/data/node.country) and DIRAC database [online]; http://www-naweb.iaea.org/nahu/dirac/default.asp)

| | Total Density of Specialized Hospitals (per 100,000 population) | Total Density of Magnetic Resonance Imaging Units (per million population) | Total Density of Computed Tomography Units (per million population) | Total Density of Positron Emission Tomography Units (per million population) | Total Density of Gamma Camera or Nuclear Medicine Units (per million population) | Total Density of Linear Accelerator (per million population) | Total Density of Telecobalt Unit (per million population) |
|---|---|---|---|---|---|---|---|
| Bulgaria | | NA | NA | NA | NA | 0.6870* | 1.3740* |
| Czech Republic | | 5.015 | 13.4054 | 0.5787 | 11.6695 | 3.5683 | 1.4466 |
| Estonia | | 8.2073 | 14.9224 | 0.7461 | 2.2384 | 2.2384 | NA |
| Hungary | | 1.401 | 6.6048 | 0.6004 | 10.2075 | 1.1008 | 0.7005 |
| Latvia | | 6.6686 | 27.11888 | 0 | 2.2229 | 4.0011 | 0.97087* |
| Lithuania | | NA | NA | NA | NA | 2.9723* | 0.6605* |
| Poland | | 3.2831 | 10.6373 | 0.3414 | 2.8103 | 2.6002 | 0.1313 |
| Romania | | 2.0212 | 5.5465 | 0.047 | 24.3782 | 0.517 | 0.6581 |
| Slovakia | | NA | NA | NA | NA | 2.9379* | 1.8362* |
| Slovenia | | 4.4552 | 12.3755 | 0.99 | 6.9303 | 2.9701 | 0.495 |

*Source:* WHO database.
*DIRAC database.

TABLE 19.7  Breast Cancer Screening in Central and Eastern European Countries

| Breast Cancer Screening | Organized Program | National Coverage | Year First Program Started | Age of Target Population | Screening Interval (years) | Coverage (%) | Participation Rate (%) |
|---|---|---|---|---|---|---|---|
| Bulgaria | No | | | | | | |
| Czech Republic | Yes | Yes | 2002 | 45 to 69 | 2 | 1.00 | 0.60 |
| Estonia | Yes | Yes | 2003 | 50 to 59 | 2 | 74.0 | 0.51 |
| Hungary | Yes | Yes | 2002 | 45 to 65 | 2 | 76.8 | 45.1 |
| Latvia | No | | | | | | |
| Lithuania | Yes | Yes | 2006 | 50 to 69 | 2 | 0.80 | NA |
| Poland | Yes | Yes | 2007 | 50 to 69 | 2 | 1.00 | NA |
| Romania | No | | | | | | |
| Slovakia | No | | | | | | |
| Slovenia | No | | | | | | |

TABLE 19.8  Colorectal Cancer Screening in Central and Eastern European Countries

| Colorectal Cancer Screening | Organized Program | National Coverage | Year First Program Started | Age of Target Population | Screening Interval (years) | Coverage | Screening test |
|---|---|---|---|---|---|---|---|
| Bulgaria | No | | | | | | |
| Czech Republic | Yes | Yes | 2001 | ≥50 | 2 | NA | FOBT |
| Estonia | No | | | | | | |
| Hungary | No | | | | | | |
| Latvia | No | | | | | | |
| Lithuania | No | | | | | | |
| Poland | Yes | No | 2000 | 50 to 65 | 10 | NA | Colonoscopy |
| Romania | No | | | | | | |
| Slovakia | No | | | | | | |
| Slovenia | No | | | | | | |

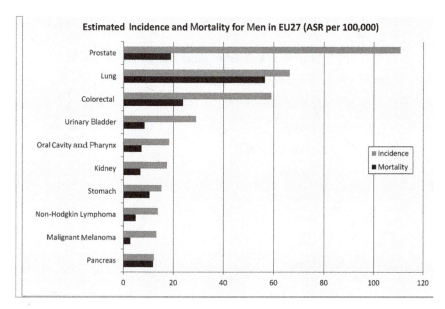

**FIGURE 19.1** Estimated incidence and mortality for men in EU27 (ASR per 100,000 individuals).

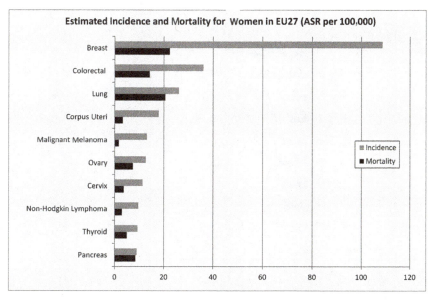

**FIGURE 19.2** Estimated incidence and mortality for women in EU27 (ASR per 100,000 individuals).

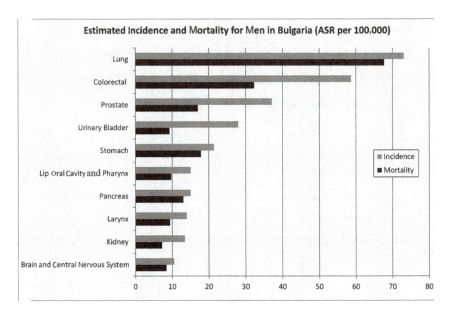

**FIGURE 19.3** Estimated incidence and mortality for men in Bulgaria (ASR per 100,000 individuals).

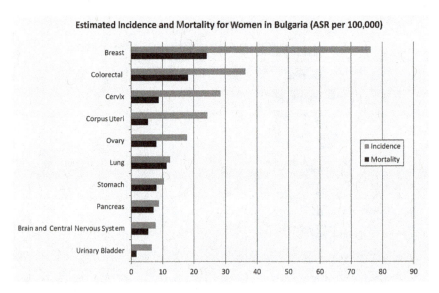

**FIGURE 19.4** Estimated incidence and mortality for women in Bulgaria (ASR per 100,000 individuals).

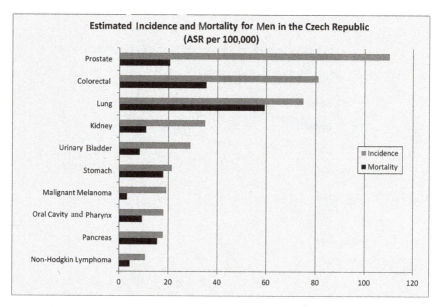

**FIGURE 19.5** Estimated incidence and mortality for men in the Czech Republic (ASR per 100,000).

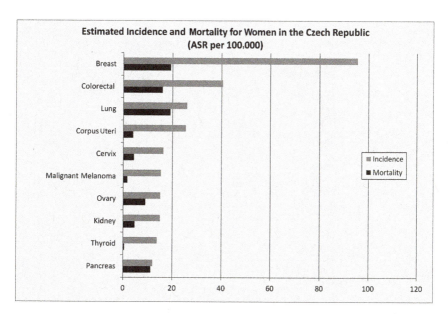

**FIGURE 19.6** Estimated incidence and mortality for women in the Czech Republic (ASR per 100,000).

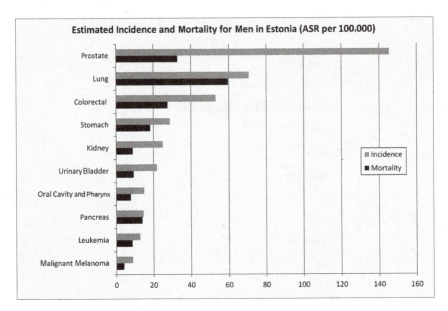

**FIGURE 19.7** Estimated incidence and mortality for men in Estonia (ASR per 100,000).

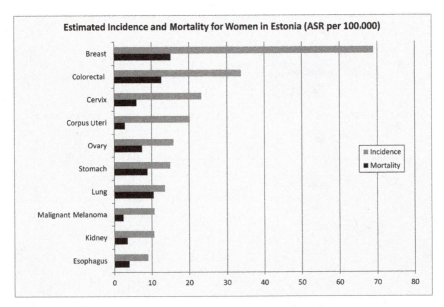

**FIGURE 19.8** Estimated incidence and mortality for women in Estonia (ASR per 100,000).

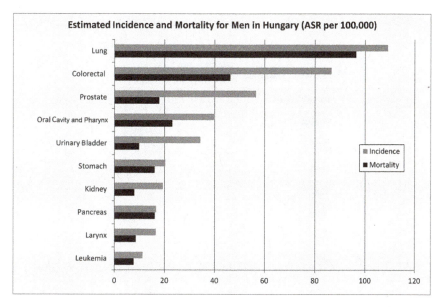

**FIGURE 19.9** Estimated incidence and mortality for men in Hungary (ASR per 100,000).

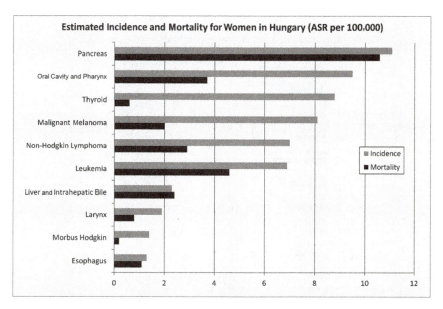

**FIGURE 19.10** Estimated incidence and mortality for women in Hungary (ASR per 100,000).

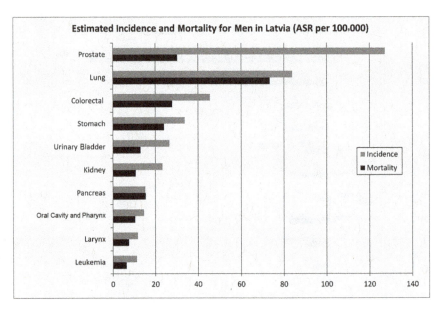

**FIGURE 19.11** Estimated incidence and mortality for men in Latvia (ASR per 100,000).

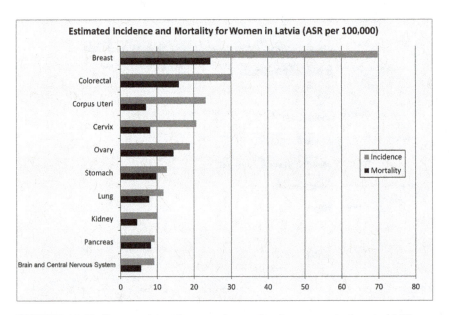

**FIGURE 19.12** Estimated incidence and mortality for women in Latvia (ASR per 100,000).

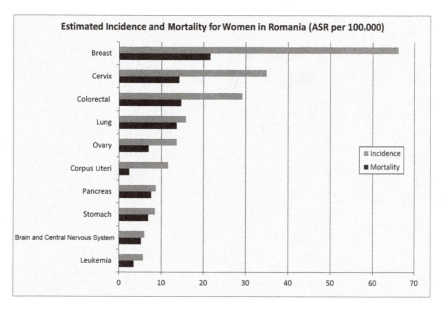

**FIGURE 19.13** Estimated incidence and mortality for women in Romania (ASR per 100,000).

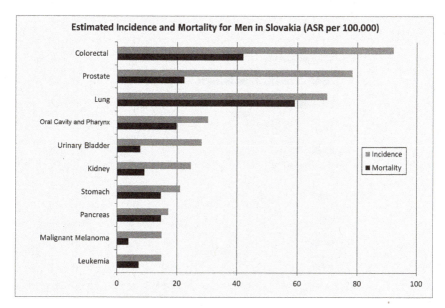

**FIGURE 19.14** Estimated incidence and mortality for men in Slovakia (ASR per 100,000).

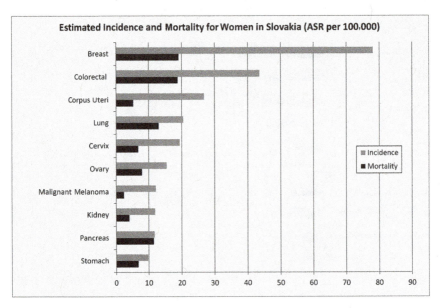

**FIGURE 19.15** Estimated incidence and mortality for women in Slovakia (ASR per 100,000).

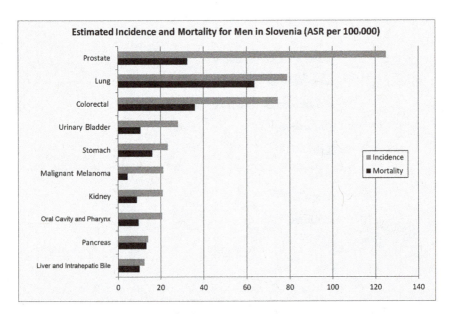

**FIGURE 19.16** Estimated incidence and mortality for men in Slovenia (ASR per 100,000).

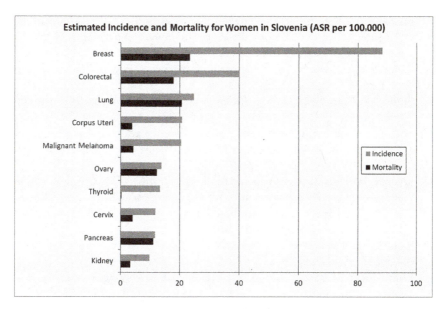

**FIGURE 19.17** Estimated incidence and mortality for women in Slovenia (ASR per 100,000).

## REFERENCES

1. Zatonski W. Closing the health gap in European Union. Warsaw: Cancer Epidemiology and Prevention Division, Maria Skłodowska-Curie Memorial Cancer Centre and Institute of Oncology, 2008. Available at http://www.hem.waw.pl/. Accessed August 30, 2011.
2. European health systems and cancer care. Closing the health gap in European Union. Executive Summary of Health Care Reform in Central and Eastern Europe: Setting the Stage for Discussion.
3. Novotny TE. HIV is not just a transitional problem. *BMJ* 2005; 331(7510): 219.
4. Quinn MJ, d'Onofrio A, Møller A, et al. Cancer mortality trends in the EU and acceding countries up to 2015. *Ann Oncol* 2003; 14: 1148–52.
5. Micheli A, Coebergh JW, Mugno E, et al. European health systems and cancer care. *Ann Oncol* 2003; 14(Suppl 5): v41–v60.
6. Pająk A, Kozela M. Cardiovascular disease in Central and East Europe. *Public Health Rev* 2012; 33(2): 416–35.
7. Allender S, Scarborough P, Peto V, et al. *European Cardiovascular Disease Statistics. 2008 Edition.* British Heart Foundation, 2008. Available at http://www.bhf.org.uk/publications/view-publication.aspx?ps=1001443.
8. World Health Organization Regional Office for Europe. European Health for All Database (HFA-DB). WHO Europe, 2011. Available at http://www.euro.who.int/en/what-we-do/data-and-evidence/databases/europeanhealth-for-all-database-hfa-db2 Accessed 23 April, 2012.

9. Global Status Report on Noncommunicable Diseases 2010. World Health Organization, Geneva, 2011. Available at http://www.who.int/nmh/publications/ncd_report2010/en/ Accessed Feb 7, 2012.

10. Zatonski WA, Bhala N. Changing trends of diseases in Eastern Europe: closing the gap. *Public Health* 2012; 126: 248–52.

11. Brown LM, Lipscomb J, Snyder C. The burden and cost of cancer. *Annu Rev Public Health* 2001; 22: 91–113.

12. Boyle P, d'Onofrio A, Maisonneuve P, et al. Measuring progress against cancer in Europe: has the 15% decline targeted for 2000 come about? *Ann Oncol* 2003; 14(8): 1312–25.

13. Zatonski W. Closing the health gap in European Union 2008. Available www.hem.waw.pl/export/download.php%3Ffn%3D0,92242A37hZ2.

14. Zatonski W, Boyle P. Commentary. Health transformations in Poland after 1988. *J Epid Biostatistics* 1996; 1(4): 183–97.

15. Zatonski W. The east-west health gap in Europe—what are the causes? *Eur J Public Heath* 2007; 17(2): 121.

16. Primic-Zakelj M, Zadnik V, Zagar T. Is cancer epidemiology different in Western Europe to that in Eastern Europe? *Ann Oncol* 2005; 16(Suppl 2): ii27–ii29.

17. Soerjomataram I, Lortet-Tieulent J, Parkin DM, et al. Global burden of cancer. *Lancet* 2012 Nov 24; 380(9856): 1840–50. doi:10.1016/S0140–6736(12)60919–2. Epub Oct 16, 2012.

18. Bray F, Tyczynski J, Parkin DM. Going up or coming down? The changing phases of the lung cancer epidemic from 1967 to 1999 in the 15 European Union countries. *Eur J Cancer* 2004; 40: 96–125.

19. Tyczynski J, Bray F, Aareleid T, et al. Lung cancer mortality patterns in selected central, eastern and southern European countries. *Int J Cancer* 2004; 109: 598–610.

20. Brennan P, Bray I. Recent trends and future directions for lung cancer mortality in Europe. *Br J Cancer* 2002; 87: 43–48.

21. Rechel B, Dubois CA, McKee M. The Health Care Workforce in Europe. Available at www.euro.who.int/document/e89156.pdf.

22. Vrdoljak E, Wojtukiewicz MZ, Pienkowski T, et al. Cancer epidemiology in Central and South Eastern European countries. *Croat Med J* 2011 Aug; 52(4): 478–87.

23. Murchiea P, Campbella NC, Delaney EK, et al. Comparing diagnostic delay in cancer: a crosssectional study in three European countries with primary care-led health care systems. *Fam Pract* 2012; 29: 69–78.

24. Verdecchia A, Baili P, Quaglia A et al. Patient survival for all cancers combined as indicator of cancer control in Europe. *Eur J Public Health* 2008; 18(5): 527–32.

25. Siegel R, DeSantis C, Virgo K, et al. Cancer treatment and survivorship statistics, 2012. *CA Cancer J Clin* 2012 July/Aug; 62(4): 220–41.

26. Hristova L, Dimova I, Iltcheva T. Projected cancer incidence rates in Bulgaria, 1968–2017. *Int J Epidemiol* 1997; 26: 469–75.

27. Bastos J, Peleteiro B, Gouveia J, Coleman MP, Lunet N. The state of the art of cancer control in 30 European countries in 2008. *Int J Cancer* 2010 Jun 1; 126(11): 2700–15.

28. Jozan PE, Prokhorkas R. *Atlas of Leading and Avoidable Causes of Death in Countries of Central and Eastern Europe.* Budapest: Hungarian Co. Publishing House, 1997, pp. 1–323.

29. Farkas I. A daganatos halalozas helyzete Magyarorszagon (Cancer mortality in Hungary, in Hungarian, English abstract). *Magyar Tudomany* 1994; 5: 524–39.

30. Holland JC. History of psycho-oncology: overcoming attitudinal and conceptual barriers. *Psychosom Med* 2002; 64(2): 206–21.

31. Grassi L, Holland JC, Johansen C, Koch U, Fawzy F. Psychiatric concomitants of cancer, screening procedures, and training of health-care professionals in oncology: the paradigms of psycho-oncology in the psychiatry field. In: Christodoulou GN (Ed). *Advances in Psychiatry,* vol II. Athens: World Psychiatric Association, 2005, pp. 59–66.

32. Plass A, Koch U. Participation of oncological outpatients in psychosocial support. *Psychooncology* 2001; 10(6): 511–20.

33. Fawzy FI. Psychosocial interventions for patients with cancer: what works and what doesn't. *Eur J Cancer* 1999; 35(11): 1559–64.

34. Fawzy FI, Fawzy NW. Group therapy in the cancer setting. *J Psychosom Res* 1998; 45(3): 191–200.

35. FAO. Food balance sheets. FAOSTAT data, 2005. Available at http://faostat .fao.org. Food and Agriculture Organizations of the United Nations, updated June 2010.

36. van Ballegooijen M, van den Akker-van Marle E, Patnick J, et al. Overview of important cervical cancer screening process values in European Union (EU) countries, and tentative predictions of the corresponding effectiveness and cost-effectiveness. *Eur J Cancer* 2000 Nov; 36(17): 2177–88.

37. Dokova KG, Stoeva KJ, Kirov PI, Feschieva NG, Petrova SP, Powles JW. Public understanding of the causes of high stroke risk in northeast Bulgaria. *Eur J Public Health* 2005; 15(3): 313–16.

38. Zatoński W. Tobacco smoking in central European countries: Poland. In: Boyle P, Gray, N, Henningfield J, Seffrin J, Zatoński W (Eds). *Tobacco and Public Health: Science and Policy.* Oxford: Oxford University Press, 2004, pp. 235–52.

39. Zatoński W, Campos H, Willett W. Rapid declines in coronary heart disease mortality in Eastern Europe are associated with increased consumption of oils rich in alpha-linolenic acid. *Eur J Epidemiol* 2008; 23(1): 3–10.

40. WHO. *The World Health Report 2004—Changing History.* Geneva: WHO, 2004.

41. Szucs S, Sarvary A, McKee M, Adany R. Could the high level of cirrhosis in Central and Eastern Europe be due partly to the quality of alcohol consumed? An exploratory investigation. *Addiction* 2005; 100: 536–42.

42. Popova S, Rehm J, Patra J, Zatonski W. Comparing alcohol consumption in Central and Eastern Europe to other European countries. *Alcohol Alcohol* 2007; 42: 465–73.

43. McKarns SC, Hansch C, Caldwell WS, Morgan WT, Moore SK, Doolittle DJ. Correlation between hydrophobicity of short-chain aliphatic alcohols and their ability to alter plasma membrane integrity. *Fundam Appl Toxicol* 1997; 36: 62–70.

44. Strubelt O, Deters M, Pentz R, Siegers CP, Younes M. The toxic and metabolic effects of 23 aliphatic alcohols in the isolated perfused rat liver. *Toxicol Sci* 1999; 49: 133–42.

45. Zatoński WA, Sulkowska U, Mańczuk M, et al. Liver cirrhosis mortality in Europe, with special attention to Central and Eastern Europe. *Eur Addict Res* 2010; 16: 193–201.

46. Vyzula R, Žaloudík J. *Cancer Prevention and Care in the Czech Republic.* Masaryk Memorial Cancer Institute Brno, Czech Republic. Available at www.cabrnoch .cz/media/RostislavVyzula15_9.pdf.

47. www.eolc-observatory.net.

48. Clark D, Wright M. *Transitions in End of Life Care: Hospice and Related Developments in Eastern Europe and Central Asia.* Buckingham: Open University Press, 2002.

49. http://www.healthobservatory.eu.

50. World Health Organization, mortality database. Available at http://www.who .int/healthinfo/statistics/mortality_rawdata/en/index.html. Accessed July 5, 2013.

51. The burden and cost of cancer. *Ann Oncol* 2007; 18(Suppl 3): iii8–iii22.

52. Sullivan R, Kowalczyk JR, Agarwal B, et al. New policies to address the global burden of childhood cancers. Available at www.thelancet.com/oncology. Published online February 20, 2013. http://dx.doi.org/10.1016/S1470-2045(13)70007-X.

53. United Nations, World Population Prospects, the 2010 Revision. Available at http://esa.un.org/unpd/wpp/index.htm.

54. Houweling TA, Kunst AE. Socio-economic inequalities in childhood mortality in low- and middle-income countries: a review of the international evidence. *Br Med Bull* 2010; 93: 7–26.

55. Kovács A, Döbrôssy L, Budai A, Cornides A, Boncz I. [The state of the organized screening in Hungary in 2006]. *Orv Hetil* 2007 Mar 11; 148(10): 435–40. Review. Hungarian.

56. Atun R, Ogawa T, Martin-Moreno JM. Analysis of National Cancer Control Programmes in Europe. Available at http://ideas.repec.org/p/imp/wpaper/4204.html.

57. Coleman MP, Quaresma M, Berrino F, et al. Cancer survival in five continents: a worldwide population-based study (CONCORD). *Lancet Oncol* 2008 Aug; 9(8):730–56.

58. Verdecchia A, Santaquilani M, Sant M. Survival for cancer patients in Europe. *Ann Ist Super Sanita* 2009; 45(3): 315–24.

59. Berrino F, De Angelis R, Sant M, et al. Survival for eight major cancers and all cancers combined for European adults diagnosed in 1995–99: results of the EUROCARE-4 study. *Lancet Oncol* 2007; 8(9): 773–83.

60. Databas-Eurocare. Available at http://www.eurocare.it/Database.

# 20

# Egypt

## Emad Shash and Mohamed Amgad

## PUBLIC HEALTH PERSPECTIVE

### Life Expectancy

The average life expectancy of Egyptians has increased over the past decade. In 2011, the life expectancy at birth was 73 years (71 for males, 75 for females), and the life expectancy at age 60 was 18 years (17 years for males, 20 years for females). In 1990, the average life expectancy at birth was only 63 years.[2]

### Communicable Diseases

The most important communicable disease causing a public health burden in Egypt is viral hepatitis.[3] Over 14,600 cases of hepatitis were reported in 2000, and the Egyptian Ministry of Health and Population set it as a priority to control the spread of the disease through its national 2008 to 2012 plan,[4] which showed some success. The other two major communicable disease burdens in Egypt are pulmonary tuberculosis and meningococcal meningitis. The number of reported cases of pulmonary tuberculosis and meningococcal meningitis in 2000 was 7,919 and 278, respectively. HIV/AIDS has a prevalence of only 0.03% among 15- to 49-year-olds. All of the diseases mentioned carry high mortality rates in Egypt. Malaria, while present in Egypt, is not considered a major public health burden. Poliomyelitis and diphtheria infections decreased dramatically due to the compulsory vaccination efforts and are now almost diminished in Egypt (polio has already been eradicated in Egypt since 2006). Prevalence of the endemic parasite *Schistosoma mansoni* and *Schistosoma haematobium* infections decreased from 14.5% and 5.4% in 1995 to 0.9% and 0.6% in 2007, respectively. Among preschool children, diarrhea and upper respiratory tract infections are the main communicable disease causes of mortality. Parasitic infestations, particularly schistosomiasis and ancylostoma, are also fairly prevalent among Egyptian children.[3,5]

## Noncommunicable Diseases

The most important causes of noncommunicable disease morbidity in Egypt are neuropsychiatric disorders (19.8%), digestive system diseases (11.5%), chronic respiratory diseases (6.9%), injuries (6.7%), and cardiovascular diseases (5.6%).[5]

## Cancer as a Public Health Problem

In 2012, more than 2,600 patients were admitted with malignant neoplasms to the Ministry of Health (MOH) hospitals and facilities.[1] The age-standardized mortality rate from cancer in 2011 was found to be 50.9 per 100,000 among males and 34.4 per 100,000 among females. That is, cancer caused more than 16,000 and 12,000 deaths among male and female Egyptians in 2011, respectively. The top causes of cancer mortality are breast, liver, lung, brain and CNS, leukemia, and bladder cancers. Among females, breast cancer is by far the comment cause of cancer mortality, and among males liver cancer takes the lead (Table 20.1).[6]

These numbers, no doubt, point to the magnitude of the problem. It should be noted that early morbidity and mortality is a burden to the state, depriving the working sector from potentially effective workforce. The economic burden of treatment and diagnosis, too, is significant. In 2012, for example, about 17,800 cancer patients were treated at the cost of the state (12.5% of all patients treated at state cost), at an average cost of 2,732 per patient.[1]

TABLE 20.1  Cancers That Cause the Highest Mortality among Egyptians, according to WHO IRAC 2011 Statistics

| Males | | | Females | | |
|---|---|---|---|---|---|
| Cancer Site | Age-Standardized Mortality Rate (per 100,000) | Rank | Cancer Site | Age-Standardized Mortality Rate (per 100,000) | Rank |
| Liver | 12.3 | 1 | Breast | 5.8 | 1 |
| Lung | 6.9 | 2 | Liver | 5.2 | 2 |
| Brain and CNS | 4.9 | 3 | Brain and CNS | 3.9 | 3 |
| Leukemia | 4.4 | 4 | Leukemia | 3.4 | 4 |
| Bladder | 4.5 | 5 | Lung | 2.8 | 5 |

## CANCER ETIOLOGY

The exact etiology of cancer formation is unknown. However, predisposing and triggering factors, whether genetic or environmental, are important determinants in cancer distribution and statistics. These affect the geographical distribution of cancers within Egypt. For example, an important study found significantly higher incidence of all cancers in urban areas and in men. Moreover, the study found that the cancer incidence varied significantly within a single governorate, possibly due to different environmental factors and exposures.[7]

## CANCER STATISTICS

The most common cancer subtypes in Egypt are breast cancer (especially infiltrating duct carcinoma and lobular carcinoma), bladder cancer (transitional cell carcinoma and squamous cell carcinoma), lymphoma (especially non-Hodgkin's lymphoma), liver cancer (especially hepatocellular carcinoma [HCC]), leukemia, colorectal cancer, and lung cancer. Among females and in both sexes combined, breast cancer far exceeds all other sites in terms of its incidence. Many of the features of Egypt's cancer profile are typical of developing countries, although some patterns are starting to emerge that indicate westernization in Egyptian cancer profile. Table 20.2 summarizes the top cancers among Egyptians.[8,9]

## HISTORY OF CANCER CARE

There were no specialized cancer care centers in Egypt before the National Cancer Institute (NCI); Cairo University was established in 1969. In 1975, the first MOH cancer center, Tanta Cancer Center, was established in the governorate of Gharbiyah. Landmarks in the history of cancer care in Egypt include the Egyptian account of schistosomiasis, the establishment of Egypt's first population-based registry, and the introduction of hepatitis B vaccine into the compulsory vaccination schedule, as which are explained in the following sections of this chapter.

## CANCER CARE INFRASTRUCTURE

Primary health care is readily available to the Egyptian population, and 95% of the population is within 5 km of a health facility. About 7.4% of the Egyptian government's expenditure is on health care, and the total expenditure on health as a percentage of Egypt's gross domestic product (GDP)

TABLE 20.2 The Most Common Cancers among Egyptians according to Egypt's Largest Hospital-Based Cancer Registry (NCI) 2004 Statistical Report,[9] as well as the Gharbiyah Population-Based Cancer Registry (GPCR) 1996 to 2001[8]

| | Males | | | | Females | | | | Combined | | | |
| | NCI 2004 | | GPCR 1996 to 2001 | | NCI 2004 | | GPCR 1996 to 2001 | | NCI 2004 | | GPCR 1996 to 2001 | |
| Site | Total Percentage | Rank | Total Percentage | Rank | Total Percentage | Rank | Total Percentage | Rank | Total Percentage | Rank | Total Percentage | Rank |
|---|---|---|---|---|---|---|---|---|---|---|---|---|
| Breast | – | – | 0.5 | – | 35.5 | 1 | 37.6 | 1 | 18.9 | 1 | 18.9 | 1 |
| Bladder | 15.1 | 1 | 16.1 | 1 | 4.6 | 4 | 4.0 | 5 | 9.7 | 2 | 10.1 | 3 |
| Lymphoma | 10.4 | 3 | 15.5 | 2 | 6.6 | 2 | 9.6 | 2 | 8.4 | 3 | 12.6 | 2 |
| Liver | 12.7 | 2 | 12.7 | 3 | 4.0 | 6 | 3.4 | 7 | 8.1 | 4 | 8.1 | 4 |
| Leukemia | 9.0 | 4 | 5.4 | 5 | 5.9 | 3 | 4.5 | 3 | 7.4 | 5 | 4.9 | 5 |
| Colorectal | 5.1 | 6 | 4.9 | 6 | 4.6 | 5 | 3.8 | 6 | 4.8 | 6 | 4.4 | 7 |
| Lungs | 5.9 | 5 | 7.0 | 4 | – | – | 2.4 | 10 | 3.6 | 8 | 4.7 | 6 |

in 2009 was 6.1%. About 2% of Egyptian national expenditure on health in 2009 came from external sources. The most important providers of external funds included the African Development Fund, the United States Agency for International Development, the Japanese Development Fund, and the World Bank.[5]

The MOH facilities, which include outpatient clinics and MOH hospitals throughout Egyptian governorates, are the most important source of free medical care in Egypt. Because MOH services are free of charge, their costs are provided by the Ministry of Finance in a decentralized manner. Besides free MOH services, there are two important health insurance programs in Egypt: the Health Insurance Organization (HIO) program and the Student Medical Insurance Program (SMIP). HIO is an insurance agency that was founded in 1964, which is funded by a compulsory payroll on all public pensioners and formal sector workers. Although the number of people benefiting from HIO increased over the years, its services remain far from covering the full population (only 45% of the population was covered by the program in 2009[5]) and are still limited to the formal sector. One of the odd things about the HIO is that its income from premiums is often less than its spending, which necessitates its receiving ad hoc subsidies from the Egyptian government. The SMIP was first started in 1993 and provides its services to enrolled students. SMIP funding comes from premiums paid by enrolled students (a small proportion of the funds) as well as other sources such as cigarette taxes and contributions from general revenue (most of the funds). Besides this, both the MOH and the Ministry of Education run a comparatively smaller number of specialized tertiary teaching hospitals. As with other MOH facilities, MOH teaching hospitals provide their services free of charge. Education Ministry Teaching Hospitals are University Hospitals that provide their services also to the general public free of charge. Compared to MOH teaching hospitals, Ministry of Education University Hospitals usually provide higher-quality medical care and receive higher government subsidies. Other health-care providers in Egypt include the Ministry of Defense hospitals, private clinics, and pharmacies. Table 20.3 summarizes the major outline of Egypt's health-care system.[10]

By 2008, Egypt had seven MOH-run specialized cancer centers (excluding specialized hospitals),[1] and in 2007, the total number of Co16 and Linear Accelerator radiotherapy devices in MOH facilities was 25 and 43, respectively.[11]

The largest specialized cancer care facility in Egypt is the NCI, which receives up to 70% to 80% of cancer patients in Egypt. The NCI contains 600 inpatient beds (which serve more than 12,000 patients a year) and receives more than 18,000 new patients a year.[12]

Other cancer care facilities in Egypt include tertiary university hospitals such as Kasr Al Ainy Hospital and recently charity-based hospitals such as the Children's Cancer Hospital Egypt, CCHE 57357, which contains over 180 inpatient beds. Just like the NCI, CCHE 57357 provides its services free

TABLE 20.3  List of the Most Important Health-Care Providers in Egypt[10]

| Health-Care Provider | Private or Public? | Fees |
|---|---|---|
| Ministry of Health facilities and services | Public | Free of charge or subsidized |
| Ministry of Health Teaching Hospitals | Public | Free of charge or subsidized |
| University Hospitals (Ministry of Education) | Public | Free of charge or subsidized. Some affiliated centers provide service at a nonsubsidized rate |
| Health Insurance Organization facilities | Public | Free to those covered by the program |
| Ministry of Defense Hospitals and similar health-care providers | Public | Variable |
| Private hospitals and clinics | Private | Fees vary depending on center and service provided |

of charge to all its patients. Currently, CCHE 57357 is building an extension to increase its capacity.[13]

## Cancer Care Disparities

In Egypt, there are disparities, both geographical and economic, in access to health care. To begin with, the HIO facilities are mostly found in urban areas and are available only to formal sector workers. The same is true for the SMIP, which is available only to students formally enrolled in schools, leaving out the poorest sectors of the population, which often drop out or do not enroll in school in the first place. Moreover, only the richer portion of the population can afford to go to private clinics, further increasing the gap between the rich and the poor in terms of health-care spending.[10]

Behavioral factors also contribute to such disparities. When different sectors of the population are asked to report on how they perceive their own health (i.e., general perception of health, activity restriction, and acute and chronic illness), the lower-income groups tend to report being better-off than the higher-income groups. That is of course paradoxical, since it is well known that the poorer sectors of the population have higher rates of illness. This paradox could be explained by lack of health awareness among the poorer sector and hence "less sensitivity" to illness.[14] This furthers the gap between the richer and the poorer sectors in terms of health-care spending. It also means that the poorer sectors are more likely to present at later stages of the disease, which may partially explain why large portions of Egyptian cancer patients get diagnosed at very late or terminal stages of the disease.[11]

## CANCER CARE WORKFORCE

In 2007, Egypt had only 560 radio oncologists and medical oncologists. Even though the data on Egyptian cancer workforce is scarce, it is known that there is a lack of sufficient numbers of specialist surgical oncologists, especially pediatric surgical oncologists. In Egypt, most of the cancer surgeries are performed by general surgeons and specialist surgeons such as neurosurgeons, without sufficient training in oncology.[11]

The Egyptian health-care workforce body has expanded significantly over the past decade. According to government reports, the number of MOH physicians, nurses, and pharmacists in 2012 per 10,000 was 8.0, 14.2, and 2.6, respectively. In 2004, the numbers were 6.3, 13.5, and 0.9.[1] It is important to realize that cancer care workforce includes the full spectrum of health-care workers, including general physicians who should be able to recognize the early signs of cancer and refer cancer patients effectively and appropriately. There have been reports showing deficient cancer knowledge among Egyptian physicians and medical students, and recommendations that cancer rotations get incorporated into the medical school curricula of Egypt and other developing countries.[15]

## CANCER CLINICAL CARE

The diagnostic and therapeutic care profile in Egypt is similar to that of developing countries. Oftentimes, clinical examination alone is substituted for expensive imaging or histopathology tests. Although this substitution may indeed be necessary in some settings due to funding constraints, it is important that national guidelines are set to standardize care.

In the following sections, we discuss the most important cancers in Egypt and analyze some of the factors involved in their high incidence and their implications on clinical cancer care.

### Breast Cancer

Breast cancer is the leading malignancy in females in Egypt. The age-standardized incidence rate of breast cancer in Egypt is 49.6 per 100,000. The most common tumor histology is infiltrative duct carcinoma and lobular carcinoma. It is particularly prevalent among the younger age groups; the age-standardized incidence rate of breast cancer among 20- to 24, 25- to 29, 30- to 34, and 35- to 39-year-old Egyptian females is 1.4, 9.8, 28.9, and 63.6 per 100,000, respectively. These values are among the highest in the world.[8] The reasons for this trend are not entirely clear. It is possible that different environmental factors acting on the younger generation lead to this. It may also be true that the delayed age of marriage (late age of first birth), smaller number of children, and declining breastfeeding (as more women in the younger generation join the workforce) is responsible for this trend.

Given these factors, it is clear why breast cancer care, whether therapeutic or preventive, has received increasing attention over the past decade. One of the important challenges facing breast cancer care in Egypt is late stage at first presentation, leading to reduced effectiveness of therapy and higher morbidity and mortality rates.[16] Several studies have been performed to assess the reasons behind delayed presentation. Among the most important reasons is the lack of health awareness among Egyptian women regarding the early warning signs of breast cancer and the importance of early consultation. In fact, as much as 85% of Egyptian women were found to have insufficient knowledge about the disease in some studies.[17] This essentially means that when a palpable breast mass develops, it is often missed.

Nevertheless, the Egyptian health-care system, too, is responsible and takes part of the blame. It was found that Egyptian women whose first consultation about worrisome symptoms was with a primary-care physician, a general surgeon, or a gynecologist were significantly likely to experience a delay in referral to Tanta Cancer Center than those who first consulted with a surgical oncologist. Moreover, the percentage of patients referred to Tanta Cancer Center was higher among women who consulted with a surgical oncologist.[18]

This sheds light on some of the issues that need to be fixed regarding the Egyptian health-care system. First of all, referral policies and integration of health-care services need improvement. Second, Continuing Medical Education (CME) of primary-care physicians and general surgeons should receive a higher priority. Indeed, CME is known to be a weak point in Egypt.[19]

## Liver Cancer

Liver cancer, particularly HCC, is a major health burden in Egypt, which ranks in the 90th percentile worldwide in terms of its liver cancer incidence.[20] The age-standardized incidence rate of liver cancer in Egypt is 12.8 per 100,000 (20.6 among males, 5.2 among females), with a male-to-female ratio of 3.8:1. Liver cancer is predominant in males presumably due to higher exposure to hepatitis C virus (HCV).[8]

The reason for these worrisome figures lies largely behind the extremely high prevalence of viral hepatitis C among the Egyptian population; the prevalence of hepatitis C in Egypt is a staggering 15%;[21] 93% of anti-HCV-positive Egyptians are found to be infected with Genotype 4 (Genotype 4a alone constitutes about 63% of hepatitis C genotypes) and are thus less responsive to interferon therapy.[22,23]

The high prevalence of viral hepatitis B and C has been largely attributed to iatrogenic transmission of infection, both historically and now.[24]

### *Schistosomiasis: A Tale of Two Cancers*

During the 1960s and 1970s the Egyptian authorities organized a national campaign to treat schistosomiasis. *Schistosoma*, the causative agent of schistosomiasis, is a parasite whose life cycle includes snail vectors in non-salty water, which is why the Nile River provided a good medium for schistosomiasis to become endemic in Egypt since ancient times. In fact, ancient Egyptians recognized schistosomiasis and even described the use of antimony in its treatment. Two major types of *Schistosoma* exist: *S. mansoni*, which causes hepatic periportal fibrosis, and *S. haematobium*, responsible for the development of Schistosoma-associated bladder cancer (SABC).

Unfortunately, the nationwide campaigns of parenteral anti-schistosomiasis treatment (i.e., before oral praziquantel was developed) did not involve effective infection control measures, and the campaigns were responsible for spreading viral hepatitis through improperly sterilized needles. Indeed, about 29.6% of HCV-positive patients received parenteral anti-schistosomiasis treatment, and a significant correlation was found between the degree of exposure to parenteral anti-schistosomiasis treatment and seroprevalence of anti-HCV antibodies.[21,25]

Being responsible for two of Egypt's main health concerns (i.e., liver fibrosis and failure and bladder cancer), it is clear why the Egyptian authorities saw it as a matter of importance to treat and control the spread of this parasite.

Environmental factors, particularly aflatoxins, have also been attributed to the high prevalence of liver cancer in Egypt[26] and have been shown to contaminate more than 20% of silage, due to improper grain storage.[27] The role of aflatoxins and other environmental factors in liver cancer highlights the importance of collaboration between different governmental sectors (in this case, the agricultural sector and the health sector) in facing national health concerns in Egypt.

### Bladder Cancer

Egypt has a very high prevalence of bladder cancer compared to other countries; in 1987, Egypt was ranked the top worldwide in terms of its bladder cancer mortality (age-specific mortality rate of 10.8 per 100,000 in males).[28] The age-standardized incidence rate of bladder cancer in Egypt is 16.6 per 100,000. Male predominance is noted in bladder cancer rates in Egypt, with an age-standardized incidence rate of 27.5 per 100,000 among males (in contrast to 6.3 per 100,000 in females), presumably due to higher rates of schistosomiasis haematobium among male farmers who get more exposed to the Nile water. While the most common bladder carcinoma subtype worldwide is transitional cell carcinoma (TCC), in Egypt squamous cell carcinoma (SCC) of the bladder is also common; SCC is more malignant and required more aggressive treatment than TCC. The age-standardized incidence rates of TCC and SCC in Egypt are 9.3 and 3.7 per 100,000, respectively.[8] The reason behind this trend lies in the endemic parasite: *S. haematobium*, as has been mentioned earlier. SABC is so different from ordinary bladder carcinoma that it is often regarded as a separate subtype of bladder cancers altogether. The eggs of *S. haematobium* trigger a chronic inflammatory response in the bladder, leading to what is known as "sandy patches." It is this chronic wear-and-tear process that leads to the release of various carcinogenic compounds. It should be noted, however, that a latent period of 20 to 30 years exists between the peak of schistosomal infestation and SABC. This explains why the age-standardized incidence rate is highest among 40- to 59-year-olds (42% of cases), while schistosomal peak is during the thirties. As mentioned earlier, Egypt has been largely successful in controlling schistosomiasis, and indeed there is an emerging trend whereby the proportion of SABC is decreasing relative to TCC. That is to say, Egypt is becoming increasingly westernized in terms of its bladder carcinoma subtypes.[8]

The levels of smoking among the Egyptian population are thought to be increasing. As is the case with lung cancer, smoking is a major risk factor for bladder carcinoma, and its prevalence could explain why bladder cancer remains to be among the top killers in Egypt.[29]

## Lung Cancer

The age-standardized incidence rate of lung cancer among Egyptians is 7.7 per 100,000 (11.9 among males, 3.7 among females).[8] As with most countries, the incidence of lung cancer in Egyptian males is higher than that in females, presumably due to the higher prevalence of smoking among males. The most important risk factor for developing lung cancer is tobacco smoking, and the most common forms of tobacco smoking in Egypt are cigarette smoking and water pipe smoking. Water pipe smoking imposes a lower risk of developing lung cancer compared to cigarette smoking.[30]

One trend reported by the MEEC report is that the age-standardized incidence rates of lung cancer showed a shift toward the younger generations. It was presumed that this shift reflected the increasing levels of smoking among younger generations in MEEC countries, although the absence of accurate data on smoking prevalence in Egypt over the past years prevented the confirmation of this hypothesis. Another important factor for lung cancer is exposure to asbestos, which acts synergistically with cigarette smoking to increase the risk of lung cancer.[31]

One peculiar finding about lung cancer in Egypt is the high proportion of large-cell carcinoma (25.6%). The reasons behind this are not clear; perhaps it stems from different environmental exposures or genetic factors. Future studies are needed to elucidate this further.[8]

## Colorectal Cancer

The age-standardized incidence rate of colorectal cancer in Egypt is 5.5 per 100,000 (6.1 among males, 4.9 among females). Colorectal cancer patterns in Egypt resemble those of developing countries, with a high proportion of rectal cancer (37.2%), such that colon-to-rectal cancer ratio is low.[32,33]

One of the interesting patterns of colorectal cancer in Egypt is that it has a relatively high prevalence among younger age groups, particularly those under 40. The age-standardized incidence rate for the age group under 40 years is 1.3 per 100,000, which is in contrast to the United States, for example. Several hypotheses have been put forward to explain this pattern. First, this pattern may reflect a changing dietary style of the younger generation, shifting to more "westernized" foods and incorporating less fruits and vegetables in their meals. Another possible explanation is that younger age groups in Egypt tend to be more exposed to environmental carcinogens, since they constitute the larger part of the workforce. Indeed, it has been found that Egyptians living in urban areas had a higher chance of developing colorectal cancer than those living in rural areas. This fact highlights the role of environmental factors (e.g., industrial pollution) and may support the aforementioned explanation for colorectal cancer incidence among the younger age groups. It may also be the case that this pattern has some genetic underpinnings, though this hypothesis has not been well supported by empirical evidence. Another peculiar pattern is the very low rate of polyps among Egyptian colorectal cancer patients. Over 97% of colorectal cancers in Gharbiyah have no polyps. This absence could be explained by dietary factors (i.e., a diet rich in fibers). Another potential explanation is the prevalence of self-medication among Egyptians, leading to high levels of intake of aspirin and aspirin-like medications, which are known to decrease polyp formation.[8,32]

## Lymphoma and Leukemia

Egypt has very high rates of lymphoma. The age-standardized incidence of lymphoma in Egypt is 16.3 per 100,000 (20.0 among males, 12.6 among females). Non-Hodgkin's lymphoma (NHL) is particularly common, and the percentage of nodal NHL is quite high (age-standardized incidence of NHL is 14.2 per 100,000; 75% of which is nodal). Leukemia in Egypt has an incidence of 6.0 per 100,000 (6.7 among males, 5.3 among females), and the most common type is chronic lymphocytic leukemia, with an incidence of 1.3 per 100,000.[8]

These rates are among the highest in the world, and thus attention is needed to explain this finding. Linking this to lymphoma-inducing viruses could provide an explanation. Examples include Epstein–Barr virus,[34] human T-cell lymphotropic virus,[35] HCV,[36] and arguably less relevant in the Egyptian context, human immunodeficiency virus (HIV).[37] HCV, as explained before, has a very high prevalence among Egyptians and could indeed be the key to understanding the abnormally high rates of NHL. Indeed, HCV has been statistically correlated with NHL in some studies on Egyptians.[38]

Chemotherapy plays a critical role in the treatment of lymphoma and leukemia, and the high incidence and mortality of these cancers among Egyptians highlights the importance of establishing a comprehensive list of essential medicines in oncology. Moreover, it stresses the importance of health-care equity and the essentiality of expanding Egypt's health insurance coverage, as chemotherapy could be very expensive and time consuming.[11]

## Childhood Cancer

As is the case in other countries, childhood cancer is relatively rare in Egypt, with an age-standardized incidence rate of 130.9 per 100,000 (150.3 in males, 110.7 in females). The most common cancers diagnosed among Egyptian children are summarized in Table 20.4. Childhood lymphoma is especially high among Egyptians and constitutes a high proportion of all childhood malignancies in Egypt (more than half of all male childhood cancers and nearly one-fifth of all female childhood cancers). This situation deserves attention and calls for careful investigation, in order to outline the factors

TABLE 20.4 The Most Common Childhood Cancers among Egyptians, according to the Gharbiyah Population-Based Cancer Registry Data between 1996 and 2001[8]

| Site | Males | | Females | | Combined | |
|---|---|---|---|---|---|---|
| | Total Percentage | Rank | Total Percentage | Rank | Total Percentage | Rank |
| Lymphoma and reticuloendothelial neoplasms | 56.7 | 1 | 17.7 | 3 | 37.7 | 1 |
| Leukemia | 33.6 | 2 | 30.2 | 1 | 31.9 | 2 |
| CNS and miscellaneous intracranial and intraspinal neoplasms | 15.7 | 3 | 18.1 | 2 | 16.9 | 3 |
| Sympathetic nervous system tumors | 11.8 | 4 | 7.0 | 5 | 9.5 | 4 |
| Malignant bone tumors | 8.0 | 6 | 9.3 | 4 | 8.6 | 5 |
| Soft tissue sarcomas | 9.0 | 5 | 6.7 | 6 | 7.9 | 6 |
| Renal tumors | 4.4 | 7 | 6.4 | 7 | 5.4 | 7 |

(whether genetic or environmental) responsible and hint at more customized chemotherapeutic options. A specialized charity-based pediatric cancer hospital, CCHE 57357, started working in July 2007. CCHE 57357 is a good example of how public awareness about health matters lead to the creation of the largest children's cancer hospital facility in the world. Children's cancer care in Egypt still needs improvement, as the number of specialized pediatric oncology facilities is not large enough to cover the needs of the population.

## Other Sites

Other important cancers among Egyptians include those of the female genital system (especially the ovary), prostate, and nervous system; their age-standardized incidence rates are 0.3, 0.3, and 0.2 per 100,000, respectively.[8] Factors governing ovarian cancer distribution are reproduction related and are mostly similar to those affecting breast cancer. It is expected that, as the population distribution shifts to a more developed outline, the incidence of prostate cancer among Egyptians will increase.

## CANCER CARE OUTCOMES

According to official government reports, the death rate of cases admitted with malignant neoplasms to MOH facilities was 1.1%.[1] The overall mortality rate at the Cairo NCI is 4.2%.[12] A surprisingly few number of studies analyze the mortality and survival statistics in Egypt. The importance of having good mortality and survival statistics cannot be overstressed. A study published in 1999 found that Egypt had higher mortality rates from liver and bladder cancers than the United States and confirmed earlier observations about the higher rates of early-onset rectal and breast cancers.[39]

Mortality data published by the WHO IARC showed that mortality due to cancer has increased over the past period (2000 to 2011) among both males and females and in almost all age groups.[6] This increase was most marked among people above 70 years (Figure 20.1). Mortality from leukemia, liver, lung, brain and CNS, and prostate cancers has increased over the same time period. One notable finding is that the age-specific mortality of bladder cancer decreased among *most* age groups and among both genders over the period 2000 to 2011 (Figure 20.2). This change is probably a result of better clinical care as well as the shifting bladder cancer subtype to TCC, which tends to be less aggressive than the schistosoma-associated SCCs.

While mortality statistics are an important indicator of the quality of cancer care, they should always be interpreted in the context of the incidence rate and stage of presentation when medical care was first sought. In other words, a particular cancer subtype could have high mortality because it

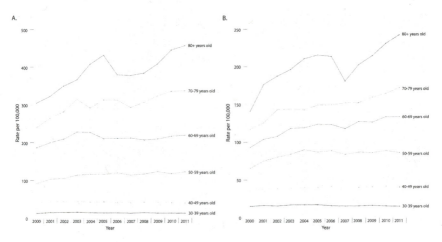

**FIGURES 20.1** Age-standardized mortality rates from cancer among (A) males and (B) females in Egypt (2000 to 2011) (reference 6).

simply has a high incidence, because of the nature of the tumor itself or because medical care was sought after the disease progressed to advanced stages. Therefore, the mortality statistics presented in Table 20.1 and Figures 20.1 and 20.2 should be interpreted with caution.

## CANCER CARE CONTINUUM

### Prevention

Two important lessons can be learned from the Egyptian experience with schistosomiasis control. First, although it is very important to implement public health screening and control programs, it is equally important to plan these programs very well and to keep in mind the risks involved. The Egyptian schistosomiasis experience, for example, provides a screaming example of large-scale iatrogenic transmission of infection. The second lesson that can be learned is that successful public health control programs can have a dramatic impact on the health profiles of the countries in which they are implemented. Just like the Western experience with PAP smear screening for cervical cancer, the Egyptian schistosomiasis prevention and control measures were largely successful in reducing the health burden imposed by the parasite. This reduction reflected most dramatically in the bladder cancer subtypes in the Egyptian population.[8]

Egypt has taken important steps so far in the fight against schistosomiasis, thereby effectively reducing SABC levels. Unfortunately, other factors counterbalanced this positive effort. In the case of bladder cancer, rising levels

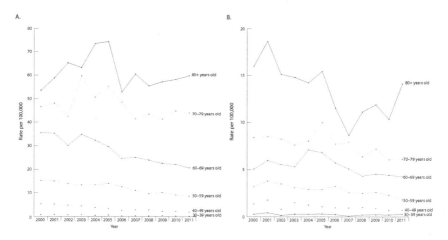

**FIGURE 20.2** Age-standardized mortality rates from bladder cancer among (A) males and (B) females in Egypt (2000 to 2011) (reference 6).

of smoking continue to keep bladder cancer among the top killers of male Egyptians.

Among people older than 15 years, the prevalence of smoking is 35% and 1.6% among Egyptian males and females, respectively.[40] It is therefore imperative that concentrated efforts be put in reducing the smoking levels among Egyptians via antismoking campaigns, higher taxes on cigarettes, prohibition of the sale of cigarettes to minors, and indoor smoking. The last two are already in the Egyptian law but are rarely enforced. The prevalence of obesity (body mass index ≥ 25) is 52.5% among Egyptian males and 67.8% among females.[41] Obesity, just like smoking, is among the important modifiable risk factors that ought to be reduced among Egyptians through public health awareness campaigns in schools and hospitals and via mass media. Hopefully, by reducing smoking and obesity levels, lung, liver, bladder, breast, ovarian, and other cancer incidence rates could be reduced.

The lack of appropriate infection control measures in Egyptian hospitals sustains Egypt's epidemic of viral hepatitis and, consequently, liver cancer. It is a top priority that Egyptian hospitals need to adhere to very strict guidelines regarding blood transfusion and any procedure involving blood access, and it is equally important that the MOH enforce these guidelines and deal sternly with any breach to them, that is, of course, besides the awareness campaigns that ought to be conducted nationwide about these issues. On the bright side, hepatitis B vaccine is on Egypt's compulsory vaccination list, and 95% of children got vaccinated in 2012.[1] While less attention is drawn to hepatitis B levels in Egypt, it is presumed that this high vaccination level marginalized HBV's role in Egypt's liver cancer in relation to HCV.

## Screening

While screening tests are available for cancers of the breast, oral cavity, colon, cervix, and prostate, the cost-effectiveness of such screening programs is highly dependent on the prevalence of these cancers in, and the economic status of, individual countries.[11]

The cost-effectiveness of a population-wide breast cancer screening program in Egypt is questionable, that is, because of the relatively low incidence rate of breast cancer in the Egyptian population. Instead, it may be argued that financial resources should be focused toward early detection of the disease. On the other hand, the type of screening program used is also an important factor affecting the cost-effectiveness of a population-wide screening program. A study published in 2010 among women in Dakahlia rural province in Egypt concluded that while a full-blown mammography-based screening program may be cost ineffective, a clinical breast assessment-based screening program with selective mammography *was* cost effective.[42]

Several initiatives have been launched to extend the outreach of breast cancer early detection among Egyptians. The most prominent ones are the BCFE (Breast Cancer Foundation in Egypt) programs and the WHOP (Women Health Outreach Program). Both programs offer free mammograms and subsidized or free treatment. WHOP was awarded the United Nations Public Service Award in 2011; its most important feature, mobile breast cancer screening units, helped extend the outreach to sectors of the Egyptian population generally not reached otherwise.

PAP smear screening for cervical cancer is arguably cost ineffective, given the relatively low rates of cervical cancer among Egyptian females compared to Western countries. Moreover, the new HPV vaccine, which was released in 2007, is very expensive, and it is unlikely that it can be incorporated into Egypt's compulsory vaccination schedule any time soon. The same could be said about colon or prostate cancer screening programs.[11]

## Psychosocial Care, Palliative Care, and Hospice

Palliative care is one aspect of cancer care that is highly dependent on national health policies and cultural factors. In 1981, Egypt's largest cancer care facility, the NCI, established a "pain clinic" for providing pain killers and opioid analgesia to terminal cancer patients. NCI's pain clinic was established as part of the department of anesthesiology, but now the NCI has, in addition, a 24/7 outpatient pain clinic. More recently, the Kasr Al Ainy Cancer Center also established a pain clinic in 2007, and so did the Children's Cancer Hospital 57357.[43,44]

Egypt's average consumption of narcotics during the period 2007 to 2009 was 49 S-DDD (sold-defined daily doses) per million inhabitants per day. This figure is very low compared with other countries; it ranks 112th. Egypt's consumption of benzodiazepines, which are used to relieve the anxiety often associated with terminal cancer, is also very low, about 2 S-DDD per million inhabitants per day.[45] This problem needs to be addressed since palliative care, just like curative care, is among the basic human rights.[46]

Several reasons could lie behind Egypt's low consumption of narcotic drugs. To begin with, Egypt lacks a national palliative care program. Moreover, injectable morphine is not available in all hospitals. Whereas injectable morphine is on the Egyptian essential drug list, oral morphine is not. Moreover, oral morphine is not available in all tertiary hospitals and is available only in some pharmacies. Lack of palliative care knowledge among physicians could also be a contributing factor. Indeed, only a few undergraduate medical programs in Egypt include pain management as part of the educational program.[43]

So far, Egypt contains very few hospice facilities, including that of the Cairo Evangelical Medical Society (started in 2001) and the Elhadra Elromany hospice in Alexandria.[43] Needless to say, more hospice facilities need to be established in Egypt in the future since many Egyptian cancer patients get diagnosed at advanced stages of the disease, making end-of-life care on the same level of importance as therapeutic cancer care.[11]

As mentioned earlier, palliative care is highly culture dependent. In fact, the same could be said about psychosocial care for cancer patients in general. The Egyptian population is composed of Sunni Muslims (the great majority), Christians (the largest minority), and other religious minorities. Nevertheless, the response of Egyptian patients and families to cancer (especially late-stage cancer) is rather similar. It is not uncommon in Egyptian culture that the patient is not told about his or her diagnosis while all the relatives know about it. This is especially true for terminal cancer patients. What gives way to this is the general lack of health awareness and the high levels of illiteracy among the elder Egyptian population (adult literacy rate in Egypt in 2009 was 71.4%[5]). Needless to say, it is this elderly age group that constitutes the larger sector of cancer patients.

This lack of disclosure of diagnosis to the patient (and the breach of patient privacy by telling the relatives) may be seen as a major flaw in the enforcement of medical ethics via strict laws. On the other hand, it could be argued that culture plays an important role in determining what we consider to be moral standards. In the Islamic culture, for example, death is often more accepted than in Western cultures, as it is generally believed that life and death matters are predetermined by God. That being said, approximately

73% of dying cancer patients spend their last hours in their homes beside their relatives rather than at cancer care facilities.[47] Given the earlier-mentioned knowledge about the Islamic conception of life and death, it should not be surprising that euthanasia (also known as "mercy killing") is forbidden by the Egyptian law and is generally considered an unacceptable practice among Egyptian families.

## CANCER RESEARCH

According to UNESCO 2010 Science Report, Egypt's Gross Domestic Expenditure on Research and Development as a fraction of GDP was only 0.23% in 2007. This is very low in comparison to developed countries such as the United Kingdom, where the fraction is 1.82%. Nearly 4,000 scientific publications were produced from Egypt in 2008, placing it in the top position among Arab countries, but in a very modest position worldwide. In fact, the number of publications *per million population* was 48.6, placing Egypt in a very low position even among Arab countries.[48]

Most of Egyptian research institutions are owned by the government and 90% of research activity is government funded. Foreign sources account for 10% of research funding in Egypt, and the role of production firms and private funds is almost negligible! This is in striking contrast with developed countries such as the United States or Japan, where production firms and private funds account for 59% and 81% of the total research funds, respectively. One of the paradoxes about research expenditure in Egypt is that higher education staff (including university professors and researchers) receive a very low proportion of national research spending despite forming over 70% of Egypt's research personnel. In 1996/1997, this proportion was as low as 0.3%. Without a doubt, the national research budget needs to increase and so does the spending on the higher education sector.[49]

A number of hospital-based cancer registries are available in Egypt, including the National Cancer Institute in Cairo, Alexandria Cancer Registry, and the Cancer Registry of MOH Cancer Centers. The largest hospital-based cancer registry in Egypt is the NCI. The NCI cancer registry was first established in 2001, over 30 years after the institution was first established.[9] The problem with hospital-based cancer registries is that they cannot be used to gain accurate incidence and prevalence data about populations. That is, they are liable to reporting bias and it would be difficult to judge their representativeness of the whole population. It is for this reason that the Gharbiyah Population-Based Cancer Registry (GPCR) was established in 1998 as the first (and so far the only) population-based cancer registry in Egypt. The Gharbiyah governorate lies about 90 km north of Cairo and has a population of about 3.4 million residents. GPCR collects data from three main cancer hospitals: Tanta Cancer Center, Tanta University Hospital, and Gharbiyah Cancer Society Hospital. In addition, it collects data from all cancer care centers and laboratories, whether private or public in Gharbiyah, as well as data on Gharbiyah patients receiving care at the NCI Cairo.[8] The data gathered by GPCR could be argued to be representative of the Egyptian populations since (1) the population of Gharbiyah has an age structure equivalent to Egypt's overall age structure and has a male-to-female ratio of 1.02:1 and (2) GPCR covers over 90% of the population of Gharbiyah.[1,8]

GPCR was established as part of the Middle East Cancer Consortium (MECC) efforts to gain accurate cancer epidemiology data about its member states. MECC is one of the very encouraging examples of regional cooperation between different countries for a common cause, in this case the establishment of high-quality, countrywide cancer statistics. MECC was first established in 1996, and current members include Egypt, Cyprus, The Palestinian Authority, Israel, and Jordan. One of the main advantages of this regional cooperation effort is that it set standards for the reporting of cancer data of its member countries, and made sure that the data is registered in such a way to make it comparable among all members, thus giving way to better analysis of the different factors affecting cancer epidemiology across member countries.[8]

## FUTURE DIRECTIONS

Cancer care in Egypt is far from optimum, and there are numerous opportunities for growth and improvement. It is of utmost importance that the fraction of the national budget allocated to health care increase and that cancer, specifically, be given a higher priority by future Egyptian policy makers.

It is important that a more comprehensive population-based cancer registry be established and that this registry cover a higher proportion of the Egyptian population. Currently, Egypt's National Cancer Registry is being established. Egypt's National Cancer Registry is population based and includes the governorates of Aswan, Menia, Sinai, and Matrouh. Its data is going to be linked with GPCR and NCI central registry data to establish national estimates. Only through large and comprehensive databases like these could informative decisions be taken.

All aspects of cancer care need improvement in Egypt, including prevention, screening, treatment, research, palliative care, and hospice.

As with most countries around the world, breast cancer continues to be the top killer among cancers in females. Egypt has taken an important step by introducing mobile breast cancer screening programs, yet it remains important that the culture of breast self-examination gets spread among Egyptian females. No matter how good the screening programs are, without breast self-examination, the likelihood of missing the disease in its earlier stages remains higher. It is simply inevitable that health awareness is the greatest first-line defense against all cancers, and there is plenty of room for improvement for Egypt in that area.

It is also important that some of the deepest convictions and misconceptions about cancer and cancer care get corrected. Having cancer is not necessarily equivalent to a death sentence, as is often perceived by the general population. Nor does the availability of narcotic analgesics for terminal cancer pain management necessarily threaten to increase addiction levels. Egyptian future policy makers need to increase the number of hospice facilities and the availability of end-of-life care for dying patients.

## REFERENCES

1. Central Agency for Public Mobilisation and Statistics (Capmas). *2013 Electronic Statistical Yearbook*, 2013. Available at http://www.capmas.gov.eg/book.aspx. Accessed September 14, 2013.

2. World Health Organization. World Health Observatory Data Repository: Life Expectancy. Available at http://apps.who.int/gho/data/node.main.688?lang=en. Accessed September 10, 2013.

3. Food and Agriculture Organization of the United Nations. The Double Burden of Malnutrition: Case Studies from Six Developing Countries, 2006. pp. 77–91. Available at ftp://ftp.fao.org/docrep/fao/009/a0442e/a0442e00.pdf. Accessed September 10, 2013.

4. National Committee for the Control of Viral Hepatitis: Ministry of Health and Population. Egyptian National Control Strategy for Viral Hepatitis 2008–2012, 2008.

5. World Health Organization. Country Cooperation Strategy: Egypt, 2009. Available at http://www.who.int/countryfocus/cooperation_strategy/ccsbrief_egy_en.pdf. Accessed September 10, 2013.

6. Number of cancer deaths: World Health Organization, mortality database. Available at http://www.who.int/healthinfo/statistics/mortality_rawdata/en/index.html. Accessed July 5, 2013). Demographic data: United Nations, World Population Prospects, the 2010 Revision. Available at http://esa.un.org/unpd/wpp/index.htm.

7. Dey S, Zhang Z, Hablas A, et al. Geographic patterns of cancer in the population-based registry of Egypt: possible links to environmental exposures. *Cancer Epidemiol* 2011; 35: 254–64.

8. Freedman LS, Edwards BK, Ries LAG, Young JL (Eds). *Cancer Incidence in Four Member Countries (Cyprus, Egypt, Israel and Jordan) of the Middle East Cancer Consortium (MECC) Compared with US SEER*. Bethesda, MD: National Cancer Institute, 2006. NIH Pub. No. 06–5873.

9. Department of Biostatistics and Epidemiology of the National Cancer Institute Cairo University. Statistical Report for NCI, 2004,2005. Available at http://www.nci.cu.edu.eg/lectures/NCI2004.ppt. Accessed September 14, 2013.

10. Rannan-Eliya RP, Blanco-Vidal C, Nandakumar AK. The Distribution of Health-care Resources in Egypt: Implications for Equity. An Analysis Using a National Health Accounts Framework. Harvard School of Public Health. Available at http://www.hsph.harvard.edu/ihsg/publications/pdf/No-81.PDF. Accessed September 8, 2013.

11. World Health Organization. Towards a Strategy for Cancer Prevention and Control in the Eastern Mediterranean Region. Intercountry Meeting on the Adoption of the Regional Cancer Control Strategy, December 15–18, 2008. Available at http://www.emro.who.int/dsaf/dsa1002.pdf.

12. National Cancer Institute Cairo University. Administrative and Statistical Report for NCI, 2002–2010. Available at http://www.nci.cu.edu.eg/lectures/NCI adminst.pdf.

13. Children's Cancer Hospital Egypt (CCHE) 57357 website. Available at http://beta.57357.com/category/about/.

14. Caldwell J, Gajanayake I, Caldwell P, Peiris I. Sensitization to illness and the risk of death: an explanation for Sri Lanka's approach to good health for all. *Soc Sci Med* 1989; 28: 365–79.

15. Amgad M, Shash E, Gaafar R. Cancer education for medical students in developing countries: where do we stand and how to improve? *Crit Rev Oncol/Hematol* 2012; 84: 122–29.

16. El-Bolkainy M. *Topographic Pathology of Cancer*. 2nd ed. Cairo: National Cancer Institute, Cairo University, 2000, p. 87.

17. Allam MF, Abd Elaziz KM. Evaluation of the level of knowledge of Egyptian women of breast cancer and its risk factors. A cross sectional study. *J Prev Med Hyg* 2012; 53: 195–98.

18. Mousa SM, Seifeldin IA, Hablas A, Elbana ES, Soliman AS. Patterns of seeking medical care among Egyptian breast cancer patients: relationship to late-stage presentation. *Breast* (Edinburgh, Scotland) 2011; 20: 555–61.

19. Soliman AS, Raouf AA, Chamberlain RM. Knowledge of, attitudes toward, and barriers to cancer control and screening among primary care physicians in Egypt: the need for postgraduate medical education. *J Cancer Educ* 1997; 12: 100–107.

20. Parkin D, Whelan S, Ferlay J, Teppo L (Eds). *Cancer Incidence in Five Continents*, vol VIII. IARC Scientific Publication No. 155. Lyon (France): International Agency for Research on Cancer, 2002.

21. El-Zanaty F, Way A. *Egypt Demographic and Health Survey, 2008*. Cairo, Egypt: Ministry of Health and Population, 2009.

22. Ray SC, Arthur RR, Carella A, Bukh J, Thomas DL. Genetic epidemiology of hepatitis C virus throughout Egypt. *J Infect Dis* 2000; 182: 698–707.

23. Abdel-Hamid M, El-Daly M, Molnegren V, et al. Genetic diversity in hepatitis C virus in Egypt and possible association with hepatocellular carcinoma. *J Gen Virol* 2007; 88: 1526–31.

24. Sievert W, Altraif I, Razavi HA, et al. A systematic review of hepatitis C virus epidemiology in Asia, Australia and Egypt. *Liver Int* 2011; 31(Suppl 2): 61–80.

25. Frank C, Mohamed MK, Strickland GT, et al. The role of parenteral antischistosomal therapy in the spread of hepatitis C virus in Egypt. *Lancet* 2000; 355: 887–91.

26. Abdel-Wahab M, Mostafa M, Sabry M, El-Farrash M, Yousef T. Aflatoxins as a risk factor for hepatocellular carcinoma in Egypt, Mansoura Gastroenterology Center study. *Hepatogastroenterology* 2008; 55: 1754–59.

27. El-Shanawany AA, Mostafa ME, Barakat A. Fungal populations and mycotoxins in silage in Assiut and Sohag governorates in Egypt, with a special reference to characteristic Aspergilli toxins. *Mycopathologia* 2005; 159: 281–89.

28. Schistosomes, Liver Flukes and Helicobacter pylori. IARC Working Group on the Evaluation of Carcinogenic Risks to Humans. Lyon, 7–14 June 1994. *IARC Monographs on the Evaluation of Carcinogenic Risks to Humans/World Health Organization, International Agency for Research on Cancer* 1994; 61: 1–241.

29. Chu H, Wang M, Zhang Z. Bladder cancer epidemiology and genetic susceptibility. *J Biomed Res* 2013; 27: 170–78.

30. Blot W, Fraumeni JJ. Cancers of the lung and pleura. In: Schottenfeld D, Fraumeni JF Jr (Eds). *Cancer Epidemiology and Prevention.* 2nd ed. New York: Oxford University Press, 1996, pp. 637–65.

31. Berry G, Newhouse ML, Antonis P. Combined effect of asbestos and smoking on mortality from lung cancer and mesothelioma in factory workers. *Br J Ind Med* 1985; 42: 12–18.

32. Veruttipong D, Soliman AS, Gilbert SF, et al. Age distribution, polyps and rectal cancer in the Egyptian population-based cancer registry. *World J Gastroenterol* 2012; 18: 3997–4003.

33. Parkin DM, Bray F, Ferlay J, Pisani P. Global cancer statistics, 2002. *CA Cancer J Clin* 2005; 55: 74–108.

34. Grywalska E, Markowicz J, Grabarczyk P, Pasiarski M, Roliński J. Epstein-Barr virus-associated lymphoproliferative disorders. *Postępy Hig Med Dosw* (Online) 2013; 67: 481–90.

35. Gallo RC. Research and discovery of the first human cancer virus, HTLV-1. *Best Pract Res. Clin Haematol* 2011; 24: 559–65.

36. Zignego AL, Giannini C, Gragnani L. HCV and lymphoproliferation. *Clin Dev Immunol* 2012; 2012: 980942.

37. Martis N, Mounier N. Hodgkin lymphoma in patients with HIV infection: a review. *Curr Hematol Malig Rep* 2012; 7: 228–34.

38. Cowgill KD, Loffredo CA, Eissa SA, et al. Case-control study of non-Hodgkin's lymphoma and hepatitis C virus infection in Egypt. *Int J Epidemiol* 2004; 33, 1034–39.

39. Soliman AS, Bondy ML, Raouf AA, Makram MA, Johnston DA, Levin B. Cancer mortality in Menofeia, Egypt: comparison with US mortality rates. *Cancer Causes Control* 1999; 10: 349–54.

40. World Health Organization. *WHO Report on the Global Tobacco Epidemic 2008. The MPOWER Package*, Geneva, 2008.

41. World Health Organization WHO Global Infobase. Available at https://apps .who.int/infobase/CountryProfiles.aspx.

42. Denewer A, Hussein O, Farouk O, Elnahas W, Khater A, El-Saed A. Cost-effectiveness of clinical breast assessment-based screening in rural Egypt. *World J Surg* 2010; 34: 2204–10.

43. Silbermann M, Arnaout M, Daher M, et al. Palliative cancer care in Middle Eastern countries: accomplishments and challenges. *Ann Oncol* 2012; 23(Suppl 3): 15–28.

44. ElShami M. Palliative care: concepts, needs, and challenges: perspectives on the experience at the Children's Cancer Hospital in Egypt. *J Pediatr Hematol/Oncol* 2011; 33(Suppl 1): S54–S55.

45. United Nations. Report of the International Narcotics Control Board on the Availability of Internationally Controlled Drugs: Ensuring Adequate Access for Medical and Scientific Purposes. 2010 Report, 2011.

46. Human Rights Watch. Global State of Pain Treatment: Access to Palliative Care as a Human Right, 2011.

47. Alsirafy SA, El Mesidy SM, Abou-Elela EN. Where do Egyptian palliative care patients with cancer die? *Am J Hosp Palliat Care* 2010; 27: 313–15.

48. Badran A, Zou'bi MR. Arab States: UNESCO Science Report 2010, pp. 251–77, 2010. Available at http://www.unesco.org/new/fileadmin/MULTIMEDIA/HQ /SC/pdf/sc_usr10_arab_states_EN.pdf.

49. Korayem K. Chapter 4: The research environment in Egypt. Research for Development in the Middle East and North Africa. Available at http://archive.idrc .ca/books/focus/930/15koraye.html.

# 21

# Honduras

## José A. Sánchez

## PUBLIC HEALTH PERSPECTIVE

Honduras has three health-care systems working independently. First, the public health-care system is under the Ministry of Health or "Secretary," which includes all state hospitals and handles 60% of the general population, where assistance is free of charge. Second, El Instituto Hondureño de Seguridad Social (IHSS) provides medical care to people who are employed in private companies or in the government. The patient pays a low-cost insurance, and this system attends to 15% of the population. Finally, in the private practice system (which handles 10% of population) the patient or the family pays 100% of the costs for medical fees, diagnostics procedures, and treatment options; 15% of the population has no access to any health-care system.

Though most people are taken care by the state public system, this is an archaic, inefficient, and corrupt system, which does not meet the population's health demands. It does not provide adequate response to the problems pertaining to radiology diagnoses and treatments because this system is outdated and inefficient because of lack of equipment and personnel, and medications are scarce, especially in the diagnosis and treatment of cancer.

### Life Expectancy

Life expectancy at birth is 70.6 years for men and 77.8 years for women, taking into account the population of 8,385,072 for 2012.

The average number of children per woman is 3.2. Infant mortality rate is 23.5 per 1,000 for boys and 19.2 per 1,000 for girls.

### Communicable Diseases

Vaccination programs on polio, measles, pertussis, and tetanus have achieved control of these diseases; however, infections remain important cause of morbidity and mortality, especially diseases such as HIV/AIDS and pulmonary tuberculosis.

Honduras has limited statistics and does not have a National Information System. This nonavailability makes it difficult to acquire details about some health problems, such as cancer.

Some diseases are considered a priority in terms of control; these diseases include chicken pox, hepatitis A, diarrhea, strep throat, pneumonia, bronchitis, asthma, malaria, syphilis, and HIV/AIDS.

## Noncommunicable Diseases

### Cancer as a Public Health Problem

Although cancer is a health problem worldwide, it is an uncontrolled one in developing countries; currently 7.6 million people die annually worldwide from cancer, with an estimated 4.8 million in developing countries alone.

The Ministry of Health had a national strategic plan to control cancer as a health problem, but this did not reach the targets set for 2013.

No studies have been conducted regarding the impact of cancer in society, in family structure, or in economical production.

Most cases of cancer occur in economically active but unemployed women, causing an economical burden to the family, because state hospitals do not provide adequate care. In many instances, patients and their families have to buy medicines or pay for laboratory tests, images, and biopsies, and because most of the population lives in poverty, cancer leads them to extreme poverty, creating a vicious circle of poverty-disease-poverty, which could lead to family breakdown and social problems.

## CANCER ETIOLOGY

Cancer etiology has not been studied in Honduras; however, some studies on papillomavirus and its relation to cervical cancer are available. Others have related stomach cancer with *Helicobacter pylori*. In general, the etiology of cancer in Honduras remains unknown.

## CANCER IN HONDURAS

### Cancer Statistics

The incidence of cancer worldwide continues to increase. Observations dating back over 20 years in Honduras show that the number of cases increases every year, and in the Main Referral Hospital for Cancer, the number of cases increased yearly. According to the International Agency for Cancer Research, Globocan 2008 estimated 8,923 new cases with a mortality of

5,723 people, representing 64% of incident cases; the reason for high mortality is that most cases are detected only in advanced clinical stages.

According to Globocan, the cancers with the highest incidence are prostate, cervical, stomach, breast, liver, uterine body, lung, colorectal, leukemia, and central nervous system tumors, as shown in Figure 21.1.

According to the health secretary of Honduras, cancer is more common in women than in men. In 2010, 5,083 new cases were reported, representing a total rate of 63.2 cases per 100,000 people, 71.5 per 100,000 for women and 54.6 per 100,000 for men.

The main types of cancers in men are leukemia, stomach, lung, and prostate cancers. For women, the main types are uterus, breast, stomach, thyroid, and ovary cancers.

The statistics vary because the National Registry of Cancer is under development and sub-registry is as high as 40%.

The incidence and mortality of the three most common cancers in men, prostate, stomach, and liver, and women, cervix, stomach, and breast, are given in Table 21.1.

## Cancer in Hospital General San Felipe

Hospital General San Felipe (HGSF) in Tegucigalpa is the main referral center for cancer in Honduras; Data from the national cancer program reveals that

**Estimated Age-Standardized Incidence and Mortality Rates: Both Sexes**

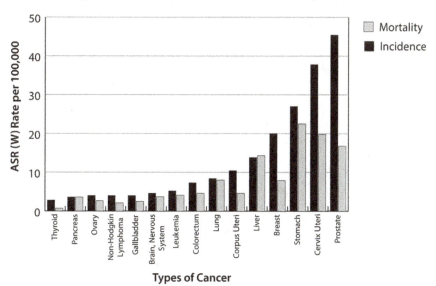

**FIGURE 21.1** Estimated age-standardized incidence and mortality rates: both sexes (Globocan 2008).

TABLE 21.1A  Incidence and Mortality of the Most Common Cancer in Men in
            Honduras

|          | Incidence | Mortality |
|----------|-----------|-----------|
| Prostate | 983       | 395       |
| Stomach  | 701       | 585       |
| Liver    | 350       | 347       |

GLOBOCAN 2008.

TABLE 21.1B  Incidence and Mortality of the Most Common Cancer in Women
            in Honduras

|         | Incidence | Mortality |
|---------|-----------|-----------|
| Cervix  | 1,014     | 490       |
| Stomach | 544       | 474       |
| Breast  | 487       | 182       |

GLOBOCAN 2008.

the number of cancer cases increases gradually. This data however is not entirely reliable, because the National Cancer Program, with support from the Pan American Health Organization, conducted a diagnosis identifying a sub-register of cases. A total of 1,763 new cases were identified in 2010, as shown in Figure 21.2; in the same year, over 13,000 hospital discharges due to cancer took place.

In HGSF, cancer is more common in women than in men; with a ratio of 3:1; around 70% of cases are women. The ratio of the frequency has been stable through the years; this stability is mainly due to the incidence of cervical cancer. The age group most affected is 40 to 54 years, but all population groups are affected, as shown in Figure 21.3.

Of the cases treated in HGSF from 2009 to 2011, cervical cancer remained the most frequent in women, but the incidence of breast cancer and thyroid increased progressively. In men, gastric cancer remained the most frequent.

The cancer statistics in Honduras are confusing because no proper National Registry of Cancer is available, but it is clear that the incidence of cancer increases every year.

## History of Cancer Care

On July 31, 1861, the government issued the decree to build The Hospital Tegucigalpa, which later became the Hospital General San Felipe, inaugurated on June 6, 1926, accommodating 285 beds.

In 1952, the Blood Bank was inaugurated, and in 1957 the first oncology service was created, introducing radiotherapy using radium and cobalt in 1961. In 1975, chemotherapy was introduced as an alternative treatment.

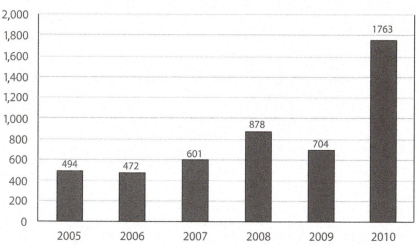

**FIGURE 21.2** Hospital Registry of Cancer: Hospital General San Felipe, 2005 to 2010.

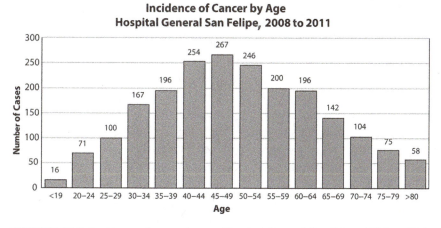

**FIGURE 21.3** Incidence of cancer by age: Hospital General San Felipe, 2008 to 2011.

In 1979, El Hospital Escuela was inaugurated in Tegucigalpa, and the staff members working in the HGSF, including the Department of Pathology and Service of Oncology, were transferred to the new hospital to provide medical and surgical oncology treatment.

Oncology staff in HGSF continued delivering service, patients' demands grew, and in 1984, the Department of Oncology was created. In 2000, the second cobalt 60 unit was established, and in 2007, a plan with the intention of converting the Department of Oncology at the National Cancer Center was created but is still in development.

## Cancer Care Infrastructure

Most patients suffering from cancer in Honduras are treated in HGSF, Hospital Escuela in Tegucigalpa, and Hospital Mario Catarino Rivas in San Pedro Sula. These are general hospitals with oncology departments; however, no hospitals dedicated exclusively to cancer's treatment exist.

A small portion of patients is treated in the hospital of the IHSS in Tegucigalpa and San Pedro Sula, and a smaller part of the population is treated in private clinics.

Currently, the Department of Oncology at HGSF is the largest in the country. It consists of 72 beds, for the services of medical oncology, surgical oncology, and radiotherapy, which together serve more than 12,000 patients and more than 2,000 discharges every year. The hospital has seven surgical oncologists, three radiotherapists, two medical oncologists, two gyneco-oncologists, and one hematologist, but no nurses specialized in oncology.

HGSF offers the only oncology-teaching program in the country, which is a surgical oncology program. With the help of Health Volunteers Overseas and the American Society of Clinical Oncology, this program has become a valuable aid for cancer education in Honduras.

The Hospital Escuela provides care through one hematologist and one surgical oncologist, and the Social Security Hospital provides care through three surgical oncologists, one medical oncologist, one hematologist, and one palliative care doctor.

Two private cancer clinics are functioning in Tegucigalpa: one provides care in medical oncology, surgery, and radiation therapy based on cobalt, and the other operates the only linear accelerator for cancer treatment in Tegucigalpa.

In San Pedro Sula, medical, surgical, and pediatric oncology services are provided in Hospital Mario Catarino Rivas for the general population, whereas two private cancer centers provide care in medical oncology and radiotherapy using cobalt, and another private center provides clinical oncology and radiotherapy using a linear accelerator.

## Cancer Care Workforce

The health secretary has developed a national strategic plan for cancer control, whose overall objectives are to reduce the incidence of cancer, to reduce mortality, and to improve the quality of life of patients and their family community through specific objectives, which include prevention, monitoring, treatment, and cancer research.

This plan has identified problems to be solved, including limited human resources, inadequate infrastructure, poor support services, obsolete radiotherapy equipment, limited availability of surgical equipment, lack of basic drugs, rehabilitation systems and palliative care, and no concrete treatment guidelines.

This plan was developed for the years from 2008 to 2013, but progress has been minimal.

## Clinical Cancer Care

No specialized units exist to handle specific forms of cancer such as breast, prostate, lymphoma, stomach, cervix, and colon. These diseases are managed in the context of general oncology, under individual care rather than institutional guidelines; there are no mandatory protocols or systematic research in the practice of oncology.

## Childhood Cancer

Cancer in children in Honduras has been increasing each year; in general, the treatment is performed at the Department of Pediatric Oncology at Hospital Escuela in Tegucigalpa. The incidence in children under 15 years is 12.7 per 100,000 individuals, and the population under 15 years corresponds to 39.1% of the total.

The reported cases up to 2009 can be observed in Figure 21.4, which shows a gradual increase yearly. The decline of cases in 2009 is probably due to the political and social crisis experienced by the country in that year.

The Department of Pediatric Oncology serves as a model in terms of organization and development for oncology in Honduras; it has specific physical areas, adequate hospitalization services, and outpatient clinics. It provides cancer care through specialized personnel in the areas of medical and surgical care, nursing, psychology, infectious diseases, epidemiology, data managers, pharmacy, radiology, and pathology, which, although not ideal, meet the minimum number necessary to overcome the challenges of pediatric cancer.

The most common cancers affecting children are acute lymphoblastic leukemia, Hodgkin's and non-Hodgkin's lymphomas, acute myelogenous leukemia, and central nervous system tumors, as shown in Table 21.2.

This department has chemotherapy, surgery, and radiotherapy with a cobalt unit elite 100 and works with management's protocols for most types of cancer. It is in collaboration with international institutions such as the

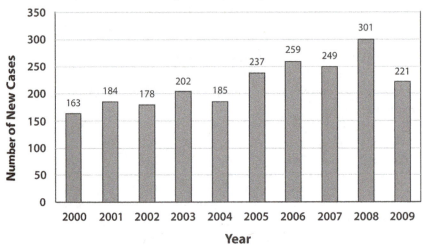

**FIGURE 21.4** Incidence of new cases in pediatric oncology: Hospital Escuela, 2000 to 2009.

**TABLE 21.2** Types of Most Frequent Cancer in Pediatric Oncology Hospital Escuela

| Diagnosis | 2000 | 2001 | 2002 | 2003 | 2004 | 2005 | 2006 | 2007 | 2008 | Total |
|---|---|---|---|---|---|---|---|---|---|---|
| Acute lymphoblastic leukemia | 69 | 64 | 69 | 71 | 74 | 88 | 96 | 95 | 101 | 727 |
| Hodgkin's lymphoma | 18 | 15 | 14 | 21 | 16 | 15 | 33 | 27 | 29 | 188 |
| Acute myeloblastic leukemia | 10 | 14 | 18 | 19 | 9 | 10 | 18 | 13 | 28 | 139 |
| Central nervous system tumors | 4 | 8 | 10 | 8 | 10 | 20 | 22 | 22 | 31 | 135 |
| Non-Hodgkin's lymphoma | 9 | 17 | 10 | 12 | 12 | 11 | 10 | 10 | 15 | 106 |
| Wilms' tumor | 8 | 10 | 6 | 8 | 8 | 19 | 11 | 8 | 7 | 85 |
| Retinoblastoma | 4 | 12 | 11 | 12 | 14 | 9 | 8 | 9 | 6 | 85 |
| Various | 2 | 11 | 6 | 5 | 5 | 10 | 16 | 14 | 12 | 81 |
| Germinal cell tumors | 4 | 4 | 10 | 8 | 5 | 8 | 5 | 9 | 14 | 67 |
| Rhabdomyosarcoma | 2 | 12 | 4 | 6 | 4 | 10 | 6 | 8 | 13 | 65 |

Hospital Saint Judes, International Union Against Cancer, Ontario Pediatric Society of Canada, and other national organizations such as Childhood Cancer Foundation, the Social Security Institute of Honduras, and The National Children's Society.

One of the problems in the management of pediatric cancer is the abandonment of treatment, which has traditionally been around 30%; however, the department has recently created peripheral clinics in different cities, including San Pedro Sula. This measure is expected to reduce the treatment abandonment to 6%.

Although work has been excellent, it still needs staff, pathological diagnosis, and availability of blood products, antibiotics, and chemotherapy agents.

## CANCER CARE OUTCOMES

There is no systematic way to bring the results of therapeutic interventions, as there are no standards for reporting results of response or survival, so the response or survival rates of different types of cancers in Honduras are unknown.

## CANCER CARE CONTINUUM

### Prevention

No systematic programs or specific interventions within cancer prevention are available in Honduras; however, recently an antismoking law, which limits the purchase and use of tobacco, was implemented in Honduras.

### Screening

Cervical cancer is the only cancer that has a screening program through Pap smear, which is available in all public hospitals; however, this facility failed to decrease the incidence and prevalence of the disease.

### Psychosocial Care

Counseling is available in reference centers, especially in pediatrics. However, the staff is limited and attendance is poor; in fact, the importance given to psychological care to the patient or his or her family is minimal. In some hospitals, like HGSF, most patients are not satisfied with the quality of medical care.

## CANCER RESEARCH

No systematic cancer research exists; publications are limited based on individual studies. There are also no institutions or groups dedicated to cancer research, nor ethics committee available in centers with research potential.

## FUTURE DIRECTION

The incidence of cancer in Honduras, as in the developing countries, continues to rise. The population is increasing, and cancer is complicated to control in terms of prevention, screening, diagnosis, treatment, and research. Problems are not solved because of a lack of financial resources, and it is unlikely that Honduras will be able to control cancer in the next few years. There is an urgent need to implement educational actions, as education is the most powerful low-cost tool available to control cancer. Education must be imparted by nurses, oncologists, surgeons, radiotherapists, medical students, and patients; in addition, research must be stimulated at all levels, and collaboration with international institutions becomes vital to implement strong educational programs.

Particular topics that must be addressed are as follows:

1. Developing a tumor registry nationwide, through staff training, implementing technology, and creating an information network to report all cancer cases from each hospital in the country
2. Establishing programs for prevention and control of the most common cancers in Honduras
3. Implementing education in nursing and medical schools
4. Strengthening the surgical oncology program and developing the programs on hematology and medical oncology
5. Conducting and promoting research
6. Creating the National Cancer Institute or the National Reference Cancer Center.
7. Modernizing existing infrastructure and creating new spaces regarding medical oncology, surgical oncology, and radiotherapy
8. Creating regional centers that allow the management of cancer for all regions of the country
9. Collaborating with international institutions such as HVO, ASCO, PAHO, WHO, and UICC
10. Creating ethics committees in each center where oncology is practiced

## REFERENCES

1. National Statistics Institute. INE 2012 Honduras CA. Available at www.INE, gob.hn.
2. Health Secretary. Department of Population Risks, address health promotion. National Program for Cancer Control, Dr. Rosa Duarte 2010.
3. National Strategic Plan for the Prevention and Control of Cancer 2009—2013, National Program for Cancer Control, Ministry of Health, Honduras, PAHO. PENCC.
4. Globocan 2008.

5. Figueroa M, Ferrera A, Barahona O, et al. Infecciones con virus papiloma en mujeres con cáncer de cuello uterino y sus controles. *Itzamná* (OPS) 1994; 1: 6–10.

6. Tábora N, Bulnes R, Toro LA, et al. Human papillomavirus infection in Honduran women with cervical dysplasia or cervical cancer. *J Low Genit Tract Dis* 2011; 15: 48–53.

7. Ferrera A, Velema JP, Figueroa M, et al. Human papillomavirus infection, cervical dysplasia and invasive cervical cancer in Honduras: a case-control study. *Int J Cancer* 1999; 82(6): 799–803.

8. Morgan DR, Dunn RL, Keku TO, et al. Gastric cancer and the high combination prevalence of host cytokine genotypes and Helicobacter pylori in Honduras. Clin Gastroenterol Hepatol 2006 Sep; 4(9): 1103–11. Epub Jul 3, 2006. PMID: 16820326 [PubMed—indexed for MEDLINE]

9. Porras C, Nodora J, Sexton R, et al. Epidemiology of Helicobacter pylori infection in six Latin American countries (SWOG Trial S0701). *Cancer Causes Control* 2012 Dec 12 [Epub ahead of print].

10. Sanchez JA, Castillo MA, Guzman OA, et al. Frecuencia de enfermedades neoplasica en familiars de pacientes con cancer. *Rev Medica Hondureña* 2005: 73: 114–21.

11. World Health Organization. Country Cooperation Strategy at a Glance. Available at www.whoint/countryfocus/cooperation_strategy/ccsbriefe_hnd_en.pdf.

12. Sanchez JA, Duarte F, Mojica R. Estado actual, prevencion y manejo del cancer en Honduras. *Rev Medica Hondureña* 1992; 60: 171–77.

13. Hospital General San Felipe. Cancer Registry, Secretaria de salud publica, programa nacional de cancer. Dra. Rosa Maria Duarte, 2012.

14. Globocan country fast sta-Globocan 2008 IARC.

15. Magazine: Health for all, N 8, March 1987. Ministry of Public Health. R. Bulnes, P. Zelaya.

16. Armando Peña Chief of Pediatric Oncology Department, Hospital Escuela, Tegucigalpa Honduras, 2013. Personal communication.

17. Ley especial para el control del tabao. Decreto N. 92–2010. La Gaceta. Diario oficila de la republica de Honduras. Sabado 21 de Agosto del 2010: A1–A12.

18. José Ángel Sánchez N, Cruz Zuniga AM, Rubio JRB, et al. Cancer patient satisfaction with medical care received at the General Hospital and Teaching Hospital San Felipe. *J Faculty Med Sci* 2009; 9: 1.

# 22

# India

## *Rohit Jain and Rutika Mehta*

## LIFE EXPECTANCY

According to the latest WHO data, life expectancy in India for males is 64 years and for females, is 67 years; total life expectancy is 65 years. India ranks 138th in life expectancy ranking among the countries of the world.

## HEALTH CARE IN INDIA

For a population of over 1.2 billion, the health-care spending of the gross domestic product is as low as 4%. The health-care system is split between public and private sectors, as in many developing countries. Interestingly, there is a far higher contribution from the private sector in health-care spending as compared to the public sector (78% vs. 20%), implying that Indian health care witnesses a large proportion of out-of-pocket pay for health. This fact accentuates health-care inequalities and delivery of appropriate care. Although most of the population is middle and upper class that live in urban areas and have access to health care, a significant proportion of population (ca. 69%) still lives in rural areas that have limited resources. After the Insurance Regulatory and Development Act was enacted in 2000, several companies in the market have begun to offer medical insurances, although most of these are in the public sector. Although it is good to see a growing number of medical insurance companies, insurance is still a commodity of rarity and availed by a minority of the population. A statement in the report of the National Commission on Macroeconomics and Health of India is that as few as 3% to 5% of Indians are covered by health insurance policies.

In addition to allopathic medicine, a mix of other traditional medicinal systems such as homeopathic, ayurveda, unani, and other folk medicine is in use. About 25% of the population in India has access to allopathic medicine, and most of this is available in the urban areas. The private sector has a network of hospitals in the urban areas because of health-care awareness and interest in investment, which is available to most of the affluent urban dwellers. Though 70% of the Indian population lives in rural areas, only 2% of the physicians are available in these areas. Access to health care becomes a challenge for such nonurban population and even if they travel to the major cities, high out-of-pocket expenditure is a major shortcoming. Rural areas are predominated by treatments such as folk remedies.

The population with health-care insurance is a minority, and most of them are within the organized labor sector. Moreover, the coverage in majority of these schemes is for primary health care, whereas secondary and tertiary care is limited, especially for surgical procedures.

For several years, the primary health concern in India has been sanitation and the resulting diseases. Although India has been able to achieve certain goals of providing clean drinking water for a large proportion of population, 814 million people are still without improved sanitation.

## COMMUNICABLE DISEASES

So far with government initiatives in public sector, there has been success in eradicating small pox and Guinea worm diseases from India. Polio is on the verge of being eradicated; leprosy, kala-azar, and filariasis are expected to be eliminated in the near future. Dengue, which was earlier limited to urban areas, is now prevalent in rural areas also. The malaria eradication program, which has been in place since the last 50 years, had initial success in controlling the disease; however, it is now becoming more widespread, with more reported deaths. Some diseases like plague, which was initially thought to be eradicated, have reemerged in recent years. The national tuberculosis control program established since 1962 has not been able to control the disease. Some of the reasons are unavailability of drugs and poor management, along with stigma of the disease, and incomplete treatment has led to the persistence of the disease. Approximately there are 2.2 million new cases every year. In pediatric population, diarrheal diseases and respiratory infections are the main killers of children below 5 years. The incidence of HIV/AIDS is increasing, with the current estimates being 3.86 million.[1]

## NONCOMMUNICABLE DISEASES

Noncommunicable diseases continue to be a major public health problem in India, accounting for major morbidity and mortality. The four leading causes are cardiovascular diseases, diabetes mellitus, chronic obstructive pulmonary disease, and cancer. Other noncommunicable diseases include stroke and accidents and injuries. Demographic changes, changes in lifestyle with sedentary work practices, and increased urbanization and industrialization are the major factors responsible for increase in these chronic diseases. In 2004, 40% of all in-hospital stays and 35% of all outpatient visits were due to non-communicable diseases.[2]

## CANCER ETIOLOGIES

Most of the causes of cancer are almost the same as in other parts of the world. Studies have shown that improper diet has been one of the major causes of colorectal cancer in India, especially high consumption of red meat. It has been postulated that during charcoal cooking, pyrolysates, which have carcinogenic effect, are produced.[3,4] Less consumption of fresh fruits and cooking foods on high temperature also deplete people of vitamin C, which increases the risk for various cancers.[5] On the other hand, the fact that the majority of Indian population practices vegetarianism, which includes beans, chickpeas, and lentils, has been associated with reductions in cancer.[6,7] Tobacco consumption is the leading cause of cancers in India. Tobacco consumption has been associated with oral cavity, pharynx, esophagus, larynx, lungs, and bladder cancers. It is usually consumed by smoking, chewing, snuffing, and so on. Most of the carcinogenic effects have been seen with the use of the unrefined form of tobacco used in India known as "bidi," which is a thin cigarette-type structure filled with tobacco flakes and wrapped in tendu leaf with a string at one end.[8] Studies have associated hookah smoking, which is a special cigar used in India using raw tobacco, with lung cancer.[9] In some states, consumption of betel, nut, pan masala, opium, and bhang (leaves and flower powder of female cannabis plant) has been associated with oral cancer.[10]

## CANCER STATISTICS IN INDIA

The International Agency for Research on Cancer estimated that over 6,00,000 people died of cancer in India in 2008, accounting for 6% deaths in India, which corresponds to 8% of cancer deaths worldwide.[11] Despite advancement in diagnosis and treatment, cancer yet remains the second most common disease after cardiovascular disorders, with the highest number of accountable deaths worldwide.[12] The Indian Council of Medical Research (ICMR) has published data on projection of prevalence rate of cancer and estimates that the number of cancer cases will increase from 9,79,786 in 2010 to 11,48,757 in 2020.[13] Majority of Indians live in rural areas, and yet most of the cancer mortality data is estimated from India's 24 urban population–based cancer registries and only 2 registries representing rural India.[14] Although ICMR projections for cancer cases in 2020 utilized the pooled data from the registries mentioned earlier, it could not adjust for the rural–urban differences at the country level.[13] Estimates in 2010 revealed that almost 70% cancer deaths in India were in the age group of 30 to 69 years and more specifically 8% deaths in males and 12.3% deaths in females also in this age group. The most common cancers in this age group were oral (22.9%), stomach (12.6%), and lung (11.4%) in males and cervical (17.1%), stomach (14.1%), breast (10.2%), and oral (9.8%) cancers in females. Tobacco-related cancers accounted for almost 20% cancer deaths in both sexes within this age group. Studies have failed to show an appreciable difference in the cancer mortality rates between urban and rural areas. However, illiteracy carried twice as much as the risk for cancer mortality than literacy.

Cancer accounts for 1.6% to 4.8% of all diseases in Indians below the age of 15 years. In comparison, the standardized incidence of childhood cancer ranges from 75 to 150 per million children per year in the developed countries and 38 to 124 per million children per year in India. There is also disparity in the incidence rates between urban and rural areas in India. For example, the highest reported incidence is in Chennai, whereas incidence rates are low in rural Ahmedabad. The reason for these differences is uncertain, but it has been postulated that rural areas may have under-ascertainment or under-reporting of cases whereas urban areas have been modernized with growing population, pollution, and exposure to carcinogens, predisposing children in these areas to cancer. The male-to-female ratio in the incidence rates is high all over the country, except for northeast India.

Leukemia is the most common childhood cancer in India accounting for up to 40% of all cancers, with the predominant type being acute lymphoblastic leukemia (almost 85%). Almost 50% of the acute lymphocytic leukemias (ALLs) are T-cell subtype, which is unlike that seen in the developed world where only 10% to 20% of these are T-cell ALL. Poor prognostic indicators such as hypodiploidy, t(1;19), t(9,22), and t(4.11) dominate the biology of ALLs seen in India. With central nervous system tumors being common in children of the developed worlds, the picture in India is different. A higher proportion of lymphomas are observed, with Hodgkin's disease (HD) more common than non-Hodgkin's lymphoma (NHL). The incidence rate of HD in male children in India could be as high as 20, whereas that in the United States and Britain is one-third this number. The incidence of HD in females and NHL in India is similar to that of the developed world.

## HISTORY OF CANCER CARE

The anticancer campaign in India started much later, as there was widespread notion that it is an incurable disease of "fate" and was considered a consequence of one's actions. In 1941 there was only one cancer hospital in India, known as the Tata Memorial Hospital in Bombay (now Mumbai).

After independence, another cancer hospital was opened in Calcutta, which started functioning in 1954. Later, by 1960 it was realized that because of late presentation of the disease, the chances of achieving cure were minimal; that's when earlier detection and treatment methods were initiated under different projects. The government of India identified it as a national problem and laid out the framework for cancer treatment and research. In 1982, the National Cancer Control Program (NCCP) and the ICMR initiated the National Cancer Registry projects in three cities, which have expanded to 26 demographic registries currently.

## CANCER INFRASTRUCTURE

The three pillars of cancer care in India are surgical oncology, medical oncology, and radiotherapy. Several cancer institutes are currently functioning in India and many more in phases of development; however, certain rural areas still lack adequate provision for cancer care. Unfortunately, most cancers are diagnosed in terminal stages, and radiotherapy is offered as palliation.

### Medical and Surgical Oncology

The ICMR has helped lay down clinical practice guidelines for 34 most common types of cancers. However, most of these guidelines are based on studies conducted in the United States or Europe, and physicians in India are now striving to establish guidelines based on evidence obtained on population studies in India. The entire cancer care scenario is evolving in India. There is a paucity of both medical and surgical oncologists in India. In the entire country, 15 surgical oncologists are trained every year, whereas the need is triple this number. Similarly, only 1,200 medical oncologists are available for a population of 1.2 billion; some states in the country do not even have one oncologist. Thus, 60% of times, cancer care is provided by non-oncologists, which makes it imperative that specific guidelines be followed. There are 15 medical colleges/institutes in India that train 55 medical oncologists each year. Similarly, 13 institutes now offer training in surgical oncology, with 58 physicians being trained per year.

### Radiation Therapy

Over 70% of patients in India mostly present in the advanced stage for diagnostic and treatment services; thus, radiotherapy is one of the main modality of treatment. In India, the NCCP has developed 27 regional cancer centers, which provide specialized radiation treatment along with research in the field of oncology. Apart from the regional cancer centers, some of the medical colleges and oncology wings have been established, which provide facilities for radiation treatment.[15] Currently, 35 linear accelerators are operating in some of the major institutes. However, with the increased cancer burden, India still depends on imported units both for cobalt-60 teletherapy and linear accelerators, which are the most preferred units of radiotherapy.[16]

## Palliative Care

Among the analgesics on the WHO step 2 ladders for pain control, those available in India are dextropropoxyphene, codeine, pentazocine, tramadol, and sublingual buprenorphine. Although considered inappropriate for severe pain caused by cancer, pentazocine is widely prescribed by physicians and used by patients in India. Although India is one of the largest producers of opium poppies, manufacturing of codeine is limited and frequently imported, making it an expensive analgesic. Tramadol is widely marketed and prescribed but remains expensive, making it difficult for patients to purchase. Morphine is the only analgesic on the WHO step 3 of analgesic ladder that is available in India. Stringent narcotic regulations prevent these from being available to the patients. However, some of these regulations have recently been liberalized in a few states of the country. Surprisingly, a more expensive transdermal fentanyl is prescribed to patients where oral morphine is not available. When it comes to palliative care delivery, most families opt for health care at home. Although India lacks the resources for daily nurse visits at home, such services may not be necessary daily as most patients have family members taking care of them. Empowering family members thus becomes a major challenge. The Institute of Palliative Medicine in Calicut, India, is a newly found organization that is experimenting such palliative care delivery methods with the help of families and volunteers.[17]

## ALTERNATIVE CANCER THERAPIES IN INDIA

Different forms of alternative medicines such as ayurveda, naturopathy, biopathy, homeopathy, home remedies, wheat-grass therapy, hydrotherapy, acupuncture, auto urine therapy, osteopathy, and vipasana therapy are being used in India. The main reason people use these medicines is limited medical therapy for patients who are diagnosed in advanced stages and for those who are in economically disadvantaged position and have limited access to medical services. Recently, some of the alternative cancer therapies, such as psonirum which is a combination of homeopathy and natural medicine, in an anecdotal report have shown to improve survival for advanced cancer. Other popular alternative medicines include herbal, tribal, and folk medicines such as Kromba and Muthu Marunthu which are combinations of different plant ingredients. Other approaches include nutritional therapy, Tulse, Reiki, religious therapy, meditation, yoga, laughter therapy, and black magic.[18]

## CANCER CARE CONTINUUM

### Prevention

The NCCP that was started in 1975 in India developed different regional cancer centers and district cancer control programs, focusing on various preventative strategies such as education and creating awareness about the harmful effects of tobacco and trying to control and discourage its use. The NCCP also created awareness about increasing physical activity, avoiding obesities, encouraging health diets, using safe sex measures, immunization against hepatitis B for avoiding cancer genesis. Deficiencies in the health system and poor resources made the execution of these strategies difficult.[19]

### Screening

Worldwide, Pap smears and mammography have been recognized as screening methods for cervical and breast cancers. However, in India these are not practical and affordable methods for cancer screening. Some of the reasons are lack of trained manpower, resources, infrastructure, logistics, quality assurance, frequency of screening, and costs involved. VIA, which is visual inspection of cervix after the application of 5% acetic acid, or VILI, visual inspection of cervix after the application of 1% Lugol's iodine, has been found to be simple and inexpensive and can be provided by trained health workers.[20] Studies have shown that these tests have a sensitivity of 64% to 75%, with a specificity of 83% to 85%.[21] It has been indicated that the combination of VIA and VILI can be used as an acceptable technological tool in countries like India with inadequate resources.[20] Routine imaging techniques like mammography are not widely practiced in India because of expenses associated with them. Clinical breast examinations (CBE) have been noted to be effective if performed by trained health professionals. Studies have suggested that due to socioeconomic restraints, CBE can be used as a screening procedure in place of mammography.[20] There have been no screening guidelines for oral cancers. They are best evaluated with early clinical exam, detecting any precancerous lesions like leukoplakia, erythroplakia, nonhealing ulcers, and oral submucous fibrosis. Smokers are also routinely investigated with plain x-ray of chest to evaluate for any pulmonary lesions.

## FUTURE DIRECTIONS AND RESEARCH

The Ministry of Health and Family Welfare in India encourages new research in cancer to find new cures. As of March 2013, close to 2,000 clinical trials were registered in India, and the government strives to get more companies interested in conducting trials in India. The government has created 12 New Drug Advisory Committees consisting of experts from the government medical colleges and eminent institutions from all over the India to ensure transparency in evaluating application for proposals of new drug substances excluding investigational new drugs. Investigational new drugs also have two similar committees instituted for evaluation. Similarly, six Medical Device Advisory Committees (MDAC) have been created for evaluating new medical devices.

## REFERENCES

1. Nongkynrih B, Patro BK, Pandav CS. Current status of communicable and non-communicable diseases in India. _J Assoc Physicians India_ 2004; 52: 118–23.
2. Mahal A, Karan A, Engelgau M. _The Economic Implications of Non-Communicable Disease for India._ Washington DC: The International Bank for Reconstruction and Development/The World Bank, 2009, pp. 13–14.
3. Lauber SN, Gooderham NJ. The cooked meat derived genotoxic carcinogen 2-amino-3-methylimidazo[4,5-b]pyridine has potent hormone-like activity: mechanistic support for a role in breast cancer. _Cancer Res_ 2007; 67: 9597–602.
4. O'Hanlon LH. High meat consumption linked to gastric-cancer risk. _Lancet Oncol_ 2006; 7: 287.
5. Chandalia M, Abate N, Cabo-Chan AV Jr, Devaraj S, Jialal I, Grundy SM.. Hyperhomocysteinemia in Asian Indians living in the United States. _J Clin Endocrinol Metab_ 2003; 88: 1089–95.
6. Jain MG, Hislop GT, Howe GR, Ghadirian P. Plant foods, antioxidants, and prostate cancer risk: findings from case-control studies in Canada. _Nutr Cancer_ 1999; 34: 173–84.
7. Mills PK, Beeson WL, Phillips RL, Fraser GE. Cohort study of diet, lifestyle, and prostate cancer in Adventist men. _Cancer_ 1989; 64: 598–604.
8. Jussawalla DJ, Jain DK. Lung cancer in Greater Bombay: correlations with religion and smoking habits. _Br J Cancer_ 1979; 40: 437–48.
9. Nafae A, Misra SP, Dhar SN, Shah SN. Bronchogenic carcinoma in Kashmir Valley. _Indian J Chest Dis_ 1973; 15: 285–95.
10. Wahi PN, Kehar U, Lahiri B. Factors influencing oral and oropharyngeal cancers in India. _Br J Cancer_ 1965; 19: 642–60.
11. Ferlay J, Shin HR, Bray F, Forman D, Mathers C, Parkin DM. Estimates of worldwide burden of cancer in 2008: GLOBOCAN 2008. _Int J Cancer_ 2010; 127: 2893–917.
12. Jemal A, Siegel R, Ward E, Murray T, Xu J, Thun MJ. Cancer statistics, 2007. _CA Cancer J Clin_ 2007; 57: 43–66.
13. Takiar R, Nadayil D, Nandakumar A. Projections of number of cancer cases in India (2010–2020) by cancer groups. _Asian Pac J Cancer Prev_ 2010; 11: 1045–49.
14. National Cancer Registry Program. _Three-Year Report of Population Based Cancer Registries 2006–2008: Incidence and Distribution of Cancer._ Bangalore: Indian Council of Medical Research, 2010.
15. Murthy NS, Chaudhry K, Rath GK. Burden of cancer and projections for 2016, Indian scenario: gaps in the availability of radiotherapy treatment facilities. _Asian Pac J Cancer Prev_ 2008; 9: 671–77.

16. Johns HE. Data on teletherapy units in India—Personal Communication BARC: High Energy Machines. *The Physics of Radiology*. 4th ed. (Chapter 4). Illinois: Charles C. Thomas Publications, 2001, pp. 102–13.

17. Rajagopal MR, Venkateswaran C. Palliative care in India: successes and limitations. *J Pain Palliat Care Pharmacother* 2003; 17: 121–28; discussion 129–30.

18. Shukla Y, Pal SK. Complementary and alternative cancer therapies: past, present and the future scenario. *Asian Pac J Cancer Prev* 2004; 5: 3–14.

19. Ali I, Wani WA, Saleem K. Cancer scenario in India with future perspectives. *Cancer Ther* 2011; 8: 56–70.

20. Dinshaw K, Shastri S, Patil S. Cancer Control Programme in India: Challenges for the New Millennium. *Health Administrator* XVIII: 10–13.

21. Sankaranarayanan R, Nene BM, Dinshaw K, et al. Early detection of cervical cancer with visual inspection methods: a summary of completed and on-going studies in India. *Salud Publica Mex* 2003; 45(Suppl 3): S399–S407.

# 23

# Jordan

## *Fadwa Ali Attiga, Maysa M. Abu-Khalaf, and Hikmat Abdel-Razeq*

## PUBLIC HEALTH PERSPECTIVE

### Life Expectancy

Jordan's performance is better among the Arab states in terms of life expectancy, infant and child mortality rates, and maternal mortality rates. Table 23.1 summarizes basic public health indicators.[1]

### Communicable Diseases

Infectious diseases remain on the list of major causes of morbidity in Jordan, despite an epidemiological shift toward noncommunicable diseases. According to reports of the Disease Control Directorate in the Ministry of Health (MOH), gastrointestinal diseases, acute respiratory infections, and hepatitis are still major causes of morbidity in Jordan, especially among children.

Vaccination coverage for polio and DPT is around 99%, for measles 95%, and for tuberculosis 29%. Vaccination for hepatitis B and *Haemophilus influenzae* has been introduced in the national vaccination program. The list of reported communicable diseases includes 40 diseases, of which one-fourth are no longer reported in Jordan (e.g., cholera, typhus, yellow fever, and plague). Furthermore, Jordan is considered among low-prevalence countries for HIV/AIDS, with an estimated prevalence of less than 0.1%.[2]

### Noncommunicable Diseases

Noncommunicable diseases (NCDs) are the leading cause of death in Jordan. The latest mortality report issued by the MOH for 2009 indicates that

**TABLE 23.1  Basic Public Health Indicators for Jordan (2011)**

|                                                              | 2011    |
| ------------------------------------------------------------ | ------- |
| Population                                                   | 624,900 |
| Life expectancy at birth (years): male/female               | 72/74   |
| Crude death rate (per 1,000 population)                      | 7       |
| Infant mortality (per 1,000 live births)                     | 23      |
| Maternal mortality (per 100,000 live births)                | 19      |
| MOH budget as a percentage of total government budget       | 6.3     |

more than one-third of deaths are attributed to cardiovascular diseases and 14.6% to cancer.[3] NCD risk factors, including mainly smoking, physical inactivity, obesity, and unhealthy diets, are considered serious public health problems in Jordan.[4]

Furthermore, the latest survey of Behavioral Risk Factor Surveillance Survey in 2007 that was conducted by the MOH in collaboration with Centers for Disease Control and Prevention showed a high prevalence of obesity, hypertension, and diabetes among Jordanian men and women.[5] In addition, smoking is highly prevalent in Jordan, and the age-standardized prevalence of type 2 diabetes is high (17.1%) and increasing.[6] Furthermore, a high percentage of people with diabetes are not diagnosed early, complicating efforts to control NCDs in Jordan.

## Cancer as Public Health Problem

Cancer is the second leading cause of death in Jordan after cardiovascular disease.[3] Cancer mortality and morbidity are expected to increase due to an increase in life expectancy that is coupled with prolonged exposure to risks factors such as tobacco use, consumption of unhealthy food, and decreased physical activity, as well as exposure to toxic environmental chemicals and industrial and agricultural carcinogens.[7]

In Jordan, the government bears the cost of treating cancer patients. Cancer treatment is offered at no cost to all Jordanian citizens through public and private hospitals, depending on their type of insurance (i.e., through public sector insurance, military insurance, or royal court sponsorship). Although average patient-level estimates of costs for treating cancer are not publically available, annual gross figures of US$169 to US$176 million to treat cancer patients have been stated by the MOH in public press.[8] Detailed cost breakdowns for all stages of cancer care are not available on a national level. However, the expected increase in cancer incidence as the population ages and the rising cost of cancer-related care make cancer screening and early detection urgent priorities for Jordan.

A national cancer control program is a public health program designed to reduce the number of cancer cases and deaths and improve quality of life of cancer patients, through the systematic and equitable implementation of evidence-based strategies for prevention, early detection, diagnosis, treatment, and palliation, making the best use of available resources. In countries where cancer control programs have been implemented, the burden of cancer is reducing, with better outcomes for patients.[9] Most cancer-related activities in Jordan currently focus on treatment, with less effort being placed on other elements of the cancer continuum. Despite several initiatives at the national level in the past decade, Jordan does not have a national cancer control plan as of 2013. Organized cancer control, as promoted by international organizations such as WHO, its regional office EMRO, and the UICC, offers the best approach for health-care systems to be more integrated, cost-effective, and efficient and to enable efforts to prevent and cure cancers and palliate symptoms and improve quality of life.

## CANCER ETIOLOGY

In Jordan, the high prevalence of smoking is associated with high incidence of lung cancer, which is the leading cause of cancer-related death in Jordan. In addition to lung cancer, tobacco use has been reported to increase the risk of more than 15 other types of cancers, including cancers of the colorectum, bladder, and acute myeloid leukemia, all of which are among the most common neoplasms in Jordan.[10]

Viral-associated cancers have low prevalence in Jordan (Table 23.2). Forty one cases of cervical cancer were registered in 2010, representing 1.6% of female cancers.[11] Cancer in the liver and biliary passages is not common, with 113 cases registered in 2010 (2.3%).[11] The HBV vaccination national program for infants started in 1995, and the WHO core health

TABLE 23.2 Number of New Cases Recorded in the National Jordan Cancer Registry for Some Types of Solid Tumors[11]

| Cancer Primary Site | 2008 | 2009 | 2010 |
|---|---|---|---|
| Breast cancer | 864 | 942 | 951 |
| Lung cancer | 356 | 299 | 379 |
| Colon cancer | 355 | 351 | 372 |
| Liver and biliary passages cancer | 109 | 97 | 113 |
| Cervical cancer | 43 | 44 | 41 |

indicators data report for 2006 presented compliance at 98% for 1-year-olds immunized with three doses of hepatitis vaccine. In addition, MOH recommends vaccinating all health workers with three doses of hepatitis B vaccine, particularly hospital staff, dental clinic staff, and emergency room staff at health centers.

Furthermore, there is no published work on the incidence of inherited familial cancer syndromes, such as hereditary breast and ovarian cancer syndrome that is associated with mutations in BRCA1 and BRCA2, or familial adenomatous polyposis in colon cancer.

## CANCER STATISTICS

Cancer registration began in 1996 with the establishment of the Jordan Cancer Registry (JCR) as a population-based registry under the jurisdiction of the MOH, and it publishes an annual incidence report, the latest is for 2010.[11] The number of new cancer cases diagnosed among Jordanians has increased 44% in the past 10 years, from 3,362 cases in 2000 to 4,849 in 2010, although the average annual population growth rate in this decade was 2.5%. The male-to-female ratio was 0.92:1, and the overall median age at diagnosis was 56 (60 years for males and 52 years for females).[11] The crude incidence rate of all cancers among Jordanians was 79.4 per 100,000 (74 for males and 85.1 for females). The age-standardized incidence rate (ASR) adjusted to the world standard population was 135.1 per 100,000, which represents an increase by 8.5% from the ASR in 2000 (124.5 per 100,000 population). Nevertheless, Jordan's ASR for cancer is similar to that of other Arab countries in the region and much lower than that in Europe and North America (Figure 23.1).

The total number of new cancer cases was 6,820, with 4,921 (72.2%) diagnosed in Jordanians and 1,899 (27.8%) diagnosed in non-Jordanians. The total number of reported invasive cancers in Jordanians was 4,849 (2,330 cases in males and 2,519 in females), whereas the number of in situ carcinoma was 72 cases.[11]

The top five cancers among Jordanian males were colorectal 332 (14.2%), lung 311 (13.3%), prostate 218 (9.4%), urinary bladder 186 (8%), and leukemia 127 (5.5%). For Jordanian females, the top five cancers were breast 941 (37.4%), colorectal 226 (9%), thyroid 136 (5.4%), non-Hodgkin's lymphoma (NHL) 130 (5.2%), and uterus 113 (3.6%).[11] This ranking has not significantly changed in the past decade.

The most common cancer-related death in males is due to neoplasms of the lung (30.2%), colorectal (10.3%), and prostate (6.2%). In females, the most common cancer-related deaths are due to cancers of the breast (22.4%), colorectal 8.9%, and lung (7%). However, it should be noted that the WHO's last rapid assessment of Jordan's civil registration and vital statistics system indicated that although it is satisfactory, the quality of cause of death data

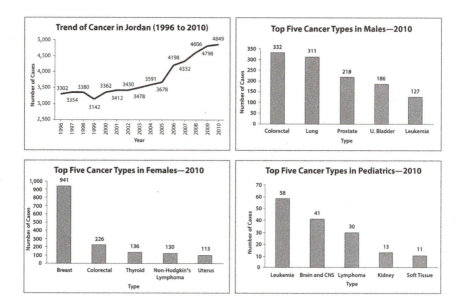

**FIGURE 23.1** Cancer incidence in Jordan and the most common cancer types in adult males and females as well as pediatrics (reference 11).

and qualification and training of coders and quality of coding are still of concern in terms of accuracy.[12]

## HISTORY OF CANCER CARE

During the 1990s, cancer care in Jordan was delivered through both public and private hospitals, including Al-Bashir Public Hospital, Royal Medical Services (RMS) for the army, Jordan University Hospital (JUH), King Abdullah University Hospital (KAUH), and King Hussein Cancer Center (formerly known as Al-Amal Hospital), as well as some private hospitals. Cancer care was delivered in a fragmented approach, with lack of coordination in the plan of care between various health-care providers from pathology, radiology, surgery, and medical oncology. In addition, there was a severe deficiency in patient support services, including nutrition, psychosocial support, and rehabilitation services.

The government is the major insurer for cancer management in Jordan. In the past, insured cancer patients were treated in public hospitals and transferred to university or private hospitals or even outside Jordan only if appropriate treatments were not available. Noninsured cancer patients, especially pediatric patients, were transferred for treatment to KHCC after approval from the MOH and at the expense of the Royal Court.

In 1997, The King Hussein Cancer Foundation and King Hussein Cancer Center (KHCF/KHCC) was established as a free-standing independent nongovernmental, not-for-profit institution founded by a royal decree to combat cancer in Jordan and the Middle East region. KHCF forged a cooperative agreement with the National Cancer Institute of the United States (National Institutes of Health) for enhancing medical sciences and improving cancer patient care in Jordan and the entire Middle East region. KHCC began a journey to transform the hospital into a comprehensive cancer center for cancer care, training, and education as well as research.[13] KHCC gained accreditation by Joint Commission International in 2006 and as an oncology center in 2009. KHCC is equipped to treat all types of adult and pediatric cancers and currently provides treatment to approximately 60% of cancer cases in Jordan. In addition, KHCC provides treatment to non-Jordanians from neighboring countries.

Currently, insured patients receive their care at the site where they are originally insured. As for uninsured patients, they receive at the MOH hospitals when available; otherwise, they are transferred to the oncology services in the RMS, to University Hospitals or to KHCC, and treated at the expenses of the Royal Court.

## CANCER CARE INFRASTRUCTURE AND WORKFORCE

In Jordan, the three major cancer treatment modalities (surgery, radiation, chemotherapy) are generally available through public and private hospitals like KHCC, KAUH, JUH, and RMS for the army as well as Al-Bashir public hospital (Table 23.3). Most services are concentrated in Amman governorate, except for KAUH which is located in the north. KHCC is the only specialized tertiary hospital in Jordan that provides multidisciplinary cancer management and related services for cancer care, including surgery, pathology, radiology, radiotherapy, chemotherapy, palliative care, and psychosocial and rehabilitative support. In addition, KHCC has a bone marrow transplantation program with multidisciplinary teams for pediatric and adult patients.

Data and studies on treatment availability, access, and patterns of care are scarce. Health-care institutions treating cancer patients tend to follow clinical practice guidelines in the management of common cancers, which is especially true for pediatric oncology. However, there are no national clinical practice guidelines for cancer management. Comprehensive guidelines and adherence to the guidelines are not well documented or monitored and sometimes research depends on the treating physician or the institution to generate data. A major exception is KHCC, which has clinical practice guidelines for the management of most types of cancers treated at the center. These were developed and implemented in the process of attaining "Disease-Specific Certification" as an Oncology Center by the Joint Commission International Accreditation in 2008.

Most of the institutions house multiple disciplines (surgery, pathology, medical oncology, radiology, nuclear medicine). However, across these institutions, variable gaps exist with regard to the availability of equipment and

**TABLE 23.3 Cancer Care: Providers and Infrastructure**

| | RMS | MOH | KAUH | JUH | Private Sector | KHCC | Total |
|---|---|---|---|---|---|---|---|
| *Specialized programs* | | | | | | | |
| Palliative program | 0 | 0 | 0 | 0 | 0 | √ | |
| Bone marrow transplantation program | √ | 0 | 0 | √ | √ | √ | |
| *Providers* | | | | | | | |
| Number of surgical and medical oncologists | 5 | 2 | 3 | 1 | 10 | 27 | **48** |
| Number of radiation oncologists | 4 | 5 | 0 | 0 | 5 | 8 | **22** |
| *Equipment* | | | | | | | |
| Radiation therapy | | | | | | | |
| Cobalt units (Theratron) | 0 | 1 | 0 | 0 | 0 | 0 | **1** |
| Linear accelerator | 2 | 2 | 0 | 0 | 2 | 4 | **10** |
| Brachytherapy unit | 0 | 0 | 0 | 0 | 0 | 1 | **1** |
| Radiology | | | | | | | |
| Mammography machine | 1 | 30 | 1 | 2 | 30 | 2 | **66** |
| Nuclear medicine | | | | | | | |
| Gamma camera | 2 | 2 | 2 | 2 | 5 | 1 | **14** |
| PET scan | 1 | 0 | 1 | 0 | 2 | 1 | **5** |

JUH, Jordan University Hospital; KAUH, King Abdullah University Hospital; KHCC, King Hussein Cancer Center; MOH, Ministry of Health; RMS, Royal Medical Services; √, available. *Source:* Personal communications with the listed institutions.

health-care providers in certain disciplines. For example, some institutions lack radiology services, and certain disciplines, such as psychological and palliative care services, are significantly under-provided. In the absence of certain medical services within an institution, referral to other institutions with the available services is common and can help address certain gaps. However, such referrals have implications with regard to interruption of patient care and furthermore may influence patient load and waiting times in the institution providing supplemental care.

Jordan hosts an adequate number of specialized medical oncologists, surgeons, and radiotherapists-oncologists who have been trained in medical schools in the Kingdom and abroad. Advanced diagnostics are available through pathologists and radiologists in addition to adult and pediatric critical care units, which collectively enhance the ability to diagnose and treat complex cases of cancer. On the other hand, there is a shortage of nurses, especially females, who are trained to meet the complex needs of a cancer patient throughout the treatment journey. There are few specialized ancillary support personnel who are trained to deliver advanced support services to enhance quality of life as well as treatment outcome, such as psychosocial and nutritional support in addition to rehabilitation.

## CANCER CLINICAL CARE

Cancer clinical care in Jordan is advanced compared to most of the Arab world, and the country hosts many Western-trained physicians who can deliver the different cancer treatment modalities. Nevertheless, coordinated multidisciplinary management of cancer patients is not optimal outside KHCC, where care is provided through multidisciplinary organized teams (MDT) or multidisciplinary organized clinics (MDC). Many of these MDTs or MDCs routinely discuss their cases through telemedicine with colleagues at rebuttable cancer centers like MD Anderson Cancer Center, St. Jude's Children Research Hospital in the United States and Hospital for Sick Children in Canada.[14] Many disease-specific workshops and conferences are carried out annually in Jordan. which provide an opportunity for health-care providers to keep up to date on advances in cancer care and collaborate on research efforts. In addition, access to advanced diagnostics and radiation therapy is available.

### Breast Cancer

Breast cancer is the most common cancer diagnosed among Jordanian women. In 2010, there were 978 cases of breast cancer in men and women, accounting for 19.8% of all newly diagnosed cancer cases and 37.4% of all female cancers (Figure 23.2). Compared to Western societies, breast cancer is

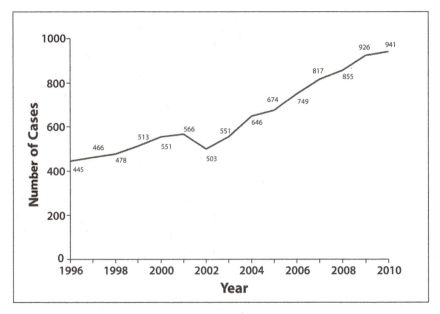

**FIGURE 23.2** Number of breast cancer cases diagnosed in Jordan since 1996 (reference 11).

diagnosed at a younger age in Jordan. The median age at diagnosis is 50 years (range 21 to 91 years), with 17% women diagnosed under the age of 40. Only 28.5% of the cases are diagnosed at 60 years or above.[11]

Ductal carcinoma is the most frequent pathological type, in 79% of breast cancer cases. More women are diagnosed at earlier stages; the most recent cancer registry report for 2010 showed that 34% of breast cancer cases were localized, 45% were regional, and 9% were distant metastasis, whereas the stage for the remainder was not available.[11]

Recently, more women are undergoing breast-conserving surgery rather than mastectomy. Special surgical techniques like nipple-sparing and skin-sparing mastectomies are offered in tertiary care centers. Moreover, sentinel lymph node sampling rather than full axillary lymph node dissection is practiced in many local hospitals. In addition, immediate and delayed breast reconstructions are routinely practiced.

Systemic therapy availability varies. Standard chemotherapy and hormonal therapy including aromatase inhibitors are widely available. Trastuzumab and lapatinib are highly restricted drugs, whereas the recently introduced medications like pertuzumab and everolimus are not registered in the Kingdom yet.

## Lung Cancer

Lung cancer is the second most common cancer diagnosed among Jordanian males but not as common as in females. With 380 cases diagnosed in 2010, the majority (82%) were among males.[11] The overall crude age-specific incidence rate for lung cancer is 6.2 per 100,000 (9.9 for males and 2.3 per 100,000 for females). Adenocarcinoma is the most common histology, whereas small cell carcinoma accounted for only 12.1%.[11]

Due to the increasing rate of smoking among Jordanians, especially among young college students and females, it is expected that lung cancer rate will remarkably increase in the coming years. Given the advanced-stage disease at presentation and its associated shortened survival, lung cancer is expected to place huge pressure on the health-care system in Jordan. Therefore, strict antitobacco efforts are warranted.

The recent years have witnessed a major shift toward personalized care that includes novel targeted antineoplastic drugs which our health-care system can't afford. Currently, most lung cancer patients are treated with standard chemotherapeutic agents, including platinum compounds, taxanes, vinorelbine, and gemcitabine. Novel drugs such as bevacizumab, erlotinib, gefitinib, and pemetrexed are not widely available in public hospitals. For example, gefitinib was recently introduced to KHCC formulary based on cost-effective studies. Patients choosing to be treated with these novel drugs can do so in private hospitals at their own expense. In addition, selecting appropriate targeted therapy for personalized care requires sophisticated lab testing for specific gene amplifications or mutations, which is expensive and can't be charged to the MOH or Royal Court. However, many private laboratories in Jordan offer such tests, which are available to those who can afford the cost.

## Colon Cancer

Colorectal cancers are the leading cancer type among males and ranked second among all cancers, with a total of 558 cases (11.9%) diagnosed in 2010.[11] The median age at diagnosis was 61 years and the overall ASR was 17.0 per 100,000. Fortunately, only 11.8% were diagnosed with advanced-stage disease. Unlike standard chemotherapy, targeted therapy is not widely available in public hospitals but routinely practiced in private hospitals and clinics.

## Prostate Cancer

Ranked sixth among male cancers, prostate cancer is not commonly encountered in Jordan, with 218 cases reported in 2010, accounting for 4.5% of all cancer cases; 28% of them presented with advanced-stage disease.[11] The median age at diagnosis was 69 years. Advanced surgical techniques like robotic surgery used in the management of early prostate surgery are not available in the Kingdom. In addition, many of the recently introduced chemotherapeutic agents used in advanced-stage disease are not available in public institutions, including KHCC.

## Lymphoma

A total of 382 cases of Hodgkin's (35%) and non-Hodgkin's (65%) lymphoma, accounting for (7.9%) of all cancer cases, were diagnosed in 2010.[11] Lymphoma ranked the third among all newly diagnosed cancer cases in both women and men. Similar to Western populations, Hodgkin's lymphoma is commonly encountered among adolescents and young adults, with a median age of 26 years. NHL is also encountered in younger age group (median age 51.5 years).

Except for the recently introduced monoclonal antibodies (e.g., the anti-CD30 brentuximab), all other medications needed in the induction or salvage therapies are widely available. High-dose chemotherapy and stem cell transplantation, both autologous and allogeneic, are widely available in Jordan.

## Childhood Cancers

In the pediatric age group, defined as <15 years in JCR, the total number of cancer cases was 194 accounting for 4% of all cancer cases in Jordan, with a male-to-female ratio 1.3:1.

The top five cancer types in the pediatric age group are shown in Figure 23.1. Comprehensive pediatric cancer therapy through MDT, MDC, bone marrow and stem cell transplantation, and specialized pediatric intensive care is offered at KHCC.

## CANCER CARE OUTCOMES

Data on cancer care outcomes is not available at a national level. However, the recent introduction of hospital-based cancer registry and research unit at KHCC enabled us to review treatment outcomes for all cancer types. The 5-year survival data was recently released and made available to clinicians, administrators, and researchers. Survival data by disease stage is also available. Despite our concerns about the difficulties in introducing many of the new chemotherapeutic medications and targeted therapies, and the increasing use of generic medications, our survival data is comparable to those observed in developed countries.

## CANCER CARE CONTINUUM

### Prevention

Cancer prevention is an essential component of the fight against cancer. Over one-third of all cancers can be prevented by addressing the known risk factors. Unfortunately, many cost-effective and inexpensive prevention measures have yet to be widely implemented in many countries, including Jordan. Four out of the 10 most common cancers in Jordan are eligible for primary prevention, including lung, colorectal, urinary bladder, and stomach cancer.[11]

Lung cancer–related death is the most preventable form of cancer-related death in Jordan. Tobacco use remains a major public health problem in Jordan through cigarette smoking and the use of water pipes called "shishas" or "nargileh." Cigarette smoking rates are high among youth (13 to 15 years), which was reported 11.5% in the 2009 WHO Global Tobacco Youth Survey,[15] and 55% of males and 8% of females smoke on a regular basis (Center of Consultation-University of Jordan). Passive smoking is a major issue in Jordan, with rates up to 80% of people being exposed to secondhand smoke.[16]

Jordan signed the Framework Convention on Tobacco Control and swiftly ratified it in 2004. Public Health Law No. 47/2008 prohibits the sale of tobacco products to minors (under the age of 18). This law created the legislative framework for 100% smoke-free public places, public transport, and health-care facilities; for building public and key decision-maker support through mass media communication and targeted advocacy; and for supporting implementation and enforcement. The smoking ban, however, is not yet adequately enforced, as it lacks an effective mechanism for implementation and adequate training of responsible staff. Smoking cessation clinics are currently available at the MOH and at KHCC, providing counseling, brochures, and antismoking drugs. Moreover, KHCC is an active partner in the Global Bridges, a health-care alliance for tobacco dependence treatment in collaboration with Mayo Clinic.[17]

In addition, Jordanians are moving toward a Western lifestyle, with increased consumption of processed food. Another major concern is the decreased levels of physical activity, resulting in an estimated 30% of the population being overweight and 35% obese. The national youth strategy for Jordan promoted recreation and encouraged youth to become more physically active and lead healthier lifestyles.[18] Implementation and impact are yet to be determined.

Larger population-based surveys on detailed elements of knowledge, attitudes, and practices associated with cancer are needed to better understand how preventive efforts can be successful. Similarly, the level of knowledge in cancer prevention and early detection among first-line health workers needs to be ascertained so that they become effective and active partners in cancer prevention.

## Screening

In a population where the majority of the cancers amenable to early detection are diagnosed in late stages, the establishment of an early diagnosis program may be the most feasible strategy to reduce the proportion of patients presenting with late-stage cancer and improve survival rates. Jordan Breast Cancer Program (JBCP) is a national program established in 2005; it includes major stakeholders and aims at downstaging the current state of diagnosis of breast cancer from its late stages to diagnosing breast cancer at its earlier stages where the disease is most curable, survival rates are highest, and treatment costs are lowest. Currently, the program offers limited screening coverage in the capital and surrounding areas.

JBCP has developed breast cancer screening and diagnosis guidelines (based on the National Comprehensive Control Network guidelines), which were published in 2008.[19] However, the feasibility of developing and sustaining a national screening program in a resource-constrained setting such as Jordan remains questionable. The country hosts more than 60 mammography units, some of which are underutilized due to lack of patients or lack of trained radiologists. Recently, KHCC and JBCP introduced a mobile mammography unit with centralized reading at KHCC to aid in increasing access of patients to breast cancer screening.

## Psychosocial Care

This area is underdeveloped in Jordan, and with the exception of KHCC, most cancer care facilities in the Kingdom lack structured programs for psychosocial support. The Psycho-Social Oncology Program at KHCC provides emotional and spiritual support to improve quality of life for patients and families and to facilitate the best possible outcome of the treatment process. Social workers interact with patients and their families as well as the health-care management team to facilitate access of patient to treatment and encourage compliance by addressing the patient's emotional and social needs.

## CANCER RESEARCH

Despite the advanced cancer care delivered to cancer patients in Jordan, clinical care is not integrated with clinical research, and one seldom sees publications emphasizing bench to bed or bed to bench applications that reflects trends seen in our patient population. Physicians are not required to do research, and recognition at the national and regional levels is not tied to the "publish or perish" rule widely known in the West. In addition, residency and fellowship programs mainly depend on clinical care and continuing medical education hours, with weak emphasis on teaching research methodology. In 2011 to 2012, Jordanian researchers published a total of 105 original articles that were mainly retrospective reviews of cancer patients' medical charts in addition to few basic research projects. The government does not have adequate funding to support research, and the ability of physicians to successfully compete for international research grants is limited due to inexperience and frail collaborative networks among individuals and institutions.

Few clinicians in Jordan lead international multi-institutional clinical trials that are sponsored by pharmaceutical companies and are conducted in clinical trial sites that are licensed by the Jordan Food and Drug Administration. Understanding the peculiarities of cancer development and treatment in our patient population in the age of personalized medicine will require commitment and coordinated efforts among all stakeholders to promote and facilitate clinical cancer research.

## FUTURE DIRECTIONS

Jordan is a currently a hub for advanced multidisciplinary cancer care in the Middle East region with satisfactory survival rates. However, cancer cases are expected to increase, reaching levels that the government and the country at large will not be able to cope with. In addition, the cost of the many recently introduced targeted cancer drugs and sophisticated technologies in radiation therapy and surgical techniques will create significant challenges for the current insurance coverage system. This should alert policy makers to plan for future strategies and seek alternatives that will address these challenges. King Hussein Cancer Center and Foundation took the lead and introduced a nonprofit cancer insurance program that partially covers the cost of cancer care at KHCC for program participants. Further planning at the national level is of paramount importance to formulate strategies for the upgrading of local laboratory capabilities and the funding of the rapidly growing list of cancer-targeted therapies in the era of personalized cancer care.

Shortage in cancer care providers will be a challenge at all levels as Jordan experiences significant difficulties in attracting and retaining highly qualified Jordanian graduates in different specialties. Financial compensation and political uncertainty in neighboring countries and the region add to the problem. KHCC has several structured training programs for physicians, nursing, and other highly needed paramedical specialties, which can become stronger through partnership with medical and nursing schools in the Kingdom.

Concrete efforts at the national level, in collaboration with all public and private stakeholders, are required to develop strategies to further strengthen the Kingdom's capabilities in cancer care, with emphasis on embracing new technologies as well as sustainability. Moreover, future strategic plans for cancer care in Jordan should address the need of integrated clinical care and clinical research programs, including research on quality, access, and treatment outcomes with links to survivorship programs.

## REFERENCES

1. Ministry of Health. *Annual Statistical Book*. Amman, Jordan, 2011.
2. Ministry of Health. *Directorate of Communicable Diseases Annual Report*. Amman, Jordan, 2008.
3. Ministry of Health, *Mortality Data in Jordan 2009*. Amman, Jordan, 2012.
4. Zindah M, Belbeisi A, Walke H, Mokdad AH. Obesity and diabetes in Jordan: findings from the Behavioral Risk Factor Surveillance System, 2004. *Prev Chronic Dis* 2008; 5(1).
5. Al-Nsour M, Zindah M, Belbeisi A, Hadaddin R, Brown D, Walke H. Prevalence of selected chronic, noncommunicable disease risk factors in Jordan: results of the 2007 Jordan Behavioral Risk Factor Surveillance Survey. *Prev Chronic Dis* 2012; 9: E25.
6. Ajlouni K, Khadr Y, Batieha A, Ajlouni H, El-Khateeb M. An increase in prevalence of diabetes mellitus in Jordan over 10 years. *J Diabetes Complications* 2007.
7. World Health Organization. *Quantifying Environmental Health Impacts: Country Profiles of Environmental Burden of Disease*, Geneva, 2004.
8. Minister of Health. *120 Million JD Annual Cost of Treating Cancer in Jordan* Anwar Al-Zayadat. Al-Arab Al-Yaum, August 19, 2009.
9. World Health Organization. *National Cancer Control Programmes: Policies and Managerial Guidelines*. 2nd ed. Geneva, 2002.
10. US Department of Health and Human Services. *The Health Consequences of Smoking—A Report of the Surgeon General*. Rockville, MD, 2004.
11. Ministry of Health, Jordan Cancer Registry. *Cancer Incidence in Jordan*. Amman, Jordan, 2010.

12. World Health Organization. *Civil Registration and Vital Statistics Systems in the Region*. Geneva, 2013.

13. Moe JL, Pappas G, Murray A. Transformational leadership, transnational culture and political competence in globalizing health care services: a case study of Jordan's King Hussein Cancer Center. *Global Health* 2007: 3–11.

14. Qaddoumi I, Mansour A, Musharbash A, et al. Impact of telemedicine on pediatric neuro-oncology in a developing country: the Jordanian-Canadian experience. *Pediatr Blood Cancer* 2007; 48(1) 39–43.

15. World Health Organization. *Global Youth Tobacco Survey Country Reports-Jordan (2009)*. Geneva, 2012.

16. King Hussein Institute for Biotechnology and Cancer (KHIBC), Center of Consultation in Univerity of Jordan. *The National Survey "Knowledge, Attitudes and Practices towards Cancer Prevention and Care in Jordan."* Amman, Jordan, 2011.

17. Global Bridges. June 14, 2013. Available at http://www.globalbridges.org.

18. Higher Council of Youth. *National Youth Strategy for Jordan (2005–2009)*. Amman, Jordan, 2004.

19. Jordan Breast Cancer Program. *Breast Cancer Screening and Diagnosis Guidelines*. Amman, Jordan, 2008.

# 24

# Lebanon

## Katia E. Khoury, Hussein A. Assi, and Nagi S. El Saghir

## PUBLIC HEALTH PERSPECTIVE

### Life Expectancy

To date, the average life expectancy at birth is 74 years for the total Lebanese population. Females have a higher life expectancy of 77 years compared to males with an estimation of 71 years.[1]

### Communicable Diseases

The Ministry of Health (MOH) in Lebanon has established a routine disease surveillance system that produces monthly reports on a number of communicable diseases. However, this system largely relies on passive reporting of diseases discovered in clinical settings or on routine screening.

The most commonly reported communicable diseases in 2012 were, in decreasing order, hepatitis A (757 cases), typhoid fever (426 cases), dysentery (176 cases), and meningitis (171 cases).[2] As for chronic communicable diseases, the incidence of tuberculosis (TB) is not high in Lebanon, with an estimated incidence of 11 per 100,000, or around 400 cases a year. The presence of multidrug resistance TB is also low, with only 1 case out of 131 positive smears in 2005. The National TB Programme of MOH has provided 11 TB clinics all over the country, which provide full TB care and were able to achieve 82% case detection and 92% treatment success in 2005. The prevalence of HIV infection is reported to be less than 0.1% in the general Lebanese population, with most reported cases being among Lebanese people travelling, working, or residing abroad. However, this might be an underestimation due to lack of a national systematic HIV surveillance.[3]

## Noncommunicable Diseases (NCDs)

According to WHO, noncommunicable diseases (NCDs) are being steered by population ageing, progressive unplanned urbanization, and globalization of trade and marketing,[4] all leading to increased exposure to risk factors for NCDs such as physical inactivity, unbalanced diet, and smoking. A national study on NCDs by the American University of Beirut research group showed that the Lebanese population is at a significant high risk for NCDs (cardiovascular, gastrointestinal, pulmonary, musculoskeletal, depression, and cancer), with lifestyle being a main risk factor.[5]

Based on a worldwide study conducted by WHO in 2008, the total death rates per 100,000 due to the diagnosis of NCDs were 12.5 for males and 9.1 for females. In addition, the number of death rates caused by NCDs in individuals under the age of 60 was 25 for males and 22 for females.[1]

### Cancer

According to data collected by the MOH in 2003, females have an age-standardized incidence rate (ASR) of 113.2 compared to males with an estimation of 151.2. It also estimated to account for 19% of the total proportional mortality rate,[1] which makes cancer a significant public health issue.

### Cardiovascular Diseases (CVDs)

Over the past few years, studies have shown CVDs to have a significant impact on mortality of the population compared to the other NCDs.[1] Based on data available from national registries, around 25,000 invasive coronary interventions are performed every year, which is nearly equivalent to 72 procedures per 10,000. In 2007, the Lebanese Interventional Coronary Registry reported 1,827 angioplasties per million people performed in Lebanon, compared to 1,601 in France the same year. This difference suggests a high prevalence of coronary and ischemic heart diseases in Lebanon, given that the Lebanese population is younger than the French population.[6]

### Diabetes

Diabetes is a very significant rising health issue. According to the data released by the International Diabetes Federation, the Arab region appears to have a higher prevalence of diabetes than the global average. Lebanon ranks number six among Arab countries with the highest prevalence of diabetes in adults aged 20 to 79 years.[7] According to WHO, Lebanon has a prevalence of non-insulin-dependent diabetes mellitus that is almost double that of industrialized countries, reaching around 13% in the adult population. These studies have also shown that there is around 6% prevalence of impaired glucose tolerance.[3]

## Cancer as a Significant Public Health Problem

In Lebanon, cancer is one of the leading causes of death with an estimated mortality of 19% in the population according to a WHO publication.[1] The number of new cancer cases in Lebanon was estimated to be 7,888 cases in 2003.[8] Progress in prevention, early detection, diagnosis, and treatment of cancer has made steady steps forward. Access to care, availability of modern management, teaching, and research has also improved.[9] Close families usually provide a large portion of supportive care needed for cancer patients.[10]

## Cancer Care Workforce

Lebanon has a fragmented health system, with multiple public insurance bodies for government employees, a growing private insurance business, and a large out-of-pocket system. The Ministry of Public Health (MOPH) oversees and partially funds numerous governmental hospitals throughout the country. It also supports designated variable numbers of MOPH beds at private hospitals for uninsured Lebanese patients. MOPH also buys and dispenses systemic therapy drugs for malignant diseases.

## CANCER STATISTICS

Like most low- and middle-income countries (LMICs), Lebanon lacks accurate and updated national vital statistics on birth, mortality, marriage, and divorce. The last official population census dates from 1932. Nevertheless, the National Survey of Household Living Conditions (The Multipurpose Survey) conducted in 2004 was used for calculating ASRs. Cancer statistics come from abstracts and publications from hospital-based registries, national surveys, and recent national collection of data published by the MOH called National Cancer Registry of Lebanon.

The first hospital-based study on cancer in Lebanon was reported by Azar[11] from the American University of Beirut Medical Center (AUBMC). The study included 2,845 cases from 1953 to 1960, and it reported 532 cases in men and 1,313 cases in women. In 1966, a national collection of data on cancer in Lebanon was published by Abou-Daoud,[12] who reported a total of 2,072 cases seen in 1 year in 1965. He collected pathology reports from the eight hospitals where pathological diagnoses were made at that time. The annual crude incidence rates per 100,000 were 102 for males and 104 for females. In 1986, Geahchan and Taleb[13] reported 2,355 cases collected from all hospitals in Lebanon. In males, 1,261 cases were reported, with bladder cancer ranking first at 16%. In females, breast cancer was the commonest (27%) among the total of 1,094 cases reported.

During the civil war that lasted from 1975 to 1990, no annual statistics were reported. In 1998, El Saghir et al.[14] reported a study of 10,220 cases diagnosed at AUBMC, which treated approximately one-third of all cancers in Lebanon from 1983 till 1995. The study showed that breast cancer was the most common cancer in women, followed by cervical cancer, colorectal cancer, lymphoma, and brain cancer. In men, lung cancer was the most common, followed by bladder cancer, larynx, lymphoma, and leukemia.

In 2004, a Lebanese Cancer Epidemiology Group (LCEG) network of physicians collected all pathology reports from the majority of hospitals and laboratories for 1998. Results were published by Shamseddine et al.[15] and showed 4,388 cases (minus an unknown number of unreported hematological malignancies). The overall crude incidence rate for all cancers combined was 141.4 per 100,000 among males and 126.8 per 100,000 among females. The most frequently reported malignancies among males were bladder (18.5%), prostate (14.2%), and lung (14.1%) cancers and among females breast (33%), colon (5.8%), and corpus uteri (4.8%) cancers. Sex differentials in incidence rates were highest for tobacco-related cancers (lung, larynx, and bladder).

In 2006, the committee of the MOH of Lebanon issued a report on National Cancer Registry (NCR).[8] The committee collected all cases with diagnosis of cancer that reached the MOH and other insurance bodies requesting chemotherapy or treatment-related reimbursements in 2003. This included collection of basic demographic information and pathology reports from various physicians, hospitals, and laboratories. Duplications were eliminated after very elaborate efforts. Of the total 7,888 cases, 51.3% were in women (4,047 cases) and 49% (3,841 cases) in men. Pediatric cases in patients less than 15 years of age accounted for 3.3% of the total. Mean age of cases was 57.1 years (SD = 17.7, median 60 years), with a significant difference on average (p < 0.05) between men (59.3 ± 18.3 years) and women (55.1 ± 16.8 years). The median age of women at diagnosis was 56 years versus 64 years for men. ASRs were calculated based on a population count roughly estimated at 4 million.

Breast cancer is the most common cancer in women in Lebanon and in most surrounding countries. Tables 24.1 and 24.2 provide lists of the 10 most common cancers in males and females, respectively, in Lebanon and select Arab countries.

## Breast Cancer

Publications from 1962 until 2004 show breast cancer was the most common cancer in women in all studies reported. The percentage of breast cancer reported in 2003 was 42.3. ASR per 100,000 women per year rose from

20 in 1966 to 30 for 1983 to 2000 to 46.7 in 1998 to 52 in 2002 (an estimate by GLOBOCAN) to 69 in 2003.[8,16] The studies mentioned earlier show an increase in incidence rates, which is probably due to improved diagnosis and a young age at presentation, with 49% to 52% of cases below the age of 50 years and a median age of 49.8 years. This increase is in line with data from other Arab countries and LMICs and differs from industrialized nations like the United States and Europe where the median age is around 63 years, with only 25% to 30% of patients under 50 years and 50% of patients above 63 years.[16]

### Prostate Cancer

Demographics and data are derived from the LCEG and the MOPH reports. According to NCR data, prostate cancer ranks number one in Lebanon, whereas it was third in LCEG study. ASR of prostate cancer rose from 21.5 in 1998 to 28.5 in 2003. This rise was attributed to a prostate screening national campaign that resulted in a high and uncontrolled serum prostate-specific antigen testing in Lebanon. In 2003, the mean age was 69.9 (SD = 8.8) and the median age was 71. There were a total of 676 cases (17.6% of all male cancers, 8.5% of all cancers).[8,15]

### Lung Cancer

Lung cancer was number one in men throughout several studies and was second to bladder cancer in the 1998 LCEG survey. According to NCR data collection, 875 (11.1% of all cancers) cases were reported in 2003 (614 [16.0%] males and 261 [4.5%] females), corresponding to an ASR of 28.3 in males and 11.9 in females. The median age was 64 for males and females.[8]

### Colorectal Cancer

According to NCR data collection, 614 (7.7% of all cancers) cases were reported in 2003 (313 [8.0%] males and 301 [7.4%] females), corresponding to an ASR of 12.9 in males and 11.9 in females. The median age was 64 for males and 62 for females.[8]

### Hodgkin's Lymphoma

According to NCR data collection, 130 (1.6% of all cancers) cases were reported in 2003 (80 [2.1%] male and 50 [1.2%] females), corresponding to an ASR of 3.5 in males and 1.8 in females. The median age was 31.5 for males and 32 for females.[8]

## Non-Hodgkin's Lymphoma

According to NCR data collection, 358 (4.5% of all cancers) cases were reported in 2003 (192 [5.0%] males and 166 [4.1%] females), corresponding to an ASR of 8.9 in males and 7.1 in females. The median age was 60 for males and 59 for females.[8]

## Childhood Cancer

According to NCR data collection, there were a total of 237 cases (133 males and 104 females). The age-specific incidence rate of all cancers in the 0 to 14 age group in 2003 was 19.8 in males, 16.5 in females, and 18.2 in total. The proportion of specific cancers were as follows: leukemia 82 (34.5%), meninges and brain 33 (13.9%), bone and cartilage 21 (8.8%), kidney 14 (5.9%), non-Hodgkin's lymphoma 13 (5.5%), soft/connective tissues 8 (3.4%), eye 7 (2.9%), testis 7 (2.9%), Hodgkin's lymphoma 7 (2.9%), lung and trachea 6 (2.5%), others 40 (16.8%).[8]

## HISTORICAL DEVELOPMENTS IN CANCER CARE

### Surgery

The treatment of cancer in earlier years was mainly surgical where general surgeons usually performed the surgery for cancers. The trend in Lebanese patients is to ask for the "best doctor" and the "best surgeon." That made it difficult for new surgeons to build practices and for subspecialty surgery to develop. Many physicians worked on establishing oncology surgery and medical oncology practices after their training abroad, especially in the United States, France, and other industrialized countries. Advances in radiology, pathology, and anesthesia as well as supportive care followed, in addition to developments in antibiotics and better treatment of infectious diseases and complications.[17]

### Radiation Therapy

Radiation therapy has had many advances since the rise of the century. Radiation therapists used to stack rice over patients' skin to reduce dermatological effects. Cobalt machines were later introduced, and in the 1990s, linear accelerators started being acquired. Currently, most radiation therapy centers in Lebanon provide state-of-the-art treatment planning and delivery.[17]

### Medical Oncology

After the end of the civil war in 1990, large numbers of medical oncologists returned to Lebanon from Europe and the United States. Subspecialties were built and research increased. Established in 1997, the Lebanese Society of Medical Oncology, in collaboration with other societies, organizes annual meetings and periodic Medical Education postgraduate updates and conferences.[17]

### Pediatric Oncology

The establishment of St. Jude's Children Cancer Center in Lebanon provided one of the most important and major steps forward in the treatment of children with cancer in Lebanon and the Middle East. The center is affiliated with St. Jude's Children Research Center, provides treatment free of charge to children with cancer, and has high cure rates as in Memphis, Tennessee, its origin of establishment, under the same motto: "No child should die in the dawn of life."[17]

## CANCER CARE INFRASTRUCTURE AND CANCER CARE WORKFORCE

The private sector (hospitals, doctors, and pharmacies) dominates the health-care system. Lebanon has are 6 medical schools, 11 nursing schools, around 100 medical oncologists, and 15 radiotherapists. This number has been on the rise since to include more hospitals, medical centers, pathology laboratories, specialized physicians, nurses, chemotherapy centers, radiation oncology centers, and radiology. Around 400 students graduate from medical schools, many of whom go for specialization overseas. University hospitals and affiliated medical centers offer training in Lebanon and provide specialized care for patients. Clinical research and basic research take place at those institutions.

Major academic institutions hold multidisciplinary tumor board conferences where they discuss their patients among different specialists. Variable numbers of physicians from community, smaller, or rural hospitals attend university hospital tumor boards periodically. When all specialists are not available, mini-tumor boards were suggested to be held between physicians caring for particular patients.[18] Postgraduate conferences are held periodically, with annual meetings organized by the Lebanese Society of Medical Oncology, as well as Best of ASCO meetings in collaboration with the American Society of Clinical Oncology.[19]

## CANCER CLINICAL CARE

Most care for cancer patients is provided at physicians' private clinics and general hospitals. There are no stand-alone cancer centers except for a Children's Cancer Center in Lebanon affiliated with St. Jude's. Naef K. Basile Cancer Institute is part of AUBMC. There are oncology divisions and oncology surgeons in several hospitals and institutions who specialize in certain types of cancer such as breast or hepatobiliary cancer. This trend started in the 1960s when surgeons began returning from their specialties and subspecialties abroad to practice in Lebanon; it was pushed further by improvements in other fields such as imaging, radiation, pathology, surgery, anesthesia, and infectious diseases.[17]

## CANCER CARE OUTCOMES

Data on outcome of cancer patients is limited. Concerning breast cancer, the majority of patients are operated by general surgeons, with a limited but growing number of oncology surgeons at major medical centers. After historical data that showed a large number of locally advanced and metastatic disease at presentation,[16] new experience shows less advanced and relatively more early breast cancer in Lebanon.[20] The rates of mastectomies fell to about 50% of cases. Survival rates of 80% to 90% in cases of early breast cancer were reported from the American University of Beirut.[20] Awareness campaigns have made a significant contribution to the relative increase of early breast cancer stages at diagnosis. As for prostate, lung, colon, lymphoma, and childhood cancers, there are no reports or data on clinical characteristics or outcome of patients from Lebanon.

## CANCER CARE CONTINUUM

In Lebanon, physicians, oncology societies, nongovernmental organizations (NGOs), and MOPH organize regular media appearances and periodic campaigns for prevention and early detection of cancer. Antismoking campaigns and dedicated NGOs and lobbying had a great influence on the implementation of an antismoking law banning ads and smoking in public places in Lebanon.[21,22] With regard to breast cancer, awareness campaigns promote awareness, monthly breast self-examination, annual clinical breast examination, and yearly mammography starting at age 40. The campaigns are run throughout the year but intensely during the international breast awareness month of October, which have had a great impact on breast cancer in Lebanon with lower rates of advanced breast cancer and less total mastectomies.[23] Innovative campaigns include lectures and support by the MOH, medical societies, and Lebanese Breast Cancer Foundation, Faire Face, May Jallad Foundation, and other NGOs. Campaigns for awareness evolved to include fighting taboos that associated cancer with inevitable death and promote celebration of survivorship from cancer. Media has proven to be very helpful for wide dissemination of historic events such as lighting in pink of Lebanese landmark Raouche Rocks in Beirut to promote awareness and celebrate survivorship against hardships.[23] Campaigns for prevention of other cancers are mostly media campaigns and periodic intervention by physicians and medical societies. More organized and systematic campaigns are needed for avoiding excessive exposures to sun and also for colorectal cancer screening by occult blood testing and colonoscopies.

## CANCER RESEARCH

Clinical and basic research is mostly done at universities and major centers. Clinical research activities include few phase II trials and participation in international phase III clinical trials, as well as prospective and retrospective studies. Many studies performed in Lebanon have resulted in data being published in both local and international peer-reviewed journals.

Concerning funding of such research, the main bulk comes from research grants from pharmaceutical companies and donations. The Lebanese government and major universities and institutions are asked to increase investment in research.[9]

## FUTURE DIRECTIONS

We provided in this chapter a summary of demographic and epidemiologic information on Lebanon. In spite of continuing political instabilities and repeated wars, the country provides advanced health care for patients with cancer. Awareness campaigns have made significant impact on prevention and early detection of certain cancers, such as downstaging of breast cancer and increased breast-conserving surgery and higher cure rates. Antismoking campaigns have resulted in banning smoking on national and satellite televisions and antismoking laws. State-of-the-art diagnostics and treatment modalities progress at a fast rate in a free market and private environment. Large numbers of oncologists and health-care professionals trained in the United States and Europe contributed to availability of state-of-the-art multidisciplinary oncology care and research in Lebanon. The five most common cancers in males, in decreasing order, are prostate, lung, bladder, colorectal, and non-Hodgkin's lymphoma. In females, the most common cancers are breast, colorectal, ovarian, lung, and bladder cancers.[8] In addition to increased public awareness and health education, more organized national screening campaigns, better access to care, patient support, and patient advocacy, future developments should focus on quality care and patient outcome both at university medical centers and at primary-care community hospitals. Efforts at better and complete collection of cancer registry data that should include demographics, clinical and pathological information, and follow-up and outcome data are needed. A reliable NCR is an essential component of

TABLE 24.1 The 10 Most Frequent Cancers among Males in Selected Arab Countries

| Country | Algeria | Egypt | Jordan | Lebanon | Oman | KSA |
|---|---|---|---|---|---|---|
| Source | Cancer Incidence in five continents 2002[24] | Middle East Cancer Consortium 2005[25] | MOH Jordan 2008[26] | MOPH Lebanon 2003[8] | MOH Oman 2006[27] | MOH KSA 2004[28] |
| Total number of cancer patients | 3,426 | 5,284 | 2,274 | 3,841 | 393 | 3,478 |
| #1 | Lung (18%) | Bladder (16.1%) | Colorectal (14.5%) | Prostate (17.6%) | Lymphoma (14.4%) | Colorectal (10.5%) |
| #2 | Bladder (11.7%) | Lymphoma (15.6%) | Lung (13.1%) | Lung (16%) | Stomach (9.8%) | NHL (9.5%) |
| #3 | Colorectal (8.3%) | Liver (12.4%) | Bladder (7.5%) | Bladder (15.2%) | Leukemia (9%) | Leukemia (6.9%) |
| #4 | Stomach (6.2%) | Leukemia (9.1%) | Prostate (7.2%) | Colorectal (8%) | Lung (6.8%) | Lung (6.7%) |
| #5 | Prostate (5.7%) | Lung (7%) | Leukemia (6.7%) | NHL (5%) | Bladder (6.6%) | Liver (6.6%) |
| #6 | Lymphoma (5.7%) | Colorectal (4.9%) | NHL (5.1%) | Stomach (3.2%) | Prostate (6.6%) | Prostate (6.2%) |
| #7 | Larynx (4.5%) | Prostate (3.7%) | Stomach (4.2%) | Larynx (2.8%) | Colorectal (5.1%) | Hodgkin (4.8%) |
| #8 | Nasoph. (3.7%) | CNS (3.1%) | CNS (3.9%) | CNS (2.7%) | Skin (4.1%) | Bladder (4.6%) |
| #9 | CNS (3.7%) | Larynx (2.5%) | Larynx (3.8%) | Testis (2.2%) | Liver (4.1%) | CNS (4.2%) |
| #10 | Larynx (3.2%) | Stomach (2.4%) | Hodgkin (2.9%) | Kidney (2.1%) | Larynx (2.4%) | Stomach (4.1%) |

TABLE 24.2  The 10 Most Frequent Cancers among Females in Selected Arab Countries

| Country | Algeria | Egypt | Jordan | Lebanon | Oman | KSA |
|---|---|---|---|---|---|---|
| Source | Cancer incidence in five continents 2002[24] | Middle East Cancer Consortium 2005[25] | MOH Jordan 2008[26] | MOPH Lebanon 2003[8] | MOH Oman 2006[27] | MOHKSA 2004[28] |
| Total number of cancer patients | 3,767 | 5,171 | 2,332 | 4,047 | 423 | 3,491 |
| #1 | Breast (25%) | Breast (37.6%) | Breast (36.7%) | Breast (42.3%) | Breast (21.5%) | Breast (22.4%) |
| #2 | Cervix (14%) | Lymphoma (9.6%) | Colorectal (9.4%) | Colorectal (7.4%) | Thyroid (8.7%) | Thyroid (9.4%) |
| #3 | Colorectal (6.9%) | Leukemia (4.5%) | Uterine (5.4%) | Ovarian (4.7%) | Cervix (6.2%) | Colorectal (8.0%) |
| #4 | Gall Bladder, etc. (5.6%) | Ovarian (4.1%) | Thyroid (4.7%) | Lung (4.5%) | Stomach (5.9%) | NHL (6.4%) |
| #5 | Thyroid (5.3%) | Bladder (4%) | NHL (4.6%) | Bladder (3.5%) | Lymphoma (5.9%) | Leukemia (5.6%) |
| #6 | Ovarian (5%) | Cervix (3.8%) | Leukemia (4.0%) | Uterine. (2.8%) | Ovarian (5%) | Skin (3.6%) |
| #7 | Stomach (4.3%) | Larynx (3.4%) | Ovarian (3.6%) | Stomach (2.6%) | Leukemia (4.3%) | Uterine. (3.4%) |
| #8 | Lymphoma (3.7%) | CNS (3.1%) | Stomach (3.1%) | Thyroid (2.4%) | Bladder (3.4%) | Ovarian (3.1%) |
| #9 | Bladder (2.4%) | Uterine (2.4%) | CNS (2.8%) | Cervix (2.3%) | Skin (3.2%) | CNS (2.9%) |
| #10 | Uterine (2.3%) | Lung (2.4%) | Lung (2.5%) | Kidney (1.5%) | Colorectal (3%) | Hodgkin (2.8%) |

a national cancer control plan that should be given a national priority. More investment in basic and clinical research related to local health issues, as well as international science, is required in Lebanon and most neighboring Arab countries, and they go hand in hand with advancement and improvement of the care of patients with cancer.

## REFERENCES

1. World Health Organization. NCD Country Profiles. 2011. Available at http://www.who.int/nmh/countries/lbn_en.pdf. Accessed February 21, 2013.
2. Ministry of Public Health—Lebanon. Communicable Disease Surveillance, 2012. Available at http://www.moph.gov.lb/Prevention/Surveillance/documents/Lebanon2012.htm. Accessed February 21, 2013.
3. World Health Organization. Communicable Disease Risk Assessment and Interventions—Middle East crisis: Lebanon, 2006. Available at http://www.who.int/diseasecontrol_emergencies/guidelines/cd_risk_assessment_leba non_. Accessed February 21, 2013.
4. World Health Organization. Noncommunicable Disease. Available at http://www.emro.who.int/entity/noncommunicable-diseases/.
5. Rady A. Is lifestyle affecting the risk of noncommunicable diseases in Lebanon? *Human Health* 2010; 13: 15–17.
6. Kronfol N. LICOR and Rates of Cardiovascular Interventions, 2009. Available at http://www.syndicateofhospitals.org.lb/magazine/apr2009/Latin 25 Report.pdf.
7. Boutayeb A, Lamlili M, Boutayeb W, Abdellatif M, Abderrahim Z, Noureddine R. The rise of diabetes prevalence in the Arab region. *Open J Epidemiol* 2012; 2: 55–60.
8. National Cancer Registry. Cancer in Lebanon 2003, 2003. Available at http://www.moph.gov.lb/Publications/Documents/NCR2003.pdf. Accessed February 18, 2013.
9. El Saghir NS. Modern cancer management and research in the Middle East. *Lancet Oncol* 2012; 13(11): 1076–78.
10. Doumit MAA, Huijer HA, Kelley JH, Nassar N. The lived experience of Lebanese family caregivers of cancer patients. *Cancer Nurs* 2008; 31(4): E36–E42.
11. Azar HA. Cancer in Lebanon and the Near East. *Cancer* 1962; 15: 66–78.
12. Abou-Daoud KT. Morbidity from cancer in Lebanon. *Cancer* 1966; 19(9): 1293–300.
13. Geahchan N, Taleb N. Epidemiological study of cancer in Lebanon. Presentation at the IARC Mediterranean Colloquium on Epidemiology and Cancer Incidence. Lyon, France, 1986.
14. El Saghir NS, Adib S, Mufarrij A, et al. Cancer in Lebanon: analysis of 10,220 cases from the American University of Beirut Medical Center. *J Med Liban* 1998; 46(1): 4–11.
15. Shamseddine A, Sibai A-M, Gehchan N, et al. Cancer incidence in postwar Lebanon: findings from the first national population-based registry, 1998. *Ann Epidemiol* 2004; 14(9): 663–68.

16. El Saghir NS, Khalil MK, Eid T, et al. Trends in epidemiology and management of breast cancer in developing Arab countries: a literature and registry analysis. *Int J Surg* (London, England) 2007; 5(4): 225–33.

17. El Saghir N, Khoury K, Bikhazi K. Cancer care in Lebanon: incidence, history, and developments of therapy. In: *The Order of Physicians . . . After Half a Century. From Pioneers . . . to a Promising Future*. 1st ed. Beirut, 2013.

18. El Saghir NS, El-Asmar N, Hajj C, et al. Survey of utilization of multidisciplinary management tumor boards in Arab countries. *Breast* (Edinburgh, Scotland) 2011; 20(Suppl 2): S70–S74.

19. El Saghir N, Kattan J, Ibrahim K. Participants Laud a Successful Best of ASCO® Lebanon 2010. ASCO Connection, 2011. Available at http://connection.asco.org/Magazine/Article/ID/2807/Participants-Laud-a-Successful-Best-of-ASCO-Lebanon-2010.aspx.

20. El Saghir N, Hatoum H, Shamseddeen W, Shamseddine A. Lymph node ratio of involved lymph nodes to the total number of removed lymph nodes from the axilla predicts prognosis and survival in early stage breast cancer. ASCO Breast Cancer Symposium. San Francisco, 2007.

21. Burki TK. Tobacco control in the Middle East. *Lancet Oncol* 2012; 13(11): 1079.

22. Anon. Tobacco Control Legislation, 2011. Available at http://www.tobaccocontrol.gov.lb/Legislation/Documents/law english pdf.pdf. Accessed February 22, 2013.

23. Khoury K, Assi H, El Saghir N. Lebanon Lights Up in Pink Its Landmark Raouché Rocks in the Middle of the Mediterranean Sea. ASCO Connection. 2012. Available at http://connection.asco.org/Magazine/Article/ID/3373/Lebanon-Lights-Up-in-Pink-its-Landmark-Raouche-Rocks-in-the-Middle-of-the-Mediterranean-Sea.aspx.

24. International Agency for Research on Cancer. Cancer Incidence in Five Continents. IX. Available at http://www.iarc.fr/en/publications/pdfs-online/epi/sp160/CI5vol9.pdf. Accessed April 30, 2013.

25. Freedman L, Edwards B, Ries L, Young J. Cancer Incidence in Four Member Countries (Cyprus, Egypt, Israel, and Jordan) of the Middle East Cancer Consortium (MECC) Compared with US SEER. National Cancer Institute. Available at http://www.mecc.cancer.gov/publication/mecc-monograph.pdf. Accessed April 30, 2013.

26. Jordan Cancer Registry. Cancer Incidence in Jordan 2008. 2008. Available at http://www.jbcp.jo/files/JRC 2008.pdf. Accessed April 30, 2013.

27. Oman National Cancer Registry. Cancer Incidence in Oman 2006. 2006. Available at http://www.moh.gov.om/en/reports/publications/Newsletter17-3.pdf. Accessed April 30, 2013.

28. Saudi Cancer Registry. Cancer Incidence Report Saudi Arabia 2004. 2004. Available at http://www.kfshrc.edu.sa/wps/wcm/connect/40dcba804a8d741fb731f7e404c39865/SCR2004W.pdf?MOD=AJPERES&lmod=1265914960&CACHEID=40dcba804a8d741fb731f7e404c39865. Accessed April 30, 2013.

# 25

# Morocco

## *Zineb Benbrahim*

## PUBLIC HEALTH PERSPECTIVE

The social protection system covers all employees: workers and retired employees from the public sector benefit via CNOPS (National Social Welfare Organisations) and employees and retired workers from the private sector benefit via CNSS (National Social Security). Since 2005, *all* Moroccan citizens are required to be members of a basic medical scheme, AMO, via their local branch.

The neediest part of the population has access to RAMED, a medical assistance scheme, which allows persons who are not members of the AMO to benefit from treatment dispensed in public medical centers.[1]

The health budget corresponds to 1.1% of the gross domestic product and 5.5% of the central government budget.

The health-care system includes 201 hospitals, 2,400 health centers, and 5 university clinics. Morocco has an inadequate number of physicians (6.46 per 10,000 people) and hospital beds (11 per 10,000 people).[2]

### Life Expectancy

The average life expectancy at birth was 72.13 years in 2011, 69.91 years for males and 74.47 years for females.[3]

### Communicable Diseases

According to 2009 estimates, approximately 92 per 100,000 inhabitants were infected with tuberculosis and 0.1% of the population between the ages of 15 and 49 was infected with human immunodeficiency virus/acquired immune deficiency syndrome (HIV/AIDS).[4]

## Noncommunicable Diseases

No national NCD mortality register is available in Morocco. WHO estimates that in 2010 the principal causes of mortality were circulatory system diseases (40%), perinatal diseases (19%), cancer (12%), endocrine, nutritional, and metabolic diseases (16%), and respiratory system diseases (5%).[5]

## Cancer as a Public Health Problem

In Morocco, about 30,000 new cancer cases are recorded every year. Patients are more often diagnosed at very advanced stages of the disease: for breast cancers the diagnosis is made at stages III and IV in 57% of cases, whereas for lung cancers 96% of the cases are diagnosed at stages III and IV.

The time length between the onset of the first symptoms and the first medical examination exceeds 6 months in 14% of cases.

The follow-up period of cancer patients is very low (below 2 years in 74% of cases), and about half of the patients are not followed up after 1 year. Therefore, no reliable data exists to estimate the patient survival after 5 years.[6]

## CANCER ETIOLOGY

Smoking prevalence in Moroccan population is 16% (30% for males and 1% for females). Passive smoking is also high: 32% of nonsmokers are exposed to smoking in their familial environment, 18% are exposed in their professional environment, and 60% are exposed in public places.

A total of 6.8% of males drink alcoholic beverages, and 2 out of 1,000 consume alcohol on a daily basis.

The prevalence of obesity is 14%, and 30% of that group is overweight.

Among the general population, 64% are usually exposed to sun during the hot time of the day (11 A.M. to 4 P.M.); one-third of them do not use any protection from the sun.

In professional environments, exposure to carcinogenic products is frequent, and the use of protective means is quite weak. For example, in the leather handicraft environment, the exposure to salt and paint is, respectively, 100% and 55%.[6]

## CANCER STATISTICS

In Morocco, two cancer registries are available. The first one is the Grand Casablanca Registry, established in 2004 and reissued in 2012.[7] The second one is the Rabat Cancer Registry, established in June 2012.[8] According to Rabat Cancer Registry, between 2006 and 2008, 2,473 new cases of cancer were recorded in this region. The median age was 62 years for men and 54 years for women. The mean age was significantly higher in men (60.1 years vs. 54.1 years). The standardized incidence of the Moroccan population between 2006 and 2008 was 110.8 out of 100,000 in men versus 100.4 out of 100,000 for women. The cumulative risk is 15.2% and 12.1%, respectively, in men and women. Lung cancer ranks first among men (19.0%) followed by prostate cancer (15.5%). In women, 40% of cases are breast cancer, followed by cervical cancer (11.4%). In both sexes, colon cancer is the most common digestive cancer and non-Hodgkin's lymphoma is the most common hematological malignancy. The observed incidence was significantly lower than the incidence reported in Western countries.

## CANCER CARE INFRASTRUCTURE AND WORKFORCE

The public sector, which provides care for the majority of Moroccans, has 10 sites for cancer care. All those centers are located in the following cities: Rabat, Casablanca, Fez, Oujda, Meknes, Houcima, Marrakesh, Agadir, Errachidia, and Beni Mellal.

In Morocco, a deficit is seen in specialized technical and human means; for instance, consider the following deficits in 2007:

- 7 mammographic units per 1 million women
- 1.3 MRI per 1 million inhabitants
- 2.8 medical oncologists per 1 million inhabitants
- 2.1 radiotherapists per 1 million inhabitants
- one simulator per 5 million inhabitants
- one cobalt-therapy unit per 3 million inhabitants
- one accelerator for about every 2.8 million inhabitants[6]

## CANCER CLINICAL CARE

The following data is given according to the Rabat Cancer Registry.[8]

*Breast cancer* is the most common cancer in women (40% of cases). The median age is 50 years, and young women under 35 account for 6.7% of cases. Infiltrating ductal carcinoma is the most frequent, accounting for 85% of cases; 58% of cases are diagnosed at stages I and II. The incidence of breast cancer in Morocco, as in other Arab and African countries, remains significantly lower than the observed incidences in Europe and North America.

*Lung cancer* is the most common cancer in males (19% of cases). Its incidence and the cumulative risk from 0 to 74 years is 10 times higher in men than in women. This incidence, especially among women, is lower than that observed in Europe and North America. It is most often adenocarcinoma (42%) or a squamous cell carcinoma (29%). At least half of the cases are at the stage of metastasis at diagnosis.

*Prostate cancer* is the second most common cancer in males after lung cancer. Its incidence increases significantly with age and exceeds 230 per 100,000 people aged 65 and over. Almost all prostate cancers are adenocarcinomas. The incidence of prostate cancer found in Rabat remains significantly lower than that reported in developed countries.

*Uterine cervix* is the second most common cancer in women (11.4%). The median age at diagnosis is 53 years; 11% of patients are younger than 40 years. Human papillomavirus infection is the main risk factor. Uterine cervix is diagnosed at stages I or II in 54% of cases and stage IV in 8% of cases in Morocco. Squamous cell carcinoma is the most common histologic type (89%). The incidence of cervical cancer in Morocco is higher than that in Europe and North America.

*Colon* is the first location of digestive cancers in Morocco (28%). The incidence of colon cancer increases with age and is significantly higher among men over 65 years; 30% of cases are diagnosed at the stage of metastasis. In Rabat, the incidence of colon cancer is higher than the incidence of rectal cancer. However, the incidence in Morocco remains much lower than that in Europe, North America, and the Far East.

## CANCER CARE CONTINUUM

### Prevention

Morocco has adopted, under the guidance of Her Royal Highness Princess Lalla Salma, president of the Association Lalla Salma against Cancer, the National Plan of Cancer Prevention and Control (NPCPC), which has the following objectives:

- Reducing active and passive smoking
- Reducing obesity
- Increasing the number of persons with a healthy lifestyle
- Reducing the number of people drinking alcohol
- Improving protective measures and practices in occupational environments
- Implementing a strategy for the surveillance of cancers and its risk factors

### Screening

Only 1 out of 10 Moroccans undergoes medical examinations on a regular basis, and about three-quarters of women have never visited a gynecologist.

NPCPC has the objective to introduce, from 2010 to 2019, a screening program for both breast and cervical cancers.

## FUTURE DIRECTIONS

The goals of NCPCP implementation for 2010 to 2019 are as follows:

- Reduce by 30% the prevalence of behavioral and environmental risks.
- Screen a minimum of 50% of women for breast and cervical cancers, representing the target population.
- Cure 50% of treated cancer patients.
- Have a nationwide palliative care network and support 100% of patients requiring palliative care.[6]

## REFERENCES

1. http://en.april-international.com/global/destination/the-healthcare-system-in-morocco.
2. "Demography. Kingdom of Morocco."
3. http://www.sesrtcic.org/oic-member-countries-infigures.php?c_code=36&cat_code=8.
4. http://www.indexmundi.com/morocco/.
5. http://www.who.int/nmh/countries/mar_en.pdf.
6. http://www.contrelecancer.ma/site_media/uploaded_files/Synthese_PNPCC_2010-1019.pdf.
7. http://www.contrelecancer.ma/fr/media/2012/05/26/le-nouveau-registre-des-cancers-de-la-region-du-grand-casablanca-est-paru/.
8. http://www.fmp-usmba.ac.ma/pdf/Documents/cancer_registry_mor_rabat.pdf.

# 26

# Pakistan

## Sheheryar Kairas Kabraji and Nehal Masood

### PUBLIC HEALTH PERSPECTIVE

The biggest challenge facing effective public health care in Pakistan is the lack of resources, which severely restricts access to health care. Total expenditure on health (TEH) constituted only 2.5% of gross domestic product in 2011. Government expenditure was 27% of TEH, with private expenditure being 73%. Of this private expenditure, 86.3% was out-of-pocket expense. Thus, individual economic status determines access to oncology care and affects outcomes in Pakistan.

#### Life Expectancy

In 2012, the life expectancy at birth was 66.35 years (64.52 years for men and 68.28 for women). Infant mortality rate was 72 per 1,000 live births, whereas adult mortality rate was 208 per 1,000 persons.

#### Communicable Diseases

Communicable diseases are responsible for 64% of years of life lost in Pakistan. In 2008, childhood mortality (0 to 14 years) was predominantly due to respiratory tract infections (106,400 deaths), diarrheal diseases (94,100 deaths), and childhood cluster diseases (pertussis, poliomyelitis, diphtheria, measles, and tetanus). Tuberculosis (TB) caused 4,200 deaths, whereas malaria caused 800 deaths. In adults (>15 years) communicable diseases caused comparatively fewer deaths: respiratory tract infections (82,500 deaths) followed by TB (26,900), diarrheal diseases (17,600), and HIV (4,600 deaths, 15 to 59 years).

## Noncommunicable Diseases

In 2011, noncommunicable diseases accounted for 46% of all deaths in Pakistan (33.4% of men and 35.4% of women). Of these, cardiovascular disease was the biggest killer (25%), followed by cancer (7%), respiratory diseases (5%), and diabetes (1%). These are likely to be underestimates since cause of death is not consistently reported in Pakistan.

## Cancer as a Public Health Problem

The public health burden of cancer in Pakistan is underestimated and underappreciated by health-care providers as well as the general public. Although regional cancer registries exist in Pakistan, there is no national cancer registry. Thus, the burden of disease is extrapolated from regional and historical data.

The annual incidence is estimated at 114.7 cases per 100,000 persons. In 2008, cancer caused 101,700 deaths in Pakistan, surpassed only by cardiovascular disease. Most of these deaths occurred in persons aged 14 to 59, reflecting Pakistan's young population. It has been estimated that between 2008 and 2030, there will be a 78% increase in cancer incidence in medium-development index countries like Pakistan, which is ill-equipped to tackle its existing cancer burden, let alone a case increase of that magnitude.

## CANCER ETIOLOGY

### Cancer Statistics

The first population-based cancer registry was established in 1995 in Karachi at Sindh Government Services Hospital. The Punjab Cancer Registry was founded in 2005 and draws data from 15 participating centers as of 2013.

In the absence of a national cancer registry, the most comprehensive reports on incidence and prevalence of cancer in Pakistan come from the World Health Organization. The data is derived from the observed incidence rates in south Karachi (1998 to 2002), the estimated rates for north India, and the national estimate for Iran (2008). Figure 26.1 shows the age-standardized incidence and mortality rates for cancers in both sexes in Pakistan. Table 26.1 shows the most common cancers in Pakistan by total cases divided by sex. Breast and cervical cancer are most common in women, whereas lung and lip, oral cavity cancers are most common in men.

The age-adjusted incidence of breast cancer in Pakistan (based on the Karachi registry) has been reported as the highest in Asia (excepting Israel). Ductal carcinoma in situ accounts for only 0.6% of cases, suggesting a greater proportion of invasive disease in Pakistani women. However, a

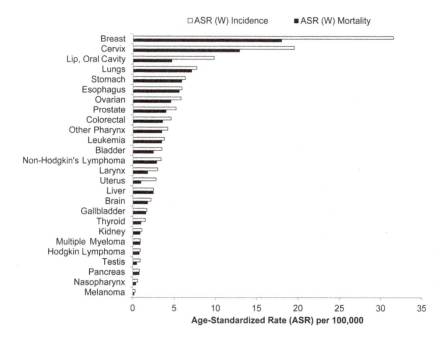

**FIGURE 26.1** Research on cancer, 2010. Available at http://globocan.iarc.fr. Accessed August 6, 2013.

**TABLE 26.1 Most Common Cancers in Pakistan by Incidence**

| Most Common Cancers by Incidence (2008) | | |
| --- | --- | --- |
| Male (number of cases) | Female (number of cases) | Both Sexes (number of cases) |
| Lung (6,844) | Breast (19,271) | Breast (19,271) |
| Lip, oral cavity (6,803) | Cervix uteri (11,688) | Lip, oral cavity (11,698) |
| Stomach (4,530) | Lip, oral cavity (4,895) | Cervix uteri (11,688) |
| Other pharynx (3,631) | Ovary (3,568) | Lung (8,282) |
| Esophagus (3,529) | Esophagus (3,115) | Stomach (7,052) |

study comparing Pakistani-Indian women living in the United States with a non-Hispanic white cohort using SEER data found no difference in the proportion of invasive to noninvasive disease. But South Asian women did present with tumors at an earlier age, with higher stage and grade and more involved lymph nodes. This suggests that the biology of breast cancer in women living in Pakistan may differ from North American populations and requires further elucidation.

Use of betel leaf and areca (betel) nut in *paan* (both with and without tobacco) has been associated with a number of squamous cell cancers, including oral, esophageal, and lung. Persons affected with oral squamous cell cancers were more likely (adjusted odds ratio 8.42; 95% CI: 2.31, 30.64) to be heavy users of *paan* than case-matched controls in an urban tertiary hospital.

The combination of areca nut with chewed tobacco has also been associated with an increased risk of squamous cell carcinoma of the esophagus (adjusted matched odds ratio 7.6; 95% CI: 4.4, 13.3) in an urban population at a tertiary center in Karachi. Areca nut extract is thought to induce carcinogenesis via effects on cell division (activation of checkpoint kinase 1/2) and invasion (activation of matrix metalloproteinase-9). Frequent use of areca nut and snuff among residents of Khyber-Pakhtunkhwa may explain the elevated rates of esophageal cancer in this population.

The countrywide age-standardized rate for hepatocellular carcinoma for both sexes is 2.5 per 100,000 persons but noted to be as high as 12.3 per 100,000 persons from the Quetta cancer registry. Between 1970 and the late 1990s, hepatitis B infection was the commonest etiology but since 2000 hepatitis C has been the predominant etiologic agent (1,569 out of 3,036 cases), with nonalcoholic fatty liver disease rising in incidence.

## HISTORY OF CANCER CARE

At independence in 1947, cancer care was delivered in general hospitals and surgery was the only available modality. Radiotherapy was introduced in 1950 at Mayo Hospital. The first hospitals dedicated to cancer care were set up by the Pakistan Atomic Energy Commission as radiation/clinical oncology faculties. The first medical oncology faculty was established at the Aga Khan University Hospital (AKUH) in 1980. Shaukat Khanum Memorial Research Center and Hospital (SKMRCH) was Pakistan's first private stand-alone cancer center, founded in 1994.

Bone marrow transplant was first performed in 1995 at the Dr. Ziauddin Hospital, Karachi, for acute myeloid leukemia. This transplant was followed by the first allogenic transplant in 1996 at the Combined Military Hospital, Rawalpindi. By 2004, bone marrow transplantation was under way at the AKUH in Karachi. In 2013, autologous bone marrow transplants were also performed at SKMRCH, with a program for allogenic transplants pending. Aplastic anemia was the commonest indication for transplant, followed by beta-thalassemia major and leukemia.

## CANCER CARE INFRASTRUCTURE

Cancer care is delivered through both public hospitals (government owned and operated) and a number of private hospitals and clinics. In 2013, there were 21 stand-alone cancer centers in Pakistan, of which SKMRCH is the largest and best known. Supportive care infrastructure for cancer patients, such as blood banks, intensive care units, and outpatient chemotherapy infusion rooms, are available at all major centers. However, some local limitations persist regardless of institution, such as expecting patients to arrange blood products from family or other institutions.

### Radiation Oncology

The use of radiotherapy to treat cancer began in Lahore in 1950 followed by Karachi in 1959. In 2009, there were 20 cobalt-60, 17 linear accelerators, 12 fluoroscopic simulators, and 4 CT simulators in Pakistan. The College of Physicians and Surgeons Pakistan has accredited 12 centers for radiotherapy: four in Karachi, three in Lahore, and one each in Faisalabad, Islamabad, Multan, Peshawar, and Rawalpindi.

### Palliative Care

The provision of high-quality palliative care is hampered by poor government support and lack of trained palliative care teams. Two centers in Pakistan, the SKMRCH and AKUH, have formal palliative care services. Inpatient hospices are few and most are run as informal charities. There is minimal formal home hospice care. Morphine is available but in order to prescribe opioids, practitioners must undergo an onerous process of bureaucratic approval involving no less than four government ministries. However, efforts are under way by the International Network for Cancer Training and Research and Association of Physicians of Pakistani Descent in North America to develop local capacity and build government support for palliative care services.

### Cancer Care Workforce

The health-care workforce in Pakistan is inadequate, with 7.8 physicians per 10,000 persons and 3.8 nurses and midwives per 10,000 persons. Although pockets of excellence exist, medical education is often out of date and systems of continuing medical education are lacking. Health-care personnel are largely undercompensated and brain drain is a pervasive problem.

### Allopathic

In 2013, there were approximately 125 oncologists in Pakistan. The majority were clinical oncologists, providing both radiotherapy and chemotherapy treatment. Given the paucity of oncologists, care is rarely subspecialized, even at academic medical centers, such that an individual oncologist may see hematologic and solid malignancies in the same clinic. The AKUH in Karachi, an urban tertiary center, reports seven oncologists and four hematologists on staff. Multidisciplinary clinics are not present in most major centers although there are moves to make this arrangement standard. Most oncological surgery is performed by organ-system generalists, and there are few specialized surgical oncologists. Nurses administer chemotherapy in both the inpatient and outpatient settings. Intermediate providers such as nurse practitioners or physician assistants are not available in Pakistan.

## Traditional, Complementary, and Alternative Medicine (TCAM)

Alternative and traditional medical practitioners form a significant source of care for Pakistanis with cancer. Up to 84% of cancer patients surveyed at four allopathic hospitals in Pakistan admitted to using TCAM in addition to allopathic therapies. Most common of these (70.4%) is *dum darood* or the practice of using prayer as part of healing; 35% of those surveyed visited a *hakeem* or traditional medical practitioner who uses herbs and minerals. Those with a college education were much less likely to use a hakeem.

## CANCER CLINICAL CARE AND OUTCOMES

### Diagnosis

Given the absence of screening and regular primary-care visits, most patients are diagnosed with late-stage disease. In one report, 67% of patients with cervical cancer presented with stages II to IV disease. Financial limitations, limited awareness of cancer risk factors, and scant preventative care practices contribute to the problem of late diagnosis.

### Staging

Available technologies for staging include plain radiography, computed tomography, and positron-emitted tomography as well as endoscopic procedures such as bronchoscopy. Pakistan's first PET scanner was installed in 2010 in Lahore, while a second facility became functional in Karachi in 2012.

### Treatment

Chemotherapeutics are widely available in Pakistan although the regimens offered vary depending on the practitioner's knowledge and patient's ability to pay. This can lead to patients' receiving second-line therapies because they are less expensive or being unable to complete treatment due to cost. In one report, one-third of patients being treated for acute myeloid leukemia could not complete or initiate treatment due to financial constraints. Certain chemotherapeutics are made more accessible by patient assistance programs. Novartis' Glivec International Patient Assistance Program makes imatinib available for treatment of chronic myeloid leukemia to patients who would otherwise be unable to afford the drug.

Treatment outcomes are often curtailed by the need for better supportive care, such as managing infections after chemotherapy. A 5-year retrospective review of 304 cases of acute lymphoblastic leukemia treated at a tertiary center found that 63 of 74 deaths were related to infection.

As much of cancer surgery is performed by generalists (fellowship training in surgical oncology started only in 2012), patients are frequently taken to surgery inappropriately, often because of inadequate staging. However, a retrospective review found that 30-day mortality after colorectal surgery at a university hospital in Karachi was comparable to a similar institution in Germany. These data suggest that good surgical outcomes are readily achievable if performed at appropriate centers in Pakistan.

## CANCER CARE CONTINUUM

### Prevention

Efforts to prevent cancers that develop from occupational, environmental, toxin, or infectious exposure are limited by lack of knowledge by both the public and health-care professionals. A 2010 study of 400 health-care professionals at two tertiary centers in Karachi found that only 37 were aware that a vaccine could prevent HPV infection and more than 25% of respondents could not identify risk factors for cervical cancer. Although a National Action Plan for Noncommunicable Diseases Prevention, Control and Health Promotion in Pakistan was proposed in 2004 with the aim of reducing exposure to carcinogenic agents in the environment, no restriction on the purchase or use of tobacco products has been instituted.

### Screening

Among surveyed Pakistanis, there is limited awareness that screening asymptomatic persons can prevent cancer. In a sample of 200 urban women in Karachi, only 30% were aware of mammography and only 25% of those over 40 years had undergone a mammogram. Surveyed physicians assumed that stigma associated with a breast cancer diagnosis was the most significant barrier to screening. In contrast, most women cited the cost and logistics of obtaining a mammogram.

Screening for cervical cancer is similarly hampered. In a survey, only 5% of women surveyed at an urban tertiary care center were aware of screening for cervical cancer. Barriers to screening for cervical cancer include poor participation (25% across women aged 15 to 59 years in urban Karachi) due to lack of husband's permission, reluctance to undergo a vaginal examination, and a failure to appreciate a benefit from screening in the absence of symptoms.

## Psychosocial Care

Cancer treatment and survival imposes a significant burden on patients and their families in Pakistan. In a study of 200 outpatients undergoing treatment, one-third had major depression. Family and religion were major sources of support, and only 11% consulted a psychiatrist. Given that the financial cost for care can be prohibitive, up to 56% of patients relied on family for financial support and 61% reported selling property or taking loans in order to afford care.

## CANCER RESEARCH

While the bulk of research from Pakistan comprises case reports or retrospective studies, prospective clinical trials (such as one demonstrating efficacy of fortnightly cetuximab in KRAS wild-type colon cancer) are increasingly common. However, extensive service obligations mean that most practitioners at academic centers struggle to find protected time for research. The training and employment of nonphysician providers such as nurse practitioners and physician assistants would free up oncologists to focus on important local research questions.

## FUTURE DIRECTIONS

Improving cancer care in Pakistan can be achieved only from increasing local knowledge, resources, and capacity. Establishing cancer registries, making large-scale investments in personnel, disseminating technology, and developing screening programs cannot occur via the private sector alone and require government investment. The focus should be on prevention via screening, reducing exposure to carcinogens like tobacco, and instituting vaccination programs (e.g., against HPV and hepatitis B). International partnerships can provide local researchers with the tools and knowledge base necessary to answer key questions about local patterns of disease. With the growing burden of cancer in Pakistan, both local and international resources will need to be mobilized to avert a crisis of care.

## BIBLIOGRAPHY

Akhtar S, Sheikh AA, Qureshi HU. Chewing areca nut, betel quid, oral snuff, cigarette smoking and the risk of oesophageal squamous-cell carcinoma in South Asians: a multicentre case-control study. *Eur J Cancer* 2012; 48: 655–61. doi:10.1016/j.ejca.2011.06.008.

Ali SF, Ayub S, Manzoor NF, et al. Knowledge and awareness about cervical cancer and its prevention amongst interns and nursing staff in Tertiary Care Hospitals in Karachi, Pakistan. *PLoS One* 2010; 5: e11059. doi:10.1371/journal.pone.0011059.

Ann-Lii Cheng GHC, Shen L, Price TJ, et al. Efficacy and safety of every-2-weeks cetuximab combined with FOLFOX or FOLFIRI as first-line therapy in patients with KRAS wild-type metastatic colorectal cancer (mCRC): an Asia-Pacific non-randomized phase II study (APEC). *J Clin Oncol* 2013; 13 (Suppl); abstr e14501. Available at http://meetinglibrary.asco.org/print/1157901.

Asim M, Zaidi A, Ghafoor T, Qureshi Y. Death analysis of childhood acute lymphoblastic leukaemia; experience at Shaukat Khanum Memorial Cancer Hospital and Research Centre, Pakistan. *J Pak Med Assoc* 2011; 61: 666–70.

Bhurgri Y. Cancer survival in South Karachi, Pakistan, 1995–1999. *IARC Sci Publ* 2011; 143–46.

Bray F, Jemal A, Grey N, Ferlay J, Forman D. Global cancer transitions according to the Human Development Index (2008–2030): a population-based study. *Lancet Oncol* 2012; 13: 790–801. doi:10.1016/s1470-2045(12)70211-5.

Butt AS, Abbas Z, Jafri W. Hepatocellular carcinoma in Pakistan: where do we stand? *Hepat Mon* 2012; 12: e6023. doi:10.5812/hepatmon.6023.

Cause-Specific Mortality, 2008: WHO Region by Country, 2013. Available at http://apps.who.int/gho/data/node.main.887?lang=en.

Chang MC, Chan CP, Wang WT, et al. Toxicity of areca nut ingredients: activation of CHK1/CHK2, induction of cell cycle arrest, and regulation of MMP-9 and TIMPs production in SAS epithelial cells. *Head Neck* 2013; 35: 1295–302. doi:10.1002/hed.23119.

CIA—The World Factbook, 2013. Available at https://www.cia.gov/library/publications/the-world-factbook/geos/pk.html.

Fadoo Z, Mushtaq N, Alvi S, Ali M. Acute myeloid leukaemia in children: experience at a tertiary care facility of Pakistan. *J Pak Med Assoc* 2012; 62: 125–28.

Ferlay J, Shin HR, Bray F, Forman D, Mathers C, Parkin DM. Estimates of worldwide burden of cancer in 2008: GLOBOCAN 2008. *Int J Cancer* 2010; 127: 2893–917. doi:10.1002/ijc.25516.

Geographical variation in th . . . [Asian Pac J Cancer Prev. 2005 Apr-Jun]—PubMed—NCBI, 2013. Available at http://www.ncbi.nlm.nih.gov/pubmed.

Imam SZ, Rehman F, Zeeshan MM, et al. Perceptions and practices of a Pakistani population regarding cervical cancer screening. *Asian Pac J Cancer Prev* 2008; 9: 42–44.

Javed A. Progress of oncology in Pakistan. *Indian J Med Paed* 2006; 27: 54–59.

Khan MR, Bari H, Zafar SN, Raza SA. Impact of age on outcome after colorectal cancer surgery in the elderly—a developing country perspective. *BMC Surg* 2011; 11, 17. doi:10.1186/1471-2482-11-17.

Life Expectancy: Life Tables Pakistan, 2013. Available at http://apps.who.int /gho/data/view.main.61230.

Maqsood B, Zeeshan MM, Rehman F, et al. Breast cancer screening practices and awareness in women admitted to a tertiary care hospital of Lahore, Pakistan. *J Pak Med Assoc* 2009; 59: 418–21.

Merchant A, Husain SS, Hosain M, et al. Paan without tobacco: an independent risk factor for oral cancer. *Int J Cancer* 2000; 86: 128–31. doi:10.1002/(SICI) 1097–0215(20000401)86:1<128::AID-IJC20>3.0.CO;2-M.

Moore MA, Ariyaratne Y, Badar F, et al. Cancer epidemiology in South Asia—past, present and future. *Asian Pac J Cancer Prev* 2010; 11(Suppl 2): 49–66..

Moran MS, Gonsalves L, Goss DM, Ma S. Breast cancers in U.S. residing Indian-Pakistani versus non-Hispanic White women: comparative analysis of clinical-pathologic features, treatment, and survival. *Breast Cancer Res Treat* 2011; 128: 543–51. doi:10.1007/s10549–011–1362–0.

Nishtar S, Mirza Z, Mohamud KB, Latif E, Ahmed A, Jafarey NA. Tobacco control: National Action Plan for NCD Prevention, Control and Health Promotion in Pakistan. *J Pak Med Assoc* 2004; 54: S31–S41.

Rashid YA, Ghafoor ZA, Masood N, et al. Psychosocial impact of cancer on adult patients. *J Pak Med Assoc* 2012; 62: 905–9.

Raza SA, Franceschi S, Pallardy S, et al. Human papillomavirus infection in women with and without cervical cancer in Karachi, Pakistan. *Br J Cancer* 2010; 102, 1657–60. doi:10.1038/sj.bjc.6605664.

Raza S, Sajun SZ, Selhorst CC. Breast cancer in Pakistan: identifying local beliefs and knowledge. *J Am Coll Radiol* 2012; 9: 571–77. doi:10.1016/j.jacr .2012.02.020.

Shad A, Ashraf MS, Hafeez H. Development of palliative-care services in a developing country: Pakistan. *J Pediatr Hematol Oncol* 2011 33(Suppl 1): S62–S63. doi:10.1097/MPH.0b013e3182122391.

Shamsi T, Hashmi K, Adil S, et al. The stem cell transplant program in Pakistan— the first decade. *Bone Marrow Transplant* 2008; 42(Suppl 1): S114–17. doi:10.1038/bmt.2008.137.

Sharan RN, Mehrotra R, Choudhury Y, Asotra K. Association of betel nut with carcinogenesis: revisit with a clinical perspective. *PLoS One* 2012; 7: e42759. doi:10.1371/journal.pone.0042759.

Tovey PA, Broom AF, Chatwin J, Ahmad S, Hafeez M. Use of traditional, complementary and allopathic medicines in Pakistan by cancer patients. *Rural Remote Health* 2005; 5: 447.

WHO | Pakistan. WHO, 2013. doi:/countries/pak/en/index.html.

Yusuf A. Cancer care in Pakistan. *Jpn J Clin Oncol* 2013; 43(8): 771–75. doi:10.1093/ jjco/hyt078.

# 27

# South Africa

*Lydia Dreosti*

## PUBLIC HEALTH PERSPECTIVE

South Africa has a dual health-care system. The majority (approximately 80%)[1] of the population have access only to health-care services provided by the government. A smaller proportion of the population has private health-care insurance (approximately 20%)[1] and can access both the public system if they so wish, or the private health-care system.

Currently, South Africa has 388 public hospitals—these hospitals are grouped into District Hospitals (64%), Regional Hospitals, and Tertiary Hospitals. The District Hospitals are the first level of referral and staffed by general practitioners. Basic services including diagnostic and therapeutic services and general anesthesia facilities exist. Regional Hospitals provide care at a specialist physician level in the following areas: surgery, medicine, orthopedics, pediatrics, obstetrics and gynecology, psychiatry, diagnostic radiology, and anesthetics. Tertiary Hospitals are those hospitals used in a teaching capacity and, as such, have a full complement of specialty and subspecialty personnel.[2]

In a survey conducted comparing 1998 and 2003, more women attended public health facilities than men, and the numbers increased across all age groups for both men and women when comparing the 2 years' figures. People who attended public hospitals expressed general dissatisfaction regarding long waiting times, staff attitudes, prescribed medicines not being available, and a general shortage of staff.[3]

### Life Expectancy

According to 2009 statistics, the current life expectancy is 53.9 years for males and 57.2 years for females.[4] This figure has decreased since the period 1985 to 1994 when the estimated life expectancy was 54.12 for males and 64.38 for females. These figures are due to diseases such as HIV, tuberculosis, and malaria. According to the South African Institute of Race Relation's annual report (2008–2009),[5] the projected life expectancy is expected to fall to 48 years for men and 51 years for women. As is to be expected, the provinces with the highest HIV rates had the lowest life expectancy.

According to IndexMundi,[6] South Africa reached its lowest life expectancy in 2007, with an expectancy of 42 years.

### Cancer as a Public Health Problem

It is estimated that in South Africa currently, 1 in 6 men and 1 in 7 women will be diagnosed with cancer. The leading pathologies are breast, cervical, and colorectal in women and prostate, lung, and esophagus in men.

Before 2001, the National Cancer Registry (NCR) kept records of the incidence of cancer in South Africa.

In April 2011, Regulations Relating to Cancer Registration (Act 61 of 2003) was promulgated, which requires every medical official making the primary diagnosis of cancer to send information regarding the histology and risk factor profile to the NCR.[7] Information gathered from this database should clearly delineate the cancer demographics of cancer in South Africa. According to the most recent National Cancer Registry of South Africa data from 2004, 55,553 new patients were reported, showing that South African males have an overall age-standardized incidence rate (ASR) of cancer of 126.43 per 100,000 population and a lifetime risk (LR) of 1 in 6 of developing cancer before the age of 74 years, whereas South African females have an ASR of 114.53 per 100,000 and an LR of 1 in 8 of developing cancer. The overall LR of developing cancer in South Africa before the age of 74 remains 1 in 4.[8] Unfortunately, information from 2004 to the present is not available.

## CANCER ETIOLOGY

Although the etiology of most malignancies is unknown, or similar to that of developed countries, certain cancers have etiologies specific to this region. The high incidence of hepatocellular carcinoma in some provinces such as Mpumalanga has been linked to a high infection rate and carrier status of hepatitis B.[9] The Eastern Cape has reported a high incidence of esophageal carcinoma possibly related to aflatoxin in maize products.[10] The epidemic of HIV infection in all regions has seen an increase of related malignancies such as lymphomas and Kaposi's sarcoma.[11]

## CANCER STATISTICS

One in four people in South Africa will be diagnosed with cancer—these figures, however, are still the lowest of all reported chronic illnesses in South Africa.[12]

According to Jemal et al.,[13] breast cancer in females (10.9%) and lung cancer (12.7) are the two leading cancers diagnosed worldwide, closely followed by colorectal cancer (9.8%).[14]

Esophagus cancer and nasopharyngeal cancer are reported to have the highest incidence in South Africa (first and second) (2011 data).[13] This incidence differs with that reported by the NCR from 2004 where breast cancer is the most common cancer in women and prostate cancer the most common in men.[8]

Kaposi's sarcoma, a relatively rare sarcoma previously, also has rising incidence due to the relationship with HIV. Prostate, cervix, and liver cancers are seen more frequently compared to the rest of the world (sixth, third, and fifth, respectively). This ranking is out of a total of 20 disease areas. Due to the HIV status of South Africans, the incidence of Hodgkin's lymphoma and oral cavity carcinoma is predicted to rise in the future.[13]

Of note, however, are the figures of incidence and mortality between developed areas and less developed areas (i.e., Africa). Although the incidence in less developed areas is about half that seen in developed areas, the mortality is about equal.[14] South Africa ranks between 8th and 10th position with the four most reported cancers worldwide, namely breast (10th), lung and Hodgkin's disease and oral cavity (11th), urinary bladder (9th), and colorectal (8th).

## HISTORY OF CANCER CARE

Departments of Radiation Oncology were established at most universities in the 1960s. The first linear accelerators were introduced at the University of the Free State during the 1960s and were the first introduced in Africa as a whole. A site for proton and neutron therapy was established in the Municipality of Faure, close to the city of Stellenbosch during the 1980s.

Departments of Medical Oncology were established first at the University of Pretoria in 1961, and later at the University of the Witwatersrand during the 1980s.

Private practices offering oncological services were established in the main centers during the 1980s starting in Gauteng.

## CANCER CARE INFRASTRUCTURE

In the public sector that provides care for the majority of South Africans, 18 sites for cancer care have been identified by the National Department of Health.[15] The level of cancer care provided by these hospitals is variable, with more advanced levels of care being available in the larger centers. Some of the smaller centers, such as Polokwane Hospital in Limpopo, are staffed mainly by medical officers/general practitioners who deliver cancer care under the supervision of a registered oncologist.

In addition, most of the centers are located in the cities. Patients from the more rural districts are referred for treatment to the larger centers for treatment. Even then, some may be referred again to larger academic centers for more specialized therapy.

This situation is in stark contrast to the private sector that provides cancer care for less than 20% of the population.[16] Here the cancer care sites are located in larger centers such as Cape Town, Stellenbosch, Durban, Johannesburg, and Pretoria, with sites concentrated in the more populated urban areas. It is estimated that there are 103 private practice oncology centers in South Africa. Some are large and a few single-oncologist practices.

The availability of chemotherapy drugs is very variable between provinces. The budget for chemotherapy allows for the use of such drugs as bevacizumab, trastuzumab, and other expensive items in one province; yet, other hospitals in other provinces have very restricted access to expensive chemotherapies; trastuzumab used for treating both adjuvant and metastatic breast cancers is generally not available. Similarly, the type of radiation machines and therefore the type of radiation therapy available are very variable between provinces.

The budget allocation from the central government for cancer care for each of the provinces depends on the population size of the province. Gauteng province, situated in the center of the country, has four large tertiary care hospitals, but has been allocated a smaller budget than KwaZulu-Natal, previously the most populated province but with only one large academic center.

## PRIVATE INSURANCE COMPANIES (MEDICAL AID SCHEMES) AND PRESCRIBED MINIMUM BENEFITS

One of the largest medical aid financial institutions reports cancer claims to comprise 60% of the total trauma claims between 2007 and 2009, a fiscal value of more than R40 million in 2008.[17] Currently (latest figures of 2009), the disparity between private and public hospitals is quite large with a per capita spending of R1.9 in the public sector versus R11.30 in the private sector. The doctor-to-patient ratio is also varied, with 4,200 patients per 1 general practitioner in the public sector versus 243 patients to 1 general practitioner in the private sector.[4]

According to a private insurance scheme (Momentum[18]), the numbers of people on an open medical aid scheme with more extensive benefits increased by 5% in 2007. Restricted-funded insurance schemes with limited benefits increased by 300%. Individual contribution costs were higher in open schemes, and of the total spent, 36% of these contribution costs were paid for hospital care.

In a census conducted by the SA Stats Department in 2012,[19] it was shown that the current workforce who have a subsidized medical aid increased from 32.1% from the first quarter of 2011 to 33% in the second quarter of 2012, but has subsequently decreased to 32.0% for the fourth quarter of 2012.[20]

In the 2011–2012 Annual Report of the Council for Medical Schemes, South Africa, it was reported that approximately 8.5 million people (average age 31 years) were members of some sort of medical aid, with only 6.6% of those on a medical aid being pensioners.[21]

Prescribed minimum benefits are minimum benefits that must legally be covered in full by a medical aid, regardless of which level of health-care plan the patient is on. According to the Government Gazette Number 20556 of 1998,[22] treatable cancers are the following:

1. Not spread to adjacent organs
2. Not metastasized
3. Not brought about irreparable damage to the organ within which they originated
4. There is a demonstrated 5-year survival rate of greater than 10% for the given therapy.

## CANCER CARE WORKFORCE

According to the Health Professions Council of South Africa (HPCSA) records, there are 33 registered medical oncologists in South Africa.[23] Also from the HPCSA records, South Africa has 260 registered oncologists; 1 oncologist per 194,000 people. It is not apparent from the HPCSA records how many of the registered oncologists are clinical oncologists, radiation oncologists, medical oncologists, gynecology oncologists, and so forth. It is also not apparent from the data how many of the registered oncologists still live and work in South Africa, as there has been a significant emigration of medical professionals from South Africa.

It must be noted that there is not a separate registration for clinical oncologists in South Africa. Many of those registered as radiation oncologists in fact practice as clinical oncologists and administer chemotherapy in addition to treating with radiation therapy. The majority of the registered oncologists practice in the private sector. There is an uneven distribution of oncologists throughout the country, with the majority of oncologists practicing in four large cities, namely Johannesburg, Pretoria, Cape Town, and Durban. Medical oncology is limited to the province of Gauteng, with oncology services in other provinces provided mainly by clinical oncologists and hematologists. This reflects the location of medical oncology training facilities.

Doctors providing cancer care are represented by three main societies, namely the South African Society for Medical Oncology, South African

Society for Clinical and Radiation Oncology, and South African Society of Haematology. The membership of these three academic societies overlaps and comprises 133, 240, and 140, members respectively. These societies represent the oncology medical fraternity at various levels, such as meeting with government, meeting with the Board of Healthcare Funders, and other societies. The biannual National Oncology Congress is organized under the umbrella of these three societies. The societies are also responsible for organizing other smaller meetings and symposia.

Very few centers offer pediatric oncology services. These are located in the main centers, and most are within academic institutions. Examples are the Red Cross Children's Hospital in Cape Town, the Charlotte Maxeke Academic Hospital in Johannesburg, the Steve Biko Academic Hospital in Pretoria, and the Universitas Hospital in Bloemfontein. Very few pediatric oncologists provide a service in the private sector.

Doctors with palliative care training are very few in number, are located mainly in the larger centers, and are often affiliated to a hospice association.

## TRAINING

Training of all oncologists in South Africa takes place in seven accredited centers, the University of Pretoria, the University of the Witwatersrand, Stellenbosch University, University of Cape Town, Walter Sisulu University, University of KwaZulu-Natal, University of the Free State and Medunsa.[24]

The University of Pretoria and the University of the Witwatersrand have separate departments of radiation and medical oncology. At the University of Cape Town, the University of the Free State, and the University of KwaZulu-Natal, there is no separation of medical oncology and radiation oncology, although doctors trained at the latter facilities are registered with the HPCSA as radiation oncologists, but act in the capacity of clinical oncologists when treating patients.

The College of Medicine, South Africa, is tasked with setting curricula and examination requirements for all specialist training in South Africa. Once the successful candidate has passed all the requirements, only then can the candidate register with the HPCSA as a specialist.

The curricular and examination requirements for radiation oncologists and medical oncologists are different from that certification in medical oncology, which is a subspecialty of internal medicine, and candidates must register as a specialist physician before being accepted into training.

It is of interest that, according to the 2008 MOSES report,[25] European countries with oncology training facilities differ from less than two facilities per million inhabitants to others with more than 10 facilities. In comparison, South Africa has only seven training facilities for 50 million inhabitants.

## CANCER CLINICAL CARE

In general, the commonly used guidelines are those of the National Comprehensive Cancer Network and the European Society of Medical Oncology. In the private sector, these guidelines are adapted per medical aid, based on health economic factors, often taking into account reports from the United Kingdom National Institute for Clinical Excellence. Access to expensive new therapies is restricted, and limited to certain options in medical aids, or dependent on individual academic hospital guidelines within the public sector.

Each training unit in the public sector has its own protocols for both chemotherapy and radiation therapy based on the availability of drugs or radiation machines at the individual centers. Due to the limited number of oncologists in the country, in contrast to many cancer care units in Europe and the United States, no specific centers are dedicated to the treatment for a specified solid tumor. All oncologists see and treat a variety of tumor types.

Clinical oncologists treat solid tumors and some treat hematological oncological malignancies as well. Medical oncologists are trained to treat both hematological malignancies and solid tumors.

Public oncology units with allogeneic transplant facilities are limited to two public sites, namely the University of the Witwatersrand and the University of Cape Town, Groote Schuur Hospital.

By contrast, transplantation facilities for allogeneic transplantation are available at two private sites, one in Gauteng in Pretoria and the other in the Western Cape, Cape Town.

## CANCER CARE OUTCOMES

No data regarding cancer care outcomes in the public sector is known , nor has it been recorded for the private sector.

## CANCER CARE CONTINUUM

### Prevention

Numerous nongovernmental organizations (NGOs) assist both patients and relatives of patients who have been diagnosed with cancer. The Cancer Association of South Africa (CANSA) remains the largest, with branches reaching all corners of South Africa. This organization not only assists financially but also has qualified nursing staff who perform home visits to assess patients and assist with daily activities.

Hospice Palliative Care Association of South Africa[26] is tasked with palliative care of all terminal patients, with inpatient facilities, community centers, and hospice home-based care.

The Cancer Research Initiative of South Africa concentrates on children who have been diagnosed with cancer and patients with prostate cancer and HIV-associated malignancies.

The Cancer Alliance (a group of nine privately run NGOs)[27] and a number of other smaller institutions privately run and tied to pharmaceutical companies also assist with cancer care and dissemination of information.

## CANCER RESEARCH

In great part, cancer research is collaborative pharmaceutical company–sponsored clinical studies. A number of sites participate in these studies. These include the large academic centers such as the University of the Witwatersrand, the University of Pretoria, and the University of Cape Town, Stellenbosch, and KwaZulu-Natal. A number of private oncology centers also participate in such studies.

Single institution or investigator-initiated studies are limited for a number of reasons. First, the practice of oncology and the treatment of malignancies have become tailored toward the genomics of the particular malignancy as well as identification of specific mutations of targets in the signaling pathways and inhibition thereof. Second, there is limited funding for investigator-initiated research. Cooperative group studies such as ECOG-ACRIN and EORTC are conducted in South Africa. The ECOG-ACRIN studies are being conducted at the University of Pretoria,[28] which is the only site in Africa to participate in such studies. EORTC studies are conducted at other sites but are limited in type of malignancy (Prof. P. Ruff, personal communication).

International Atomic Energy Agency (IAEA) supports clinical trials involving radiotherapy. Several large academic centers conduct IAEA-approved research.[29]

All studies in South Africa are overseen by the Medicine Control Council Clinical Trials Committee (MCC CTC). No study involving therapy may be conducted without the approval of the MCC CTC in addition to local ethic review boards at the individual sites such as the Witwatersrand University's Human Research Ethics Committee (Medical). The MCC CTC places a great deal of emphasis on capacity building in the recognition that investigators who were disadvantaged during the apartheid era receive training in the conduct of clinical studies. To this end, studies conducted at academic centers such as the University of the Witwatersrand and the University of Pretoria are preferred.[30] All investigators and members of the study team at all sites are required to undergo training and obtain a certificate in accordance with the Good Clinical Practice (GCP) requirements of South Africa.[31] This training cannot be done online. In many respects, it is more rigorous than elsewhere in the world. In addition to obtaining a GCP certificate, 1-day in-depth training is required. GCP certification must be updated every 2 years with a further half day of training. The South African GCP guidelines incorporate the following:

1. ICH Guideline for Good Clinical Practice, ICH Harmonised Tripartite Guideline
2. The Declaration of Helsinki
3. International Guidelines for Ethical Review of Epidemiological Studies, Council for International Organizations for Medical Sciences
4. World Health Organization Technical Report Series and Operational Guidelines for Ethics Committees
5. MEDSAFE, New Zealand Regulatory Guidelines for Medicines
6. Association of the British Pharmaceutical Industry Clinical Trial Compensation Guidelines
7. The Institutional Review Board Guidebook, Office for the Protections from Research Risks, NIH

Due to lack of funding, laboratory-based research is still being conducted about on a lesser scale than in previous years. This is mainly in the large academic centers.[32]

Research, both clinical and laboratory, is supported and funded by such organizations as the Medical Research Council and NGOs, in particular, the CANSA. At least 70 studies are currently being supported by CANSA.[33] In 2011, at the National Health Research Summit attended by 271 delegates, several main issues requiring action to promote research in South Africa were recognized.[34] As regards noncommunicable diseases (including cancer), a further factor recognized was the heavy clinical service load of many of the investigators. Of the recommendations made to the Department of Health and the Minister of Health, the first four related to funding. The slow administrative processes of the MCC were also recognized, and a process of restructuring of the MCC has been put into place.[30]

## FUTURE DIRECTIONS

The Green Paper for Health Care in South Africa was tasked in Parliament in 2011, by the Minister of Health, the Honorable Dr. Pakishe Aaron Motsoaledi. This paper outlined the direction health care will take in South Africa in the future. It included a proposal for the 10 large academic hospitals to be declared national assets and to be managed directly from the Minister's Office, National Department of Health. Also included in this was the proposal that a National Quaternary/Tertiary Grant be established, allowing equal access of the 10 institutions to a larger budget from the National

Treasury than occurs at present. Improvement of facilities and supply of drugs including oncological services will result.

A National Health Insurance Plan was also proposed and will be implemented over the next approximately 14 years. This will improve the access to health care for all South African citizens, also improving access to cancer care.

## ACKNOWLEDGMENTS

I would like to thank the following people for their contribution.

Prof. P. Ruff: Chair: South African Society of Medical Oncology and University of Witwatersrand

Prof. R. Lakier: Department Head: University of Pretoria

Prof. J. Mahlangu: Chair: South African Society of Haematology and University of Pretoria

Prof. S. Fourie: Chair: South African Society for Clinical and Radiation Oncologists

Dr. C.F. Slabber: Medical Oncologist in private practice

## REFERENCES

1. Board of Healthcare Funders. Available at http://www.bhfglobal.com/. Accessed March 4, 2013.
2. Cullinan K. Health Services in South Africa: A Basic Introduction. Health-e News Service, January 2006.
3. South African Demographic and Health Survey, 2003. Available at http://www .info.gov.za/view/DownloadFileAction?id=90143.
4. Delivery Agreement for Outcome 2: A Long and Healthy Life for All South Africans. Available at http://www.info.gov.za/view/DownloadFileAction?id=135747.
5. South Africa: Life Expectancy Drops. Available at http://www.plusnews.org /Report/87144/SOUTH-AFRICA-Life-expectancy-drops.
6. Available at http://www.indexmundi.com/g/g.aspx?c=sf&v=30.
7. Government Notice, Department of Health, National Health Act, 2003 (Act No 61 of 2003): Regulations Relating to Cancer Registration, April 26, 2011.
8. National Cancer Registry, 2004. Available at http://www.cansa.org.za/files/2012 /05/Cancer_Registry_2004.pdf. Accessed February 27, 2013.
9. Di Bisceglie AM. Hepatitis B and hepatocellular carcinoma. *Hepatology* 2009; 49(Suppl 5): S56–S60.
10. Williams JH, Grubb JA, Davis JW, et al. HIV and hepatocellular and esophageal carcinomas related to consumption of mycotoxin-prone foods in sub-Saharan Africa. *Am J Clin Nutr* 2010; 92: 154–60.
11. Available at http://www.cancer.gov/cancertopics/factsheet/Risk/hiv-infection. Accessed February 11, 2013.

12. South African Demographic and Health Survey, 2003. Available at http://www.mrc.ac.za/bod/sadhs.htm.
13. Jemal A, Bray F, Center MM, Ferlay J, Ward E, Forman D. Global cancer statistics. CA *Cancer J Clin* 2011; 61: 69–90.
14. GLOBOCAN 2008 database (Version 1.2). Available at http://globocan.iarc.fr/factsheets/populations/factsheet.asp?uno=900.
15. Information obtained from the Department of Health, South Africa.
16. Council of Medical Schemes Annual Report, 2011–2012.
17. Available at http://www.sanlam.co.za/wps/wcm/connect/Sanlam_EN/sanlam/media+centre/media+releases/cancer+stats+show+south+africans+cant+take+chances. Accessed October 2012.
18. Available at http://www.southafrica.co.za/about-south-africa/health/s.
19. Department of Statistics, Quarterly Labour Force Survey, Quarter 1, 2012, P0211, issued May 8, 2012.
20. Available at http://www.statssa.gov.za/publications/P0211/P02114thQuarter2012.pdf. Accessed March 13, 2013.
21. Council for Medical Schemes, Annual Report: 2011–2012. Available at http://www.medicalschemes.com/files/Press%20Releases/PressRelease14Of2012.pdf.
22. Government Notice 20556, Number R.1262. Regulations in Terms of the Medical Schemes Act 1998 (Act No 131 of 1998), Chapter 3 and annexures.
23. Information supplied by the South African Society of Medical Oncology.
24. Information supplied by the College of Medicine, South Africa.
25. Medical Oncology Status in Europe Survey (MOSES), Phase III, September 2008.
26. Available at http://www.hospicepalliativecaresa.co.za/. Accessed March 13, 2013.
27. Available at http://www.health24.com/news/Cancer/1-898,79241.asp. Accessed February 16, 2013.
28. Available at www.up.ac.za. Accessed February 15, 2013.
29. IAEA website: www-naweb.iaea.org/nahu/ARBR/programmeactivities.html. Accessed March 7, 2013.
30. MCC website: http://www.mccza.com/.
31. Good Clinical Guidelines, South Africa, 2006. Available at http://www.kznhealth.gov.za/research/guideline2.pdf.
32. Available at http://www.doh.gov.za/docs/reports/2012/summitreport.pdf. Accessed March 13, 2013.
33. Available at http://www.cansa.org.za/research-projects/. Accessed February 15, 2013.
34. 2011 National Health Research Summit published by the Department of Health. Available at http://www.doh.gov.za/docs/reports/2012/summitreport.pdf.

# 28

# Tunisia

## *Yazid Belkacemi and Hamouda Boussen*

## PUBLIC HEALTH PERSPECTIVE

The Tunisian health system is well developed; it is based mainly on an extended network of first-line general practitioners; this network aids in reducing the rate of many transmissible diseases such as tuberculosis and managing many chronic diseases such as hypertension and diabetes.

As a consequence of the efforts of first-line practitioners, specialists, and academic hospitals that positively influenced mortality rates of newborns and mothers, life expectancy increased significantly, reaching 75.2 years for the whole population, 73.2 years for males, and 77.4 years for females, according to a 2012 estimation.[1] The total expenditure on health is 5.8% of the gross domestic product (rank 97 of 185), and the rate of prevalence of communicable diseases decreased significantly, especially for tuberculosis and other infectious-parasitic entities, because of the extended national campaigns started since the 1970s.[1] However, since 2005 the incidence of cancer has been rapidly increasing exponentially, which is becoming a public health problem that has motivated the start of a national cancer plan.

## CANCER ETIOLOGY IN TUNISIA

The Cancer profile in Tunisia has been rapidly occidentalized, especially in the past 10 years, and its etiologies related to "classical" causes, such as tobacco and alcohol consumption, diet occidentalization (e.g., overweight), and viral infectious (e.g., Epstein–Barr virus [EBV], human papillomavirus), have been rarely implicated in nasopharyngeal carcinomas, Hodgkin's disease, and cervical cancer.[2,3] In the absence of genetic oncology studies, hereditary causes are estimated at less than 5% of cases.[4]

## CANCER STATISTICS IN TUNISIA

Age-standardized incidence rate data is available from the three Tunisian cancer registries installed in 1997 for the north (CRNT), center, and south of the country.[5] Recent data report 14,000 cases annually, mainly from lung cancer (around 2,000 cases) in males and breast cancer (BC) in females (around 2,000 cases).[5,6] However, most of the cases remain diagnosed at locally advanced-metastatic stages because of a frequent delay in consultation and diagnosis and the absence of a structured screening program. Improvements in socioeconomic level, urbanization, modern diet, and habits have led to an epidemiological transition to an occidentalization tumor profile with more colorectal and prostate cancers, whereas some classical Tunisian entities, such as undifferentiated EBV-linked nasopharyngeal carcinomas, are decreasing and low-economic patients' immunoproliferative small intestinal disease (IPSID), also called "Mediterranean lymphoma," has disappeared.[5,7] The evolution of BC epidemiology is interesting, because the mean age at diagnosis in Tunisia is around 50 years, 10 years younger than that in Western countries. Ten percent of cases occur in females aged less than 35 years, and 10% of cases of BC have initial metastases.[5,8] Due to the lack of structured mammography screening, mean clinical tumor size is around 30 mm, with a high rate of node positive lesions and high-grade tumors and, consequently, a low rate (30%) of breast-conserving surgery.[6,8] This occidentalized profile of cancers in Tunisia and the age effect will lead, in the next 15 years, to the doubling of cases of breast and lung cancers, an increase of mean ages at cancer diagnosis, a decrease of cancers in young patients (especially for BC in females younger than 35 years), and an impressive decrease of inflammatory BC due to improvement in socioeconomic level.[9]

## HISTORY OF CANCER CARE IN TUNISIA

Institut Salah Azaiez (ISA), the unique Tunisian comprehensive cancer center (CCC), was created in 1969 by local oncologists to improve the multidisciplinary management of malignancies. Most of them have been trained in France at the Institut Gustave Roussy. They applied a multidisciplinary approach based on the therapeutic committee's collegial decisions and worked with international teams from France, Italy, and the United States. This international collaboration is led by Pr Najib Mourali, the first ISA director, who has headed many collaborative projects and publications focused on IBC, nasopharyngeal cancer (NPC), and IPSID.[10–12]

## CANCER CARE INFRASTRUCTURE

Tunisia has one CCC, four medical oncology and radiotherapy units in university hospitals, and six medical oncology units in regional hospitals as well as oncologists and organ specialists in private practice. The CCC, located in Tunis, functions on the concept of multidisciplinary spirit in cancer diagnosis, workup, and treatment, involving at every step of the decisions surgical oncologists, medical oncologists, and radiotherapists make. CCC treats around 5,000 patients annually, including 400 BC patients and around 250 cervical cancers patients.[5] The ISA, since its creation in 1969, acquired a great deal of experience in BC, especially IBC, and gynecologic oncology as well as NPC and ear, nose, and throat oncology. Since 1992, most of the patients of Sousse and Sfax have been managed locally by medical oncologists and radiotherapists practicing in university hospitals, and since 2011 patients have been treated by medical oncologists from regional hospitals located in Gabes, Gafsa, Jendouba, and Bizerta. Most of the university hospitals diagnose and treat cancer cases. Oncology is also covered by four private clinics devoted to oncology.

Tunisia has 5 linear accelerators and 10 cobalt machines for radiotherapy treatment, the coverage per inhabitant remaining low.[13]

## ONCOLOGY SOCIETIES

Many specialty societies, such as the Tunisian Society of Medical Oncology (STOM), the Tunisian Society of Hematology, and the Tunisian Society of Radiotherapy Oncology, are functioning in collaboration with many organ specialist scientific societies to improve cancer knowledge, to organize national and international congresses, to develop education for medical and paramedical professionals, and to adapt international guidelines to local Tunisian socioeconomic capacities.[14,15] The task force of specialists in Tunisia is composed of 70 medical oncologists, 60 radiotherapists, and 30 surgical oncologists working mainly in ISA and academic hospitals, with a huge pool of fellows currently training in oncology. Nongovernmental organizations/ societies located in Tunis, Sousse, and Sfax, such as Association tunisienne de lutte contre le cancer, Association Tunisienne d'Assistance aux maladies de Cancers du sein, Association des maladies du Cancer, Association Dar El Amal, and Epidémiologie Prévention et Information sur le Cancer, aim to cover fields of action such as cancer education and social coverage.

## CANCER TREATMENT

In ISA, treatment protocols are decided by multidisciplinary teams in accordance with guidelines devised by the local specialty society STOM and international recommendations from consensual conferences such as European and U.S. conferences; that is, European Society for Medical Oncology (ESMO), American Society of Clinical Oncology (ASCO), and National Comprehensive Cancer Network (NCCN).[14] Most of the drugs used,

TABLE 28.1 Epidemiological (North Tunisia Cancer Registry), Clinical, and Histological Features and Therapeutic Protocols of Cancers in Tunisia

| Site | ASR | Annual Cases | Mean Age | Percentage of Young People | In Metastases (%) | Treatment |
|---|---|---|---|---|---|---|
| BC | 31.8 | 785 | 51.5 | 7 (<35 years) | 12.2 | A, T, Tra, Cap, Vin, Gem, Bip |
| Lung cancer | 32.5 | 734 | 62.2 | 13.9 (<50 years) | 31.4 | Gem, Pem, Tax, Vin |
| Colorectal cancer | 6 | 550 | 60 | | | Bev, Cet, Folfox-Folfiri |
| Prostate cancer | 11.8 | 286 | 72 | | 14 | HT, Tax, Bip |
| Nasopharyngeal cancer | 2 | 125 | 45 | | | Tax, Pl |
| Hodgkin's disease | 1.8 | 95 | 48 | | | BEACOPP, ABVD |
| Non-Hodgkin's lymphoma | 4 | 225 | 45 | 3.6 | | R-CHOP-ACVBP |
| Renal cancer | 1.5 | 97 | 60 | | 16 | Sun, Soraf |
| Cervical cancer | 4,2 | 299 | 55 | | 4.4 | Pl, RT |
| Ovarian cancer | 4.1 | 296 | 51 | | 21.6 | Tax, Pl, Gem |
| Gallbladder | 2 | 99 | 72 | | 21.9 | Gem, Pl, Elox |
| Pediatric cancer | 10 | 115 | 10 | | | SIOP, NCCN |

MA, mean age; ASR, adjusted standardized incidence; A, anthracyclines; El, Eloxatin; Cp, campthothecin; Cet, cetuximab; Ri, rituximab; Fl, Fludarabine; Im, imatinib; Sun, sunitinib; CML, chronic myeloid leukemia; GIST, gastrointestinal stromal tumor; ENT, ear nose throat Gem, gemcitabine; Pl, cisplatin; Elox, oxaliplatin; Bip, bisphosphonates; Vin, vinorelbine; Tra, trastuzumab; Bev, bevacizumab; Cet, cetuximab; Pem, Pemetrexed; Tax, Taxol; HT, hormone therapy.

both classical and targeted therapies, are available in the list of Ministry of Health–approved medications, and few of them are delivered outside this approval and protocols are mostly in accordance with the international recommendations. An important work in terms of good clinical practices in oncology has to be, however, performed outside of the academic centers to improve diagnosis and treatment. Table 28.1 details adjusted standardized rates, clinical features, and treatment capacities/protocols for breast, prostate, lung, colorectal, lymphomas, nasopharyngeal, and pediatric cancers.

## SUPPORTIVE CARE

An approach to supportive care, concerned with cancer pain management, was started 20 years ago, which led to the creation of scientific societies devoted to pain study (Association Tunisienne pour l'étude de la douleur) and palliative care (Association Tunisienne des Soins Palliatifs) as well as the creation of a department of pain treatment in a university hospital in Tunis in 2000. Pain is studied at the Faculty of Medicine of Tunis at a postgraduate level, and many institutions that treat cancer have consultations oriented for pain and supportive care; STOM edited one chapter devoted to pain in 2013 national guidelines.[14]

## HEALTH SOCIAL COVERAGE

For the administrative aspect, 55% of patients affected by cancer are covered by two national security agencies (Caisse Nationale de Sécurité Sociale and Caisse Nationale de Retraite et Prévoyance Sociale) unified 5 years ago under CNAM (Caisse Nationale d'Assurance Maladie), and this agency provides access to public and private health-care providers. For these "insured" patients, coverage is full in public hospitals/clinics and partial in private clinics. The remaining patients, 45%, with a low socioeconomic level are considered as indigents and have free access to the public health-care system. Drug approvals are controlled by Direction de la Pharmacie et du medicament, linked to the Ministry of Health, and are decided in accordance with international guidelines recommended by ASCO and ESMO and Institut National du Cancer of France. Chemotherapy drugs and targeted therapies are provided by insurance and local authorities to insured and indigent patients.[16]

## CANCER CARE OUTCOMES

Cancer registries provide only descriptive data, and survival data is available from retrospective monocentric studies. However, data about a retrospective series of 1,150 BC cases treated in Sousse showed an overall 5-year survival of 70% after multidisciplinary treatment by surgery, anthracylin-taxanes CT, and locoregional radiation therapy.[17]

## CANCER CARE CONTINUUM

### Prevention

Few prevention campaigns have been conducted, and despite the existence of legal limitations on tobacco use, few are used to prohibit smoking in public areas, such as train stations, airports, and public administration offices. Audiovisual initiatives are also rare in the field of tobacco and alimentation of life habits.

### Screening

Most of the cancers diagnosed remain discovered more frequently at advanced stages because of late consultations and lack of availability of diagnosis tools like mammographs in hospitals. Until now no structured programmed screening was available for breast or colorectal cancer, and a great deal of effort has to be taken to improve early detection. However, a confined experience concerned a large-scale mammography campaign in Ariana state, conducted by the structures of Office National de la Famille et la Population (ONFP). This initiative covered less than 10% of the targeted population and detected smaller tumors with a mean tumor size of 11 mm, compared to the more than 3 cm mean clinical size usually reported.[18] Unfortunately, this campaign remained confined to Ariana state because of the high cost of screening, and the authorities decided to focus more on early detection. The first-line structures of ONFP remain involved in Pap-smear samples for cervical cancer detection realized by nurses.

## Psychosocial Care

Psychosocial care remains an orphan parent in cancer management in Tunisia, with patients and their families having to solve by themselves the management of socioeconomic problems occurring at disease diagnosis, treatment, and after the patient's death. Tunisia has to develop more initiatives in the field of psycho-oncology and work on patients coping skills.

## CANCER RESEARCH

From basic and applied research to prevention and treatment, the field of cancer research, although insufficient, has enjoyed a great interest from the Tunisian research stakeholders. This interest focused on cancers that affect women and children, such as cervical cancer and BC. To limit the damages caused by cancer in Tunisia, a better understanding of local risk factors is required. In fact, more data on the epidemiological and biological features of each disease will allow the implementation of efficient prevention strategies. Although uncoordinated, several ongoing research projects aim to assess the etiology of several cancers to improve population-preventive measures and identify specific biomarkers for early diagnosis of the most prevalent cancers, such as lung cancer, NPC, or BC.[19–21]

To contribute to mechanisms that would transform research breakthroughs into innovative products, Tunisian research teams work in partnership with international cancer comprehensive centers mostly in Europe. A primary aim is to create synergies with existing local institutions involved in innovation and economic development.

Clearly, a need exists to set up a national scientific program to foster interactions between scientists from academia and industry, which involves a multidisciplinary approach of basic scientists, clinicians, and epidemiologists.[22]

## FUTURE DIRECTIONS

The number of cancer cases will double in the next 15 years, especially breast, lung, colorectal, and prostate cancers. A national cancer plan was started in 2007 but with only partial application in training and improving/increasing specialized care units. Programmed screening is absent, excluding cervical cancer initiatives by cytologic studies in primary care. Before locoregional guidelines are outlined, like in the Association of Radiotherapy and Oncology for Mediterranean Area, one should assess the available technical and socioeconomic capacities.[23]

## REFERENCES

1. http://www.nationmaster.com/country/ts-tunisia/health. Accessed August 11, 2013.
2. Boussen H, Ghorbal L, Naouel L, et al.. Nasopharyngeal cancer (NPC) around the Mediterranean area: standard of care. *Crit Rev Oncol Hematol* 2012 Dec; 84(Suppl 1): e106–9.
3. Hassen E, Chaieb A, Letaief M, et al. Cervical human papillomavirus infection in Tunisian women. *Infection* 2003 Jun; 31(3): 143–48.
4. Troudi W, Uhrhammer N, Sibille C, et al. Contribution of the BRCA1 and BRCA2 mutations to breast cancer in Tunisia. *J Hum Genet* 2007; 52(11): 915–20.
5. http://www.emro.who.int/noncommunicable-diseases/information-resources/cancer-registration.html. Accessed August 13, 2013.
6. North Tunisia Cancer Registry. *2004–2006 Data.* Tunis: Ministry of Health, 2012.
7. Belaid I, Mezlini A, Rais H, et al. Primary small intestinal lymphoma: epidemiological, histological and therapeutic transition in Tunisia. *Bull Cancer* 2012 Apr 1; 99(4): 425–30.
8. Maalej M, Hentati D, Messai T, et al. Breast cancer in Tunisia in 2004: a comparative clinical and epidemiological study. *Bull Cancer* 2008; 95: E5–E9.
9. Boussen H, Bouzaiene H, Hassouna JB, et al. Inflammatory breast cancer in Tunisia: epidemiological and clinical trends. *Cancer* 2010; 116(11 Suppl): 2730–35.
10. Mourali N, Tabbane F, Muenz LR, et al. Ten-year results utilizing chemotherapy as primary treatment in nonmetastatic, rapidly progressing breast cancer. *Cancer Invest* 1993; 11: 363–70.
11. Lê MG, Arriagada R, Contesso G, et al. Dermal lymphatic emboli in inflammatory and noninflammatory breast cancer: a French-Tunisian joint study in 337 patients. *Clin Breast Cancer* 2005; 6: 439–45.
12. Ben-Ayed F, Halphen M, Najjar T, et al. Treatment of alpha chain disease. Results of a prospective study in 21 Tunisian patients by the Tunisian-French Intestinal Lymphoma Study Group. *Cancer* 1989; 63(7): 1251–56.
13. Abdel-Wahab M, Bourque JM, Pynda Y, et al. Status of radiotherapy resources in Africa: an International Atomic Energy Agency analysis. *Lancet Oncol* 2013; 14: e168–75.
14. Available at http//www.stom-Tunisie.org/.

15. Available at www.radiothérapietunisie.org/.

16. Available at http//www.ins.tn.

17. Landolsi A, et al. Retrospective Study about 1200 Cases Treated in the Center of Tunisia from 1999 to 2004 (personal data).

18. Bouchlaka A, Ben Abdallah M, Ben Aissa R, et al. Results and evaluation of 3 years of a large scale mammography program in the Ariana area of Tunisia. *Tunis Med* 2009; 87: 438–42.

19. Mahfoudh W, Bouaouina N, Gabbouj S, Chouchane L. FASL-844 T/C polymorphism: a biomarker of good prognosis of breast cancer in the Tunisian population. *Hum Immunol* 2012 Sep; 73(9): 932–38.

20. Mahfoudh W, Bouaouina N, Ahmed SB, et al. Hereditary breast cancer in Middle Eastern and North African (MENA) populations: identification of novel, recurrent and founder BRCA1 mutations in the Tunisian population. *Mol Biol Rep* 2012; 39(2): 1037–46.

21. Laantri N, Jalbout M, Khyatti M, et al. XRCC1 and hOGG1 genes and risk of nasopharyngeal carcinoma in North African countries. *Mol Carcinog* 2011; 50: 732–37.

22. Chouchane L, Mamtani R, Dallol A, Sheikh JI. Personalized medicine: a patient-centeredparadigm.*J TranslMed*2011Dec1;9:206.doi:10.1186/1479–5876-9-206.

23. AROME. Guidelines, minimal requirements and standard of cancer care around the Mediterranean Area: report from the Collaborative AROME (Association of Radiotherapy and Oncology of the Mediterranean Area) working parties. *Crit Rev Oncol Hematol* 2011; 78: 1–16.

# 29

# Cancer Care in the United States: Progress and Challenges

*Amitoj S. Gill, Rahul Gosain, Rekha Chandran, Bella Nadler, Miklos Simon, Cara Miller, and Kenneth D. Miller*

## CANCER IN THE UNITED STATES: AN OVERVIEW

Over 13 million people in the United States have either been treated or are currently undergoing cancer therapy, and it is estimated that in 2014, 1.6 million Americans will be diagnosed with and 580,350 (36%) are expected to die of cancer. Over a 30-year period, 5-year survival rates have improved significantly from 49% in 1977 to 68% in 2008 because of improved screening and detection, newer therapeutic agents, and better supportive care. However, the 5-year survival rates for some cancers, for example, pancreatic and lung cancers, continue to be dismal.[2] Cancer is second only to heart disease as a cause of mortality among American people, and in 2008, direct cancer care costs and total costs in the United States were $77 billion and $201.5 billion, respectively.[2]

## THE WAR ON CANCER: HISTORY OF CANCER IN THE UNITED STATES

In the 19th and 20th centuries, Theodor Billroth, Vincenz Czerny, and William Halstead developed innovative surgery to treat cancer. In 1947, aminopterin was introduced by Dr. Sidney Farber to treat acute leukemia followed by 6-mercaptopurine, nitrogen mustard, and methotrexate. In 1955, the Cancer Chemotherapy National Service Center at the National Cancer Institute (NCI) was formed to test potential anticancer agents.[3] During this era the American Cancer Society (ACS) and other organizations helped to advocate for and support cancer research (Figure 29.1).

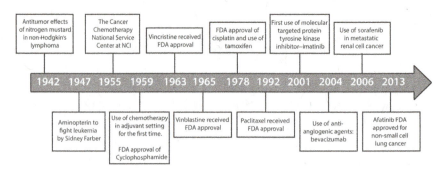

**FIGURE 29.1** Timeline of major events in the history of cancer.

**TABLE 29.1 NCI Budget**

| Year | Budget in Billion Dollars |
|------|---------------------------|
| 1980 | 0.99 |
| 1985 | 1.17 |
| 1990 | 1.68 |
| 1995 | 1.93 |
| 2000 | 3.32 |
| 2005 | 4.81 |
| 2010 | 5.11 |
| 2012 | 5.06 |
| 2013 | 5.8 |

The Nixon government passed the National Cancer Act of 1971, which authorized the NCI to further enhance national cancer programs by establishing national cancer research centers and control programs.[3] Since 1971, approximately $200 billion has been spent on cancer research, and currently, two-thirds of the drugs approved by the Federal Drug Administration are discovered by NCI-sponsored institutions.[4] From 2005 through 2013, the NCI budget averaged $4.9 billion per year.[4] In 2012, NCI's budget for the year was $5.067 billion and then to $5.8 billion in 2013 (Table 29.1).[4]

## UNDERSTANDING THE ETIOLOGY

With an increasing focus on eradicating cancer, there has been an intense focus on defining its etiology and pathogenesis. Several environmental, lifestyle, and infectious factors have been identified in the pathogenesis of specific cancer types, leading to public education campaigns (tobacco use), vaccination (HPV [human papillomavirus] vaccines), and programs to promote weight loss and a healthy lifestyle.

Tobacco use is by far the leading preventable cause of cancer death. In 2013, the ACS predicted that 174,100 cancer deaths will be related to tobacco, including lung, head and neck, esophagus, stomach, pancreas, kidney, bladder, and cervix cancers as well as acute myeloid leukemia. Over 200 compounds in tobacco smoke have been classified as carcinogens, including hydrogen cyanide, ammonia, and carbon monoxide. Radon (a radioactive gas) has been implicated as the second most common cause of lung cancer. Radon is released from the decay of uranium and radium and causes damage to the endobronchial endothelium when inhaled in large amounts or over a period of time.[2,5] Other contributory lifestyle factors include obesity, decreased physical activity (colorectal, breast), alcohol consumption (breast, colorectal), use of oral contraceptives, diet high in red meat and low in vegetables and fruits (colorectal cancer [CRC]), exposure to benzene, viral infections including hepatitis B and C and HPV, and hormone replacement therapy.[2,5,6]

Dietary intake of certain carcinogens and other exposures has been linked to cancer pathogenesis with varying degrees of evidence, including the following:

Acrylamide, a carcinogen found in potato chips and French fries that have attained temperatures greater than 120 degree F.

Heterocyclic amines and polycyclic aromatic hydrocarbons are formed when meat is cooked, at high temperatures or directly over flames.[5,6]

Sugar substitutes or artificial sweeteners such as saccharin, aspartame, acesulfame potassium, sucralose, neotame, and cyclamate).

Cell phones have raised concerns because of the effect of radiofrequency energy that could potentially damage brain tissue.[6] Ambient radiation has also been linked to an increase in the risk of breast cancer.

## TRENDS IN CANCER INCIDENCE AND MORTALITY

Cancer is the second most common cause of death in the United States following heart disease.[2] The SEER 13 data demonstrates that incidence for all cancer types combined has been relatively stable from 2000 to 2009.[8] Men have a higher lifetime probability of developing invasive cancer (45%) than women (38%), but cancer incidence among men has decreased on an average of 0.6% annually from 1994 to 2009. More specifically, incidence of prostate, lung, colon, stomach, rectum, and larynx decreased, whereas the incidence of kidney, liver, melanoma, and myeloma is on the rise.[8] For men in the United States., the cancers with the highest incidence include prostate

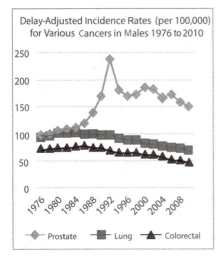
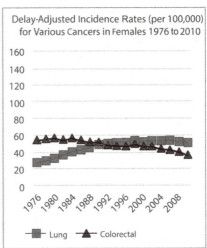

**FIGURE 29.2** Delay-Adjusted Incidence Rates (per 100,000) in Males and Females from 1976 to 2010 (adapted from SEER cancer data at seer.cancer.gov).

cancer, lung, bladder cancer, melanoma, non-Hodgkin's lymphoma, kidney, head and neck, leukemia, and pancreas.

For women the overall incidence of cancer decreased at a rate of 0.5% annually from 1998 to 2006 but has been stable from 2006 to 2009. The incidence for lung, colorectal, bladder, cervix, ovary, and oral cavity has declined, whereas the incidence of cancer of thyroid, melanoma, kidney, pancreas, leukemia, liver, and uterus has increased.[7,8] Presently, among women the most common cancers are breast, lung, colorectal, uterine, thyroid and ovarian malignancies, melanoma, lymphoma, kidney, leukemia, and pancreatic.

In the United States, cancer-related mortality rates have declined even more significantly than incidence, at 1.8% per year in men and 1.5% per year in women from 2000 to 2009. Mortality rates among men decreased for lung, prostate, colorectal, leukemia, non-Hodgkin's lymphoma, kidney, stomach, myeloma, oral cavity and pharynx, and laryngeal cancers but increased for liver, pancreas, and melanomas. For women, the mortality rate has increased only for pancreatic, liver, and uterine cancers (Figure 29.2).

## TRENDS FOR MAJOR CANCER TYPES

### Breast

There has been a decrease of 7% in the incidence of breast cancer in women from 2002 to 2003, with further decline subsequently. Breast cancer is the second most common cause of cancer death in women (after lung cancer), though there has been a steady decrease in breast cancer mortality since 1989; the largest rate of decline is between 2005 and 2009 (Figure 29.3).[2]

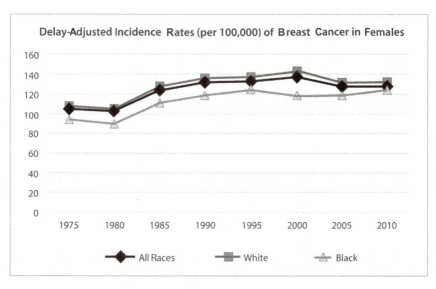

**FIGURE 29.3** Delay-adjusted incidence rates (per 100,000) of breast cancer in females (adapted from SEER cancer data at seer.cancer.gov).

## Colon and Rectum

Incidence of CRC has been decreasing during the past two decades due to increased awareness, screening, and earlier detection, as well as removal of polyps before they progress to cancer. From 2005 to 2009, incidence rates declined by 4.1% per year among adults 50 years and older, which is the age at which screening is recommended. At the same time, the incidence increased by 1.1% per year among those younger than age 50;[2] 9% of all cancer deaths are from CRC. Similarly, there has been a decline in CRC deaths of 2.4% per year in men and 3.1% per year in women from 2005 to 2009.[2]

## Lung Cancer

Lung cancer is the most common cause of cancer death and accounts for 27% of all cancer deaths. The incidence of lung cancer in men has decreased by 1.9% per year, whereas the decline in women has been more recent and only at 0.3% per year.[2] Lung cancer mortality decreased in men since 1991 and in women since 2003. From 2005 to 2009 the death rates have been declining in men by 2.8% per year and in women by 1% per year. Gender differences in lung cancer incidence and mortality patterns reflect historical differences in the reduction of cigarette smoking over the past 50 years.[2]

## Prostate

Prostate cancer is the most frequently diagnosed cancer in men. Incidence rates spiked in the mid-1990s due to the increased of prostate-specific antigen screening. The incidence rate has decreased by 1.9% per year from 2005 to 2009. Due to better treatment options, the mortality rate associated with prostate cancer has also declined at approximately 3.5% per year during this same time period.[2] Unfortunately, prostate cancer incidence is 70% higher in African Americans than in Caucasian men.

## PROGRESS IN CANCER TREATMENT

Progress in cancer research has led to a decrease in cancer incidence and improved the 5-year survival rates of cancer to 66%, which was in part due to the invention of drugs, which target specific molecular changes, and vaccines that can prevent cancers. The impact of these advances has already been substantial in the treatment of some cancers (such as chronic myelogenous leukemia) but not in others (such as lung cancer) when comparing survival data across three decades, 1980–1989, 1990–1999, and 2,000–2010 (Figures 29.4 and 29.5).

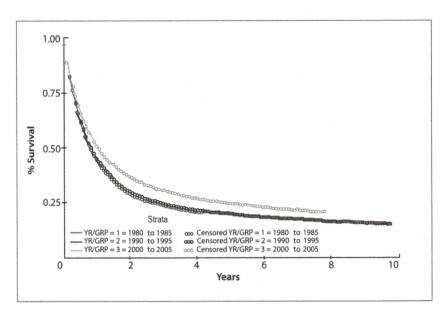

**FIGURE 29.4** Survival of lung cancer patients over the past three decades (reference 19).

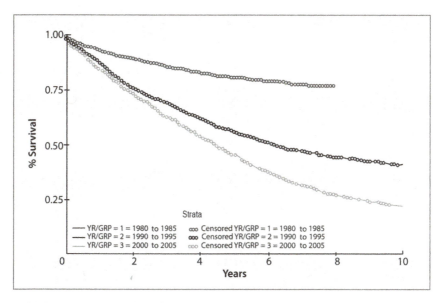

**FIGURE 29.5** Survival of chronic myeloid leukemia patients over the past three decades (reference 19).

## CHALLENGES TO PROGRESS: THE ONCOLOGY WORKFORCE

The Association of American Medical Colleges specialty data book in 2012 indicates that the number of medical oncologists practicing in the United States was 12,743, with 81% involved primarily in patient care, 1.2% in teaching, and 7.4% in research.[9] Since 2000, there has been a 26.8% increase in the number of medical oncologists, as of 2010.[9,10] The ratio of oncologists to population is 1:24,253, which is dramatically higher than the ratio of 1:4 million in Ethiopia and 1:10 million in Uganda. Similarly, there has been a 16.9% increase in the number of radiation oncologists from 2000 to 2010.[9]

In 2010, there were 560 fellowship positions in hematology/oncology, which was an increase of 19% compared to 2005.[11] Radiation oncology residencies increased by 16.9% for radiation oncology from 2005.[11] It is projected that the demand for oncologists will increase by 48% and the required patient visit capacity will increase by 14% by 2020. This situation will leave a projected shortage of 9.4 to 15.1 million patient visits, translating into a shortage of 2,550 to 4,080 oncologists in the coming years.

## CHALLENGES TO PROGRESS: CANCER DISPARITIES

Many groups across the United States suffer disproportionately from cancer. Among women, breast cancer incidence is greater in white as compared to the black women but the mortality rate is higher in blacks. Moreover, recent research suggests increased prevalence of aggressive tumors in younger black and Hispanic population living with low socioeconomic groups.[13]

There is also a greater burden of cervical cancer among black and Hispanic population perhaps due to inadequate screening among these groups.[14] Easier accessibility to the HPV vaccination may also reduce this disparity.

In men, the higher risk and burden of prostate cancer among black males are linked both to the genetics and to behavioral differences.[14] Lack of health care and insurance coverage is an obstacle to early detection. More research needs to be conducted to figure out the genetic link with the disease. Asian American men and Pacific islanders have a higher incidence of stomach cancer, may be linked to higher chances of infection with *Helicobacter pylori*. This population group has also been linked to higher rates of liver and bile duct cancers. The incidence of kidney cancer is higher in Alaskan and American Indian population.[15]

NCI and its divisions have been proactive in promoting research programs that address the issues which contribute to cancer health disparities. The Centers for Population Health and Health Disparities was established in 2003 and comprises eight centers. The NCI and other national institutions collectively back them up. Five of these centers address health disparities in cancer (Figure 29.6).

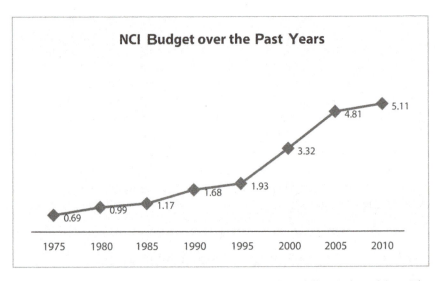

**FIGURE 29.6** NCI budget over the past years in billion dollars (adapted from The annual NCI Fact Book, reference 8).

## CONCLUSION

Cancer is a leading cause of death and disability in the United States. Public health initiatives, including smoking cessation, cervical and breast cancer screening, and HPV vaccination, have each had a significantly favorable impact. Similarly, improved treatment continues to reduce cancer mortality. Ultimately, it is the combination of both preventative and treatment initiatives that hold the greatest promise for improving cancer care outcomes. As a result of ongoing efforts in cancer control, overall cancer incidence and mortality in the United States have continued to decrease in the past two decades. Notably, the reported 5-year relative survival for all pediatric cancer sites is close to 90%, which is a 25% improvement from three decades ago.[1] Nonetheless, cancer is still a major public health problem, and despite these achievements there are significant racial and ethnic disparities in cancer incidence and mortality.

## REFERENCES

1. Murphy SL, Xu J, Kochanek KD. National Vital Statistics Reports (NVSS). 2013 May 8; 61: 4

2. American Cancer Society. *Cancer Facts & Figures 2013*. Atlanta, GA: American Cancer Society, 2013.

3. 150 Years of Advances against Cancer—National Cancer Institute at the National Institute of Health. Last updated June 1, 2011.

4. The NCI Annual Fact Book: Office of Budget and Finance, National Cancer Institute, Accessed December 9, 2013.

5. National Cancer Institute. Cancer Causes and Risk Factors. Available at http://www.cancer.gov/cancertopics/causes. Accessed December 9, 2013.

6. Carcinogens, 2010. Available at http://www.atsdr.cdc.gov/risk/cancer/cancer-substances.html. Accessed December 9, 2013.

7. Jemal A, Simard EP, Dorell C, et al. Annual report to the nation on the status of cancer, 1975–2009, featuring the burden and trends in HPV-associated cancers and HPV vaccination coverage levels. *J Natl Cancer Inst* 2013 Feb 1; 105(3): 175–201.

8. Jemal A, Siegel R, Xu J, Ward E. Cancer statistics, 2010. *CA Cancer J Clin* 2010; 60(5): 277–300.

9. AMA Physician Masterfile (December 2010) and Annual Estimates of the Population of the United States, Regions, States and Puerto Rico: April 2001–July 2010 (NST_PEST2010–01). Population Division, U.S. Census Bureau.

10. Physician Characteristics and Distribution in the US, 2002–2003 Edition and Physician Characteristics and Distribution in the US, 2012 Edition.

11. 2010 AAMC/AMA National GME Census as reported in JAMA 2006; 296(9): 1154–69 and JAMA 2011; 306(9): 1015–30.

12. Miller K. Available at http://www.valuebasedcancer.com/opm/article/seasons-survival.

13. Carey LA, Perou CM, Livasy CA, et al. Race, breast cancer subtypes, and survival in the Carolina Breast Cancer Study. JAMA 2006; 295(21): 2492–502.

14. The Excess Cervical Cancer Mortality: A Marker for Low Access to Health Care in Poor Communities report. Available at http://crchd.cancer.gov/attach ments/excess-cervcanmort.pdf. Accessed December 9, 2013.

15. Annual Report to the Nation on the Status of Cancer 1975–2004, Featuring Cancer in American Indians and Alaska Natives. Available at http://www.in terscience.wiley.com/cancer/report2007.

# 30

# West Africa

## *Verna D.N.K. Vanderpuye, Kofi Mensah Nyarko, and Pippa Newell*

## PUBLIC HEALTH PERSPECTIVE

West Africa's enormous disease burden can be viewed within a broader context of poverty, underdevelopment, conflict, and weak management of governmental institutions. Though infectious diseases remain a predominant health challenge in Africa, the incidence of chronic noncommunicable diseases such as cardiovascular diseases, diabetes, cancer, and respiratory conditions is increasing rapidly. Most of the health budgets in these countries are donor driven, and since donor attention is focused primarily on infectious diseases, funding is allocated to acute communicable diseases rather than noncommunicable diseases. Rather than competing for the limited available funds, policy interventions should consider joint approaches such as integration in disease control.

## COMMUNICABLE DISEASES AND CANCER

The major communicable diseases in the subregion that have attracted the most attention are HIV/AIDS, tuberculosis, and malaria. Unfortunately, hepatitis B virus is also endemic in West Africa and is the most common cause of liver cancer there. Hepatitis B infection is preventable by vaccination. Mass vaccination for hepatitis B in China has resulted in a significant decline in liver cancer rates there. Hepatitis B and liver cancer represent potential examples in which public health resources in West Africa could be expended to reduce simultaneously both a communicable disease and a deadly cancer.

## CANCER AS A PUBLIC HEALTH PROBLEM

The burden of cancer is increasing in West Africa. However, the level of awareness is very low, even among health workers, which is due, in part, to lack of national programs that provide health education in the communities. Another reason is that patients often present with late-stage disease, particularly those patients from rural areas and those who lack resources to pay for medical care. An important goal of public health efforts is to provide education and medical care within the confines of local cultural beliefs: patients may understand disease as spiritual, rather than biological in nature. Patients will often seek care from a traditional healer, which can delay diagnosis and treatment.

## CANCER STATISTICS

### Morbidity

Cancer is not a rare disease in Africa. The overall incidence is 13% to 17%, similar to other countries and regions.[1] Lack of organized cancer registries is detrimental to the development of strategies for effective national cancer control programs. However, a few population- and institutional-based registries are available, which are supported by the African Cancer Registry Network and funded by international agencies (Table 30.1). Most of the data available is based on Globocan 2008 estimates and other less substantiated local data sources. Poor patient follow up contributes to inaccurate survival statistics.

The Globocan estimates that about 184,071 new cases of cancer, excluding non-melanoma skin cancer, occur in West Africa annually. It is estimated that 5-year prevalence of cancer in adults is 317.4 per 100,000 in women and 149.7 per 100,000 in men.[2]

The most common cancers in men are prostate, liver, colorectal, non-Hodgkin's lymphoma (NHL), stomach, and bladder, whereas those common in women are breast, cervical, liver, colorectal, ovarian, and stomach. An estimated number of 139,255 individuals (77,993 females and 61,262 males) die annually from cancer in West Africa (Table 30.2).

**TABLE 30.1 Cancer Registries Updated in West Africa, 2013**

| Country | Population Based | Institutional Based |
| --- | --- | --- |
| Nigeria | 3 (Ibadan, Calabar, Maiduguiri) | 21 |
| Ghana | 1 (Kumasi Cancer Registry) | 1 Korle Bu Cancer Registry |
| Senegal | 1 | – |
| Cote D'Ivoire | 1 | – |
| Togo | 1 | – |
| Gambia | 1 | – |
| Guinea | 1 | – |
| Mauritius | 1 | – |
| Niger | 1 | – |

TABLE 30.2  Summary Statistics of Cancer Morbidity and Mortality in West Africa

| Western Africa | Male | Female | Both Sexes |
|---|---|---|---|
| Population (thousands) | 145,979 | 145,290 | 291,270 |
| Number of new cancer cases (thousands) | 72.5 | 111.6 | 184.1 |
|     Age-standardized rate (W) | 92.0 | 123.5 | 107.6 |
|     Risk of getting cancer before age 75 (%) | 10.1 | 13.1 | 11.6 |
| Number of cancer deaths (thousands) | 61.3 | 78.0 | 139.3 |
|     Age-standardized rate (W) | 80.1 | 91.2 | 85.3 |
|     Risk of dying from cancer before age 75 (%) | 8.7 | 10.3 | 9.5 |
| Five-year prevalent cases, adult population (thousands) | 123.9 | 265.9 | 389.8 |
|     Proportion (per 100,000) | 149.7 | 317.4 | 234.1 |

## CANCER ETIOLOGY

Up to 32% of cancers in sub-Saharan Africa are related to infections, compared to 7.4% in developed countries.[3] Chronic infections lead to the development of several common cancers, including liver, cervix, anal, penile, oropharyngeal, and squamous cell carcinoma of the bladder. The second leading cause of cancer-related death is liver cancer, which is associated with hepatitis B and C viral infections and the aflatoxin fungus. The leading cancer in females is cervical cancer, which is strongly related to infection with human papillomavirus (HPV 18, 16, and 31). *Helicobacter pylori* infection of the stomach and duodenum is known to play a role in the initiation and progression of cancers of the upper gastrointestinal tract. High HIV prevalence is a contributing factor to the cancer burden, especially with Kaposi's sarcoma, lymphoma, and cervical cancer, particularly in countries such as Cote d'Ivoire where HIV is the number one cause of death.[4] The incidence of Burkitt's lymphoma is higher in the *Plasmodium falciparum* malaria belt of West Africa and has decreased with malaria prophylaxis.[5] Epstein–Barr virus is also associated with Burkitt's lymphoma and nasopharyngeal cancer.

Lifestyle changes have resulted in increasing rates of obesity, low intake of fruits and vegetables, and high fat and meat intake. These may account for the increased incidence of breast, colorectal, and prostate cancers compared to a decade ago. Head and neck cancers are associated with alcohol intake and tobacco smoking, as well as HPV infections, especially in younger people. Areas where tobacco chewing is practiced have high rates of oral cancers. Common food preparation methods in the region, such as salting and smoking of fish, curing of meats, and cooking at high temperatures, lead to high nitrate and nitrosamine levels, and the use of food dyes may be associated with increased gastrointestinal cancer risk.[6]

Genetic associations in cancer are not properly studied or documented. A few studies indicate BRCA 1 and 2 expressions are associated with aggressive breast cancer in some West African countries.[7]

## HISTORY OF CANCER CARE

For many decades, surgical specialists were at the forefront of cancer management in most West African countries. The general surgeon was often the first to see the patient for tumor removal and also administered available anticancer drugs.

The first radiotherapy unit was set up in Lagos, Nigeria, in 1981. With increasing availability of radiotherapy services in more countries, cancer specialists are being trained locally. Radiotherapy facilities now exist in Ghana, Nigeria, Senegal, and, most recently, Mauritania (Table 30.3). The quality of radiation delivered, maintenance of equipment, and labor force training are supported by the International Atomic Energy Agency (IAEA). New centers are planned for Cote D'Ivoire, Niger, Burkina Faso, and Mali under the Programme of Action for Cancer Therapy mission of the IAEA. The implementation of the African Virtual University on Cancer Control, spearheaded by the International Atomic Energy Commission, will hopefully improve skilled labor force to fight the cancer epidemic.

## BREAST CANCER

Breast cancer is a very common cancer and the cause of death in females in the region, second only to cervical cancer. There is an unusually high incidence of male breast cancer (2% to 15%) compared with 1% worldwide.[8] The reason for this is unclear, but the trend is mirrored in African American males, who are 3 times as likely to die from breast cancer as white American

TABLE 30.3 Radiotherapy Facilities in West Africa

| Country | Radio-therapy Centers | Linear Accelera-tor Units | Cobalt 60 Units | Low-Dose Rate Brachy-therapy | Low-Dose Rate Brachy-therapy | Ra-diation Oncolo-gist | Ra-diation Thera-pist |
|---|---|---|---|---|---|---|---|
| Ghana | 3 | 1 | 2 | 2 | 0 | 6 | 16 |
| Mauritania | 1 | 1 | 0 | 0 | 1 | 2 | 4 |
| Nigeria | 9 | 8 | 5 | 2 | 1 | 30 | 27 |
| Senegal | 1 | 0 | 1 | 0 | 0 | 2 | 1 |
| Total | 15 | 10 | 8 | 4 | 2 | 40 | 48 |

*Source:* www.iaea.org.

males. High mortality from breast cancer in West Africa can be attributed to late presentation, limited access to care, younger age at presentation, and aggressive nature of disease.

The use of screening mammography is limited due to poor accessibility and cost. About 50% to 70% of patients present with advanced stage. The median age at presentation ranges between 42 and 49 years, compared with >60 years for other races. Average size of breast lumps is 7 to 10 cm despite improved awareness programs.

Histologically, estrogen receptor (ER) positivity is between 20% and 60% irrespective of age, and >75% of tumors are high grade.[9] Studies involving women of African ancestry and indigenous West African women have shown relatively high incidence of triple negative breast cancer subtypes (estrogen, progesterone, Her2Neu-negative receptor expression) 50% to 86% versus 26% in other races and are associated with poorer outcomes.[10,11] Adebamawo et al. disputed the high negative ER status found in the subregion and attributed this finding to poor tissue fixation practices.[12] Available data suggests Her2Neu receptor status positivity to be 15% to 19% across the subregion, not different from other countries.[13] The cost involved with immunohistochemistry testing is a limiting factor in obtaining accurate data within the subregion.

Most patients with advanced-stage presentation require neoadjuvant chemotherapy to improve resectability. Breast conservation is increasingly being employed compared to a decade ago for early-stage disease. Adherence to strict criteria is important to achieve good results, and breast conservation requires the presence of radiotherapy facilities. Chemotherapy protocols are adapted from international guidelines; however, cost and availability of drugs as well as expertise in managing side effects lead to frequent modifications of protocols. For example, trastuzumab for HER-2 positive breast cancer is available only in teaching and private hospitals, as less than 1% of patients requiring the drug can afford it. The use of radiotherapy in the adjuvant and palliative setting depends on availability of services. Even where the facilities are available, delays in referral and initiating treatment are of grave concern. According to Globocan 2008 estimates, West Africa has one of the highest breast cancer mortality rates in the world.

## CERVICAL CANCER

West African countries have highest incidence and mortality rates from cervical cancer in the world.[14] Poverty, multiparity (average 6.8), risky sexual practices, and the culture of polygamy are associated with poor control of cervical cancer in the region.[15] The crude incidence rates are 19.9 per 100,000 for western Africa versus 15.8 per 100,000 for the world. HPV 16, 18, and 31 are prevalent in West Africa (21.5% vs. 11.4% in the world) (WHO 2010) and associated with at least two-thirds of cervical cancer cases. HPV 45 is common (18.6%) in Mali, Gabon, and Senegal, necessitating different vaccination strategies.[16] High HIV prevalence rates in the region are also associated with higher occurrence rates, although a direct association has not been established.[17]

Papanicolaou smear testing is not routine even in urban areas in West Africa, due to cost, access to kits, and limitations with pathology expertise. The Visual Inspection Acetic Acid test using vinegar or Lugol's iodine requires less logistics, and immediate treatment of precancerous lesions was considered cost effective in pilot studies conducted in some West African countries.[18] In combination with cryotherapy, the risk of developing cervical cancer can be reduced by half with this intervention.[19] However, the lower sensitivity rate compared to Pap smear reduces its overall effectiveness.[20]

The success rate of surgery for early disease depends on availability of resources and surgical expertise. Patients with advanced disease are offered radiation therapy with or without chemotherapy where available. Cisplatin as a radiosensitizer is less beneficial in very advanced disease and can be detrimental in patients with poor renal function and performance status.[21] Unfortunately, many of our patients fall within this category and receive only radiation treatments. In the absence of brachytherapy facilities, available only in Senegal and some centers in Nigeria, treatment of cervical cancer with external beam radiotherapy alone typically results in poor outcomes.

## PROSTATE CANCER

Although prostate cancer is the most common cancer, and the most common cause of cancer mortality,[3] West Africa has a lower incidence of this cancer compared with other African regions.[22] Incidence per 100,000 ranges from 4 in the Gambia to 19.8 in Ghana to 127 in Nigeria.[23]

The high mortality rates in the region could be related to genetic factors, diets low in fruits and vegetables and high in fats and red meats, and late presentation.[24]

Studies from Ghana, Senegal, and Nigeria show that the mean age at presentation ranges from 60 to 68 years, and more than 90% of men present in late stages.[25] Prostate cancer in men from West African ancestry is aggressive in nature. Initial prostate-specific antigen (PSA) level >20 ng/dL was found in 73% of patients, and the mean PSA was 39.0 ng/dL in Ghana and 72 ng/dL in Senegal.[26] Factors contributing to late presentation include low levels of awareness, lack of structured screening programs, use of alternative medications, poor health facilities, and cultural beliefs.[27]

Management of curable disease depends on surgical or urological expertise. Hormonal manipulation is used in low-risk groups as an easier treatment option in contradiction to evidence-based guidelines.[28] Preoperative lymph node assessment in moderate- to high-risk patients, attainment of negative surgical margins, and lymph node dissection remain a challenge because of lack of surgical expertise and available pathologists. Use of radiation therapy is limited by availability and finances: most radiation therapy centers in West Africa lack the expertise and techniques needed to deliver high doses without profound normal tissue injury. Brachytherapy services for prostate cancer are available only in Ghana. Most patients presenting with very high PSA values and clinically advanced or metastatic disease are treated with palliative radiotherapy and/or hormonal manipulation.

Stilbestrol is prescribed in place of leuprolide and goserelin as a cheaper option. Surgical castration is a cheaper and frequently performed procedure compared to medical castration. In Ghana, however, most men preferred medical castration despite the high cost. They considered orchiectomy as loss of manhood and authority and not necessarily related to fertility or sexual function. Total androgen blockade is rarely prescribed due to cost limitations. Duration of hormonal manipulation depends on cost rather than risk category. Hormone refractory prostate cancer has a dismal outcome due to the limited availability and high cost of effective drugs.

## COLORECTAL CANCER

Africa has the lowest incidence rates of colorectal cancer worldwide. The West African diet is considered protective from colorectal carcinogenesis. Low-protein diets, lactose intolerance, high maize fiber, use of spices such as turmeric, onions, red pepper, and high vitamin D levels related to sunshine exposure are thought to be protective.[29] Unfortunately, recent data from the Ibadan cancer registry records colorectal as the 4th most common cause of cancer compared to 10th most common a decade ago;[30] this could be attributable to lifestyle changes, including obesity and physical inactivity. Data from Ghana, Nigeria, and Senegal[31,32] indicates 75% have advanced disease at presentation and one-third are below the age of 40 years.[33]

With the increased utilization and improved expertise in endoscopic and radiological procedures in urban health facilities, more cases are being diagnosed. They are often diagnosed in advanced stages, as rectal discomfort and bleeding are presumably diagnosed as hemorrhoids: average time from initial symptoms to presentation is 1 year.[34]

Surgical resection including lymph node dissection is an essential step in the treatment of non-metastatic or symptomatic tumors, yet the availability of competent surgeons is usually limited to urban areas. Liver resections for metastatic lesions are rarely performed. Locally advanced rectal tumors may receive chemotherapy and radiation therapy as adjuvant, neoadjuvant, or palliative treatment. Pain management, diverting colostomy, and nutritional support are paramount in managing advanced disease. Drugs such as oxaliplatin and irinotecan and targeted therapies are expensive, and their use is limited to a few specialized centers.

## PEDIATRIC CANCER

Cancer in children accounts for 5% to 15% of all malignancies in West Africa. At least 85% present with advanced and incurable disease, resulting in an overall cure rate of 5% compared to 85% in developed countries.[35]

Data from Ghana (L. Renner, personal communication) shows that of 495 patients seen over a 3-year period, 2008 to 2011, the most prevalent cancer was lymphoma (30%); 75% of lymphomas were Burkitt's type; 19% were leukemia. Retinoblastoma and Wilms' tumor constituted 15.8% and 12.3%, respectively. Soft tissue sarcoma accounted for 6.5%, with greater than 80% being rhabdomyosarcoma. Neuroblastoma accounted for 5.9%, followed by central nervous system and nasopharyngeal tumors.

There is some regional variability in incidence and mortality rates. Lower incidence rates of Burkitt's lymphoma are found in Nigeria, Mali, and the Gambia compared with other Africa countries and reflect the role of variable cofactors in the development of the disease. Childhood cancer mortality data from Ghana demonstrated that NHL accounts for the highest rate of deaths from cancer in children (54%), whereas in Guinea, higher incidence rates were observed for Hodgkin's lymphoma, Burkitt's lymphoma, and retinoblastoma.[36] A 26-year retrospective and descriptive study from Ivory Coast cancer registry shows that the most common childhood cancers are Burkitt's lymphoma (33%), retinoblastoma (10.9%), and nephroblastoma (5.9%).[37] Even within individual countries, there are variations by regions: in northern Nigeria, for example, retinoblastoma (30.6%) is the most common cancer in children (Kano), whereas Burkitt's lymphoma is the most common in eastern Nigeria.[38] In summary, the most common pediatric cancers in West Africa are Burkitt's lymphoma, retinoblastoma, leukemia, and nephroblastoma.[39-41]

International collaboration research is aimed at improving diagnosis, knowledge of health personnel, development of clinical trials, and access to expensive medication. Local capacity building should be the ultimate goal of these collaborative efforts to ensure sustainable improvements in outcomes. The Franco-African Childhood Cancer Group[42] developed protocols for Burkitt's lymphoma in West Africa and achieved 61% survival rate. Another protocol developed for unilateral neuroblastoma using single-agent cyclophosphamide increased survival to 73%. The role of pediatric palliative care cannot be overemphasized in improving quality in end of life and requires training and resources for broader implementation. The major challenge is identifying children in poorer rural communities, providing free sustainable health care, and educating all parents about common childhood cancers.

## LYMPHOMA

Lymphoma is one on the top 10 cancers in the region according to Globocan estimates. The increasing incidence of lymphoma is attributed to the HIV epidemic. Paucity of reliable data and inadequate pathology services in many poor areas probably mean that the burden of disease is underestimated. Sub-Saharan Africa is postulated to have over 30,000 new cases a year, with a majority being NHL of B-cell origin.

Hodgkin's disease is relatively rare in West Africa (0.5 to 0.7 per 100,000), mostly occurring in patients under age 30.[3] Adequate treatment and improved outcomes are limited by cost, management of related toxicities, and HIV status.

Burkitt's lymphoma is a disease of the tropics, affecting mostly children between ages 5 and 9 years. The higher prevalence in the tropical malaria belt, proliferation of the Epstein–Barr virus, and exposure to the *Euphorbia tirucalli* plant lead to these factors being causal agents of the disease. Facial presentation is the most common type, but there is an increase in presentation of the abdominal type and a combination of both. The facial type is highly chemosensitive and therefore curable with early presentation. Cure rates in Africa, even though still comparatively low compared to other continents (40% vs. 80%), have improved over the years through international collaborative and translational research partnerships such as that supported by the French African Pediatric Oncology Group.[43] Poorer survival in HIV-positive patients could be a contributing factor to lower survival rate despite improved access to care and treatment protocols.

Diffuse large B-cell type is the most common lymphoma in adults and tends to be high grade. The prevalence of HIV in the subregion contributes to high incidence and poor outcomes.[44] Many patients present with advanced disease and poor performance status and therefore cannot tolerate chemotherapy. Palliative radiotherapy is prescribed where available.

## HEPATOCELLULAR CARCINOMA

Globocan estimates that hepatocellular carcinoma (HCC), or primary liver cancer, is the second most fatal cancer in West Africa, with a mortality of 16.5 per 100,000; it is the deadliest cancer in men in some countries, such as the Gambia. Patients tend to present at a relatively young age compared to their white or Asian counterparts, and there the disease grows more aggressively: patients who present with symptoms have an average life expectancy of less than 3 months in West Africa.[45] Although the viral etiologies of HCC are similar to those in other parts of the world, the younger age at presentation and the relatively low incidence of cirrhosis in patients with HCC in West Africa suggest that there may be additional environmental and genetic factors at play.

A well-known environmental factor present in West Africa is aflatoxin B1, a mycotoxin produced by *Aspergillus* and found to contaminate stored food. It is thought that aflatoxin B1 can bind DNA and cause somatic mutations of tumor suppressor gene TP53, thereby rendering cells less able to repair the damage wrought by chronic viral infections.[46] Observational and molecular studies show that the effects of aflatoxin exposure and hepatitis B virus infection are synergistic risk factors for cancer, including seasonal variability in TP53 mutations.[47,48]

The most common cause of HCC in West Africa is chronic infection with hepatitis B virus. The predominant genotypes there are A, D, and E.[49] Horizontal, rather than vertical (mother to child), transmission is predominant in West Africa, where most of the population is exposed to the virus.[50] Vaccination programs have been effective at reducing the rates of chronic infection in West Africa.

The Gambia Hepatitis Intervention Study (GHIS) aimed to study whether immunization could reduce the incidence of HCC in collaboration with the International Agency for Research on Cancer, the Government of the Republic of the Gambia, and the Medical Research Council of the United Kingdom. The program was launched in 1986 with the objective of evaluating the efficacy of hepatitis B vaccination in childhood for the prevention of HB infection, chronic liver disease, and HCC in a population at high risk.[52] By February 1990, a cohort of 124,577 children had been recruited, 61,065 of whom had received HB vaccine. Since the start of the GHIS, a population-based National Cancer Registry was set up to evaluate the protectiveness of the hepatitis vaccination against HCC.[53] Assuming that in the Gambia the risk of HCC attributable to HBV is about 70%, the final stage of evaluation of efficacy of HBV vaccination in preventing HCC will be possible in 2015 to 2017.[54] The effects are expected to be impressive and will ideally boost investment in vaccination programs in the entire region.

Although hepatitis C is less of a risk factor here than in other parts of the world, the World Health Organization estimates that sub-Saharan Africa, including West Africa, is home to the highest seropositivity rate for HCV in the world, at 5.8%.[55] Hepatitis C infection is present in 19% of all patients with HCC in West Africa.[54] Coinfection with hepatitis B and C can increase rates of cirrhosis and liver cancer. Unfortunately, no vaccination for hepatitis C is available at present.

## CANCER CARE OUTCOMES

The gross national income of a country is directly proportional to the mortality rate in West Africa. For example, the Gambia is one of the least developed countries and records the lowest overall 5-year survival rate for cancer (22%).[56] Incidence and mortality rates for the most common cancers almost mirror each other throughout the region. Survival data from even accredited cancer registries is skewed, as the majority of patients are not captured in their databases.

### Prevention

For low-resource countries, primary and secondary cancer prevention measures are more likely to have positive impact compared to tertiary prevention methods that involve treatment and palliation.

The role of education is underestimated in the control of preventable diseases. The media could be employed to disseminate educative programs on cancer prevention, especially on the risks of obesity, sedentary lifestyles, high-risk sexual behaviors, and alcohol and tobacco use. Incorporating educational programs into school curricula could have an enormous impact. Training community health workers has also been very cost effective in many areas of the world, including some areas of West Africa.[57]

Infections play a vital role in cancer etiology and can be effectively controlled to minimize the subsequent development of cancer:

(a) Hepatitis B vaccination integration into childhood immunization programs in almost all of West Africa is currently supported by the Global Alliance for Vaccines and Immunizations, Merck Vaccine Network for Africa, and Program for Appropriate Technology in Health. This intervention is expected to reduce chronic HBV carrier rates and eventually reduce liver cancer rates.

(b) Aflatoxin biocontrol can be explored to reduce contamination, as was done in Burkina Fasso, Senegal, Guinea, and Nigeria at the subsistence farm level.[58] Control of schistosomiasis and prompt treatment of the infection in areas affected are practiced in Ghana, Niger, and Senegal. These interventions may reduce liver and bile duct cancer rates.

(c) HPV vaccination in girls should be available and accessible to all. Nigeria and Ghana are taking the lead on this initiative. Senegal, the Gambia, Cameroon, and Mali have received donations of HPV vaccines by manufacturers, and ideally, the program will be expanded to other countries.

### Screening

The integration of national screening programs into health-care systems has not materialized in most countries. Mammography for breast cancer screening is not considered cost effective in some of these countries and may not be effective in detecting cancers in young patients with dense breast tissue.[59] Clinical breast exams are therefore promoted as an ad hoc measure in place of mammography despite the lack of evidence to support this screening method.

Cultural and religious beliefs can hinder the success of screening programs. For example, visual inspection cervical screening methods were introduced into most West African countries as pilot projects to help lower the high incidence and mortality rates from cervical cancer. Spousal permission to participate in screening programs that involve the reproductive organs can be an obstacle.[60] These methods were found to be cost effective but have lower sensitivity compared with other screening methods such as Pap smear and HPV DNA testing.[61] Less expensive HPV DNA tests will make cervical cancer screening more cost effective.

Colorectal cancer screening is not considered relevant in West Africa as the incidence rates are relatively low. However, the 1:1 ratio of mortality to incidence of colorectal cancer in this region infers that cost-effective screening methods have potential for making a positive impact; fecal occult blood method may be a more appropriate method for screening than endoscopy.

Liver cancer screening for patients with cirrhosis and/or chronic hepatitis B using biannual liver ultrasound imaging is standard of care in the United States, Europe, and parts of Asia, but ultrasounds are expensive and a significant percentage of patients in West Africa develop HCC through aflatoxin exposure, who are negative for hepatitis B or C; these patients would be missed under the international screening guidelines.[62] Alpha-fetoprotein has been proposed as a cheaper alternative, but has a poorer sensitivity.

## CANCER CARE WORKFORCE

West African countries have low health spending budgets compared to South and East Africa. Multidisciplinary care, especially for breast cancer, is established in most teaching hospitals with cancer treatment facilities. Investment in education and training for health-care providers is limited. The scarcity of cancer care specialists of all types is a huge challenge in the region. Undergraduate and postgraduate training programs have been established in West Africa to improve the cancer care workforce. Factors leading to a high attrition rate of skilled workers will also need to be addressed, such as poor remuneration, difficult working conditions, outmoded infrastructure, and lack of political will to support cancer control as a whole.

Pathology expertise in the diagnosis and stratification of cancer is lacking in the region. The few services available are located in urban centers with limited personnel and suboptimal resources, which affect the accuracy of diagnosis. Recent inroads toward improvement of this pivotal discipline in cancer management across Africa have been made possible through collaborations with the African Organization for Research and Treatment of Cancer.[63]

The need for palliative care services for cancer patients should not be underestimated. With the aid of international hospice groups such as Hospice Africa, Africa Oxford Cancer Foundation, and American Society of Clinical Oncology and other civil society groups, palliative care for cancer is gradually being integrated into health-care practices, especially at the community level. The rate-limiting steps are government participation, the willingness of health providers to prescribe the drugs, and the availability and affordability of narcotic pain medication.

Counseling for and follow-up of cancer patients and their caregivers is vital to survivorship, particularly in light of cultural understanding of diseases. Psychologists skilled at helping patients and families deal with the stigmata of cancer and infection are lacking; the practice of psycho-oncology is rare in West Africa. Nigeria and Senegal are making headway by recruiting psycho-oncologists in their cancer care programs. Most families receive psychosocial support from their spiritual leaders who lack basic knowledge about cancer. Nursing staff and pharmacists often embrace the role of counselors. Finally, cancer care specialists themselves also would benefit from increased psychological support to cope with the stress of helplessness when treating large patient loads with the scant resources available.

## CANCER RESEARCH

Searchable data on cancers from West Africa published entirely by local researchers is relatively sparse. Due to lack of funding opportunities and research infrastructure, clinical trials are not regularly conducted in the region; Nigeria and Senegal record the highest number of international clinical trials conducted. Lack of cancer care specialists and national regulatory bodies may contribute to the impression that unreliable data and poor adherence to trial protocols conducted in West Africa could violate trial results. The prohibitive cost of conducting and publishing research in peer-reviewed international journals and the lack of financial commitment by academic institutions are likely contributory factors to this phenomenon.[64]

Major research collaborators are the National Cancer Institute, USA, Mel and Belina Gates Foundation, World Health Organization, pharmaceutical industries, IAEA, ASCO, and FRANCE. Research areas highly patronized are pediatric, lymphoma, breast, cervix, and prostate cancers.

## FUTURE DIRECTIONS

Collaborative work in cancer care with our development partners needs to be encouraged and strengthened. Support of local cancer research capabilities to determine and strategize preventive, curative, and palliative programs for cancers will invariably reduce the high cancer mortality rates. International collaborations may be necessary for the expansion of radiotherapy, which represents a relatively expensive undertaking.

The development and implementation of national cancer control program for each country is an absolute necessity. The focus of these programs should be on cost-effective measures such as public education, immunization programs in HPV and HBV, and training of community health workers able to perform simple data collection, screening, and psychosocial support.

## REFERENCES

1. Sitas F, Parkin M, Chirenje Z, Stein L, Mqoqi N, Wabinga H. Cancers. In: Jamison DT, Feachem RG, Makgoba MW et al. (Eds). *Disease and Mortality in Sub-Saharan Africa*. Washington DC: The International Bank for Reconstruction and Development/The World Bank, 2006.
2. Ferlay J, Shin HR, Bray F, Forman D, Mathers C, Parkin DM. GLOBOCAN 2008 v2.0, Cancer Incidence and Mortality Worldwide: IARC CancerBase No. 10 [Internet]. Lyon, France: International Agency for Research on Cancer, 2010. Available at http://globocan.iarc.fr.
3. de Martel C, Ferlay J, Franceschi S, et al.. Global burden of cancers attributable to infections in 2008: a review and synthetic analysis. *Lancet Oncol* 2012; 13(6): 607–15.
4. Tanon A, Jaquet A, Ekouevi DK, et al.. The spectrum of cancers in West Africa: associations with human immunodeficiency virus. *PLoS One* 2012; 7(10): e48108. doi:10.1371/journal.pone.0048108.
5. Geser A, Brubaker G, Draper CC. Effect of a malaria suppression program on the incidence of African Burkitt's lymphoma. *Am J Epidemiol* 1989; 129(4): 740–52.
6. Marques-Vidal P, Ravasco P, Camilo ME. Foodstuffs and colorectal cancer risk: a review. *Clin Nutr* 2006; 25(1): 14–36. doi:http://dx.doi.org/10.1016/j.clnu.2005.09.008.
7. Fackenthal JD, Zhang J, Zhang B, et al. High prevalence of BRCA1 and BRCA2 mutations in unselected Nigerian breast cancer patients. *Int J Cancer* 2012; 131(5): 1114–23. doi:10.1002/ijc.27326.
8. Rachid S, Yacouba H, Hassane N Male breast cancer: 22 case reports at the National Hospital of Niamey, Niger. *Pan Afr Med J* 2009; 3: 15.
9. Adisa CA, Eleweke N, Alfred AA, et al. Biology of breast cancer in Nigerian women: a pilot study. *Ann Afr Med* 2012; 11(3): 169–75. doi:10.4103/1596-3519.96880.
10. Huo D, Ikpatt F, Khramtsov A, et al. Population differences in breast cancer: survey in indigenous African women reveals over-representation of triple-negative breast cancer. *J Clin Oncol* 2009; 27(27): 4515–21. doi:10.1200/jco.2008.19.6873.

11. Stark A, Kleer CG, Martin I, et al. African ancestry and higher prevalence of triple-negative breast cancer: findings from an international study. *Cancer* 2010; 116(21): 4926–32. doi:10.1002/cncr.25276.

12. Adebamowo CA, Famooto A, Ogundiran TO, Aniagwu T, Nkwodimmah C, Akang EE. Immunohistochemical and molecular subtypes of breast cancer in Nigeria. *Breast Cancer Res Treat* 2008; 110(1): 183–88. doi:10.1007/s10549–007–9694–5.

13. Yarney J, Vanderpuye V, Clegg Lamptey JN. Hormone receptor and HER-2 expression in breast cancers among Sub-Saharan African women. *Breast J* 2008; 14(5): 510–11. doi:10.1111/j.1524–4741.2008.00636.

14. Singh GK, Azuine RE Siahpush M. Global inequalities in cervical cancer incidence and mortality are linked to deprivation, low socioeconomic status, and human development. *Int J MCH AIDS* 2012; 1(1): 17–30.

15. Bah E, Parkin DM, Hall AJ, Jack AD, Whittle H. Cancer in the Gambia: 1988–97. *Br J Cancer* 2001; 84(9): 1207–14. doi:10.1054/bjoc.2001.1730.

16. Keita N, Clifford GM, Koulibaly M, et al. HPV infection in women with and without cervical cancer in Conakry, Guinea. *Br J Cancer* 2009; 101(1): 202–208.

17. Adjorlolo-Johnson G, Unger ER, Boni-Ouattara E, et al.. Assessing the relationship between HIV infection and cervical cancer in Cote d'Ivoire: a case-control study. *BMC Infect Dis* 2010; 10: 242. doi:10.1186/1471–2334–10–242.

18. Blumenthal PD, Gaffikin L, Deganus S, Lewis R, Emerson M, Adadevoh S. Cervical cancer prevention: safety, acceptability, and feasibility of a single-visit approach in Accra, Ghana. *Am J Obstet Gynecol* 2007; 196(4): 407.e1–407.e9. doi:http://dx.doi.org/10.1016/j.ajog.2006.12.031.

19. Goldie SJ, Gaffikin L, Goldhaber-Fiebert JD, et al. Cost-effectiveness of cervical-cancer screening in five developing countries. *N Engl J Med* 2005; 353(20): 2158–68. doi:10.1056/NEJMsa044278.

20. Gravitt PE, Paul P, Katki HA, et al. Effectiveness of VIA, Pap, and HPV DNA testing in a cervical cancer screening program in a peri-urban community in Andhra Pradesh, India. *PLoS One* 2010; 5(10): e13711. doi:10.1371/journal.pone.0013711.

21. McArdle O, Kigula-Mugambe J. Contraindications to cisplatin based chemoradiotherapy. *Rad Oncol* 2007; 83(10): 94–96.

22. Chu LW, Ritchey J, Devesa SS, Quraishi SM, Zhang H, Hsing AW. Prostate cancer incidence rates in Africa. *Prostate Cancer* 2011.

23. Kheirandish P, Chinegwundoh F. Ethnic differences in prostate cancer. *Br J Cancer* 2011; 105(4): 481–85. doi:10.1038/bjc.2011.273.

24. Yarney J, Vanderpuye V, Mensah J. Clinicopathologic features and determinants of Gleason score of prostate cancer in Ghanaian men. *Urol Oncol Semin Original Investig* 2013; 31(3): 325–30. doi:http://dx.doi.org/10.1016/j.urolonc.2011.01.018.

25. Yamoah K, Beecham K, Hegarty SE, Hyslop T, Showalter T, Yarney J. Early results of prostate cancer radiation therapy: an analysis with emphasis on research strategies to improve treatment delivery and outcomes. *BMC Cancer* 2013; 13: 23. doi:10.1186/1471–2407–13–23.

26. Gueye SM, Zeigler-Johnson CM, Friebel T, et al. Clinical characteristics of prostate cancer in African Americans, American whites, and Senegalese men. *Urology* 2003; 61(5): 987–92.

27. Olapade-Olaopa EO, Obamuyide HA, Yisa GT. Management of advanced prostate cancer in Africa. *Can J Urol* 2008; 15(1): 3890–98.

28. NCCN.org. Prostate cancer, Version 2.2014. *J Natl Compr Canc Netw* 2014; 12: 686–718.

29. Irabor DO. Colorectal carcinoma: why is there a lower incidence in Nigerians when compared to Caucasians? *J Cancer Epidemiol* 2011. doi:10.1155/2011/675154.

30. Iliyasu Y, Ladipo JK, Akang EE, Adebamowo CA, Ajao OG, Aghadiuno PU. A twenty-year review of malignant colorectal neoplasms at University College Hospital, Ibadan, Nigeria. *Dis Colon Rectum* 1996; 39(5): 536–40.

31. Dakubo JC, Naaeder SB, Tettey Y, Gyasi RK. Colorectal carcinoma: an update of current trends in Accra. *West Afr J Med* 2010; 29(3): 178–83.

32. Dem A, Kasse AA, Diop M, et al. [Epidemiological and therapeutic aspects of rectal cancer in Senegal: 74 cases at the Cancer Institute of Dakar]. *Dakar Med* 2000; 45(1): 66–69.

33. Ibrahim OK, Afolayan AE, Adeniji KA, Buhari OM, Badmos KB. Colorectal carcinoma in children and young adults in Ilorin, Nigeria. *West Afr J Med* 2011; 30(3): 202–5.

34. Vanderpuye V. (unpublished data).

35. Hadley LG, Rouma BS, Saad-Eldin Y. Challenge of pediatric oncology in Africa. *Semin Pediatr Surg* 2012; 21(2): 136–41. doi:10.1053/j.sempedsurg.2012.01.006.

36. Koulibaly M, Kabba IS, Cissé A, et al. Cancer incidence in Conakry, Guinea: first results from the cancer registry 1992–1995. *Int J Cancer* 1997; 70(1): 39–45. doi:10.1002/(SICI)1097–0215(19970106)70:1<39::AID-IJC6>3.0.CO;2–7.

37. Effi AB, Koffi KE, Aman NA, et al. Descriptive epidemiology of cancers in Cote d'Ivoire. *Bull Cancer* 2013. doi:10.1684/bdc.2013.1695.

38. Ochicha O, Gwarzo AK, Gwarzo D. Pediatric malignancies in Kano, Northern Nigeria. *World J Pediatr* 2012; 8(3): 235–39. doi:10.1007/s12519–012–0363–3.

39. Garba SM, Zaki HM, Arfaoui A, et al. Epidemiology of cancers in Niger, 1992 to 2009. *Bull Cancer* 2013; 100(2): 127–33. doi:10.1684/bdc.2013.1699.

40. Ka AS, Imbert P, Moreira C, et al. Epidemiology and prognosis of childhood cancers in Dakar, Senegal. *Med Trop (Mars)* 2003; 63(4–5): 521–26.

41. Amegbor K, Darre T, Ayena KD, et al. Cancers in togo from 1984 to 2008: epidemiological and pathological aspects of 5251 cases. *J Cancer Epidemiol* 2011; 2011:319872. doi:10.1155/2011/319872.

42. Lemerle J, Barsaoui S, Harif M, et al. Treatment of childhood cancer in Africa. Action of the Franco-African childhood cancer group. *Med Trop (Mars)* 2007; 67(5): 497–504.

43. Traore F, Coze C, Atteby JJ, et al. Cyclophosphamide monotherapy in children with Burkitt lymphoma: a study from the French-African Pediatric Oncology Group (GFAOP). *Pediatr Blood Cancer* 2011; 56(1): 70–76. doi:10.1002/pbc.22746.

44. Lucas SB, De Cock KM, Peacock C, Diomande M, Kadio A. Effect of HIV infection on the incidence of lymphoma in Africa. *East Afr Med J* 1996; 73 (5 Suppl): S29–S30.

45. Mendy M, Walton R. Molecular pathogenesis and early detection of hepatocellular carcinoma—perspectives from West Africa. *Cancer Lett* 2009 Dec 1; 286(1): 44–51.

46. Gouas DA, Villar S, Ortiz-Cuaran S, et al. TP53 R249S mutation, genetic variations in HBX and risk of hepatocellular carcinoma in the Gambia. *Carcinogenesis* 2012 Jun; 33(6): 1219–24.

47. Villar S, Le Roux-Goglin E, Gouas DA, et al. Seasonal variation in TP53 R249S-mutated serum DNA with aflatoxin exposure and hepatitis B virus infection. *Environ Health Perspect* 2011 Nov; 119(11): 1635–40.

48. Kirk GD, Turner PC, Gong Y, et al. Hepatocellular carcinoma and polymorphisms in carcinogen-metabolizing and DNA repair enzymes in a population with aflatoxin exposure and hepatitis B virus endemicity. *Cancer Epidemiol Biomarkers Prev* 2005; 14: 373–79.

49. Dumpis U, Holmes EC, Mendy M, et al. Transmission of hepatitis B virus infection in Gambian families revealed by phylogenetic analysis. *J Hepatol* 2001; 35: 99–104.

50. Plymoth A, Viviani S, Hainaut P. Control of hepatocellular carcinoma through hepatitis B vaccination in areas of high endemicity: perspectives for global liver cancer prevention. *Cancer Lett* 2009 Dec 1; 286(1): 15–21.

51. Coursaget P, Leboulleux D, Soumare M, et al. Twelve-year follow-up study of hepatitis B immunization of Senegalese infants. *J Hepatol* 1994); 21: 250–54.

52. Hall A, Inskip H, Loik F, et al. The Gambia Hepatitis Intervention Study. The Gambia Hepatitis Study Group. *Cancer Res* 1987; 47: 5782–87.

53. Bah E, Hall AJ, Inskip HM. The first 2 years of the Gambian National Cancer Registry. *Br J Cancer* 1990; 62: 647.

54. Kirk GD, Lesi OA, Mendy M, et al. The Gambia liver cancer study: infection with hepatitis B and C and the risk of hepatocellular carcinoma in West Africa. *Hepatology* 2004; 39: 211.

55. Madhava V, Burgess C, Drucker E. Epidemiology of chronic hepatitis C virus infection in sub-Saharan Africa. *Lancet Infect Dis* 2002; 2: 293–302.

56. Sankaranarayanan R, Swaminathan R, Brenner H, et al. Cancer survival in Africa, Asia, and Central America: a population-based study. *Lancet Oncol* 2010; 11(2): 165–73. doi:10.1016/s1470–2045(09)70335–3.

57. ASBEF Senegal, 2007; Sarli L, Enongene E, Bulgarelli K, Sarli A, Renda A, Sansebastiano G, Diouff M. Training program for community health workers in remote areas in Senegal. First experience. *Acta Biomed* 2010 Dec;81(1):54–62.

58. Turner, PC, Sylla A, Gong YY, et al. Reduction in exposure to carcinogenic aflatoxins by postharvest intervention measures in West Africa: a community-based intervention study. *Lancet* 2005; 365(9475): 1950–56. doi:10.1016/s0140–6736 (05)66661–5.

59. Zelle SG, Nyarko KM, Bosu WK, et al. Costs, effects and cost-effectiveness of breast cancer control in Ghana. *Trop Med Int Health* 2012; 17(8): 1031–43. doi:10.1111/j.1365–3156.2012.03021.x.

60. Williams MS, Amoateng P. Knowledge and beliefs about cervical cancer screening among men in Kumasi, Ghana. *Ghana Med J* 2012; 46(3): 147–51.

61. Denny L. Cervical cancer prevention: new opportunities for primary and secondary prevention in the 21st century. *Int J Gynaecol Obstet* 2012; 119(Suppl 1): S80–S84. doi:10.1016/j.ijgo.2012.03.023.

62. Umoh NJ, Lesi OA, Mendy M, et al. Aetiological differences in demographical, clinical and pathological characteristics of hepatocellular carcinoma in the Gambia. *Liver Int* 2011 Feb 31(2): 215–21.

63. Williams CK, Cristina Stefan D, Rawlinson F, Simbiri K, Mbulaiteye SM. The African Organisation for Research and Training in Cancer and its conferences: a historical perspective and highlights of the Ninth International Conference,

Durban, South Africa, November 21-24, 2013. *Ecancermedicalscience* Feb 3 2014;8:396. doi: 10.3332/ecancer.2014.396. eCollection 2014. www.aortic.org.

64. Muula AS. Medical journals and authorship in low-income countries. *Croat Med J* 2008; 49(5): 681–83.

# 31

# Western Europe

## *Dirk Schrijvers*


## INTRODUCTION

Western Europe is the region comprising the westerly countries of Europe, including Andorra, Austria, Belgium, Cyprus, Denmark, Faroe Islands, Finland, France, Germany, Gibraltar, Greece, Guernsey, Iceland, Ireland, Isle of Man, Italy, Jersey, Liechtenstein, Luxembourg, Malta, Monaco, the Netherlands, Norway, Portugal, San Marino, Spain, Sweden, Switzerland, and the United Kingdom. As of 2013, its estimated number of inhabitants is 415,580,161, and it is considered to be a high-income developed region with democratic political systems, mixed economies, and a social security ensuring health care for most of its inhabitants.[1] Its population has a life expectancy of around 80 years. The population structure shows an increasing number of elderly people, and as of 2013, 18.7% of the population is older than 65 years.

Projections indicate that in 2025 there will be a slight increase in the number of inhabitants, namely to 428,178,608, while the number of people aged 65 and more will constitute 22.1% of the entire population and life expectancy will rise to 82 years.


## HEALTH-CARE PROVISION

In most Western European countries, health care is ensured for 60% to 80% by social health insurance organized by governmental organizations, while private insurance companies cover a minority of inhabitants. Health-care insurance is mainly based on the principle of equity and solidarity: "everybody invests in the health (care) of all." Health-care coverage is almost 100%, and most inhabitants have readily access to health-care facilities, including those ensuring cancer care. At the moment around 9% to 12% of the gross domestic product (GDP) is spent on health care in different Western countries,[2] and the amount spent has been increasing between 2001 and 2009 with 2% to 4%.[3] In future, health-care costs will further increase due to the demographic shift, putting even more stress on the GDP.

Western European health-care provision is spread over a number of governmental and nongovernmental organizations with specific tasks in relation to health care. Most emphasis is given to treatment of different diseases while disease prevention by healthy living environment and food safety is not a core business of the health-care system. Health care is directed at prevention, treatment and care for injury, communicable and noncommunicable diseases (NCDs).

Prevention is covered by different programs of primary and secondary prevention. Primary prevention (e.g., tobacco and alcohol prevention, vaccination) to decrease the occurrence of disease by healthy living style promotion is organized by governmental and nongovernmental organizations. Secondary prevention or screening programs are mainly organized by governmental bodies and may be the responsibility of national (e.g., the Netherlands) or regional (e.g., Belgium) governments. Most Western European countries have an organized screening of the population for cervical and breast cancers and are starting to screen for colorectal cancer, based on a European Union recommendation. Opportunistic screening is present in certain countries, but is being discouraged by the authorities.

Curative and palliative treatment and care is ensured in most Western European countries by a social health insurance body (European observatory). In many Western European countries, sickness funds play a key role in the financial organization of health care. They are funded by governmental organizations (via income taxes) or (possible) health-care consumers (e.g., personal contributions) and their organizations (e.g., employers) to reimburse parts of the costs made by health-care consumers. Health-care providers, being individual health-care professionals, groups, or institutions, receive payment directly from health-care consumers, sickness funds, or governmental organizations. National governmental bodies in collaboration with the sickness funds and representatives of professional health-care providers regulate the criteria for funding and reimbursement.

## Health-Care Providers

Several groups of recognized health-care providers (e.g., general practitioners, medical specialists, dentists, nurses, dieticians, physiotherapists, nursing helpers) are involved in practical health care, and care can be provided at home, in home-replacing environments (e.g., nursing homes, palliative care units), in day-care centers, in special institutions (e.g., cabinets, revalidation centers), or in hospitals.

Western European countries base their primary-care systems largely on general practitioners (GPs), who deal mainly with disease but in some countries also play a role in prevention. GPs work mostly in solo practices or in an increasing number in group practices and can involve other professionals to organize care or can refer patients to specialist care. In many but not all Western European countries, GPs have a gate-keeping role for access to secondary care.

Secondary care can be given by private or public organizations. The health authorities have strict regulation for recognition of individual specialists and institutions (e.g., hospitals) for providing care and receiving public funding.

In 2010, the number of practicing medical physicians ranged from 219 per 100,000 inhabitants in the United Kingdom to more than 478 per 100,000 in Austria and Greece.[4,5] The number of nurses per 100,000 inhabitants in 2010 varied between 587 per 100,000 (Spain) and 2,468 per 100,000 inhabitants (Norway).[4,5] Projections of the World Health Organization[6,7] show that the health-care professionals will have to increase from 7,450,000 in 2005 to 1,135,000 in 2050 to maintain the current level of care only due to the demographic shift. This means that the percentage of health-care professionals among economically active people will have to increase from 8.42% to 13.80% in that same time span.[8]

## MORTALITY IN WESTERN EUROPE

The majority of deaths in Western Europe are due to NCDs followed by injuries and communicable diseases. On average the crude death rate equals 1,032 deaths per 100,000 inhabitants.[4] Almost 80% of all deaths occur in people aged 65 years or older.

### Noncommunicable Diseases in Western Europe

Noncommunicable diseases (NCDs), including cardiovascular diseases, cancer, respiratory diseases, and diabetes are the principal causes of death in Western Europe. Cardiovascular system diseases are the main cause of death due to NCDs and account for 42% of all deaths. On average, the male age-standardized death rate due to cardiovascular diseases varies between 151 and 1,500 per 100,000 inhabitants and for women these figures are 97 and 1,054 per 100,000, respectively. The second most important NCD mortality cause is cancer. The average standardized death rate equals 243 per 100,000 for men and 137 per 100,000 for women.

### Injuries

Injuries is defined as physical damage that results when a human body is suddenly or briefly subjected to intolerable levels of energy; it is the second cause of death in Western Europe. It ranges from 23 per 100,000 inhabitants in France to 116 per 100,000 in Luxemburg.

## Communicable Diseases in Western Europe

Death rate due to communicable diseases has dramatically decreased in Western Europe. Death and disability from infectious and parasitic diseases decreased due to improvements in sanitation and water quality and the development and widespread use of antibiotics and vaccines. However, Western Europe has been challenged in communicable disease control due to the emergence of new infectious agents such as human immunodeficiency virus, the reemergence of old infectious agents such as tuberculosis, and the spread of antimicrobial-resistant organisms. Mean mortality due to infections in 2009 was 8.3 per 100,000 inhabitants, ranging from 2.1 per 100,000 in Malta to 17.1 per 100,000 in Portugal.[4]

## CANCER AS A PUBLIC HEALTH PROBLEM

Cancer constitutes a major health problem in Western Europe. The age-standardized incidence rates of cancer in Western Europe are 335.3 per 100,000 in men and 250.5 per 100,000 in women.[9] Mortality figures range from 243 per 100,000 for men and 137 per 100,000 for women.

The three most frequently diagnosed cancers in men are prostate cancer (93.1 per 100,000); lung cancer (44.8 per 100,000), and colorectal cancer (41.3 per 100,000), whereas for women these are breast cancer (89.7 per 100,000), colorectal (26.3 per 100,000), and lung cancer (16.9 per 100,000). Most frequent causes of death due to cancer in men are lung (37.1 per 100,000), colorectal (15.1 per 100,000), and prostate (12.4 per 100,000), and in women breast (17.5 per 100,000), lung (12.9 per 100,000), and colorectal (9.3 per 100,000).[10]

Smoking is an important cause of cancer in Western Europe, and 27% of all cancer deaths in this region are attributed to smoking.[11] Lung cancer is the leading cause of smoking-related cancer mortality with a contribution of 60% to 70% in Europe. Other smoking-related cancers are upper gastrointestinal and genitourinary cancers.[11]

Alcohol use is related to upper respiratory, upper gastrointestinal, liver, and breast cancers. Among men and women in selected Western European countries, 10% and 3% of the incidence of cancer were attributable to former and current alcohol consumption. It was 44% and 25% for upper aerodigestive tract, 33% and 18% for liver, 17% and 4% for colorectal cancer for men and women, respectively, and 5.0% for female breast cancer.[12]

Another important cause of cancer in Western Europe is viral infections (e.g., hepatitis B and C, human papillomavirus [HPV], Epstein–Barr virus).

Among these HPV is the most frequent cause of virus-related cancer in Western Europe compared to other regions (e.g., Southeastern Asia, China), where hepatitis B and C are the main causes of viral-related cancers such as hepatocellular cancer. HPV is involved in cervical (incidence ranging from around 5 to 10 per /100,000 women), vulvar, vaginal, oropharyngeal, and anal cancers in women and in penile, oropharyngeal, and anal cancers in men and accounts for 7.7% of cancer cases in developed regions.[13]

The incidence of cancer has been increasing while mortality did not decrease until the mid-2000s. Since then, there has been a steadily decrease in cancer mortality in both men and women (Tables 31.1 and 31.2).

Western European cancer care has a tradition since a long time. However, discrepancies exist in relation to the cancer care planning among different Western European countries in relation to national cancer plans, implementation of cancer programs, infrastructure, and health-care professionals involved in cancer treatment and care.

Since the mid-2000s, most Western European countries have a national cancer plan (Table 31.3). The infrastructure in some Western European countries is insufficient (e.g., day-care centers, hospitals, radiotherapy units, and infrastructure for palliative care and revalidation) to provide optimal cancer care.

- In Western Europe there has been a trend to decrease the number of hospital beds, putting stress on the possibility to hospitalize patients for treatment and care.[4] At the same time, there was a tendency to treat more and more oncology patients in an ambulatory setting. This trend is going on and most cancer patients in need of medical treatment are treated in ambulatory or day-care centers. Another trend is that care and treatment is given at home or in home-replacing environments (e.g., chemotherapy or other parenteral cancer treatments given at home by trained nurses).
- In Western Europe, there is on average 1 radiotherapy machine per 250,000 inhabitants. However, in several Western Europe countries there are too few radiotherapy units to guarantee that cancer patients in need of radiotherapy receive treatment: in Italy around 16% of need is unmet, in Portugal 19%, Austria 20%, and the United Kingdom and Germany 21%. However, these possible gaps in treatment supply may be compensated by more effective organization of radiotherapy provision.

Several groups of professional oncology health-care providers are involved in cancer care, including organ specialists, medical oncology, clinical oncologists, oncological surgeons, radiotherapists, palliative care specialists, and oncology nurses.

Medical oncology and radiation oncology are recognized specialties by the European Union, although the term "medical oncologist" is not accepted by

TABLE 31.1  Cancer Mortality in Selected Western European Countries in Men over Time (per 100,000 Inhabitants)

| Geo\Time | 1999 | 2000 | 2001 | 2002 | 2003 | 2004 | 2005 | 2006 | 2007 | 2008 | 2009 | 2010 |
|---|---|---|---|---|---|---|---|---|---|---|---|---|
| Belgium | 267.5 | 260.4 | | | | 235.3 | 236.6 | 227.1 | 223.7 | 226 | 217.1 | |
| Denmark | 258.4 | 239.7 | 253.1 | 244.7 | 241.5 | 247.8 | 241 | 245.9 | 227.7 | 225 | 219.4 | |
| Germany | 243.3 | 246.4 | 231 | 228.8 | 225.3 | 219.3 | 215.3 | 210.9 | 206.4 | 206.2 | 201.9 | 199.2 |
| Ireland | 248.7 | 222.7 | 241 | 235.3 | 228.3 | 230.8 | 218.9 | 226.3 | 214.6 | 214.5 | 221.3 | 199 |
| Greece | 222.4 | 248.8 | 223.8 | 215.1 | 217.9 | 219 | 217.5 | 207.3 | 211.2 | 210.1 | 207.3 | 197.7 |
| Spain | 253.8 | 270 | 250.9 | 245 | 243.9 | 240 | 232.7 | 228.8 | 227.3 | 222 | 219.4 | 217.5 |
| France | 276.4 | 244.6 | 266.6 | 263.9 | 259.7 | 251.7 | 249.9 | 242.6 | 238.2 | 232.1 | 229.8 | 222.7 |
| Italy | 250.2 | | 247.4 | 239.6 | 238 | | | 223.5 | 219.6 | 215.2 | 212.1 | 207.6 |
| Cyprus | | | | | | 164.3 | 149.1 | 145.7 | 147.3 | 150.8 | 153.1 | 148.7 |
| Luxembourg | 236.7 | 259.9 | 225.8 | 225.6 | 235.9 | 229.6 | 209.4 | 205.9 | 218.8 | 194.4 | 206.9 | 211.7 |
| Malta | 236 | 202.8 | 217.2 | 211.8 | 192 | 189 | 183.4 | 198 | 194.7 | 205.8 | 197.2 | 184.3 |
| The Netherlands | 270.2 | 261.4 | 254 | 250.5 | 246.3 | 244 | 240.1 | 234.6 | 232 | 227.9 | 227.2 | 226.9 |
| Austria | 232.3 | 225.4 | 220.4 | 227 | 227.9 | 223.6 | 215.7 | 212.3 | 202.2 | 211.2 | 203.9 | 198.4 |
| Portugal | 222 | 223.2 | 222.6 | 223.5 | 224.7 | 216.2 | 215.6 | 210.4 | 215.5 | 218 | 216.4 | 215.9 |
| Finland | 208.4 | 198.5 | 199.2 | 192.8 | 190.2 | 188.9 | 183.7 | 183.9 | 177.6 | 171.9 | 171.4 | 174.4 |
| Sweden | 190.2 | 186.1 | 185.3 | 182.4 | 186.3 | 181.9 | 182.4 | 178.4 | 172 | 170.4 | 168.1 | 163.6 |
| United Kingdom | 234.2 | 222 | 233.6 | 231.8 | 226 | 221.5 | 216.9 | 215.6 | 212.3 | 209.1 | 205.7 | 202.1 |
| Iceland | 221.9 | 186.7 | 205.4 | 189.6 | 166.7 | 180.7 | 192.8 | 182.2 | 180.1 | 170.8 | 185.9 | |
| Liechtenstein | | | | | | | | | | | | 154.7 |
| Norway | 224.6 | 217 | 214.6 | 217.1 | 212.3 | 207.2 | 203.9 | 197 | 199.8 | 195.9 | 190.9 | 192.5 |
| Switzerland | 201.5 | 213.4 | 214 | 199.9 | 198.8 | 193.3 | 191.7 | 186.6 | 187.2 | 183.2 | 176.8 | 177 |

TABLE 31.2 Cancer Mortality in Selected Western European Countries in Women over Time (per 100,000 Inhabitants)

| Geo\Time | 1999 | 2000 | 2001 | 2002 | 2003 | 2004 | 2005 | 2006 | 2007 | 2008 | 2009 | 2010 |
|---|---|---|---|---|---|---|---|---|---|---|---|---|
| Belgium | 142.4 | | | | | 130.7 | 130.7 | 129.4 | 131.8 | 131 | 130.3 | |
| Denmark | 201.4 | 198 | 197.3 | 188.6 | 184.6 | 181.8 | 184.6 | 182.2 | 178.6 | 175.7 | 168.2 | |
| Germany | 147.3 | 144.2 | 140.4 | 140.1 | 137.5 | 135.4 | 134.7 | 131.9 | 130.1 | 130.7 | 128.8 | 128.1 |
| Ireland | 169.6 | 173.4 | 168.8 | 158.1 | 162.1 | 160.2 | 163 | 163.6 | 154.5 | 158.3 | 148.1 | 147.6 |
| Greece | 115.3 | 114.7 | 116.5 | 116.5 | 113.2 | 114.8 | 113 | 110.9 | 113.4 | 113.2 | 108.9 | 108.8 |
| Spain | 111.1 | 110.1 | 110.2 | 108.3 | 107.9 | 105.6 | 103.3 | 103.4 | 102.4 | 102.2 | 101.2 | 101.6 |
| France | 126.7 | 124.3 | 123.9 | 124.4 | 124.1 | 122 | 121.5 | 120.2 | 116.1 | 117.6 | 116.7 | 114.2 |
| Italy | 127.9 | 131.2 | 131.9 | 129.1 | 128.4 | | | 122.6 | 123.4 | 122.1 | 122.2 | 119.9 |
| Cyprus | | | | | | 90.6 | 99.4 | 94.2 | 102.2 | 98.5 | 99 | 91.7 |
| Luxembourg | 135.2 | 142.3 | 141.2 | 129.3 | 133.3 | 111.8 | 117.9 | 122.5 | 133.6 | 121.8 | 133.1 | 120 |
| Malta | 136.3 | 149.1 | 122.6 | 128.4 | 135 | 125.6 | 119.9 | 127.1 | 129.9 | 121 | 122.4 | 127.7 |
| The Netherlands | 161.6 | 157.9 | 156.1 | 157.1 | 155.2 | 156.1 | 156.7 | 154.3 | 151.3 | 155.4 | 151.3 | 152 |
| Austria | 140.3 | 140.9 | 135.7 | 134.2 | 136.8 | 135.5 | 132.5 | 127.5 | 126.5 | 127.7 | 125.5 | 125.4 |
| Poland | 153.2 | 158.4 | 158 | 156.8 | 157.5 | 154.9 | 155.3 | 154.8 | 154.4 | 152 | 150 | 146.8 |
| Portugal | 115.6 | 116.2 | 117.1 | 115.8 | 114.4 | 110.7 | 111.4 | 103.4 | 109.1 | 108.5 | 110.8 | 106.3 |
| Finland | 121.6 | 124.9 | 121.3 | 117.9 | 119.3 | 116.2 | 116.9 | 113.4 | 113.2 | 113.9 | 110.8 | 114.4 |
| Sweden | 137 | 138.9 | 140.5 | 137.2 | 135.5 | 139 | 136.5 | 135.2 | 134.1 | 131.5 | 129.5 | 126.3 |
| United Kingdom | 164.4 | 159.2 | 163.2 | 161.7 | 159.4 | 157.4 | 156.7 | 153.8 | 153.7 | 151.9 | 148.4 | 147.2 |
| Iceland | 160.6 | 168 | 134.6 | 151.2 | 157.9 | 147.4 | 133.5 | 132.8 | 157.6 | 151.8 | 133.6 | |
| Liechtenstein | | | | | | | | | | | | 103.3 |
| Norway | 146.3 | 148 | 148.5 | 147.8 | 145.1 | 142.4 | 142 | 138.5 | 139.9 | 137.4 | 132.8 | 136.7 |
| Switzerland | 115.7 | 125.9 | 121.1 | 121 | 119.4 | 118.1 | 113.9 | 116.6 | 117.3 | 111.8 | 113.3 | 111.1 |

TABLE 31.3  National Cancer Plans in Western Europe

| Country | National Cancer Plan 2010 | Year of Launching Cancer Plan |
| --- | --- | --- |
| Andorra | No | |
| Austria | No | |
| Belgium | Yes | 2008 |
| Cyprus | No | |
| Denmark | Yes | 2005 |
| Faroe Islands | | |
| Finland | Yes | |
| France | Yes | 2003 |
| Germany | Yes | |
| Gibraltar | | |
| Greece | No | |
| Guernsey | | |
| Iceland | | |
| Ireland | Yes | 2006 |
| Isle of Man | | |
| Italy | Yes | 2006 |
| Jersey | | |
| Liechtenstein | | |
| Luxembourg | No | |
| Malta | Yes | 2007 |
| Monaco | Yes | |
| The Netherlands | Yes | 2004 |
| Norway | Yes | 2006 |
| Portugal | Yes | 2008 |
| San Marino | | |
| Spain | Yes | 2006 |
| Sweden | Yes | |
| Switzerland | Yes | 2005 |
| United Kingdom | Yes | 2001 to 2007 |

all Western countries. Although the European scientific organizations have defined curricula for their respective specialties, these have not yet been fully implemented in Western Europe.

The number of physician specialists in oncology ranges from 1 to 5.7 per 100,000 inhabitants across Western European countries.[4] However, due to the diversity of the professional involved in cancer care, it is difficult to give an exact figure of each specialist group.

## REFERENCES

1. Census. Available at http://www.census.gov/population/international/data/idb /region.php. Consulted January 19, 2013.

2. Roland Berger Strategy Consultants, Germany. Trends in European Health care, 2007. Available at http://www.arengufond.ee/upload/Editor/teenused/Ter vise%20lugemine/RB_Trends_in_European_healthcare_20070901.pdf. Consulted January 19, 2013.

3. Eucomed Medical Technology. Futureproofing Western Europe's Healthcare. Available at http://www.eucomed.org/uploads/Modules/Publications/111005_ eiueucomedfutureproofing_healthcarefinalv2web_51011.pdf. Accessed January 19, 2013.

4. European Commission. Eurostat. Available at http://epp.eurostat.ec.europa.eu /portal/page/portal/health/public_health/data_public_health/main_tables.

5. HOPE. Hospitals in Europe Health Care Data 2011. Available at http://www .hope.be/03activities/quality_eu-hospitals/eu_country_profiles/00-hospi tals_in_europe-synthesis_vs2011-06.pdf.

6. World Health Organisation. Primary Health Care. Available at http://www.euro .who.int/en/what-we-do/health-topics/Health-systems/primary-health-care /facts-and-figures.

7. World Health Organization, Geneva, March 2006. Available at http://www.who .int/hrh/resources/workforce_implications.pdf.

8. Matthews A, Channon A, Van Lerberghe W. Will there be enough people to care? Notes on workforce implications of demographic change 2005–2050. Evidence and Information for Policy. World Health Organization, 2006.

9. Globocan. Available at http://globocan.iarc.fr/factsheets/cancers/all.asp. Accessed January 19, 2013.

10. Atun R, Ogawa T, Martin-Moreno J. Analysis of National Cancer Control Programmes in Europe. Available at https://spiral.imperial.ac.uk/bit stream/10044/1/4204/1/Cancer%20Control%20vf2.pdf. Accessed January 19, 2013.

11. Ezzati M, Henley SJ, Lopez AD, Thun MJ. Role of smoking in global and regional cancer epidemiology: current patterns and data needs. *Int J Cancer* 2005 Oct 10; 116(6): 963–71.

12. Schütze M, Boeing H, Pischon T, et al. Alcohol attributable burden of incidence of cancer in eight European countries based on results from prospective cohort study. *BMJ* 2011 Apr 7; 342: d1584. doi:10.1136/bmj.d1584.

13. Parkin DM, Bray F. The burden of HPV-related cancers. *Vaccine* 2006 Aug 31; 24(Suppl 3): S3/11–25.

# About the Editors

**KENNETH D. MILLER, MD**, is a medical oncologist and hematologist. While on the faculty of the Yale Cancer Center, he was a Johnson and Johnson International Scholar at the Uganda Cancer Institute in Kampala and has returned there to teach and assist in ongoing research efforts. Miller was also instrumental in shipping two retiring mammography vans to Uganda to promote breast and cervical cancer awareness. He has also taught oncology in Ethiopia when he was the coordinator of ASCO's International Cancer Corp efforts there. Miller is an expert on cancer survivorship, was the founding director of the Yale Cancer Center Survivorship Program, and later was the director of the Adult Survivorship Program at the Dana-Farber Cancer Institute. He has written two textbooks on cancer survivorship along with one on breast cancer. He also lectures on the role of empathy in medicine.

**MIKLOS SIMON, MD,** is a medical oncologist at Compass Oncology, Portland, Oregon. As a recipient of grants from the European Union and the Soros Foundation, he started studying international medicine during medical school. After completing his fellowship at Yale University, his interest in global oncology led him to volunteer in India, Ethiopia, and Bhutan as an educator. Simon is currently a board member of the Oregon Society of Medical Oncology and an active participant in international educational symposiums. He is a steering committee member of the oncology section at Health Volunteer Overseas and program director of the American Society of Clinical Oncology's International Cancer Corps program in Bhutan.

# About the Contributors

DR. HIKMAT ABDEL-RAZEQ, MD, is the chief medical officer and deputy director general of King Hussein Cancer Center in Amman, Jordan. He also chairs the Department of Internal Medicine and the Section of Hematology and Medical Oncology in the same institution. He conducted his medical studies at the University of Jordan in Amman and had his postgraduate training at the Cleveland Clinic Foundation and the New York Medical College.

MAYSA M. ABU-KHALAF, MD, is associate professor of medicine (medical oncology) at Yale University School of Medicine. The focus of Dr. Abu-Khalaf's clinical practice is the treatment and management of patients with early and advanced stages of breast cancer. Dr. Abu-Khalaf is a member of the Southwest Oncology Group and Yale Cancer Center Developmental Therapeutics Program. Her major research interest is designing and conducting phase I and II clinical trials evaluating novel treatments for breast cancer, with a focus on therapies that target the PI3K/mTOR pathway.

MOHAMED AMGAD is a final year medical student at Cairo University in Cairo, Egypt. He has participated in multiple research projects, including basic lab research, clinical research, epidemiology research, and systematic review projects, some of which were published in international journals and conferences. Amgad is interested in promoting the issue of undergraduate medical research and is the former vice president of the Medical Research Society for Undergraduates, an NGO registered at the Egyptian Ministry of Social Affairs, aimed at promoting and conducting undergraduate medical research projects and organizing research education courses.

HUSSEIN A. ASSI is a medical oncologist at American University of Beirut Medical Center, Lebanon.

FADWA ALI ATTIGA, PHD, is the chief scientific officer at King Hussein Cancer Center in Amman, Jordan. She has been leading several initiatives and programs in cancer research development, cancer registry, and capacity building in cancer control. She led the National Cancer Control Planning Taskforce in Jordan as part of a collaboration between the Ministry of Health and King Hussein Institute for Biotechnology and Cancer. Dr. Attiga holds a doctoral degree in cellular and molecular oncology from the George Washington University, and she is a professional in project management as well a certified professional in health-care quality.

YAZID BELKACEMI is head of the Department of Radiation Oncology and coordinator of the Henri Mondor Breast Center, Région de Paris, France.

ZINEB BENBRAHIM, MD, is a medical oncologist at Hassan II University Hospital in Morocco. He is a European Society of Medical Oncology–certified member and a member of the American Society of Medical Oncology, the Moroccan Society of Cancer, the Moroccan Association for Training and Research in Medical Oncology, and Founding Member of the Association "Chifae" for Research and Prevention of Cancer Diseases.

GYÖRGY BODOKY, MD, PHD, is professor of clinical oncology and heads the Clinical Oncology Department at St. Laszlo Teaching Hospital in Budapest, Hungary. He is the honorary president of the Hungarian Society of Clinical Oncology. He is a member of the Academic Research on Cancer for Answers and Directions Foundation, the Swiss Group for Clinical Cancer Research, and the European Society of Medical Oncology CRC consensus working group and a founding member of South-Eastern European Research Oncology Group.

HAMOUDA BOUSSEN is professor in medical oncology in Faculte de medecine de Tunis, has been a founding member of the Mediterranean Oncology Society(MOS) since 2003, has been vice president and founding member of the Tunisian Society for Study of Pain (ATED) since 1995, and has been a member of the directory of Tunisian society for Medical Sciences Societe since 1994, the American Society of Clinical Oncology since 1987, the International Association for Study of Pain (IASP) since January 1999, the French Society of Cancer since 200, and the European Society of Medical Oncology since 2005.

EDUARDO CAZAP, MD, PHD, FASCO, is an Argentinean medical oncologist, founder and first president of the Latin American & Caribbean Society of Medical Oncology, immediate past president of the Union for International Cancer Control (Geneva, Switzerland), and member of the executive board of the National Cancer Institute of Argentina. He also serves as chairman of the Executive Committee of the Breast Health Global Initiative, Fred Hutchinson Cancer Research Center (Seattle, Washington, DC). He was elected cochair of the Civil Society Taskforce to advise the president of the United Nations General Assembly on the 2011 United Nations High-Level Meeting on Noncommunicable Diseases. He is current chairman of the International Clinical Trials Working Group-American Society of Clinical Oncology (ASCO).

HARLEEN CHAHIL, MD, is a clinical observer at Sinai Hospital Internal Medicine Program. She completed her medical school at Christian Medical College, Ludhiana, India.

REKHA CHANDRAN, MD, attended medical school in India and completed residency training at John H. Stroger Hospital of Cook County, Chicago, Illinois. Chandran is currently a fellow in hematology and oncology at the Medical College of Wisconsin.

EDWARD CHU, MD, is professor of medicine, pharmacology and chemical biology, and clinical and translational science at the University of Pittsburgh School of Medicine. He is also chief of the Division of Hematology-Oncology and deputy director of the University of Pittsburgh Cancer Institute. For the past 25 years, his research has focused on identifying mechanisms of resistance in colorectal cancer and on developing novel agents and therapeutic strategies for the treatment of metastatic colorectal cancer.

LINUS CHUANG, MD, MPH, MS, is director of gynecologic oncology, Sound Shore Medical Center, and director of the Division and Fellowship in Gynecologic Minimally Invasive Surgery, Ichan School of Medicine at Mount Sinai in New York. He is associate professor of obstetrics, gynecology and reproductive science.

MATTHEW M. COONEY, MD, is board certified in medicine, oncology, and hematology. He is assistant professor of medicine at Case Western Reserve University, Cleveland, Ohio. Dr. Cooney is the vice chief for clinical affairs for the Division of Hematology and Oncology at the University Hospitals Case Medical Center. He is the program leader for genitourinary oncology at the Seidman Cancer Center. Dr. Cooney is also involved with collaborative research and teaching projects with the Uganda Cancer Institute.

JONATHAN DANIEL, MD, is an attending thoracic surgeon at Providence Health System in Portland, Oregon. Prior to this position, he was assistant professor of surgery and chief of the Section of Thoracic Surgery at the University of Arizona. He completed his general surgery training at the Baylor College of Medicine at the Texas Medical Center and his thoracic surgery training at Brigham and Women's Hospital/Harvard Medical School under the direction of Dr. David Sugarbaker—world-renowned pioneer in mesothelioma surgery. Daniel is a member of the Society of Thoracic Surgeons and the European Association of Cardiothoracic Surgery.

LYDIA DREOSTI, MD, is a medical oncologist and department head at the Mary Potter Oncology Center, Little Company of Mary Hospital, at Groenkloof, Pretoria, Gauteng, South Africa.

CHRISTY M. DUNST, MD, is an esophageal surgeon with The Oregon Clinic in Portland. She joined the practice in 2006 after completing an Esophageal Surgery Fellowship at the University of Southern California, Thoracic Foregut Division. Currently, she is co-program director for the Advanced GI Foregut Surgery Fellowship Program at Providence Portland Medical Center and director of Research and Education for the GMIS Surgery Division of The Oregon Clinic. She is affiliate professor at Oregon Health and Science University and executive director for the nonprofit Foundation for Surgical Education and Innovation.

NAGI S. EL SAGHIR, MD, FACP, is professor and director, Breast Center of Excellence, Naef K. Basile Cancer Institute, American University of Beirut Medical Center, Beirut, Lebanon. He is founding-president of the Lebanese Society of Medical Oncology and the Lebanese Breast Cancer Foundation. He served on many committees, meetings, consensus panels, research groups, and editorial boards, including the American Society of Clinical Oncology (ASCO), the European Society of Medical Oncology, the EORTC Breast Cancer Group, the European Arab School of Oncology, the Arab Medical Association against Cancer, Breast Health Global Initiative, Advanced Breast Cancer, NCCN-MENA, JCO, The Breast, and chair of ASCO International Affairs Committee. His research is focused on breast cancer and young women. In addition to peer-reviewed publications, he is the author of *ABC of Breast Diseases* published in Arabic.

ERIN GILBERT, MD, is assistant professor of surgery at Oregon Health and Science University in Portland, Oregon. She received her MD from Louisiana State University Health and Sciences Center and subsequently completed her general surgery residency in Seattle at the University of Washington. Her clinical practice focuses on esophageal and gastric cancers as well as solid organ surgery for both benign and malignant indications. She is involved in both clinical and translational academic research, including the effects of tissue oxygenation on healing and on the surgical management and early detection of pancreatic cancer.

AMITOJ S. GILL is a second-year resident at the Johns Hopkins University/ Sinai Hospital of Baltimore Internal Medicine Residency Program. Graduated from Christian Medical College, India, he spent his time as a researcher at BC Cancer Research Agency in Vancouver, Canada, before he joined Sinai Hospital for his residency.

RAHUL GOSAIN, MD, is a second-year internal medicine resident at Johns Hopkins University/Sinai Hospital of Baltimore, Maryland. He was awarded "Outstanding Intern of the Year" and "Outstanding Performance Award— Ambulatory Internal Medicine" in his first year of residency. Gosain graduated from the University of Medicine and Health Sciences, St. Kitts, after finishing his undergraduate degree in Bachelors of Science at McMaster University, Hamilton, Canada. He holds a keen interest in hematology and medical oncology and aims to specialize in this field after his initial training in medicine.

ROHIT GOSAIN, MD is a computer engineer and a resident physician in internal medicine at Sinai Hospital of Baltimore.

WILLIAM P. HARRIS, MD, is assistant professor in the Division of Medical Oncology at the University of Washington School of Medicine and assistant member in the Division of Clinical Research at the Fred Hutchinson Cancer Research Center. Dr. Harris is a gastrointestinal medical oncologist with a clinical and research focus on hepatobiliary malignancies. He serves as the lead medical oncology consultant to the university.

FRANCISCO J. HERNANDEZ-ILIZALITURRI, MD, is associate professor in the Department of Medicine and assistant professor in the Department of Immunology at Roswell Park Cancer Institute. He is a member of the American Society of Hematology, American Society of Clinical Oncology, and the National Comprehensive Cancer Network's Hodgkin's Panel. He has a significant interest in the development of novel therapies for Hodgkin and T-cell lymphomas.

FRANKLIN W. HUANG, MD, PHD, is a senior hematology/oncology fellow at Dana-Farber Cancer Institute and Massachusetts General Hospital and a clinical fellow in medicine at Harvard Medical School in Boston, Massachusetts. He is also the cofounder and codirector of the Global Oncology Initiative (www.globa lonc.org). He conducts translational cancer research at the Broad Institute with a focus on cancers in underserved populations.

JOHN G. HUNTER, MD, is the Mackenzie Professor and Chair, Department of Surgery at Oregon Health and Science University in Portland, Oregon. Dr. Hunter spent 9 years at Emory University School of Medicine in Atlanta (1992 to 2001), where he was professor of surgery, clinical vice chairman of the Department of Surgery, chief of the Division of Gastrointestinal Surgery, director of the Emory Swallowing Center, and director of the Emory Endosurgical Center. Dr. Hunter codirects the OHSU Digestive Health Center, one of a very few fully integrated digestive health programs in the United States. In July 2004 Dr. Hunter became the editor in chief of the *World Journal of Surgery*.

ROHIT JAIN, MBBS, MPH, is currently pursuing his internal medicine residency at Johns Hopkins University/Sinai Hospital of Baltimore. He graduated from Topiwala National Medical College in Mumbai, India, following which he completed a master of public health from Indiana University. He has also worked as a postdoctoral fellow primarily on translational research in breast cancer and thymoma.

POTJANA JITAWATANARAT, MD, is a clinical instructor of medical oncology and hematology at Roswell Park Cancer Institute. She is a member of the American Society of Clinical Oncology and the American Society of Hematology. Her area of interest is hematologic malignancies, especially B-cell lymphoma.

SHEHERYAR KAIRAS KABRAJI, BM, BCH, MA, is a clinical fellow in hematology and oncology at the Dana Farber/Partners Cancer Care Program in Boston, Massachusetts.

KATIA E. KHOURY, MD, is a graduate of the American University of Beirut (AUB) in Beirut Lebanon. She earned a BS in biology, followed by a medical degree, both from AUB. She is pursuing a postdoctoral research fellowship in breast oncology since 2012 under the mentorship of Dr. Nagi El Saghir, professor of clinical oncology, and director of the Breast Center of Excellence, at the Naef K.

Basile Cancer Institute at AUB-Medical Center. She has an interest in women's health and breast cancer.

TAE W. KIM, MD, is professor of medicine at Asan Medical Center, University of Ulsan College of Medicine in Korea, and adjunct professor in the Department of Medicine at the University of Pittsburgh in the United States. He has served as director of the Clinical Research Center at Asan Medical Center.

CHRISTOPHER S. LATHAN, MD, MS, MPH, is the faculty director of the Cancer Care Equity Program at the Dana-Farber Cancer Institute, as well as the director of the Dana Farber Community Cancer Clinic at Whittier Street Health Center in Roxbury. He is a medical oncologist in the Lowe Center for Thoracic Oncology at Dana Farber Cancer Institute. Dr. Lathan is also assistant professor of medicine at Harvard Medical School. His primary research interests are centered on racial/ethnic disparities in cancer care.

JAMES J. LEE, MD, PHD, is assistant professor of medicine at the University of Pittsburgh School of Medicine in Pittsburgh, Pennsylvania. He is a board-certified medical oncologist.

XINSHENG MICHAEL LIAO, MD, PHD, is a medical oncologist practicing near Seattle, Washington. He graduated from a medical school in China and trained in science and clinical medicine in the United States. Prior to his current position, he was a tenure track faculty at the University of Texas MD Anderson Cancer Center. He served as adjunct professor at the Beijing University School of Medicine and affiliated investigator of the Fred Hutchinson Cancer Research Center.

GREGORY MACLENNAN, MD, is director of the Human Tissue Procurement Facility at University Hospitals of Cleveland, director of the Tissue Procurement and Histology Core of the Ireland Cancer Center, and director of surgical pathology in the Department of Pathology. He is professor of pathology, urology, and oncology at Case Western Reserve School of Medicine. MacLennan has a particular interest in genitourinary pathology. Much of his time is committed to diagnostic surgical pathology and cytopathology. His research has been predominantly clinically oriented, but has also involved collaborations with basic scientists.

NEHAL MASOOD, MD, is associate professor, section chief, and consultant hematologist/oncologist at the Aga Khan University (AKU) Hospital, Karachi, Pakistan. He is currently the director of Oncology Fellowship Program at AKU. Earlier, he was a faculty member at the University of Washington Seattle/Fred Hutchinson Cancer Research Center and Seattle Cancer Care Alliance in Seattle.

KINSEY A. MCCORMICK, MD, is a senior fellow in hematology/oncology at the University of Washington/Fred Hutchinson Cancer Research Center with a specific clinical and clinical research interest in gastrointestinal malignancies.

RUTIKA MEHTA, MBBS, MPH, is currently pursuing internal medicine residency at Johns Hopkins University/Sinai Hospital of Baltimore. She graduated from Topiwala National Medical College in Mumbai, India, following which she completed a master of public health from Indiana University. She has also worked as a postdoctoral fellow primarily on translational research in breast cancer.

MANOJ P. MENON, MD, MPH, is a senior fellow in hematology/oncology at the University of Washington/Fred Hutchinson Cancer Research Center with a focus on global health and malignancy. He works with colleagues at the Uganda Program on Cancer and Infectious Diseases in Kampala, Uganda. He previously served as a medical officer with the Centers for Disease Control Center for Global Health, where he worked on malaria and waterborne disease prevention efforts.

CARA MILLER recently received her PhD in clinical psychology from Gallaudet University.

BELLA NADLER is a master's degree candidate at the Johns Hopkins School of Public Health.

PIPPA NEWELL, MD, is the medical director of the Liver Cancer Program at Providence Cancer Center in Portland, Oregon. She is also a hepatobiliary surgeon at the Oregon Clinic and studies hepatocellular carcinoma as a clinical research scientist at the Earle A. Chiles Research Institute in Portland. She was a Fulbright Scholar to Senegal, West Africa.

KOFI MENSAH NYARKO, MB, CHB, MPH, PHD, is a public health physician and program manager for Noncommunicable Diseases Control Program and for the Focal Point for Cancer Control in the Ghana Health Service. He is an epidemiologist and heads the Ghana Field Epidemiology and Laboratory Training Program in the Department of Epidemiology and Disease Control at the School of Public Health, University of Ghana. He is a member of Ghana's National Cancer Steering Committee.

FRED OKUKU, MBCHB, MMED, is a medical oncologist and Uganda Cancer Institute Head, Solid Tumor Treatment Center, at the Uganda Cancer Institute. Okuku has completed a Fogarty Training Program in conjunction with the University of Washington and the Fred Hutchinson Cancer Center. He is interested in studying prostate cancer in men in sub-Saharan Africa.

AMAN OPNEJA, MBBS, is a first-year resident at Johns Hopkins University/Sinai Hospital of Baltimore Internal Medicine Program. He completed his medical school from Maulana Azad Medical College, India.

RADU PESCARUS, MD, is currently the Foregut Fellow at Providence Portland Medical Center in Portland, Oregon. Following his general surgery at Universitie de Montreal in Montreal, Canada, he trained for 1 year in minimally invasive surgery at McMaster University, Hamilton, Canada.

ÁGOTA PETRÁNYI, MD, is a clinical oncologist at the Oncology Department of St. Laszlo Teaching Hospital in Budapest, Hungary.

FREDRIC V. PRICE, MD, is director of Gynecologic Oncology and Minimally Invasive Gynecology at the Allegheny Health Network in Pittsburgh, Pennsylvania. He is adjunct associate professor of obstetrics and gynecology at Temple University School of Medicine.

JOSÉ A. SÁNCHEZ, N.MD, is professor at the Faculty of Medical Sciences at the Autonomous National University of Honduras, and internist, hematologist oncologist, attending physician at the Oncology Department, Hospital General San Felipe, Tegucigalpa, Honduras. He is local coordinator of the academic activities for Health Volunteers Overseas/American Society of Clinical Oncology (ASCO) in Honduras, as well as a researcher, writer, and ASCO member.

DIRK SCHRIJVERS, MD, PHD, is head of the Department of Medical Oncology at the Ziekenhuisnetwerk Antwerpen-Middelheim, Antwerp, Belgium. He is a member of the cancer prevention workgroup of the European Society of Medical Oncology, in which he was former board member and chairman of the educational committee. He is currently the chairman of the educational committee of the European Cancer Organisation.

AZIZA SHAD, MD, is the Amey Distinguished Professor of Neuro-Oncology and Childhood Cancer and director of the Division of Pediatric Hematology Oncology, Blood and Marrow Transplantation at the Lombardi Comprehensive Cancer Center, Georgetown University Hospital in Washington, DC. She is also the director of the Leukemia Lymphoma Program and director of the Cancer Survivorship Program. Shad is actively involved in the development of Pediatric Oncology Programs in Developing Countries, particularly in Asia, the Middle East, Africa, and Latin America. She is the president of the U.S. branch of INCTR (International Network for Cancer Treatment and Research), chair of the Pediatric Oncology Education Committee, and member of the Governing Council of the INCTR. She is also chair of the Palliative Care Committee for Middle East Cancer Consortium and Pediatric Oncology in Developing Countries, International Society for Pediatric Oncology. She has spoken at numerous scientific meetings, both nationally and internationally, and is widely published in the field of pediatric lymphomas, pediatric oncology in developing countries, and late effects in cancer survivors, a major area of her research. She is the author of two books.

ROLA SHAHEEN, MD, FRCPC, is acting chair of radiology and chief of Women's Imaging at Mafraq Hospital, a major governmental hospital in Abu Dhabi, where she is spearheading the planning of breast imaging services and interventions through a multidisciplinary approach. She completed her radiology residency at the University of Toronto, and a women's imaging fellowship at BIDMC-Teaching Hospital of Harvard Medical School. In 2011, she was appointed regional director for the Middle East by Susan G. Komen Foundation for the Cure. She is leading a study on comparative baseline needs assessment for breast cancer awareness and management in the Middle East sponsored by Susan G. Komen for the Cure in collaboration with EMRO/WHO. Shaheen serves on multiple national and international advisory committees including the technical committee for the global task force for Harvard Global Equity Initiative, and the Jordan Breast Cancer Program. She is an elected member of the American Registry for Diagnostic Medical Sonography for the global task force (EDTF) for breast examination in the United States.

EMAD SHASH, MD, MSC, is currently the coordinating research physician for the gynecologic oncology and radiation oncology groups at the European Organization for Research and Treatment of Cancer, Brussels, Belgium. He is also associate lecturer and faculty member at the National Cancer Institute, Cairo University. He earned his medical degree at Cairo University in 2004 and completed specialization in medical oncology from the National Cancer Institute, Cairo University, in 2009. Besides being a peer reviewer and specialty editor in many well-known international scientific journals, Shash holds memberships in professional societies including, the European Society of Medical Oncology (panel member), the European Association of Cancer Education, the American Society of Clinical Oncology (committee member of the International Affairs Activity), the European Arab School of Oncology, and the Arab Medical Association against Cancer.

MIYA SHITAMA graduated with distinction from the University of North Carolina at Chapel Hill in 2011. She holds a BA in international studies with a focus on global health and a minor in medical anthropology. She currently works as a program assistant for the board on Health Policy Educational Programs and Fellowships at the Institute of Medicine. She is a volunteer in the communications department at The Aslan Project, a U.S. organization dedicated to transforming pediatric cancer in the developing world.

TANIA SIERRA, MD, is a senior resident in the Department of Obstetrics, Gynecology and Reproductive Science, Ichan School of Medicine at Mount Sinai in New York. She received her bachelor's degree from Massachusetts Institute of Technology and her MD from Icahn School of Medicine at Mount Sinai. She is a member of Global Medicine at Icahn School of Medicine at Mount Sinai.

SANDRA M. SWAIN, MD, FACP, is medical director of the Washington Cancer Institute, of MedStar Washington Hospital Center, in Washington, DC. She is professor of medicine at Georgetown University and adjunct professor of medicine at F. Edward Hebert School of Medicine. She was previously the deputy branch chief of the Medicine Branch, Center for Cancer Research, National Cancer Institute (NCI), National Institutes of Health (NIH), and was a tenured principal investigator. She was also the chief of the Breast Cancer Section and chief of the Cancer Therapeutics Branch. She obtained an undergraduate degree in chemistry from the University of North Carolina in 1975 and an MD degree from the University of Florida in Gainesville in 1980. She completed her residency in internal medicine at Vanderbilt University in 1983 followed by a fellowship in medical oncology at the National Cancer Institute, National Institutes of Health in 1986. Swain's current research interests include translational research to identify novel and targeted therapeutics for metastatic and inflammatory breast cancer. She has a strong interest in the development of adjuvant therapy for breast cancer and the effect of chemotherapy on ovarian function. She is the chair of three international phase III randomized studies focused on adjuvant treatment of breast cancer. She was instrumental in the approval of dexrazoxane for cardioprotection, with anthracyclines for breast cancer treatment. She has published over 200 journal and review articles and has been the featured speaker at hundreds of presentations regarding breast cancer and breast health both domestically and internationally. She has received an NIH Challenge grant to study health disparities in African Americans in clinical trials. She has also received several Susan G. Komen for the Cure grants to study health disparities. For her work, she received the Susan G. Komen for the Cure Community Global Award of Distinction in 2012. She was the recipient of the National Cancer Institute's Mentor of Merit Award for 2 years as well as the National Institutes of Health Merit Award. She also received the Claude Jacquillat Award for Clinical Cancer Research in 2012. She is a member of the American Society of Clinical Oncology (ASCO), where she served on numerous committees including the nominating committee and as chair of that committee. For 2005 to 2007 she served as the chair of the education committee. She has served as a member of the ASCO board and is currently a member of the Conquer Cancer Foundation Board. Dr. Swain is currently ASCO immediate past president for 2013 to 2014.

LUCA SZALONTAY, MD, graduated with honors from the University of Pecs, Medical, and Health Sciences Centre in Hungary, in 2009. After graduation she joined the research group of the Nobel laureate professor, Andrew V. Schally at the University of Miami, Miller School of Medicine, where she was working on the development of hormone-based chemotherapeutic agents and conducting preclinical studies. She currently works at Medstar Georgetown University Hospital as a second-year resident in pediatrics. She is involved in clinical research and global health projects.

VERNA D.N.K. VANDERPUYE, MD, graduated from medical school at the Kwame Nkrumah University of Science and Technology, Kumasi, Ghana, in 1990. She won an IAEA Fellowship in radiation oncology at the Howard University Hospital, Washington, DC, and the Union for International Cancer Control Audrey Meyer Mars Fellowship in medical oncology at the University of Chicago Hospitals. Since 2000, she has been a consultant clinical oncologist working at the Korlebu Teaching Hospital, Accra, Ghana. She serves on international committees for the American Society of Clinical Oncology, is ESMO regional representative for sub-Saharan Africa, and a member of the African Organisation of Research and Treatment in Cancer.

TASHI DENDUP WANGDI, MBBS MS FICS, is surgical oncologist and head of the Department of Surgery at the Jigme Dorji Wangchuck National Referral

Hospital, Thimphu, Bhutan. Wangdi is associate professor of surgery and head of surgery of the newly founded University of Medical Sciences of Bhutan. Wagdi is also former secretary general of the South Asian Federation of Oncologist and currently national secretary for the South Asian Surgical Society, and is South Asian editorial board member for *the South Asian Journal of Cancer*.

TAMNA WANGJAM, MBBS, is a resident in internal medicine at the Johns Hopkins Internal Medicine Program at Sinai Hospital of Baltimore. She completed her medical training at Lady Hardinge Medical College, New Delhi, India, and received her medical degree from the University of Delhi, India.

LORI J. WIRTH, MD, is the medical director of Head and Neck Oncology at Massachusetts General Hospital and assistant professor of medicine at Harvard Medical School in Boston, Massachusetts. She is also secretary of the International Thyroid Oncology Group and a member of the National Cancer Institute's Task for Recurrent and Metastatic Head and Neck Cancer. She conducts clinical research in both head and neck cancers and advanced thyroid cancer.

XIAOHUA WU, MD, PHD, is professor and chair of the Department of Gynecologic Oncology, Fudan University Shanghai Cancer Center in Shanghai China. He is a board member for the Chinese Society of Gynecologic Oncology.

HAN-KWANG YANG, MD, FACS, is professor of surgery and director of Gastric Cancer Center, Seoul National University Hospital, and Seoul National University College of Medicine and is involved in several large-scale randomized controlled trials for gastric cancer treatment (CLASSIc trial, KLASS trials, etc.). He is Korean PI of REGATTA study (phase III study for the role of gastrectomy in stage IV gastric cancer; JCOG and KGCA) as well as the Korean PI of a phase II study for the role of neoadjuvant imatinib treatment in large gastric GIST (a collaborator study between Japan and Korea). He is also active in translational research of gastric cancer.

# Index

Note: Page numbers followed by *f* indicate a figure on the corresponding page. Page numbers followed by *t* indicate a table on the corresponding page.